Child Obesity and Nutrition Promotion Intervention

Child Obesity and Nutrition Promotion Intervention

Editor

Ana Isabel Rito

MDPI • Basel • Beijing • Wuhan • Barcelona • Belgrade • Manchester • Tokyo • Cluj • Tianjin

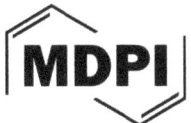

Editor
Ana Isabel Rito
WHO Collaborating Center for
Nutrition and Childhood
Obesity
Instituto Nacional de Saúde Dr
Ricardo Jorge, IP
Lisboa
Portugal

Editorial Office
MDPI
St. Alban-Anlage 66
4052 Basel, Switzerland

This is a reprint of articles from the Special Issue published online in the open access journal *Nutrients* (ISSN 2072-6643) (available at: www.mdpi.com/journal/nutrients/special_issues/Child_Obesity).

For citation purposes, cite each article independently as indicated on the article page online and as indicated below:

LastName, A.A.; LastName, B.B.; LastName, C.C. Article Title. *Journal Name* **Year**, *Volume Number*, Page Range.

ISBN 978-3-0365-1354-6 (Hbk)
ISBN 978-3-0365-1353-9 (PDF)

© 2021 by the authors. Articles in this book are Open Access and distributed under the Creative Commons Attribution (CC BY) license, which allows users to download, copy and build upon published articles, as long as the author and publisher are properly credited, which ensures maximum dissemination and a wider impact of our publications.
The book as a whole is distributed by MDPI under the terms and conditions of the Creative Commons license CC BY-NC-ND.

Contents

About the Editor vii

Julianne Williams, Marta Buoncristiano, Paola Nardone, Ana Isabel Rito, Angela Spinelli, Tatjana Hejgaard, Lene Kierkegaard, Eha Nurk, Marie Kunešová, Sanja Musić Milanović, Marta García-Solano, Enrique Gutiérrez-González, Lacramioara Aurelia Brinduse, Alexandra Cucu, Anna Fijałkowska, Victoria Farrugia Sant'Angelo, Shynar Abdrakhmanova, Iveta Pudule, Vesselka Duleva, Nazan Yardim, Andrea Gualtieri, Mirjam Heinen, Silvia Bel-Serrat, Zhamyla Usupova, Valentina Peterkova, Lela Shengelia, Jolanda Hyska, Maya Tanrygulyyeva, Ausra Petrauskiene, Sanavbar Rakhmatullaeva, Enisa Kujundzic, Sergej M. Ostojic, Daniel Weghuber, Marina Melkumova, Igor Spiroski, Gregor Starc, Harry Rutter, Giulia Rathmes, Anne Charlotte Bunge, Ivo Rakovac, Khadichamo Boymatova, Martin Weber and João Breda
A Snapshot of European Children's Eating Habits: Results from the Fourth Round of the WHO European Childhood Obesity Surveillance Initiative (COSI)
Reprinted from: *Nutrients* **2020**, *12*, 2481, doi:10.3390/nu12082481 1

Ayoub Al-Jawaldeh, Mandy Taktouk and Lara Nasreddine
Food Consumption Patterns and Nutrient Intakes of Children and Adolescents in the Eastern Mediterranean Region: A Call for Policy Action
Reprinted from: *Nutrients* **2020**, *12*, 3345, doi:10.3390/nu12113345 15

Ana Isabel Rito, Sofia Mendes, Mariana Santos, Francisco Goiana-da-Silva, Francesco Paolo Cappuccio, Stephen Whiting, Ana Dinis, Carla Rascôa, Isabel Castanheira, Ara Darzi and João Breda
Salt Reduction Strategies in Portuguese School Meals, from Pre-School to Secondary Education—The Eat Mediterranean Program
Reprinted from: *Nutrients* **2020**, *12*, 2213, doi:10.3390/nu12082213 43

Narae Yang and Kirang Kim
Is the Perceived Fruit Accessibility Related to Fruit Intakes and Prevalence of Overweight in Disadvantaged Youth: A Cross-Sectional Study
Reprinted from: *Nutrients* **2020**, *12*, 3324, doi:10.3390/nu12113324 55

Chishinga Callender, Denisse Velazquez, Meheret Adera, Jayna M. Dave, Norma Olvera, Tzu-An Chen, Shana Alford and Debbe Thompson
How Minority Parents Could Help Children Develop Healthy Eating Behaviors: Parent and Child Perspectives
Reprinted from: *Nutrients* **2020**, *12*, 3879, doi:10.3390/nu12123879 69

Ana Catarina Moreira, Patrícia Almeida Oliveira, Rute Borrego, Telma Nogueira, Raquel Ferreira and Daniel Virella
Development of RisObIn.Com, a Screening Tool for Risk of Childhood Obesity in the Community
Reprinted from: *Nutrients* **2020**, *12*, 3288, doi:10.3390/nu12113288 81

Rikke Højer, Karen Wistoft and Michael Bom Frøst
Play with Your Food and Cook It! Tactile Play with Fish as a Way of Promoting Acceptance of Fish in 11- to 13-Year-Old Children in a School Setting—A Qualitative Study
Reprinted from: *Nutrients* **2020**, *12*, 3180, doi:10.3390/nu12103180 99

Abina Chaudhary, František Sudzina and Bent Egberg Mikkelsen
Promoting Healthy Eating among Young People—A Review of the Evidence of the Impact of School-Based Interventions
Reprinted from: *Nutrients* **2020**, *12*, 2894, doi:10.3390/nu12092894 123

Carola Ray, Rejane Figuereido, Henna Vepsäläinen, Reetta Lehto, Riikka Pajulahti, Essi Skaffari, Taina Sainio, Pauliina Hiltunen, Elviira Lehto, Liisa Korkalo, Katri Sääksjärvi, Nina Sajaniemi, Maijaliisa Erkkola and Eva Roos
Effects of the Preschool-Based Family-Involving DAGIS Intervention Program on Children's Energy Balance-Related Behaviors and Self-Regulation Skills: A Clustered Randomized Controlled Trial
Reprinted from: *Nutrients* **2020**, *12*, 2599, doi:10.3390/nu12092599 157

Gonzalo Colmenarejo
Machine Learning Models to Predict Childhood and Adolescent Obesity: A Review
Reprinted from: *Nutrients* **2020**, *12*, 2466, doi:10.3390/nu12082466 175

Irma J. Evenhuis, Suzanne M. Jacobs, Ellis L. Vyth, Lydian Veldhuis, Michiel R. de Boer, Jacob C. Seidell and Carry M. Renders
The Effect of Supportive Implementation of Healthier Canteen Guidelines on Changes in Dutch School Canteens and Student Purchase Behaviour
Reprinted from: *Nutrients* **2020**, *12*, 2419, doi:10.3390/nu12082419 207

Karolina Zarychta, Anna Banik, Ewa Kulis, Monika Boberska, Theda Radtke, Carina K. Y. Chan, Karolina Lobczowska and Aleksandra Luszczynska
Do Parent–Child Dyads with Excessive Body Mass Differ from Dyads with Normal Body Mass in Perceptions of Obesogenic Environment?
Reprinted from: *Nutrients* **2020**, *12*, 2149, doi:10.3390/nu12072149 223

Anna Dzielska, Joanna Mazur, Hanna Nałecz, Anna Oblacińska and Anna Fijałkowska
Importance of Self-Efficacy in Eating Behavior and Physical Activity Change of Overweight and Non-Overweight Adolescent Girls Participating in Healthy Me: A Lifestyle Intervention with Mobile Technology
Reprinted from: *Nutrients* **2020**, *12*, 2128, doi:10.3390/nu12072128 241

Valerie Hruska, Gerarda Darlington, Jess Haines and David W. L. Ma
Parent Stress as a Consideration in Childhood Obesity Prevention: Results from the Guelph Family Health Study, a Pilot Randomized Controlled Trial
Reprinted from: *Nutrients* **2020**, *12*, 1835, doi:10.3390/nu12061835 259

Jiaxi Yang, Yukako Tani, Deirdre K. Tobias, Manami Ochi and Takeo Fujiwara
Eating Vegetables First at Start of Meal and Food Intake among Preschool Children in Japan
Reprinted from: *Nutrients* **2020**, *12*, 1762, doi:10.3390/nu12061762 271

Eliza Wasilewska, Sylwia Małgorzewicz, Marta Gruchała-Niedoszytko, Magdalena Skotnicka and Ewa Jassem
Dietary Habits in Children with Respiratory Allergies: A Single-Center Polish Pilot Study
Reprinted from: *Nutrients* **2020**, *12*, 1521, doi:10.3390/nu12051521 281

Sigrid Skouw, Anja Suldrup and Annemarie Olsen
A Serious Game Approach to Improve Food Behavior in Families—A Pilot Study
Reprinted from: *Nutrients* **2020**, *12*, 1415, doi:10.3390/nu12051415 295

About the Editor

Ana Isabel Rito

Ana Isabel Rito, MMSc, PhD, is a researcher at the National Institute of Health Dr. Ricardo Jorge-Portugal and co-leads the WHO Collaborating Center for Nutrition and Childhood Obesity. Since 2007, A.I.R. has been the principal investigator of the Obesity Surveillance Initiative—WHO/Europe"(COSI) for Portugal, a member of its advisory board, and a consultant for the WHO. Additionally, she is the director of CEIDSS.com, where she has developed and coordinated several (more than seven) community-based programs tackling childhood obesity at the national and European levels, including the EU H2020 CoCreate. She was the head of the Bachelor Degree in Nutrition Sciences (Univ. Atlantica 2005–2014) and has collaborated as a professor with other universities at the national and international levels. Besides her vast published literature, she has been involved with European networks such as EPHNA, with the WHO, and with EASO and has developed scientific research in collaboration with more than 29 international institutions.

Article

A Snapshot of European Children's Eating Habits: Results from the Fourth Round of the WHO European Childhood Obesity Surveillance Initiative (COSI)

Julianne Williams [1,*], Marta Buoncristiano [1], Paola Nardone [2], Ana Isabel Rito [3], Angela Spinelli [2], Tatjana Hejgaard [4], Lene Kierkegaard [5], Eha Nurk [6], Marie Kunešová [7], Sanja Musić Milanović [8], Marta García-Solano [9], Enrique Gutiérrez-González [9], Lacramioara Aurelia Brinduse [10], Alexandra Cucu [10], Anna Fijałkowska [11], Victoria Farrugia Sant'Angelo [12], Shynar Abdrakhmanova [13], Iveta Pudule [14], Vesselka Duleva [15], Nazan Yardim [16], Andrea Gualtieri [17], Mirjam Heinen [18], Silvia Bel-Serrat [18], Zhamyla Usupova [19], Valentina Peterkova [20], Lela Shengelia [21], Jolanda Hyska [22], Maya Tanrygulyyeva [23], Ausra Petrauskiene [24], Sanavbar Rakhmatullaeva [25], Enisa Kujundzic [26], Sergej M. Ostojic [27], Daniel Weghuber [28], Marina Melkumova [29], Igor Spiroski [30], Gregor Starc [31], Harry Rutter [32], Giulia Rathmes [1], Anne Charlotte Bunge [1], Ivo Rakovac [1], Khadichamo Boymatova [33], Martin Weber [34] and João Breda [1]

1. WHO European Office for the Prevention and Control of Noncommunicable Diseases, 125009 Moscow, Russian Federation; buoncristianom@who.int (M.B.); giuliarathmes@icloud.com (G.R.); anne-charlotte.bunge@charite.de (A.C.B.); rakovaci@who.int (I.R.); rodriguesdasilvabred@who.int (J.B.)
2. Italian National Institute of Health (Istituto Superiore Di Sanità), 00161 Rome, Italy; paola.nardone@iss.it (P.N.); angela.spinelli@iss.it (A.S.)
3. National Institute of Health Dr. Ricardo Jorge, 1600 560 Lisbon, Portugal; ana.rito@insa.min-saude.pt
4. Danish Health Authority, 2300 Copenhagen S, Denmark; thv@sst.dk
5. National Institute of Public Health, University of Southern Denmark, 1455 Copenhagen K, Denmark; leki@sdu.dk
6. Department of Nutrition Research, National Institute for Health Development, 11619 Tallinn, Estonia; eha.nurk@tai.ee
7. Institute of Endocrinology, Obesity Unit, 116 94 Prague, Czechia; mkunesova@endo.cz
8. Croatian Institute of Public Health, University of Zagreb, School of Medicine, 10000 Zagreb, Croatia; sanja.music@hzjz.hr
9. Spanish Agency for Food Safety and Nutrition, 28014 Madrid, Spain; mgarcias@mscbs.es (M.G.-S.); egutierrez@mscbs.es (E.G.-G.)
10. Department of Public Health and Management, University of Medicine and Pharmacy Carol Davila, 030167 Bucharest, Romania; lbrinduse@gmail.com (L.A.B.); alexandra.cucu@insp.gov.ro (A.C.)
11. Department of Cardiology, Institute of Mother and Child, 01-211 Warsaw, Poland; anna.fijalkowska@imid.med.pl
12. Primary Health Care, Ministry for Health, 1940 Floriana, Malta; victoria.farrugia-santangelo@gov.mt
13. National Center of Public health, Ministry of Health of the Republic of Kazakhstan, 010000 Nur-Sultan City, Kazakhstan; shynar_a@mail.ru
14. Centre for Disease Prevention and Control, LV-1005 Latvia, Riga; iveta.pudule@spkc.gov.lv
15. National Center of Public Health and Analyses, 1431 Sofia, Bulgaria; v.duleva@ncpha.government.bg
16. Turkish Ministry of Health, Public Health General Directorate, 34400 Istanbul, Turkey; nazan.yardim@saglik.gov.tr
17. Health Authority, Department of Health and Social Security, 47893 San Marino, San Marino; andrea.gualtieri.authority@pa.sm
18. National Nutrition Surveillance Centre, University College Dublin, Dublin, Ireland; mirjam.heinen@ucd.ie (M.H.); silvia.belserrat@ucd.ie (S.B.-S.)
19. Republican Center for Health Promotion and Mass Communication, 720040 Bishkek, Kyrgyzstan; jama.usupova@mail.ru
20. Institute of Paediatric Endocrinology, National Medical Research Centre for Endocrinology of the Ministry of Health of the Russian Federation, 117036 Moscow, Russian Federation; peterkovava@hotmail.com

21. National Center for Disease Control and Public Health of Georgia, 0198 Tbilisi, Georgia; l.shengelia@ncdc.ge
22. Institute of Public Health, 1007 Tirana, Albania; lhyska2002@yahoo.it
23. Internal Diseases Department of the Scientific Clinical Centre of Mother and Child Health, 744036 Ashgabat, Turkmenistan; ovezmyradovag@who.int
24. Department of Preventive Medicine, Lithuanian University of Health Sciences, 44307 Kaunas, Lithuania; ausra.petrauskiene@lsmuni.lt
25. Department for Organization of Health Services to Children, Mothers, Adolescents and Family Planning, Ministry of Health and Social Protection of Population, 734025 Dushanbe, Tajikistan; sanavbar2010@list.ru
26. Institute of Public Health of Montenegro, Podgorica, Montenegro; enisa.kujundzic@ijzcg.me
27. Applied Bioenergetics Lab, University of Novi Sad, 21000 Novi Sad, Serbia; sergej.ostojic@chess.edu.rs
28. Department of Pediatrics, Paracelsus Medical University, 5020 Salzburg, Austria; d.weghuber@salk.at
29. Arabkir Medical Centre-Institute of Child and Adolescent Health, 0014 Yerevan, Armenia; mmelkumova@mail.ru
30. Institute of Public Health, Faculty of Medicine, Ss. Cyril and Methodius University, 1000 Skopje, North Macedonia; i.spiroski@iph.mk
31. Faculty of Sport, University of Ljubljana, 1000 Ljubljana, Slovenia; gregor.starc@fsp.uni-lj.si
32. Department of Social and Policy Sciences, University of Bath, Bath BA2 7AY, UK; hr526@bath.ac.uk
33. WHO Country Office for Tajikistan, 734019 Dushanbe, Tajikistan; boymatovak@who.int
34. WHO Child and Adolescent Health and Development, WHO Regional Office for Europe, 2100 Copenhagen, Denmark; weberm@who.int

* Correspondence: williamsj@who.int

Received: 3 July 2020; Accepted: 4 August 2020; Published: 17 August 2020

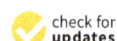

Abstract: Consuming a healthy diet in childhood helps to protect against malnutrition and noncommunicable diseases (NCDs). This cross-sectional study described the diets of 132,489 children aged six to nine years from 23 countries participating in round four (2015–2017) of the WHO European Childhood Obesity Surveillance Initiative (COSI). Children's parents or caregivers were asked to complete a questionnaire that contained indicators of energy-balance-related behaviors (including diet). For each country, we calculated the percentage of children who consumed breakfast, fruit, vegetables, sweet snacks or soft drinks "every day", "most days (four to six days per week)", "some days (one to three days per week)", or "never or less than once a week". We reported these results stratified by country, sex, and region. On a daily basis, most children (78.5%) consumed breakfast, fewer than half (42.5%) consumed fruit, fewer than a quarter (22.6%) consumed fresh vegetables, and around one in ten consumed sweet snacks or soft drinks (10.3% and 9.4%, respectively); however, there were large between-country differences. This paper highlights an urgent need to create healthier food and drink environments, reinforce health systems to promote healthy diets, and continue to support child nutrition and obesity surveillance.

Keywords: nutrition; child; obesity; surveillance; health; noncommunicable diseases; children; fruit; vegetables; soft drinks

1. Introduction

It is important for a child to eat a healthy diet in order to prevent malnutrition (stunting, wasting, micronutrient deficiencies, obesity) and noncommunicable diseases (NCDs) [1,2]. Low-quality diets are now believed to be the single biggest risk factor for the global burden of disease [3]. In recent decades, changes in dietary patterns and physical activity behaviors have been identified as likely contributors to a rise in childhood obesity [4,5]. Research from the latest round of the WHO European Childhood Obesity Surveillance Initiative (COSI) carried out in 2015–2017 indicates that 29% of boys and 27% of girls aged seven to nine years had overweight and there was a prevalence of obesity of 12% in boys and 9% in girls [6]. At the same time, in certain parts of the WHO European Region, there is a double burden of malnutrition, characterized by the coexistence of undernutrition (being underweight for one's age, too short for one's age (stunted), too thin for one's height (wasted), or deficient in vitamins and minerals (micronutrient malnutrition)), along with overweight, obesity, or noncommunicable diseases, within individuals, households, and populations, and across the life course [7,8].

The prevalence of overweight and obesity is increasing worldwide [9]. According to the WHO Global Monitoring Framework for NCDs, which is a set of 25 indicators and 9 voluntary targets are used to track progress toward reaching global targets in 2015–2020, not a single country in the WHO European Region is likely to meet Global Monitoring Target 7, which aims to "halt the rise in diabetes and obesity" [10].

Ensuring that children consume healthy diets is important for achieving the UN Sustainable Development Goals (SDGs) related to no hunger (SDG Goal 2), good health and well-being (SDG Goal 3), quality education (SDG Goal 4), no poverty (SDG Goal 1), economic growth (SDG Goal 8), and more [11,12]. Food preferences and eating habits established in childhood and adolescence tend to be maintained into adulthood [13], making nutrition in childhood an important public health issue.

A healthy diet includes adequate quantities and appropriate proportions of fruit, vegetables, legumes (e.g., lentils and beans), nuts, and whole grains [14], and limits the intake of free sugars [15,16], salt [17], saturated fats, and highly processed foods. A healthy diet eliminates trans fats of all kinds. Consumption of sugar-sweetened beverages should be limited, as it has been associated with increased body weight [18] and dental caries [19].

The WHO European Childhood Obesity Surveillance Initiative provides data on the eating behaviors of children across the WHO European Region. Established in 2007, COSI collects high-quality data on the childhood obesity prevalence and energy-balance-related behaviors [20]. These data enable countries to set national targets, monitor trends over time, make comparisons between countries, and over time, to evaluate the effectiveness of obesity prevention efforts. In addition to collecting high-quality anthropometric measurements from primary-school-aged children, COSI also collects information on children's dietary and physical activity patterns, screen time, sleep, and more.

Given the importance of nutrition in childhood, alongside the rising trend in childhood obesity, this study used the most recent results from the COSI study to describe the eating behaviors of children aged 6–9 years from across the WHO European Region.

2. Materials and Methods

Data were collected between 2015 and 2017, as part of COSI round four. Among the thirty-six countries participating in round four, 23 of them collected information on children's dietary behaviors using parental reports on a "family form". These countries were: Albania, Bulgaria, Croatia, Czechia, Denmark, Georgia, Ireland, Italy, Kazakhstan, Kyrgyzstan, Lithuania, Latvia, Malta, Montenegro, Poland, Portugal, Romania, Russian Federation (Moscow only), San Marino, Spain, Tajikistan, Turkey, and Turkmenistan. Children's parents or caregivers were asked to complete a questionnaire that contained indicators of energy-balance-related behaviors (including diet) and family socioeconomic status. Completion of the form was voluntary and participants could opt out or choose not to participate at any time.

The COSI study follows the International Ethical Guidelines for Biomedical Research Involving Human Subjects [21]. Local ethics approval was also granted. Details for this approval are found in Supplementary Box S1. More details on the data collection procedures are provided elsewhere [20,22,23].

Parents were asked: "over a typical or usual week, how often does your child eat or drink the following kinds of foods or beverages"? This was followed by a tick box, where parents answered "never", "less than once a week", "some days (1–3 days)", "most days (4–6 days)", or "every day". Parents were asked to report on a number of food items, shown in Supplementary Figure S1. For this paper, we reported on the consumption of fresh fruits, vegetables (excluding potatoes), savory snacks (e.g., potato crisps, corn chips, popcorn, peanuts), sweet treats (e.g., candy bars or chocolates), and sugar-containing soft drinks. These questions were selected because they provided a summary that was related to common sources of nutrients of interest [24]. Countries chose country-specific examples for the food examples for "savory snacks (like potato crisps, corn chips, popcorn, peanuts)", or "sweets (like candy bars or chocolate)". These examples were identified by leading nutrition experts within the country and approved by the government-appointed principal investigator of the study. All questionnaires were translated from English into the local language, and then back-translated into English to check for discrepancies with the original English form.

For each country, we calculated the percentage of children who consumed these foods "every day", "most days (four to six days per week)", "some days (one to three days per week)", or "never or less than once a week". We reported these results stratified by country, sex, and region. Geographic regions were based on the United Nations Standard Geographical regions, which are based on continental regions and are further subdivided into sub-regions and intermediary regions that are drawn to obtain greater homogeneity in the sizes of the population, demographic circumstances, and accuracy of demographic statistics [25]. We did not include sub-regional pooled estimates because these subregions include countries that are not participating in COSI, and therefore a sub-regional estimate would not provide an accurate assessment of the situation in that geographical area.

For each variable, we calculated the frequency of consumption according to country and sex. We tested for differences between sex in the distribution of the responses using the Rao–Scott chi-square test, a design-adjusted version of the Pearson's χ^2 test. We applied post-stratification weights to adjust for the sampling design, oversampling, and nonresponse proportions in order to infer results from the sample of the population. These were available and applied for all countries, with the one exception of Lithuania, where an unweighted analysis was carried out. All analyses took account of the complex survey nature of the data (i.e., multiple stages, clustering, and stratification). Pooled estimates were calculated, including only one target age group per country in order to balance the contribution of each country to the pooled estimates and to limit the differences in children's age as much as possible. An adjusting factor was applied to the post-stratification weights to take account of differences in the population sizes of the countries involved. The adjusting factor was based on the number of children belonging to the targeted age group according to Eurostat figures or national official statistics for 2016.

A p-value of 0.05 was used to define statistical significance. All statistical analyses were performed in the statistical software package Stata version 15·1 (StataCorp LLC, College Station, TX, USA).

3. Results

A total of 132,489 children from 23 countries were included in the analysis. The number of participants per country varied widely, from 306 children in San Marino to 43,696 in Italy (Table 1). Most of the children (75.2%) were seven years of age and 51.3% were boys.

The pooled estimates indicated that most children (78.8%) consumed breakfast every day, but around 2.3% consumed breakfast "never or less than once a week" and 8.6% consumed breakfast only on "some days" (one to three days a week). The pooled estimates indicated that 42.5% of children consumed fresh fruit "every day" and 7.5% "never consumed it or consumed it less than once a week". Around a quarter (22.6%) of all children consumed vegetables "every day", and 14.0% consumed it "never or less than once a week." The pooled estimates indicated that 5.2% of children consumed savory snacks "every day", but 57.9% consumed savory snacks "never or less than once a week". Around one in ten children (10.3%) consumed sweets "every day" and a third (32.8%) consumed sweets "never or less than once a week". Around one in ten (9.4%) children consumed soft drinks every day.

Table 1. Number of children invited to participate in COSI/WHO Europe Round 4 (2015–2017), the number of children included in the analysis, and the percentage of children participating by sex, age, and country.

Country [a]	Children Invited to Participate [b]		Children Included in the Analysis [c]			Percentage of Children Participating by Sex and Age (%) [d]					
	Total Number	Proportion Whose Family Form Was Filled in (%)	Boys (n)	Girls (n)	Total (n)	Boys (%)	6-Year-Olds	7-Year-Olds	8-Year-Olds	9-Year-Olds
Albania	7113	36.2	1315	1212	2527	52.5	0.1	24.2	52.0	23.7
Bulgaria	4090	83.1	1702	1698	3400	51.5	0	100.0	0	0
Croatia [e]	7220	76.0	1318	1333	2651	51.1	0	0	100.0	0
Czechia	n.a.	n.a.	670	736	1406	50.7	49.5	50.5	0	0
Denmark	3202	29.9	511	446	957	52.7	27.4	70.2	2.4	0
Georgia	4143	78.4	1667	1579	3246	51.2	1.6	85.1	13.0	0.3
Ireland	2704	32.4	438	436	874	52.6	38.2	60.2	1.6	0
Italy	50,902	95.2	22,425	21,271	43,696	51.5	0	0.5	66.3	33.1
Kazakhstan	6026	82.3	2149	2162	4311	50.6	0	0.4	51.0	48.6
Kyrgyzstan	8773	86.6	3798	3769	7567	50.7	10.5	43.5	39.5	6.5
Lithuania	5527	69.8	1930	1882	3812	50.6	0.4	66.4	33.0	0.2
Latvia	8143	71.5	2752	2955	5707	48.2	7.9	43.8	9.1	39.3
Malta	4329	73.4	1589	1590	3179	50.0	0.1	69.7	30.1	0.1
Montenegro	4094	66.8	1441	1295	2736	52.8	31.2	48.4	20.1	0.2
Poland	3828	76.9	1451	1494	2945	50.2	0	0	100.0	0
Portugal	7475	85.6	3167	3224	6391	50.7	25.2	49.0	24.0	1.7
Romania	9094	73.6	3312	3298	6610	49.1	0.4	28.4	47.5	23.8
Russian Federation	3900	52.6	1006	1046	2052	50.2	18.8	72.8	8.3	0.1
San Marino	329	93.6	138	168	306	45.1	0	0	64.7	35.3
Spain	14,908	70.1	5290	5163	10,453	50.9	25.4	25.2	24.9	24.6
Tajikistan	3502	93.5	1623	1647	3270	51.6	7.7	90.8	1.4	0.2
Turkmenistan	4085	95.3	1944	1947	3891	49.9	0	79.9	20.1	0
Turkey	14,164	81.7	5335	5167	10,502	50.9	11.4	82.3	6.0	0.3
Total	198,683	79.5	66,971	65,518	132,489	51.3	0	75.2	18.2	6.6

n.a.—not available. [a] Figures refer to primary school children from Albania (ALB), Bulgaria (BUL), Croatia (CRO), Czechia (CZH), Denmark (DEN), Georgia (GEO), Ireland (IRL), Italy (ITA), Kazakhstan (KAZ), Kyrgyzstan (KGZ), Lithuania (LTU), Latvia (LVA), Malta (MAT), Montenegro (MNE), Poland (POL), Portugal (POR), Romania (ROM), Moscow city (RUS), San Marino (SMR), Spain (SPA), Tajikistan (TJK), Turkmenistan (TKM), and Turkey (TUR). [b] Total figures were calculated including only countries with available information about the number of children invited to participate in the surveillance. [c] All children with complete information on sex, whose age was between six and nine years old and with information on eating habits from the family form. [d] Pooled values were estimated, including the following age groups/countries: 7-year-olds from Bulgaria, Czechia, Denmark, Kyrgyzstan, Georgia, Ireland, Latvia, Lithuania, Malta, Montenegro, Portugal, Spain, Tajikistan, Turkey, and Turkmenistan; 8-year-olds from Albania, Croatia, Poland, and Romania; and 9-year-olds from Kazakhstan. The figures were estimated by applying post-stratification weights. [e] For Croatia, only data on 8-year-olds were available for comparison at the European level. The proportion of children whose parents or caregivers filled in the family form was calculated in the whole sample (not only for 8-year-olds).

3.1. Consumption of Breakfast

The percentage of children who consumed breakfast every day ranged from 48.9% in Kazakhstan to 96.4% in Portugal (Figure 1). Between-country and between-region differences in breakfast consumption were not tested for significance, although there were visible between countries and no clear patterns according to region. There were no significant differences in breakfast consumption between boys and girls (Supplementary Table S1).

3.2. Consumption of Fresh Fruit

The frequency of consuming fresh fruit everyday ranged widely between the regions. The consumption of fresh fruit every day was highest in the Southern European countries, with 80.8% in San Marino, 72.6% in Italy, and 63.1% in Portugal (Figure 1, Supplementary Table S2). Meanwhile, the daily fresh fruit consumption was low in the Central Asian countries—Kyrgyzstan 18.1%, Kazakhstan 33.3%, and Tajikistan 33.5%—with an exception of Turkmenistan with 70.1%. The same trend was visible for differences in the proportion of children who consumed fresh fruit "never or less than once a week", ranging from 3.0% in San Marino, 3.3% in Portugal, and 2.2% in Montenegro to 21.4% in Tajikistan and 22.6% in Kyrgyzstan.

There were significant differences in fresh fruit consumption between sexes, with girls more likely to eat fruit on a daily basis compared to boys (Supplementary Table S2).

3.3. Consumption of Vegetables

Daily vegetable consumption ranged from 9.1% in Spain to 68.1% in Turkmenistan and 74.3% in San Marino (Figure 2). The percentage of children who consumed vegetables "never or less than once a week" was higher in Western Asian countries, with 20.4% in Turkey and 17.1% in Georgia compared with 1.3% in Czechia and 1.4% in Turkmenistan. There were significant between-sex differences, with boys tending to eat vegetables less frequently than girls (Supplementary Table S3).

3.4. Consumption of Savory Snacks (Like Potato Crisps, Corn Chips, Popcorn, or Peanuts)

We observed large differences between countries and regions of Europe in the frequency of consuming savory snacks like potato crisps, corn chips, popcorn, or peanuts. Low values for the daily consumption of savory snacks were observed in the Northern European countries, where Denmark reported 0%, Lithuania and Latvia 0.6%, and Ireland 1.5% (Figure 2). In contrast, in the Southern European and Asian countries, daily consumption of savory snacks was more frequently reported. Albania reported a percentage of 21.5% of children who consumed savory snacks every day, as well as Tajikistan with 11.3% and Montenegro and Turkmenistan with 9.0% (Table S4). In Malta, only 7.7% of the children never or less than once week, while in the Russian Federation, 90.8% of children consumed these foods "never or less than once a week". Similar results were seen in Lithuania (83.1% consumed savory snacks "never or less than once a week") and in Latvia (80.2% never or less than once a week). There were no significant differences in the consumption of savory snacks between boys and girls (Supplementary Table S4).

3.5. Consumption of Sweets (Like Candy Bars or Chocolate)

Daily consumption of sweet snacks like candy bars or chocolate ranged from 0.4% in Denmark to 21.1% in Turkmenistan and 22.8% in Bulgaria (Figure 2). The percentage of children who never or less than once a week consumed sweet snacks ranged from 3.9% in Malta to 56.7% in Spain and 67.8% in Portugal. There were no clear regional trends in the distribution of daily sweet snack consumption and there were no significant sex differences (Supplementary Table S5).

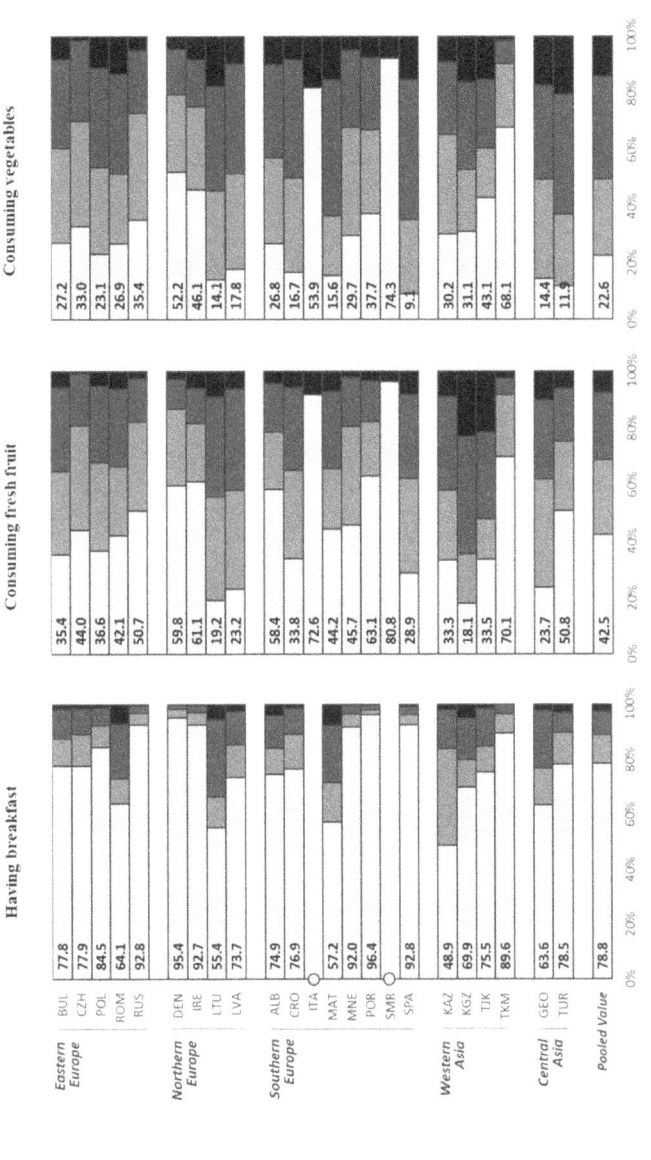

Figure 1. Frequency of consuming breakfast, fresh fruit, and vegetables among boys and girls by country [a]. COSI/WHO Europe round 4 (2015–2017). [a] Pooled values were estimated, including the following age groups/countries: 7-year-olds from Bulgaria, Czechia, Denmark, Kyrgyzstan, Georgia, Ireland, Latvia, Lithuania, Malta, Montenegro, Portugal, Spain, Tajikistan, Turkey, and Turkmenistan; 8-year-olds from Albania, Croatia, Poland, and Romania; and 9-year-olds from Kazakhstan.

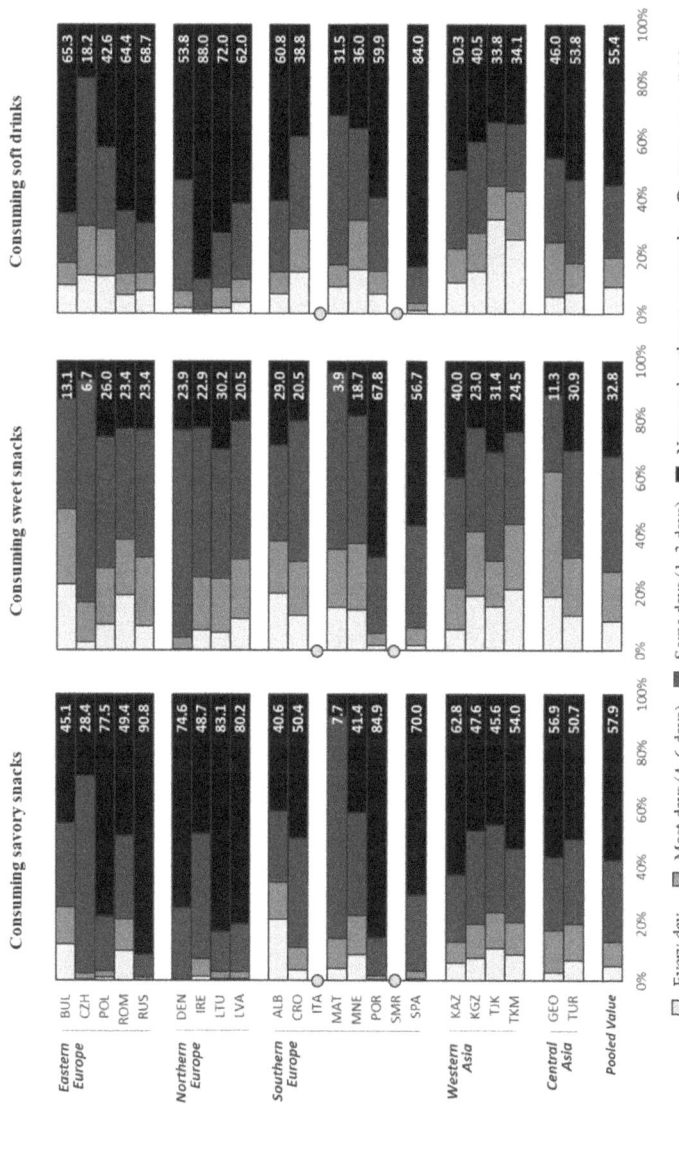

Figure 2. Frequency of consuming savory snacks, sweet snacks, and soft drinks among boys and girls by country [a]. COSI/WHO Europe round 4 (2015–2017). [a] Pooled values were estimated, including the following age groups/countries: 7-year-olds from Bulgaria, Czechia, Denmark, Ireland, Kyrgyzstan, Georgia, Latvia, Lithuania, Malta, Montenegro, Portugal, Spain, Tajikistan, Turkey, and Turkmenistan; 8-year-olds from Albania, Croatia, Poland, and Romania; and 9-year-olds from Kazakhstan.

3.6. Consumption of Soft Drinks

The frequency of consuming soft drinks every day was lowest in Northern European countries, with a value of 0.4% in Ireland, 2.0% in Lithuania, and 2.1% in Denmark (Figure 2). In comparison, in the Central Asian countries of Tajikistan (32.8%) and Turkmenistan (25.8%), daily soft drink consumption was relatively high among some children. There was a lower percentage of children who never or less than once a week consumed soft drinks in the Central Asian countries (33.8% in Tajikistan, 34.1% in Turkmenistan, 40.5% in Kyrgysztan, 50.3% in Kazakhstan) compared to the Northern European countries (88.0% in Ireland, 72.0% in Lithuania, 62.0% in Latvia, 53.8% in Denmark). We observed no significant differences between boys and girls (Supplementary Table S6).

4. Discussion

The purpose of this study was to provide a snapshot that updates the general picture of the dietary habits of European children. Our data present a largely confirmatory picture of the current understanding, with some bright spots in terms of dietary habits but also many areas of opportunity.

The bright spots include high levels of breakfast consumption, with around 80% of children consuming breakfast every day. Daily breakfast consumption was the lowest in Kazakhstan, with fewer than half of the children consuming it every day, whilst almost all the children consumed it every day in Portugal and Denmark. The pooled results align with findings from another systematic review of 286,804 children and adolescents (2 to 18 years) living in 33 countries, which found that the prevalence of skipping breakfast ranged from 10–30%, with an increasing trend in adolescents, especially girls [26]. However, there is also evidence to suggest that breakfast consumption may decrease as children get older. A recent report from the Health Behaviour in School-Aged Children (HBSC) survey of findings from 227,441 young people aged 11, 13, and 15 years living in 45 countries/regions found that more than four out of 10 adolescents do not eat breakfast every school day, and that girls across all ages tend to skip breakfast and eat fewer meals with their family than boys [27].

The areas of opportunity for improving children's diets are related to increasing the consumption of fruits and vegetables. We found that only 42.5% of children consumed fruit and 22.6% consumed vegetables on a daily basis, but there were wide between-country differences. Daily fruit consumption ranged from 80.8% in San Marino to only 18.1% in Kyrgyzstan and 19.2% in Lithuania. Three-quarters (74.3%) of the children in San Marino consumed fresh vegetables every day compared to 9.1% of children in Spain, 11.9% in Turkey, 14.1% in Lithuania, and 14.4% in Georgia. Data on fruit and vegetable consumption trends from 33 countries participating in the HBSC surveys from 2002, 2006, and 2010 indicate that many adolescents do not consume fruit and vegetables on a daily basis, but there was an increase in daily fruit and vegetable consumption between 2002 and 2010 in the majority of countries [28]. Even so, findings from the latest HBSC report (2017/2018) found that almost two in three adolescents do not eat enough nutrient-rich foods, such as fruits and vegetables [27]. A recent review on dietary patterns found that among adolescents, the average fruit and vegetable consumption is below recommended levels in almost all populations [29].

This study also highlights the need for continued efforts to discourage the consumption of foods that are high in salt, sugar, and fat, and low in nutritional value. The pooled estimates related to the frequency of consuming savory snacks, sweets, and soft drinks suggest that 5.2%, 10.3%, and 9.4% of children consume these foods daily, respectively, but there was a wide between-country variation. The percentage of children consuming savory snacks every day ranged from 0% in Denmark and 0.1% in the Russian Federation to 21.5% in Albania. Daily consumption of sweet snacks ranged from 0.4% in Denmark to 21.1% in Turkmenistan and 22.8% in Bulgaria. Consumption of daily soft drinks ranged from 0.4% in Ireland to 32.8% in Tajikistan. This aligns with similar findings from the latest results from the HBSC, which also indicates that one in four adolescents eat sweets and one in six consume sugary drinks at least once a day [27]. Few available data have been found on savory snack consumption or sodium intake among children, but for the majority of the included populations, levels were far above the recommended five grams per day [29].

Based on the data from 23 countries, this study found wide between-country differences in children's healthy and unhealthy eating habits, but few clear patterns according to region. These differences were likely due to a complex range of factors. Eating patterns and food preferences in childhood are shaped by individual, interpersonal, and environmental factors, including a child's family, cultural background, social environment, socioeconomic status, and school environment [30]. Children today are increasingly exposed to environments where energy-dense and nutrient-poor foods are promoted [31] and readily available, which can make eating a healthy diet challenging. Other factors to consider include cultural differences, differences in school food environments, differences in home food environments, differences in family traditions and mealtimes, differences in the level of adherence to national dietary guidelines, price differences (which may affect the affordability and accessibility of healthy or unhealthy foods and differences in the availability of fruit or vegetables), and more.

These data lend further support to existing calls for urgent action to improve child nutrition. Schools may improve nutrition by following quality standards for school meals and providing students with access to healthy foods and beverages (such as fresh fruits, vegetables, and fresh water), and nutrition education [32]. Examples of successful initiatives include the European Union's School Fruit and Vegetable Scheme [33] and the WHO's Nutrition-Friendly Schools Initiative [34].

Another possible action to improve nutrition is through fiscal incentives or subsidies to promote better nutrition, both for encouraging the consumption of healthy foods (such as fruit or vegetables, or discouraging the consumption of unhealthy foods, such as sugary drinks). The United States Department of Agriculture provides reimbursement to states that operate nonprofit breakfast programs in schools [35]. Taxation on sugar-sweetened beverages has been shown to be effective in the reduction of sugar consumption [36,37]. Another potential intervention is the reformulation of processed foods [38], which has shown promise for the reduction of both sugar [39] and salt [40,41].

Current food and beverage marketing practices predominantly promote low-nutrition foods and beverages, and have a direct effect on children's nutrition knowledge, preferences, purchase behavior, consumption patterns, and diet-related health [42]. Governments should restrict the marketing of unhealthy foods to children, particularly in the digital world, where advertising may be especially persuasive [43]. Implementation of the WHO recommendations on the marketing of foods and non-alcoholic beverages to children is one indicator in the Global Monitoring Framework [44].

A comprehensive approach involving action at many levels is required to improve children's diets [45]. In addition to improving food environments (within schools, at home, and in other places where children gather), action is needed to engage parents and other adults who care for children [46]. Parents or caretakers often play a key role in ensuring the availability of nutritious foods, not only at home but also at school (in instances when children bring a packed lunch to school). Parents or caregivers can also help to ensure that children consume appropriate portion sizes, and there may be opportunities for governments to provide better guidance and support for parents and caregivers [47]. Front-of-pack labeling can help provide parents with information to support healthier eating choices and food purchases [48], although a recent Cochrane review suggests that more research may be needed regarding the effects that food labeling may have on consumer choices [49]. Nutritious diets may be more expensive, and this may contribute to socioeconomic disparities in health [50]; therefore, efforts must be made to ensure access to healthy and affordable foods, especially for vulnerable groups. Results from COSI indicate that the prevalence of obesity and severe obesity among children in Europe was common among children whose mothers had a lower level of education [51].

This study had several limitations. First, this study used a dietary questionnaire that has not been validated and which did not collect information on the portion sizes of foods. Future work is needed to validate this questionnaire and identify possible methods of assessing portion sizes of various foods that are consumed per day in order to identify the prevalence of children meeting certain nutrition recommendations (such as consuming five portions of fruits and vegetables per day). Further work is needed to validate questions about "sweets" and "savory snacks" where there may be cultural variation in the ways that these categories are understood. Another limitation is that the dietary indicators used in this paper are not comprehensive. For example, we reported here on "sweet treats, such as candy bars or chocolate" but there are other sweet foods, such as "biscuits, cakes, or doughnuts" (Supplementary Figure S1) that were assessed in a separate question but not reported in this paper.

This study was limited by a cross-sectional study design and a reliance on parental reports of children's diet behaviors, which may have limited accuracy [52,53]. Other limitations include possible social desirability bias or non-response bias. We do not know how the responders in this study varied from non-responders, but previous research indicates that healthier individuals with a higher socioeconomic status are more likely to respond to health surveys [54] or dietary surveys [55], and this may result in an overestimation of the prevalence of healthy behaviors. Another limitation is that this study did not account for seasonal differences in the availability of fruit and vegetables; responses to this questionnaire were collected during the autumn, winter, or spring months when fruit and vegetable availability may have been lower than during the summer months, particularly in Central Asia.

One of the main strengths of this study was that it collected data from a large sample of children across a diverse range of countries using nationally-representative sampling methods and following a common protocol.

This project is an ongoing one and will be updated in future years. It is a valuable dataset that represents the collaboration of many committed experts and provides important visibility into the habits of European children. Accurate data on children's weight status, eating habits, and other energy-balance-related behaviors provide a vital underpinning for government actions to implement and evaluate effective and appropriate strategies to combat under-nutrition and obesity. Investment in high-quality surveillance is essential to ensure more children can benefit from good nutrition and improved health during childhood and onward through the life course.

Supplementary Materials: The following are available online at http://www.mdpi.com/2072-6643/12/8/2481/s1, Box S1: Description of national ethics approval for countries featured in this paper who were participating in the WHO European Childhood Obesity Surveillance Initiative (COSI) Round 4 (2015-2017), Table S1: Frequency of breakfast consumption among boys and girls, by country. COSI/WHO Europe Round 4 (2015-17), Table S2: Frequency of fresh fruit consumption among boys and girls, by country. COSI/WHO Europe Round 4 (2015-17), Table S3: Frequency of vegetable consumption among boys and girls, by country. COSI/WHO Europe Round 4 (2015-17), Table S4: Frequency of savory snack consumption among boys and girls, by country. COSI/WHO Europe Round 4 (2015-17), Table S5: Frequency of sweet snacks consumption among boys and girls, by country. COSI/WHO Europe Round 4 (2015-17), Table S6: Frequency of soft drinks consumption among boys and girls, by country. COSI/WHO Europe Round 4 (2015-17), Figure S1: Description of the WHO European Childhood Obesity Surveillance Initiative question related to child dietary habits, COSI Round 4 (2015-17).

Author Contributions: Conceptualization, J.B., M.B., and J.W.; formal analysis: M.B. and J.W.; data curation, M.B. and J.W.; writing—original draft preparation, J.W., G.R., P.N., M.B., and A.C.B.; writing—review and editing, J.W., M.B., P.N., G.R., A.C.B., A.I.R., A.S., T.H., L.K., E.N., M.K., S.M.M., M.G.-S., E.G.-G., L.A.B., A.C., S.M.O., D.W., M.M., H.R., G.R., A.C.B., I.R., S.A., M.H., S.B.-S., J.H., S.R., I.S., G.S., K.B., M.W. and J.B.; supervision, J.B., I.R., A.S., T.H., M.K., S.M.M., A.F., V.F.S., I.P., V.D., N.Y., A.G., Z.U., V.P., L.S., Y.H., M.T., A.P., Z.A., and E.K. All authors have read and agreed to the published version of the manuscript.

Funding: These activities were partially funded through a grant from the Russian Government in the context of the WHO European Office for the Prevention and Control of Noncommunicable Diseases. The authors gratefully acknowledge support from the Danish Ministry of Health, the Italian Ministry of Health and Italian National Institute of Health, the National Institute for Health Development in Estonia, the Health Service Executive in the Republic of Ireland, the Ministry of Health in Bulgaria, the Poland National Health Program (grant no. 6/1/3.1.12/NPZ/2016/106/1401, the Czech Republic (grants AZV MZČR 17-31670 A and MZČR—RVO EÚ 00023761), and the Ministry of Health in Latvia. The Spanish study was funded by the Spanish Agency for Food Safety and Nutrition (AESAN). COSI Austria was supported by a grant from the Federal Ministry of Social Affairs, Health, Care and Consumer Protection, Republic of Austria. COSI Turkey gratefully acknowledges the World Bank for the survey credit. COSI Lithuania gratefully acknowledges the WHO representative in Lithuania, Ingrida Zurlyte, for printing the COSI questionnaires. The study in Kazakhstan was funded by the Ministry of Health of the Republic of Kazakhstan within the scientific and technical program.

Acknowledgments: We gratefully acknowledge support from Liza Villas and Gerben Rienk for making the COSI project possible. We also acknowledge the leadership of the principal investigators from Ireland (Cecily Kelleher), Kyrgyzstan (Gulmira Aitmurzaeva), Romania (Constanta Huidimac Petrescu), and Tajikistan (Zulfiya

Abdurrahmonova). The authors alone are responsible for the views expressed in this article and they do not necessarily represent the views, decisions or policies of the institutions with which they are affiliated.

Conflicts of Interest: The authors declare no conflict of interest.

References

1. Park, M.H.; Falconer, C.; Viner, R.M.; Kinra, S. The impact of childhood obesity on morbidity and mortality in adulthood: A systematic review. *Obes. Rev.* **2012**, *13*, 985–1000. [CrossRef] [PubMed]
2. Wijnhoven, T.M.; van Raaij, J.M.; Spinelli, A.; Starc, G.; Hassapidou, M.; Spiroski, I.; Rutter, H.; Martos, E.; Rito, A.I.; Hovengen, R.; et al. WHO European Childhood Obesity Surveillance Initiative: Body mass index and level of overweight among 6-9-year-old children from school year 2007/2008 to school year 2009/2010. *BMC Public Health* **2014**, *14*, 806. [CrossRef]
3. Afshin, A.; Sur, P.J.; Fay, K.A.; Cornaby, L.; Ferrara, G.; Salama, J.S.; Mullany, E.C.; Abate, K.H.; Abbafati, C.; Abebe, Z. Health effects of dietary risks in 195 countries, 1990–2017: A systematic analysis for the Global Burden of Disease Study 2017. *Lancet* **2019**, *393*, 1958–1972. [CrossRef]
4. Freemark, M. Determinants of Risk for Childhood Obesity. *N. Engl. J. Med.* **2018**, *379*, 1371–1372. [CrossRef] [PubMed]
5. Freemark, M. Childhood obesity in the modern age: Global trends, determinants, complications, and costs. In *Pediatric Obesity*; Springer: Berlin/Heidelberg, Germany, 2018; pp. 3–24.
6. WHO. *WHO European Childhood Obesity Surveillance Initiative: Report of the Fourth Round of Data Collection (2015–2017)*; WHO: Geneva, Switzerland, 2020.
7. WHO. The Double Burden of Malnutrition. Available online: https://www.who.int/nutrition/double-burden-malnutrition/en/#:~{}:text=Double%20burden%20of%20malnutrition,populations%2C%20and%20across%20the%20lifecourse (accessed on 1 June 2020).
8. Djordjic, V.; Jorga, J.; Radisavljevic, S.; Milanovic, I.; Bozic, P.; Ostojic, S.M. Thinness in young schoolchildren in Serbia: Another case of the double burden of malnutrition? *Public Health Nutr.* **2018**, *21*, 877–881. [CrossRef] [PubMed]
9. Global Burden of Disease Collaborators Health effects of overweight and obesity in 195 countries over 25 years. *N. Engl. J. Med.* **2017**, *377*, 13–27. [CrossRef]
10. WHO. World Health Organization Global Monitoring Framework for NCDs: Target 7: Halt the Rise in Obesity. Available online: https://www.who.int/nmh/ncd-tools/target7/en/ (accessed on 1 June 2020).
11. United Nations. Sustainable Development Goals. Available online: https://sustainabledevelopment.un.org/?menu=1300 (accessed on 28 June 2020).
12. Sachs, J.; Schmidt-Traub, G.; Kroll, C.; Lafortune, G.; Fuller, G. *Sustainable Development Report 2019*; Bertelsmann Stiftung and Sustainable Development Solutions Network (SDSN): New York, NY, USA, 2019; Volume 2.
13. Mikkilä, V.; Räsänen, L.; Raitakari, O.T.; Pietinen, P.; Viikari, J. Longitudinal changes in diet from childhood into adulthood with respect to risk of cardiovascular diseases: The Cardiovascular Risk in Young Finns Study. *Eur. J. Clin. Nutr.* **2004**, *58*, 1038–1045. [CrossRef]
14. WHO. *Increasing Fruit and Vegetable Consumption to Reduce the Risk of Noncommunicable Diseases*; World Health Organization: Geneva, Switzerland, 2014.
15. WHO. *Diet, Nutrition and the Prevention of Chronic Diseases: Report of a Joint WHO/FAO Expert Consultation*; WHO Technical Report Series, No. 916; World Health Organization: Geneva, Switzerland, 2003.
16. WHO. *Guideline: Sugars Intake for Adults and Children*; World Health Organization: Geneva, Switzerland, 2015.
17. Mozaffarian, D.; Fahimi, S.; Singh, G.M.; Micha, R.; Khatibzadeh, S.; Engell, R.E.; Lim, S.; Danaei, G.; Ezzati, M.; Powles, J.; et al. Global sodium consumption and death from cardiovascular causes. *N. Engl. J. Med.* **2014**, *371*, 624–634. [CrossRef]
18. Malik, V.S.; Pan, A.; Willett, W.C.; Hu, F.B. Sugar-sweetened beverages and weight gain in children and adults: A systematic review and meta-analysis. *Am. J. Clin. Nutr.* **2013**, *98*, 1084–1102. [CrossRef]
19. Moynihan, P.J.; Kelly, S.A.M. Effect on caries of restricting sugars intake: Systematic review to inform WHO guidelines. *J. Dent. Res.* **2014**, *93*, 8–18. [CrossRef]
20. Wijnhoven, T.M.; van Raaij, J.; Breda, J. *WHO European Childhood Obesity Surveillance Initiative. Implementation of Round 1 (2007/2008) and Round 2 (2009/2010)*; WHO Regional Office for Europe: Copenhagen, Denmark, 2014.

21. Council for International Organizations of Medical Sciences, Council for International Organizations of Medical Sciences, World Health Organization. *International Ethical Guidelines for Biomedical Research Involving Human Subjects*; World Health Organization: Geneva, Switzerland, 2002.
22. Wijnhoven, T.M.; van Raaij, J.M.; Spinelli, A.; Rito, A.I.; Hovengen, R.; Kunesova, M.; Starc, G.; Rutter, H.; Sjoberg, A.; Petrauskiene, A.; et al. WHO European Childhood Obesity Surveillance Initiative 2008: Weight, height and body mass index in 6-9-year-old children. *Pediatr. Obes.* **2013**, *8*, 79–97. [CrossRef] [PubMed]
23. WHO. *European Childhood Obesity Surveillance Initiative: Overweight and Obesity among 6–9-year-old Children. Report of the Third Round of Data Collection 2012–2013*; WHO: Geneva, Switzerland, 2018.
24. WHO. Healthy Diet: Key Facts. Available online: https://www.who.int/news-room/fact-sheets/detail/healthy-diet (accessed on 29 June 2020).
25. United Nations. Statistical Division Standard Country or Area Codes for Statistical Use (M49). Available online: https://unstats.un.org/unsd/methodology/m49/ (accessed on 6 August 2020).
26. Monzani, A.; Ricotti, R.; Caputo, M.; Solito, A.; Archero, F.; Bellone, S.; Prodam, F. A systematic review of the association of skipping breakfast with weight and cardiometabolic risk factors in children and adolescents. What should we better investigate in the future? *Nutrients* **2019**, *11*, 387. [CrossRef] [PubMed]
27. Inchley, J.; Currie, D.B.; Budisavljevic, S.; Torsheim, T.; Jåstad, A.; Cosma, A.; Kelly, C.; Arnarsson, Á. *Spotlight on Adolescent Health and Well-Being: Findings from the 2017/2018 Health Behaviour in School-Aged Children (HBSC) Survey in Europe and Canada*; WHO Regional Office for Europe: Copenhagen, Denmark, 2020.
28. Vereecken, C.; Pedersen, T.P.; Ojala, K.; Krølner, R.; Dzielska, A.; Ahluwalia, N.; Giacchi, M.; Kelly, C. Fruit and vegetable consumption trends among adolescents from 2002 to 2010 in 33 countries. *Eur. J. Public Health* **2015**, *25*, 16–19. [CrossRef]
29. Rosi, A.; Paolella, G.; Biasini, B.; Scazzina, F.; Alicante, P.; De Blasio, F.; dello Russo, M.; Paolella, G.; Rendina, D.; Rosi, A. Dietary habits of adolescents living in North America, Europe or Oceania: A review on fruit, vegetable and legume consumption, sodium intake, and adherence to the Mediterranean Diet. *Nutr. Metab. Cardiovasc. Dis.* **2019**, *29*, 554–560. [CrossRef] [PubMed]
30. Scaglioni, S.; De Cosmi, V.; Ciappolino, V.; Parazzini, F.; Brambilla, P.; Agostoni, C. Factors Influencing Children's Eating Behaviours. *Nutrients* **2018**, *10*, 706. [CrossRef] [PubMed]
31. Smith, R.; Kelly, B.; Yeatman, H.; Boyland, E. Food marketing influences children's attitudes, preferences and consumption: A systematic critical review. *Nutrients* **2019**, *11*, 875. [CrossRef] [PubMed]
32. Micha, R.; Karageorgou, D.; Bakogianni, I.; Trichia, E.; Whitsel, L.P.; Story, M.; Penalvo, J.L.; Mozaffarian, D. Effectiveness of school food environment policies on children's dietary behaviors: A systematic review and meta-analysis. *PLoS ONE* **2018**, *13*, e0194555. [CrossRef]
33. European Commission. School Fruit, Vegetables and Milk Scheme. Available online: https://ec.europa.eu/info/food-farming-fisheries/key-policies/common-agricultural-policy/market-measures/school-fruit-vegetables-and-milk-scheme (accessed on 25 May 2020).
34. WHO. Nutrition-Friendly Schools Initiative (NFSI). Available online: https://www.who.int/nutrition/topics/nutrition_friendly_schools_initiative/en/ (accessed on 25 May 2020).
35. U.S. Department of Agriculture. School Breakfast Program. Available online: https://www.fns.usda.gov/sbp/school-breakfast-program (accessed on 26 May 2020).
36. WHO. *Taxes on Sugary Drinks: Why Do It?* World Health Organization: Geneva, Switzerland, 2017.
37. Colchero, M.A.; Rivera-Dommarco, J.; Popkin, B.M.; Ng, S.W. In Mexico, Evidence of Sustained Consumer Response two Years after Implementing a Sugar-Sweetened Beverage Tax. *Health Aff. (Millwood)* **2017**, *36*, 564–571. [CrossRef]
38. van Raaij, J.; Hendriksen, M.; Verhagen, H. Potential for improvement of population diet through reformulation of commonly eaten foods. *Public Health Nutr.* **2009**, *12*, 325–330. [CrossRef]
39. Goiana-da-Silva, F.; Cruz, E.S.D.; Gregorio, M.J.; Miraldo, M.; Darzi, A.; Araujo, F. The future of the sweetened beverages tax in Portugal. *Lancet Public Health* **2018**, *3*, e562. [CrossRef]
40. Griffith, R.; O'Connell, M.; Smith, K. The Importance of Product Reformulation Versus Consumer Choice in Improving Diet Quality. *Economica* **2017**, *84*, 34–53. [CrossRef]
41. Macgregor, G.A.; Hashem, K.M. Action on sugar–lessons from UK salt reduction programme. *Lancet* **2014**, *383*, 929–931. [CrossRef]

42. Cairns, G.; Angus, K.; Hastings, G.; Caraher, M. Systematic reviews of the evidence on the nature, extent and effects of food marketing to children. A retrospective summary. *Appetite* **2013**, *62*, 209–215. [CrossRef] [PubMed]
43. WHO. *Monitoring and Restricting Digital Marketing of Unhealthy Products to Children and Adolescents*; World Health Organization Regional Office for Europe: Copenhagen, Denmark, 2019.
44. WHO. *Noncommunicable Diseases Progress Monitor*; World Health Organization: Geneva, Switzerland, 2017.
45. Hodder, R.K.; O'Brien, K.M.; Tzelepis, F.; Wyse, R.J.; Wolfenden, L. Interventions for increasing fruit and vegetable consumption in children aged five years and under. *Cochrane Database Syst. Rev.* **2018**, *2018*, CD008552. [CrossRef]
46. Mazarello Paes, V.; Hesketh, K.; O'Malley, C.; Moore, H.; Summerbell, C.; Griffin, S.; Van Sluijs, E.M.F.; Ong, K.K.; Lakshman, R. Determinants of sugar-sweetened beverage consumption in young children: A systematic review. *Obes. Rev.* **2015**, *16*, 903–913. [CrossRef]
47. Kairey, L.; Matvienko-Sikar, K.; Kelly, C.; McKinley, M.C.; O'Connor, E.M.; Kearney, P.M.; Woodside, J.V.; Harrington, J.M. Plating up appropriate portion sizes for children: A systematic review of parental food and beverage portioning practices. *Obes. Rev.* **2018**, *19*, 1667–1678. [CrossRef]
48. WHO. *Report of the Commission on Ending Childhood Obesity*; World Health Organization: Geneva, Switzerland, 2016.
49. Crockett, R.A.; King, S.E.; Marteau, T.M.; Prevost, A.T.; Bignardi, G.; Roberts, N.W.; Stubbs, B.; Hollands, G.J.; Jebb, S.A. Nutritional labelling for healthier food or non-alcoholic drink purchasing and consumption. *Cochrane Database Syst. Rev.* **2018**, *2*, CD009315. [CrossRef]
50. Monsivais, P.; Aggarwal, A.; Drewnowski, A. Are socio-economic disparities in diet quality explained by diet cost? *J. Epidemiol. Community Health* **2012**, *66*, 530–535. [CrossRef]
51. Spinelli, A.; Buoncristiano, M.; Kovacs, V.A.; Yngve, A.; Spiroski, I.; Obreja, G.; Starc, G.; Pérez, N.; Rito, A.I.; Kunešová, M. Prevalence of severe obesity among primary school children in 21 European countries. *Obes. Facts* **2019**, *12*, 244–258. [CrossRef]
52. Pérez-Rodrigo, C.; Artiach Escauriaza, B.; Artiach Escauriaza, J.; Polanco Allúe, I. Dietary assessment in children and adolescents: Issues and recommendations. *Nutr. Hosp.* **2015**, *31* (Suppl. 3), 76–83. [CrossRef]
53. Medin, A.C.; Hansen, B.H.; Astrup, H.; Ekelund, U.; Frost Andersen, L. Validation of energy intake from a web-based food recall for children and adolescents. *PLoS ONE* **2017**, *12*, e0178921. [CrossRef] [PubMed]
54. Cheung, K.L.; Peter, M.; Smit, C.; de Vries, H.; Pieterse, M.E. The impact of non-response bias due to sampling in public health studies: A comparison of voluntary versus mandatory recruitment in a Dutch national survey on adolescent health. *BMC Public Health* **2017**, *17*, 276. [CrossRef] [PubMed]
55. Berg, C.; Jonsson, I.; Conner, M.T.; Lissner, L. Sources of bias in a dietary survey of children. *Eur. J. Clin. Nutr.* **1998**, *52*, 663–667. [CrossRef] [PubMed]

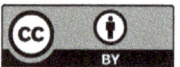

© 2020 by the authors. Licensee MDPI, Basel, Switzerland. This article is an open access article distributed under the terms and conditions of the Creative Commons Attribution (CC BY) license (http://creativecommons.org/licenses/by/4.0/).

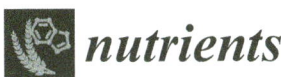

Review

Food Consumption Patterns and Nutrient Intakes of Children and Adolescents in the Eastern Mediterranean Region: A Call for Policy Action

Ayoub Al-Jawaldeh [1], Mandy Taktouk [2] and Lara Nasreddine [2,*]

1. World Health Organization (WHO), Regional Office for the Eastern Mediterranean (EMRO), Cairo 7608, Egypt; aljawaldeha@who.int
2. Nutrition and Food Sciences Department, Faculty of Agriculture and Food Sciences, American University of Beirut, Beirut 11-0236, Lebanon; mrt07@mail.aub.edu
* Correspondence: ln10@aub.edu.lb; Tel.: +961-1-350000 (ext. 4547)

Received: 8 October 2020; Accepted: 29 October 2020; Published: 30 October 2020

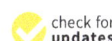

Abstract: The Eastern Mediterranean Region (EMR) has witnessed significant social and economic changes that may have influenced the diet of children and adolescents, and increased the risk for obesity and malnutrition in this age group. This review aims to characterize and assess food consumption patterns and nutrient intakes amongst school-aged children (5–10 years) and adolescents (10–19 years) in countries of the EMR. Electronic databases (MedLine, PubMed, Scopus, and Google Scholar) were searched for relevant articles published between 2005 and 2020; international organizations and governmental websites were also searched. Available studies documented low intakes of fruits, vegetables and fiber, inadequate consumption of water, milk and dairy products, coupled with high intakes of fat, saturated fat, and sugar sweetened beverages, as well as a frequent consumption of energy-dense, nutrient poor foods such as sweet and savory snacks. Micronutrient inadequacies were also observed, particularly for calcium, iron, zinc and vitamins A, D, C, and folate. Acknowledging the impact that nutrition may have on building societies and transforming the lives of children, adolescents and their families, there is a crucial need for a food system approach in developing and implementing national and regional policies and interventions aimed at improving the diet of children and adolescents.

Keywords: food consumption patterns; dietary intakes; macronutrients; micronutrients; children; adolescents; Eastern Mediterranean Region; review

1. Introduction

The health and well-being of children and adolescents are essential prerequisites for achieving the Sustainable Development Goals (SDGs), particularly those focusing on poverty, health security, education and the reduction of inequalities [1]. The World Health Organization (WHO) acknowledged the importance of adequate nutrition to "enable children and adolescents to enjoy good health while playing a full role in contributing to transformative change and sustainable development", in alignment with the SDGs [2]. Good nutrition during childhood and adolescence is in fact indispensable for growth and development, health and well-being, and the prevention of obesity and several chronic diseases [3].

Unhealthy diets in childhood and adolescence are associated with immediate as well as long-term health impacts. In the short term, inadequate dietary intakes of energy, protein, or certain micronutrients will result in slower growth rates, delayed sexual maturation, lower reserves of micronutrients, and inadequate bone mass [4]. Dietary intakes of children and adolescents may also affect their risk of developing a number of health problems, such as iron deficiency and dental caries, while also lowering their resistance to infectious diseases and adversely affecting their ability to function at peak mental and physical capacity [3]. Poor diets in these critical periods of the life course are also linked with pediatric obesity and its related metabolic abnormalities, such as high blood pressure, type 2 diabetes (T2D), metabolic syndrome, sleep disturbances, orthopedic problems, and psychosocial problems [5–8], which all tend to track into adulthood [9].

Dietary practices of children and adolescents may also carry long-term health ramifications, increasing the risk for several non-communicable diseases (NCDs), and contributing significantly to the burden of preventable diseases and premature deaths [3]. In the Eastern Mediterranean region (EMR), which has witnessed over the past few decades important social, economic, and political changes [10], three of the ten leading causes of death are related to dietary factors, including ischemic heart disease, strokes, and diabetes. Urbanization, technological development, and modernization, have in fact instigated significant demographic and epidemiologic changes in most countries of the region, with parallel shifts in diet, physical activity, and body composition [11]. These shifts represent the basis of the multidimensional phenomenon of the nutrition transition, which is characterized by increases in the intakes of energy, fat, added sugars, and salt [11,12]. Some states in the region are classified as countries in advanced nutrition transition, such as the Gulf Cooperation Council (GCC) countries, the Islamic Republic of Iran, and Tunisia, while others are classified in early nutrition transition, such as Jordan, Lebanon, Egypt, Libya, and Morocco [13]. In contrast, political turmoil and economic challenges have adversely impacted the availability of food in some EMR countries such as Iraq, Pakistan, occupied Palestinian territory, and Yemen, while some states are categorized as countries in emergency and humanitarian crisis, such as Afghanistan, Somalia, and Sudan [13,14].

Amidst the threat of transitioning to high-energy, nutrient-poor diets and the parallel hazard of food insecurity, children and adolescents may be amongst the most vulnerable population groups to the ongoing societal, lifestyle, and dietary changes in countries of the region [15]. Available evidence indicates that the region harbors one of the highest rates of pediatric and adolescent obesity worldwide, while the burden of undernutrition and micronutrient deficiencies persists in many of its countries [16]. Overcoming pediatric and adolescent malnutrition in all of its forms (overnutrition, undernourishment, and micronutrient deficiencies) entails the development of evidence-based interventions and the design of related health policies to ensure the availability of and access to healthy diets. Effective planning for such interventions should be guided by accurate, up-to date and comprehensive data on food consumption patterns and nutrient intakes. The objective of this review is to characterize and assess food consumption patterns and nutrient intakes amongst school-aged children (5–10 years) and adolescents (10–19 years) in countries of the EMR. Findings from this review will characterize food consumption patterns amongst children and adolescents in the EMR and identify prevalent nutrient excesses or inadequacies. It will also contribute to the prioritization of research to address current gaps in knowledge and inform policies and interventions aimed at developing healthy eating habits in these critical periods of the lifecycle.

2. Approach

The literature search covered the EMR, which according to the WHO, includes 21 countries that comprise Afghanistan, Bahrain, Djibouti, Egypt, Iran (Islamic Republic of), Iraq, Jordan, Kuwait, Lebanon, Libyan Arab Jamahiriya, Morocco, Oman, Pakistan, Qatar, Saudi-Arabia, Somalia, Sudan, Syrian Arab Republic, Tunisia, United Arab Emirates (UAE), and Yemen [17].

Dietary intake data including food group, energy, macronutrient, and micronutrient intakes were evaluated and compared with reference intake values and/or guidelines (when available). A comprehensive literature review was conducted, including individual studies and review articles published between 2005 and 2020, which reported on dietary intakes in children and adolescents aged 5–19 years in any country of the EMR. Electronic databases (MedLine, PubMed, Scopus, and Google Scholar) were searched between 15 July 2020, and 15 August 2020. The search was restricted to the English, French, and Arabic languages, and the key terms used in the search strategy were as follows: EMR countries and/or each country alone AND "Diet" OR "Dietary" OR "Nutritional" OR "Nutrient" AND "Intake" OR "Consumption" AND "Children" OR "Child" OR "Adolescent". In addition, for the dietary intake, a narrower search was performed while including the following key terms: "Energy", "Macronutrient", "Carbohydrate", "Fat", "Saturated Fat", "trans-fat" "Protein", "Fiber", "Sugar", "Meats", "Milk", OR "Dairy", "Fruits", "Vegetables", "Candy", OR "Candies", OR "Sweets", "Chips", "Water", "Sugar Sweetened Beverage", "Juice". A parallel search strategy was also adopted for micronutrient intake (including iron, iodine, zinc, copper, calcium, sodium, thiamin, riboflavin, folate, vitamin B12, vitamin A, vitamin D, and vitamin C). The reference lists of the specific studies were also reviewed to identify additional data sources. Studies were retained if they reported on children aged 5 to 18 years; studies reporting on under-five children were excluded. The global school-based student health survey (GSHS) database [18] was also reviewed to obtain data on the consumption of fruits, vegetables, and carbonated beverages.

Data was presented separately for school-aged children (5–10 years) and adolescents (10–19 years). Food groups were classified based on the categories proposed by Keats et al. [19] in their systematic review of dietary intakes amongst adolescent girls in low and middle income countries. Accordingly, the following food categories were adopted: (1) fruits; (2) vegetables; (3) pulses (beans, peas, lentils); (4) grains; (5) dairy; (6) meat, poultry, and fish; (7) fast foods; (8) sweet snacks; (9) salty and fried snacks, and (10) sugar-sweetened beverages (SSBs). Dietary intakes were compared, when possible, with the WHO recommendations. The recommendations of the WHO for a healthy diet include the consumption of at least 400 g, or 5 portions, of fruits and vegetables/day to reduce the risk of NCDs and ensure an adequate daily intake of dietary fiber (>25 g); reducing sodium intake to less than 2 g/day (5 g of salt), total fat intake to less than 30% of energy intake (EI), reducing saturated fat (SFA) intake to less than 10% EI, and trans fat (TFA) to less than 1% EI [20], and replacing them with unsaturated fats including polyunsaturated fats (PUFAs) (6–10% EI), n-6 PUFAs (5–8% EI), and n-3 PUFAs (1–2% EI); consuming protein in the range of 10–15% EI, carbohydrates 55–75% EI, and free sugars (FS) less than 10% EI.

3. Results

3.1. Food Consumption Patterns Amongst Children and Adolescents in the EMR

3.1.1. School-Aged Children

A striking scarcity is noticed with respect to studies investigating food consumption patterns amongst school-aged children in the EMR. Many of the available studies were conducted with the aim of investigating the relationship between dietary factors and health outcome, such as dental caries [21–23], overweight [24,25], elevated blood pressure [26], or anemia [27], in small samples of children. The majority of available studies have reported on whether the child consumes a certain food group (Yes/No) or on only the frequency of intake (per day or per week), which limits the interpretability of the findings.

In the Levant, a national study conducted in Lebanon showed that fast food alone contributed to around 11.3% of daily EI, and this was coupled with a high intake of sweets and SSBs, which provided 10.8% and 6.5% EI, respectively [24]. In the GCC, a study conducted amongst children aged six years and above in the 11 regions of Bahrain ($n = 496$) reported that only half of the children reported daily consumption of milk and its products and one fourth reported daily consumption of fruits and vegetables [28]. In contrast, daily consumption of soft drinks was reported by 50% of the children and daily consumption of sweets and snacks was reported by 64% of girls and 47% of boys [28]. A study conducted in all the seven emirates of the UAE showed that amongst 6–8 year old children, more than 90% did not meet the MyPyramid recommendations for vegetables and milk/dairy products, 72–89% did not meet the recommendations for fruits, 49–68% did not meet the recommendations for grains, and 64–75% did not meet the recommendations for meat and beans [29]. In the Kingdom of Saudi-Arabia (KSA), a study conducted amongst 7–12 year old children in Al-Baha city indicated that, 69% and 71% of children did not report daily consumption of fruits and vegetables, respectively, and that only 0.9% met the recommended intake levels of fruits and vegetables [30]. This study also showed that 32% of children did not consume milk/dairy products on a daily basis, with only 1.9% adhering to dairy intake recommendations [30]. In Qatar, a study investigating snack consumption amongst 9–10 year old students in Doha showed that the most commonly consumed snacks in the study sample included fruit drinks (consumed by 98.8% of students), and a high percentage of children reported the consumption of potato chips (81.5%), candy and chocolates (41.7%), and pizzas and pies (39.8%), while the least consumed snacks were milk (37.1%) and nuts (0.8%) [31].

Studies conducted in Iran reported a relatively high consumption of fruits and vegetables amongst school-aged children, in the range of 400 g/day [20,32], with more than 60% of children being adherent to the WHO recommendations [33]. In contrast, the consumption of milk and dairy products was reported to be low (0.8 servings/day) [34]. A high consumption of sweet snacks (two servings/day) [32], fats and oils (6.2 servings/day) [34], and salty snacks (1.3–1.4 servings/day) [32] was also noted. The average consumption of grains met the recommendations (7.4 servings/day) [34], but approximately 60% of children reported to consume grains in their refined form [35].

3.1.2. Adolescents

The GSHS database provides country-specific information on the consumption of fruits, vegetables, and carbonated beverages amongst adolescents aged 13–17 years [18]. Figure 1 summarizes data available from EMR countries. Amongst 13–15 year old adolescents, the percentage of students who reported the consumption of fruits and vegetables at least five times/day during the month preceding the survey was low, ranging between 12.6% in Libya and 38.1% in Djibouti. In contrast, higher proportions of adolescents reported the consumption of carbonated soft drinks once or more times/day. These proportions ranged between 30.8% and 66.6% amongst 13–15 year old adolescents and between 31.5% and 56.9% in those aged 16 to 17 year old (Figure 2).

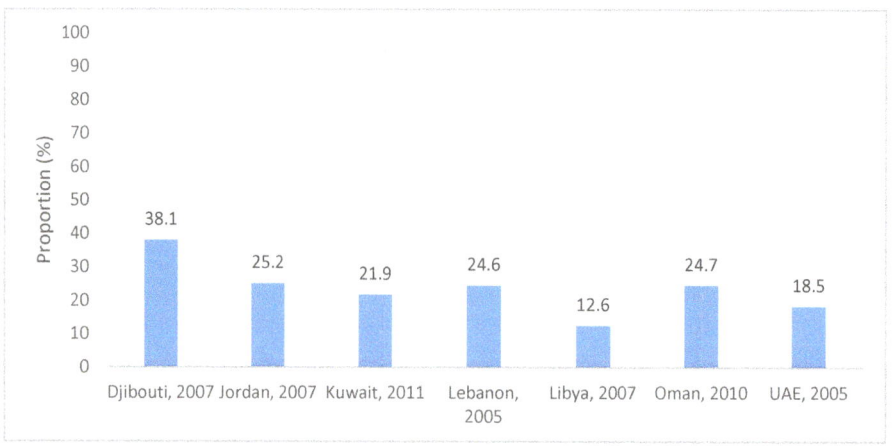

Figure 1. Proportion of students (aged 13–15 years) who had fruits and vegetables at least five times/day during the 30 days preceding the survey, based on the global school-based student health survey (GSHS) database [18].

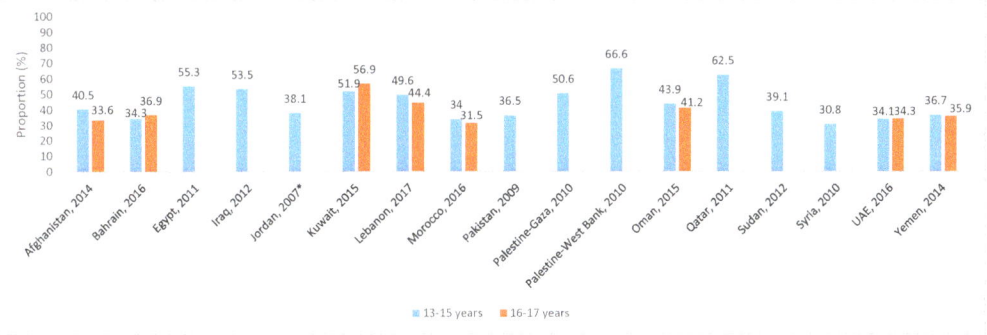

Figure 2. Proportion of students (aged 13–17 years) who drank carbonated soft drinks once or more times per day during the 30 days preceding the survey, based on the global school-based student health survey (GSHS) database [18]. *: This data represents the proportion of students (13–15 years) who drank carbonated soft drinks twice or more times per day during the 30 days preceding the survey in Jordan.

Research studies have also documented suboptimal dietary practices amongst adolescents in the EMR. Table 1, shows that the proportions of adolescents reporting daily intake of fruits ranged between 11% and 33.5% in most countries, except for studies conducted in Iraq [36] and Palestine [37] where higher estimates were reported. The proportions of adolescents reporting daily consumption of vegetables ranged between 20% and 43% in countries like Bahrain, Jordan, Kuwait, Morocco, Qatar, and KSA, while higher estimates were reported from Egypt (78.2%), Iraq (46–62%), Palestine (73%), and Sudan (70%) (Table 1). In Lebanon, a study investigating the diets of adolescents from contrasting socioeconomic backgrounds (n = 209, aged 17–19 years) [38] documented low intakes of vegetables, ranging between 1.4 and 1.9 servings/day, while fruits intake was reported as adequate. Studies conducted in Oman showed that, amongst adolescents, 52–57% consumed less than three servings of vegetables/day [39], and more than a third of adolescents consumed less than two servings of fruits/day [39]. In the UAE, Makansi et al. (2018) indicated that only 28% of adolescents from grades 10–12 (n = 620) met the recommended daily fruit and vegetable intake [40]. In a study conducted amongst 12–16 year old adolescents in Shiraz (Iran), the intake of fruits and vegetables together was estimated at 3.27 servings/day [41].

Food consumption patterns amongst adolescents in the region are also characterized by inadequate intakes of dairy: the proportions reporting daily intake did not exceed a third of adolescents in EMR countries, except for Egypt and Morocco [42–44]. In Muscat, Oman, 76% of adolescent boys and 83% of girls were found to consume less than two servings of dairy/day [39], and in Lebanon, the intake of dairy was estimated to range between 0.5 and 0.7 servings/day [38]. In Iran, Shokrvash et al. (2015) reported that only 14.2% of adolescents met the recommended daily dairy serving consumption, with the average being estimated at 1.64 servings/day [45].

Few studies have assessed the intake of grains and pulses amongst adolescents. In Lebanon and Syria, grains (breads and cereals) were the highest contributor to daily EI, being estimated at 32.7% [24] and 18.4–22% EI [46], respectively. In KSA, the most frequently consumed food items amongst adolescents were grains (rice and breads), with more than 50.5% of adolescents reporting to consume rice at least once daily [47]. Studies conducted in Egypt [42], Iran [48], KSA [49], and Sudan [50], showed that 87–96% of adolescents reported daily consumption of grains (bread, rice, and other cereals). In Muscat, Oman, Waly et al. showed that the proportion of boys and girls consuming less than six servings of grains/day did not exceed one fourth of adolescents [39]. Evidence on the consumption of pulses is scarce. The proportions of adolescents reporting daily consumption of pulses were high in some countries such as Iran (53.8%) [48] and Sudan (64.9%) [51], while estimates from Bahrain [52], Palestine [53], and Jordan [54] ranged between 4% and 19%.

Evidence on the intake of meat, poultry, and fish is also scarce in the region. In Oman, the proportions of adolescents reporting to consume more than three servings of meat, poultry, and fish/day was high, ranging between 68–78% [39]. In Syria, the meat, poultry, and fish group was the second largest contributor to EI (18–21%) [46], while in Lebanon this food group provided 10.2% EI [24]. Despite the fact that the consumption of meat and poultry is frequent in this population group (Table 1), available studies suggest that the intake of fish is suboptimal. Studies conducted in KSA [47,55] reported that half of adolescents did not consume any fish or seafood during the week preceding the survey. In Syria, fish was reported to be rarely consumed by adolescents in Damascus [56], with only 6% consuming it for two times or more/week.

The consumption of high fat, high sugar, high salt foods (HFSS) is common amongst adolescents in the EMR. Table 1 shows that the proportions of adolescents reporting daily intake of SSBs ranged between 37.5% and 80%, except for Palestine and Egypt where these proportions were lower than 20%. A national study in Kuwait [57] has even reported that 43% of adolescents consumed SSBs more than once/day. Country-specific disparities were observed in the proportions of adolescents reporting daily consumption of fast foods, which ranged between 9% and 64% (Table 1). For salty and fried snacks such as potato chips and fries, the proportions of adolescents reporting daily consumption reached as high as 84% in some countries such as Iran (Table 1). Sweet snacks (Cakes/pastries and sweets/chocolates) were also found to be frequently consumed, with the proportions of adolescents reporting daily consumption ranging between 21% and 49% for sweets/chocolates, and exceeding 40% for cakes/pastries in some countries such as Sudan. In Kuwait, Honkola et al. (2006) reported that large proportions of 11–13 years adolescents consumed sweets (42%), SSBs (43%), and cakes (42.5%) several times a day, and that almost every fourth child reported consuming all of these sugary products more than once a day [58]. The frequent consumption of these HFSS suggests that these foods may have significant contributions to EI in adolescents. In Lebanon, fast foods alone were found to contribute 17% EI amongst adolescents [24], and the caloric contribution of sweets and SSBs was estimated at 10% EI and 6.5% EI, respectively [24]. In Syrian adolescents, potato chips alone provided 5% EI and the same was observed for chocolates (5% EI), while sweets and SSBs together provided close to 8% EI [46].

Studies examining water intake amongst adolescents showed that in KSA, close to 60% of 12–15 year old adolescents consumed less than 6 cups of water per day [59] and that water provided only 37% of mean daily fluid intake in 12–13 year old adolescents [60]. Similarly, in Jordan, 74% of 6–18 year olds had fewer than four cups of water daily [61]. A study conducted in Lebanon estimated mean total water intake (TWI) at 1698 mL/day amongst 9–13 years old, and showed that, compared to the adequate intake (AI) level proposed by the Institute of Medicine (IOM) [62], only 5% met the recommendations for daily TWI [63]. In the UAE, mean total daily water intake was estimated at 1116.9 mL amongst 14–18 year old adolescents compared to 922.2 mL amongst 9–13 year olds [64]. The proportion of participants who met the IOM recommendations ranged between 23% and 24% for 9–13 year olds and between 1% and 21% for 14–18 year olds [64].

3.2. Macronutrient Intakes Amongst School-Aged Children and Adolescents in the EMR

3.2.1. School-Aged Children

Studies reporting on macronutrient intakes amongst school-aged children in the EMR are scarce. Close to 88% of 6–12 year old children in Cairo met the Recommended Dietary Allowances (RDA) for protein and [71], in Jordan, mean intake of protein ranged between 73% and 85% of the RDA amongst 5–10 year old children from Bedouin or underprivileged communities [27,72]. Another study conducted amongst five year old children from two cities in Jordan reported a high intake of total fat (34.3% EI in boys and 33.8% EI in girls) as well as a high intake of SFA (13.7–14.2% EI) [73]. Fat intake was also found to be high in Lebanese school-aged children, ranging between 35.8% and 39.7% EI, with more than half of the children exceeding the upper level for SFA intake [24,74,75]. In contrast, more than 90% of Lebanese school-aged children did not meet the recommended intakes of alpha-linolenic acid [24,74,76]. In Sudan, Alredaisy and Ibrahim (2011) showed that carbohydrates contributed 58.2% EI amongst rural school-aged children, while noting a high intake level of total fat (32.3% EI) [77]. As for countries of the GCC, a study conducted amongst 6–12 year old girls in KSA [25] showed that protein intake contributed 20.5% EI, while carbohydrates and fat provided 55% and 25.9% EI, repsectively. In the UAE, carbohydrates were reported as the main source of energy in 6–10 year old children (60% of EI) [78]. This level of carbohydrate intake was confirmed by another national study amongst children aged 6 to 13 years in the UAE, where carbohydrates provided 57.4–60.4% of daily EI [29]. It was also reported that 75–92% of participating children had fiber intakes below the requirements [74], 3.7–23% did not meet the protein requirements [74], while 28–46% exceeded the upper level for SFA [29,74].

3.2.2. Adolescents

Macronutrient intakes amongst adolescents in the EMR are displayed, by country, in Table 2.

Average protein intakes reported by the various studies were within the 10–15% range suggested by the WHO. Few countries exceeded this range, and this was particularly true for Oman [79]. In many countries of the region, the intake of total fat exceeded the upper limit of 30% EI, and this was at the expense of carbohydrates.

Table 1. Proportions of adolescents reporting daily consumption (unless otherwise indicated) of various food groups * in countries of the Eastern Mediterranean Region.

Country	Fruits	Vegetables	Dairy	Meat, Poultry, and Fish	Fast Foods	SSBs	Sweet Snacks (Including Confectionary) Cakes/Pastries	Sweet Snacks (Including Confectionary) Sweets/Chocolates	Salty and Fried Snacks
Bahrain [52] (National)	25.3%	26.3%	37.1%	Meat: 20% Fish: 6.9% Poultry: 18.2%	14.4%	42.2%	–	Sweets: 31.4% Chocolates: 32%	–
Egypt [42]	29%	78.2%	58.9%	–	64.6%	19.7%	–	–	–
Iran [48]	16.2%		16.3%	Meat: 31.9%	–	75.4%	–	45.5%	84.7%
Iraq [36]	M: 24.3% F: 46.3%	M: 46.1% F: 62.3%	Milk: M: 37.2% F: 35.2%	–	>3 days/w: M: 37.1% F: 24.9%	>3 days/w: M: 66.9% F: 60.4%	>3 days/w: M: 46.1% F: 55%	>3 days/w: M: 43.5% F: 52.2%	>3 days/w: M: 51% F: 64.6%
Jordan [54]	20%	43%	–	1–3 times/w: Meat: 47% Fish: 54% 4–6 times/w: Poultry: 40%	1–3 times/w: 57%	–	–	Chocolates: 40%	–
Kuwait [57]	M: 17.5% F: 11.8%	M: 26% F: 22.1%	M: 36.3% F: 25.3%	–	M: 9.4% F: 10.4%	M: 42.2% F: 37.5%	M: 7% F: 14.7%	M: 21.1% F: 35.6%	Potato fries/chips: M: 9.4%; F: 12.4%
Kuwait [58] (National)	–	–	–	–	–	>1 time/d: 43%	>1 time/d: 42.5%	>1 time/d: 42%	–
Morocco [43,44]	M: 18.7% F: 20.4%	M: 33.1% F: 42.5%	M: 78.1% F: 76.9%	–	>3 times/w: M: 15% F: 12.9%	>3 times/w: M: 37.5% F: 41.9%	>3 times/w: M: 66.9% F: 79%	3 times/w: M: 66.9% F: 72%	>3 times/w: Potato fries/chips: M: 18.8%; F: 29%
Palestine [53]	M: 11.6% F: 16.2%	M: 27.6% F: 34.1%	Milk: M: 33.7% F: 29.9% Yogurt: M: 19.8% F: 20.8%	>3 times/w: Meat: M: 7.3% F: 7.9% Poultry: M: 3.4% F: 3.8%	–	M: 6.2% F: 9.3%	Cookies: M: 14.6% F: 19.6%	Chocolates: M: 10.7% F: 17%	–

Table 1. Cont.

Country	Fruits	Vegetables	Dairy	Meat, Poultry, and Fish	Fast Foods	SSBs	Sweet Snacks (Including Confectionary) Cakes/Pastries	Sweet Snacks (Including Confectionary) Sweets/Chocolates	Salty and Fried Snacks
Palestine [65] (National)	31%	45%	Milk: 22%	Meat and poultry: 16%	–	24%		35%	–
Palestine [37]	M: 58.9% F: 55.2%	M: 72.8% F: 73.8%	Milk: M: 32.9% F: 18.3% Yogurt: M: 31.8% F: 28.3%	Meat: M: 11.4% F: 10.7% Poultry: M: 11.9% F: 12.2%	–	M: 39.6% F: 28.4%		M: 42.3% F: 49.2%	Salty snacks: M: 50.3% F: 61.5% Fried potatoes: M: 20.5% F: 23.8%
Qatar [66]	13.9%	20.3%	24.1%	–	≥4 days/w: 27.3%	≥4 days/w: 48.8%	≥4 days/w: 24.5%	≥4 days/w: 49.4%	≥4 days/w: 28.7%
Saudi [67]	M: 16% F: 9.6%	M: 23.3% F: 22.3%	Milk: M: 33.2% F: 25.1%	–	>3 days/w: M: 30.2% F: 24.9%	>3 days/w: M: 67.3% F: 57.4%	>3 days/w: M: 24.8% F: 28.8%	>3 days/w: M: 37.3% F: 52.6%	>3 days/w: M: 25% F: 30.7%
Sudan [50]	M: 33.5% F: 31.9%	M: 70.1% F: 69.7%	–	Meat: M: 55.7% F: 60.7%	–	M: 43.9% F: 44.8%	Sweets: M: 55.4% F: 60.6%	–	Crisps: M: 38.7% F: 39.2% Other salty snacks: M: 42.9% F: 32%
Sudan [51]	>4 times/w: 30.1%	>4 times/w: 63.9%	>4 times/w: 58.1%	>4 times/w: Meat: 59.1% Fish: 11.4% Poultry: 27.8%	>4 times/w: 26.6%	>4 times/w: 43.4%	>4 times/w: 37.1%	>4 times/w: Chocolates: 30.1%	–
Sudan [68]	–	–	–	–	–	80.6%	Dessert: 69.3% Sweet biscuits: 65.3%	Chocolates: 80% Popsicles: 61.4% Sweets: 48.7%	–
UAE [40]	–	–	–	–	≥1 time/w: M: 77.3% F: 81.4%	≥1 time/d: M: 41.1% F: 34%		–	–

Abbreviations: SSBs: sugar-sweetened beverages; M: males; F: females; w: week; d: day; UAE: United Arab Emirates. Salty snacks may include potato chips, French fries, popcorn, crackers. *: Food items categorization was adopted and modified based on a review by Keats et al., 2018 [19,69,70]. The following categories were not included in the table due to limited data: Grains, white roots, tubers and plantains; Pulses (beans, peas, lentils); Nuts and seeds; Eggs; Oils and fats.

Adequacy of macronutrient intake was investigated in some of the reviewed studies. In Iran, average protein intake was found to represent 165.4% of the RDA for protein and 154.7% of the WHO recommendations, highlighting an adequate dietary protein intake [80]. In KSA, mean nutrient adequacy ratio (NAR) of protein was estimated at 1.84, which indicates that protein intake met the dietary requirement in the majority of subjects [81]. Another study in KSA showed that mean protein intake (70.8 ± 40.6 g/day) amongst 13–18 year adolescents in Jeddah, was around 1.6 times higher than that recommended by the Academy of Nutrition and Dietetics (44 and 59 g/day for males and females respectively) [82]. In Bahrain, adolescent boys and girls consumed 1.5 times the United Kingdom's (UK's) Reference Nutrient intake (RNI) for protein [28,83], and in Kuwait, 86–92% of adolescents met the Acceptable Macronutrient Distribution range (AMDR) of 10–35% EI for protein [74,84]. In contrast, in Palestine, inadequate protein intake (<80% RDA) was observed amongst 15.1% of boys and 43.1% of girls aged 11–16 years [85], and in Northern Sudan, 50% of adolescents aged 13–18 years had inadequate protein intake (<80% of RDA) [86].

As for the adequacy of intake for the various subtypes of fat intake, a study conducted amongst 10–19 year old adolescents in Iran [87], showed that the average intake of SFA (10.3% EI) was close to the upper limit set by the WHO (10%) [88]. Another study in Iran reported that only a third of 6–18 year old participants, adhered to the WHO recommendations on SFA and half adhered to the recommendations related to PUFAs intakes [33]. Mirmiran et al. (2019) also reported on TFA, estimating its average intake at 2.2% EI, with only 6% of the study participants adhering to the TFA WHO recommendations of less than 1% EI [20,33]. In Lebanon, the average intake of SFA (10.7%) exceeded the WHO upper limit, while the intakes of Linoleic acid (4.8% EI) and Linolenic acid (0.13% EI) were short of the respective AMDRs of 5–10% and 0.6–1.2% EI [74,88,89]. In Palestine, the average intake of SFA amongst 11–16 year old adolescents (10.3% EI) exceeded the WHO maximal intake recommendations particularly amongst boys (12% EI) [85], while the intake of MUFAs (12.2% EI) was below the WHO recommendations of 15–20% EI [85,90]. In the UAE, Ali et al. (2013) showed that amongst 14–18 year old subjects, 12–13% of adolescents exceeded the AMDR for total fat, while 40% of girls and 60% of boys exceeded the 10% upper limit for SFA [29,74]. Similarly, in KSA, the average intake of SFA was high (11.3% EI), while that of MUFAs (10.5% EI) and PUFAs (5.8% EI) were suboptimal [82]. In Kuwait, 31–40% of adolescents exceeded the AMDR for total fat (i.e., 20–35% EI), but only 2–6% of adolescents met the AMDR for n-3 fatty acids, and 16–29% met the AMDR for n-6 fatty acids [74,84]. In Bahrain, the intakes of MUFAs and PUFAs were found to be inadequate, estimated at approximately 9–9.2% EI and 5.2–6.2% EI, respectively [28]. The PUFAs to SFA ratio of 0.6 for both girls and boys in Bahrain, was lower than the usually recommended value of 1, suggesting higher consumption of SFA compared to PUFA sources [28]. In contrast to the previous studies, the intakes of dietary fat subtypes in Tunisia were not far from recommendations, with SFA representing 9% EI, MUFAs 14% EI, and PUFAs 11% EI [91].

The majority of available studies have reported inadequate intake of dietary fiber amongst adolescents. Average dietary fiber intake was estimated at 7.5 g/day in Lebanon [89], 9 g/day in Libya [92], 11.6 g/day in Iran [41], 12.6 g/day in KSA [82], and 12.4–13.5 g/day in Bahrain, which are all considerably lower than the recommendation of the Food and Agriculture (FAO)/WHO of more than 25 g/day [90]. In countries of the GCC, average dietary fiber intake was estimated to range between 16 and 20 g/day amongst adolescents in Kuwait and between 13.6 and 20.7 g/day in the UAE [29,74,84]. The majority of adolescents (81–91% in Kuwait and 95% in UAE) did not meet the AI for fiber. Higher estimates were reported from Northern African countries in the EMR. In Morocco, fiber intake was estimated at 39.6 g/day in adolescent boys and 33.5 g/day in girls, which represented 18.8 g/1000 kcal in boys and 17.7 g/1000 kcal in girls [93,94]. These estimates are considered adequate when compared with the recommendation of 14 g fiber/1000 kcal for optimal cardiovascular health [95]. Similarly, in Tunisia, the average intake of dietary fiber intake was estimated at 36 g/day, thus exceeding the recommended level of >25 g/day [90,91].

Evidence on sugar intake amongst adolescents is very limited. A study conducted in Libya [92] reported that total sugars and FS contributed 20.4% and 12.6% of the daily EI, the latter being above the upper limit set by the WHO (10% EI) [90]. In Bahrain, the mean daily intake of total sugars was estimated to range between 98–114.6 g/day for boys and 85.5–93.8 g/day for girls, which were reported as high when compared with the maximum recommended intake of 60 g/day by the Dietary Reference Values of UK [28,83]. Adolescents aged 10–13 years from KSA were reported to consume high levels of total sugar, providing 26% EI [96]. In Iran, FS intake was estimated at close to 7% EI amongst 6–18 year old children and adolescents, with 81% of boys and 84% of girls adhering to the FS WHO recommendations [20,33].

3.3. Micronutrient Intakes Amongst School-Aged Children and Adolescents in the EMR

3.3.1. School-Aged Children

In Jordan, a study conducted amongst 5–6 year old children [73] showed that mean intakes of several vitamins were below their respective Dietary Reference Intakes (DRIs). More specifically, vitamins A and B12 represented 60–70% of the respective DRIs and similar values were observed for folate (73–75% DRI) and vitamin C (57–60% DRI). Inadequate intakes of calcium (64–68% DRI), iron (66–73% DRI), and zinc (56–60% DRI) were also reported [73]. Other studies conducted in Jordan, especially amongst Bedouins and children from underprivileged areas, reported that mean intakes of iron, calcium, and vitamin A represented 50%, 70%, and 65–80% of their respective RDAs [27,72,102,103]. Similarly, in school-aged children in Lebanon, 84–95%, 73–88%, and 35% did not meet two-thirds of the RDA for vitamin D, calcium, and iron, respectively [76,102,104]. In KSA, mean calcium intakes in children aged 7–12 years old did not exceed 60% of the RDA, and mean vitamin D intake represented only 23% of RDA [102,105]. In the UAE, a national study showed that more than 76% of 6–8 year old children did not meet the respective Estimated Average Requirement (EAR) level for vitamin A, while for vitamin D and vitamin E, more than 93% of 6–8 year old children did not meet the EAR value [29]. In addition, 26% of boys and 43% of girls did not meet the EAR intake level for folate [29]. In Lebanon, a study conducted amongst 5–12 year olds showed that 23% and 95% did not meet 2/3rd of the RDA for vitamin E and D, respectively [76]. In Egypt, 44–76% of 6–12 years old children did not meet 50% RDA for vitamin A [71], and close to a third did not meet 50% RDA for iron and calcium.

High intakes of sodium (Na) coupled with low intakes of potassium (K) were reported by studies in the region. In Iran, mean intakes of Na and K amongst 3–10 year old children were 2017 mg/day and 1119 mg/day, respectively [26], while the recommended intakes in this age group ranged from <1500 to <1900 mg/day and 3000–3800 mg/day, respectively [9]. In Kuwait, 64% of girls and 71% of boys aged 4–8 years, exceeded the Tolerable Upper Intake Level for Na (1900 mg/day) of the IOM [84]. In Morocco, average intake of Na was estimated at 1800 mg/day amongst 6–8 year old children, with 46.7% exceeding the IOM upper limit [106].

3.3.2. Adolescents

Figure 3 illustrates the proportions of adolescents not meeting the recommended intake levels of vitamins A, C, E, D and folate [29,48,85,99]. It is important to note that the data reported by the various studies is not readily comparable given that different studies have used different benchmarks to define nutrient adequacy. Taken together, the data underline suboptimal intakes for the micronutrients in Iran, Pakistan, Palestine and the UAE, with high proportions of adolescents not meeting the recommended nutrient intake levels. Similarly, in KSA, 63% and 87% of adolescents (9–18 year olds) had intakes below EAR for vitamin A and E, respectively [107]. In Lebanon 55.3% of Lebanese children and adolescents (6–19 year olds) did not meet 2/3rd the RDA for vitamin A, with 23–26% also not meeting 2/3rd the RDA for vitamins C and E [89]. Inadequate intakes for thiamin, riboflavin, pyridoxine, vitamin B12 were also reported by some studies in the region [29,48,85].

Table 2. Macronutrients intakes amongst adolescents in countries of the Eastern Mediterranean region.

Country	Study Area	Study Population	Dietary Assessment	CHO (%EI)	Protein (%EI)	Fat (%EI)
Bahrain [28]	11 regions of Bahrain	11–18 year old children and adolescents; n = 496	24-HR	M: 45–52.5; F: 52–53	M: 15.5–15.9; F: 15–15.4	M: 31.1–32.5; F: 32.7–33.9
Egypt [97]	Sohag	12–18 year old adolescents; n = 300	24-HR	59.1–61.3	15.7–15.9	26.9–28.5
Iran [80]	Lahijan, Northern Iran	14–17 year old girls; n = 400	24-HR	59.3	11.9	28.8
Iran [87]	Tehan	10–19 year old girls; n = 717	FFQ	–	–	30.6
Iran [48]	Sistan and Baluchistan	14–18 year old girls; n = 753	2-day 24-HR	54	14	31.9
Iran [33]	Tehan	6–18 year old; n = 424	FFQ	M: 57.2; F: 56.8	M: 12.9; F: 13.2	M: 32.1; F: 32.4
Iran [34]	Isfahan	Primary school and junior high school pupils; n = 4700	FFQ	64.1	12	23.8
Kuwait [98]	Different regions in Kuwait	8, 13 and 17 year old students; n = 588	Questionnaire	60.6	13	32.2
Kuwait [84]	National	9–18 year old children and adolescents; n = 614	24-HR	M: 53–54; F: 53	M: 15; F: 14–15	M: 31–32; F: 32–33
Lebanon [24]	National	12–19 year old adolescents; n = 498	24-HR	51.1	13.5	36.2
Lebanon [89]	National	12–19 year old children and adolescents; n = 3394	24-HR	51.4	13.4	36
Libya [92]	Benghazi	12 year old adolescents; n = 180	3-day food record	54	15.7	30.2
Morocco [93,94]	Ouarzazate	15–18 year old adolescents; n = 327	3-day food record	M: 58.8; F: 56.6	M: 12.9; F: 12.1	M: 28.3; F: 31.3
Oman [79]	Muscat	15–18 year old adolescents; n = 802	FFQ	M: 55.5; F: 51.1	M: 22.5; F: 18.7	M: 30.4; F: 22.6
Pakistan [99]	Sialkot	Mean age: 14.3 years; n = 328	3-day food record	51.5	12.5	36.3
Pakistan [100]	National	6–16 year old children and adolescents; n = 237	24-HR	60–74	10–12	18–32
Palestine [85]	East Jerusalem	11–16 year old adolescents; n = 313	24-HR	54	12.7	34.7
Saudi-Arabia [101]	Riyadh and Dawadami	17–19 year old adolescents; n = 600	24-HR	R: 54.4; U: 54.3	R: 16.9; U: 15.1	R: 29.5; U: 32.8

Table 2. *Cont.*

Country	Study Area	Study Population	Dietary Assessment	CHO (%EI)	Protein (%EI)	Fat (%EI)
Saudi-Arabia [82]	Jeddah	13–18 year old adolescents; $n = 239$	3-day 24-HR	56.6	13	30.5
Sudan [86]	Northern State	10–19 year old adolescents; $n = 401$	24-HR	77.4	12.6	9.9
Tunisia [91]	3 regions in Tunisia	15–19 year old adolescents; $n = 1019$	FFQ	52	12	36
UAE [78]	National	11–18 year old adolescents; $n = 276$	24-HR	M: 59.1; F: 58.2	M: 16; F: 14.9	M: 25.8; F: 27.8
UAE [29]	National	11–18 year old adolescents; $n = 276$	24-HR	–	M: 15–16; F: 14.7–15.3	M: 25.2–26.7; F: 27.6–27.9

Abbreviations: CHO: carbohydrates; EI: energy intake; M: males; F: females; R: rural; U: urban; 24-HR: 24-hr dietary recall; FFQ: food frequency questionnaire.

Figure 4 displays the proportions of adolescents not meeting the recommended intake levels of iron, calcium and zinc. The data suggest that high proportions of adolescents do not meet the recommendations for these nutrients in Iran, Pakistan, Palestine and KSA [48,85,99,107]. A study conducted in Lebanon of 6–19 year old children and adolescents showed that 27% and 36% do not meet 2/3rd the RDA for zinc and iron, respectively, while 77% do not meet two-thirds of the RDA for calcium [89].

Available evidence suggests that sodium (Na) intakes are high in this age group. In Kuwait, 46–61% of females and 73–80% of males aged 9–18 years exceeded the Tolerable Upper Intake Level for Na (2200–2300 mg/day) set by the IOM [84]. Mean Na intakes amongst adolescents in KSA ranged between 2209 and 2250 mg/day, exceeding the AI level (1700 mg/day) and the WHO Upper limit (2000 mg/day) [82,107]. In Morocco, Na intake was estimated at 2193.4 mg/day and 2138.0 mg/day in those aged 9–13 years and 14–18 years, respectively with 26.7–49.3% exceeding the upper intake level set by the IOM [106]. In parallel, low potassium intakes (K) were reported. In Pakistan, 45% of boys and 51% of girls had intakes below the EAR for potassium [99]. In KSA, mean intakes of K ranged between 1530 mg and 1961 mg/day, thus being inferior to the AI of 4500–4700 mg/day [82,107], and 87% of adolescents had intakes less than the AI level for K [107]. In Tunisia, mean K intake was estimated at 1044.5–1053.8 mg/day amongst 15–19 year adolescents [91], and in Morocco, 75% of children and adolescents aged 6–18 year old children and adolescents [106] consumed less than the AI of K [106]. Low intakes of phosphorous, magnesium, manganese, copper and selenium have also been reported by some studies in the region [76,85,99,107].

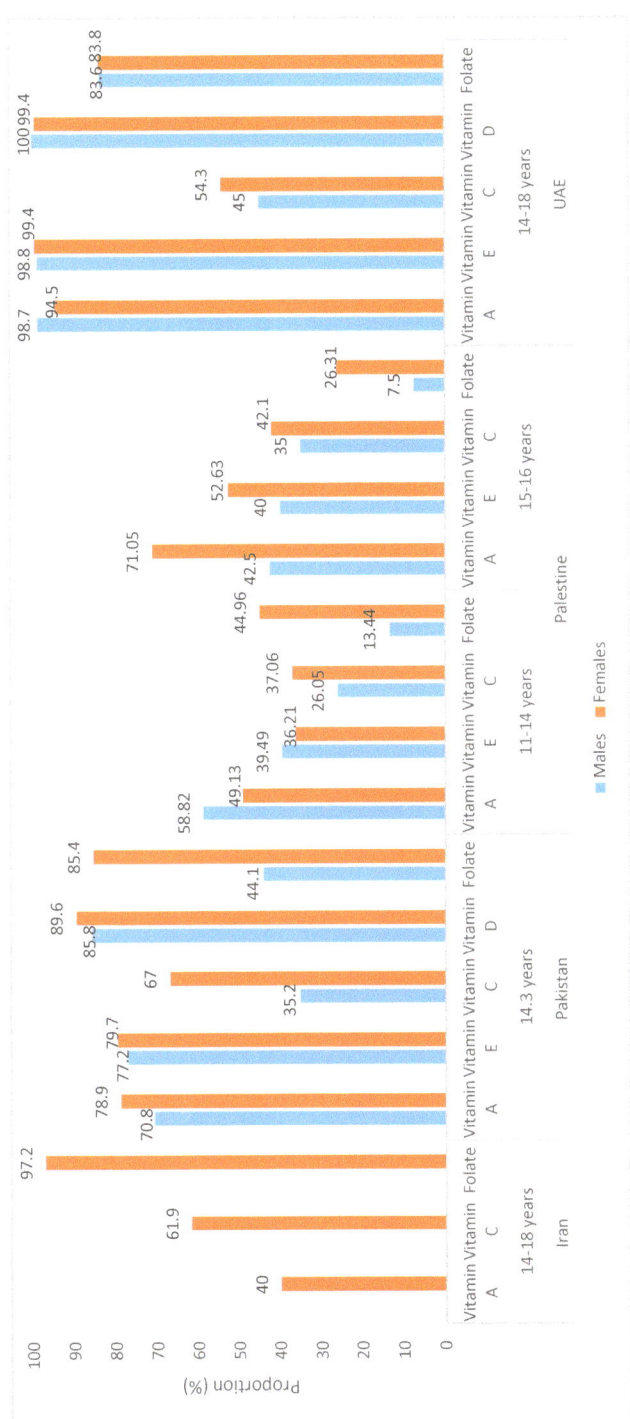

Figure 3. Proportion of adolescents not meeting the recommendations for vitamins A, E, C, D and folate. The criteria used to assess the proportion of adolescents not meeting the recommendation, are as follows: Iran, Recommended Dietary Allowances (RDAs); Pakistan, Estimated Average Requirement (EAR)/Average Intake (AI); Palestine, <80% RDA; United Arab Emirates (UAE), <EAR.

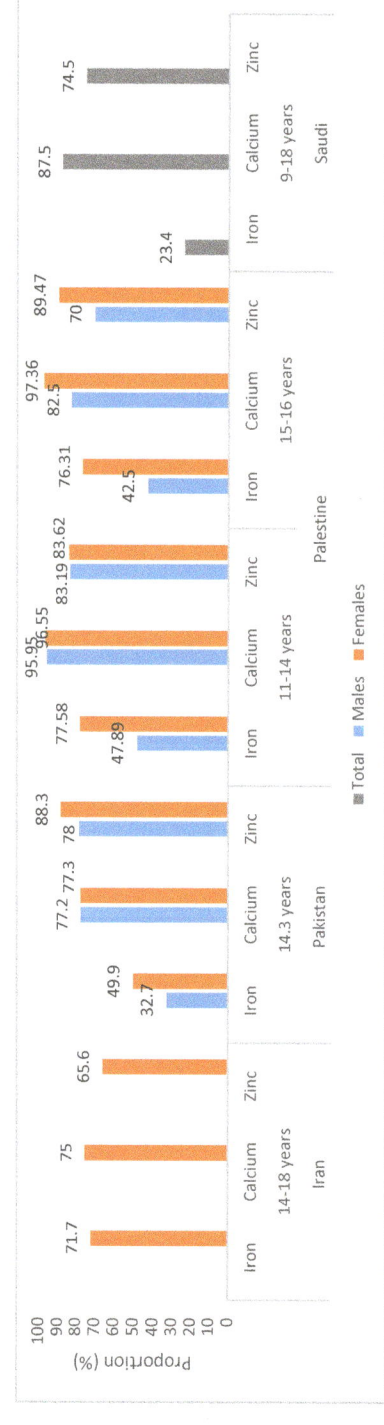

Figure 4. Proportion of adolescents not meeting the recommendation for iron, calcium and zinc. The criteria used to assess the proportion of adolescents not meeting the recommendations, are as follows: Iran, Recommended Dietary Allowances (RDAs); Pakistan, Estimated Average Requirement (EAR)/Average Intake (AI); Palestine, <80% RDA; United Arab Emirates (UAE), <EAR.

4. Discussion

The majority of available studies amongst children and adolescents in the EMR have documented a low intake of fruits, vegetables and fiber, inadequate consumption of water, milk and dairy products, coupled with a high intake of SSBs, and a frequent consumption of energy-dense, nutrient poor foods such as sweet and savory snacks. High intakes of fat and SFA were also observed in several studies conducted in the region, coupled with a number of micronutrient inadequacies, particularly low intakes of calcium, iron, and zinc and vitamins A, D, C and folate.

These food consumption and dietary intake patterns may be linked with suboptimal nutritional status and increased risk for obesity and cardiometabolic risk factors. This is of concern to the EMR given that the region harbors a "triple" burden of malnutrition in children and adolescents, characterized by the persistence of undernutrition, an alarming escalating burden of overweight and obesity, and a high prevalence of micronutrient deficiencies [108,109]. A recent review showed that the estimated weighted regional averages for stunting, wasting and underweight were 28%, 8.69% and 18%, respectively [109]. The prevalence of anemia was found to range between 16% and 81% amongst school-aged children and adolescents in countries of the region, while that of vitamin D deficiency ranged between 21% and 83% [109]. Several countries in the EMR reported an increasing trend in the prevalence of overweight and obesity amongst school-aged children and adolescents, the highest increases being reported from Iran [110,111], Lebanon [112], Qatar [113,114], Saudi Arabia [115–117], Tunisia [118] and Bahrain [119,120]. The prevalence of obesity amongst school-aged children and adolescents reached as high as 29.6% in Kuwait [121] and 21.7% in Bahrain [122]. The escalating and high prevalence of child and adolescent obesity raises questions about its implications for disease burden in the region, given its association with metabolic syndrome, insulin resistance, hypertension, dyslipidemia and hyperglycemia [121,123]. Studies conducted in various EMR countries reported a high prevalence of metabolic syndrome in obese children and adolescents, ranging between 15% and 30% in countries of the Levant and reaching as high as 44% in countries of the GCC, such as the UAE [7,8,124–126]. With those younger than 14 years representing approximately 30% of the population of the EMR, these estimates do not bode well for the future health and well-being of the population, and the development and building of productive societies [108].

The faulty dietary practices documented in this review, and which are in many instances similar to those reported by Keats et al. in low and middle income countries [19], may at least partially explain the increase in pediatric and adolescent adiposity and the persistence of undernutrition in the EMR. For instance, low intakes of fruit and vegetables may be a risk factor for obesity. In fact, available evidence suggests that adequate consumption of fruits and vegetables is usually associated with lower EI and higher intakes of dietary fiber which, through colonic, intrinsic, and/or hormonal effects may be associated with increased satiety, increased fat oxidation, and increased insulin sensitivity, all of which may contribute to the prevention of obesity and metabolic abnormalities [95,127–129]. In addition, high intake of SSBs can promote weight gain through their low satiety, incomplete compensatory reduction in EI at subsequent meals and high content of added sugar [130]. On average, SSBs provide approximately 140–150 calories and 35.0–37.5 g of sugar per 12-oz serving [131]. In addition, fructose from sucrose or from high corn fructose syrup has been linked with the development of visceral adiposity and ectopic fat deposition [132–135]. Several societies and organizations including the American Academy of Pediatrics and the WHO have advocated for reductions in the intake of SSBs to help prevent obesity and enhance overall health [136]. The observed high intakes of fat and SFA may also be linked with the burden of obesity in the region, given their high energy density and the promotion of adipogenesis [137]. The overall food consumption pattern that is low in fruit and vegetables, while being high in high fat, high sugar foods and beverages, is a hallmark of the western dietary pattern, which has been repetitively shown to be associated with increased adiposity risk [138]. At the same time, such food consumption and dietary patterns are associated with low dietary diversity, insufficient consumption of nutrient dense foods and suboptimal micronutrient intakes, which may at least partially explain the persistent burden of undernutrition and micronutrient deficiencies in countries of the EMR. The observed high intake of sodium, coupled with low intakes of potassium, is recognized as a risk factor for raised blood pressure in childhood and adolescents, and may increase the risk for hypertension and cardiovascular disease later in life [139].

Numerous factors may influence the diets of children and adolescents. These comprise both individual and socio-cultural factors as well as economic and environmental factors [140]. At the individual level, poor nutritional knowledge may be associated with unhealthy dietary practices. Studies conducted in countries of the region have documented significant nutrition knowledge gaps in children and adolescents, especially in what relates to nutrient sources, the identification of healthy snacks and diet-disease relationships [38,141,142]. Other factors such as personal likings, taste preferences, self-efficacy, and body image [143–146] may also play an important role in shaping the dietary practices in this age group [140]. Children and adolescents are also highly affected by the food environment, including the affordability, availability, and access to foods [140,147–151]. Marketing and advertising of ultra-processed foods with a high content of fat, sugar and/or salt to children and adolescents was also recognized as a factor that promotes suboptimal diets amongst children and adolescents [140,152]. Studies conducted in countries of the region have shown that the marketing of ultra-processed, nutrient-depleted foods is highly common on television, during children's programs and/or children's viewing time [153,154].

The WHO developed several standards and guidelines for health policies, strategies and interventions aimed at improving the nutrition status of children and adolescents. Aligned with the SDGs, and guided by the Global Strategy for Women's Children's and Adolescent's Health (2016–2030), the WHO Child and Adolescent Health and Nutrition program aims to translate global nutrition guidelines into actions to address the double burden of malnutrition in various countries of the world, build capacity for the monitoring of health and nutrition status, and develop evidence-based policies that contribute to the improvement of health and nutrition of children and adolescents [2]. The WHO has also established the nutrition-friendly school initiative that provides a framework for ensuring integrated school-based programs that address the double-burden of nutrition-related ill health [155], and has further articulated priorities related to adolescent nutrition in the Global Accelerated Action for the Health of Adolescents [156]. In line with its mandate, the regional office of the WHO has been active in shaping the policy environment in Member States, emphasizing the need for policies and initiatives that promote a healthier food environment for the population, with a focus on children and adolescents. The WHO EMR published, in 2018, a set of recommendations on the marketing of food and non-alcoholic beverages to children in the region [157]. The recommendations aim to guide Member States on the promotion of responsible marketing and the regulation of the marketing of foods and beverages that are high in saturated fat, trans fat, free sugar or salt to children [157]. Countries that have adopted legislation that contributes to the implementation of these recommendations include Egypt, Iran and Saudi Arabia. The WHO Regional Strategy (2020–2030) [158] also provides a comprehensive framework for regional and national efforts to reach the various targets on nutrition, including the promotion of healthier diets amongst children and adolescents. It has mapped existent nutrition policies in the region and showed that the main action areas included in nutrition policies across the region are infant and young child nutrition (84%), school health and nutrition programs (84%), healthy diet awareness (84%), vitamin and mineral nutrition (79%), acute malnutrition (53%) and nutrition and infectious diseases (37%). In addition, the Regional framework for action on obesity prevention 2019–2023 [159] provides a set of strategic interventions and progress indicators related to fiscal measures, public procurement, food supply and trade, food labeling, physical activity promotion, mass media campaigns, and product reformulation, coupled with continuous assessment and monitoring to help Member states in their obesity prevention efforts. Moreover, the WHO EMR office has issued several policy statements related to lowering sugar, fat and salt intakes in countries of the EMR [160–162], providing a road map for countries of the region for the progressive and sustainable reduction in national intakes of sugar, fat and salt. Despite the active policy response in several countries of the EMR, recent reports [140,163] are highlighting the need for a broader food system approach in order to improve the diets of children and adolescents. To better address the nutritional needs of children and adolescents, the food system should be leveraged and aligned along its four determinants (food supply chains, external food environments, personal food environments, and behaviors of caregivers, children and adolescents) to improve the quality of the diet in this age group [140].

5. Missing Knowledge and Future Research

Although this review has provided valuable insight into food consumption patterns and dietary intakes amongst school-aged children and adolescents in the EMR, it has identified several challenges and gaps in the existing dietary assessment studies. In particular, findings on food consumption patterns were often limited by the scarcity of data, particularly in school-aged children. This knowledge gap has been reported by the United Nations Children's Fund (UNICEF) [140], stating that the age group of school-aged children is often missing from health and nutrition surveys. The fact that most of the available studies have reported on daily or weekly frequency of intake, rather than quantifying consumption, has also often limited the interpretability of the data. Another challenge stemmed from the fact that most of the available studies were conducted at a small or regional scale, with only few countries having conducted national surveys on food consumption in children and adolescents. Political instabilities and turmoil, coupled with limited research funding, are amongst the challenges that some countries of the region are facing and that may contribute to the scarcity of nationally representative data. It is also important to mention that dietary assessment in many countries of the region may be limited by the availability of complete and up-to-date food composition tables, particularly for traditional foods and composite dishes, highlighting the crucial need for concerted efforts in this domain. The findings of this review may also be limited by the fact that different dietary assessment methods (food frequency questionnaires, FFQ; 24-hr recalls, 24-HR; dietary records) were used by the various countries/studies, which may impact the comparability of the generated food consumption data [108].

Based on the work undertaken in this paper, opportunities for future research include regional collaborations to: (1) consolidate and update food composition tables, with a focus on culture-specific foods and composite dishes; (2) conduct nationwide dietary surveys on children and adolescents using validated and standardized approaches and methodologies; (3) contribute to a better characterization of food consumption patterns and dietary intakes in under-represented age groups, such as school-aged children; (4) assess the intake and sources of free sugar; (5) assess the intake and sources of trans fat; and (6) gain a better understanding of factors that may be associated with unhealthy food consumption patterns in the EMR. These priorities may guide policy makers, researchers, funding agencies, and non-governmental organizations in tackling the identified knowledge gaps and developing culture specific and evidence-based intervention strategies aimed at improving the nutritional status of children in the EMR.

6. Conclusions

This review contributes toward the characterization of food consumption patterns and dietary intakes amongst children and adolescents in the EMR. The findings highlighted poor dietary habits in these age groups characterized by low intakes of fruit, vegetables, and dairy coupled with high intakes of SSBs and frequent consumption of sweets and savory snacks. High intakes of fat and saturated fat were observed, while the intakes of several micronutrients were inadequate. These suboptimal food consumption and dietary intake patterns represent a public health concern, given that the triple burden of malnutrition continues to plague most countries of the region. The findings of this review have therefore broad implications for developing public health strategies and policies to improve the diet of children and adolescents in the EMR. Acknowledging the impact that nutrition may have on building societies and transforming the lives of children, adolescents and their families, there is a crucial need for a food system approach in developing and implementing national and regional policies and interventions aimed at improving the diet of children and adolescents. Such interventions will not only enhance the diet and nutritional status of young people, but will also pave the way towards the achievement of many sustainable development goal targets, including ensuring healthy lives, promoting life-long learning, improving economic growth and building inclusive societies [164].

Author Contributions: Conceptualization, A.A.-J. and L.N.; methodology, L.N.; investigation, A.A.-J. and L.N.; resources, A.A.-J. and L.N.; data curation, M.T.; writing—original draft preparation, L.N.; writing—review and editing, M.T. and A.A.-J.; supervision, A.A.-J. and L.N.; project administration, A.A.-J.; funding acquisition, A.A.-J. All authors have read and agreed to the published version of the manuscript.

Funding: This research was funded by the World Health Organization.

Conflicts of Interest: The authors alone are responsible for the views expressed in this publication and they do not necessarily represent the official position, decisions, policy or views of the World Health Organization. We declare no competing interests.

References

1. World Health Organization Regional Office for Europe. *Fact Sheets on Sustainable Development Goals: Health Targets: Child and Adolescent Health*; WHO: Copenhagen, Denmark, 2017.
2. World Health Organization Regional Office for Africa. Child and Adolescent Health and Nutrition (CAN) Program. Available online: https://www.afro.who.int/about-us/programmes-clusters/CAN (accessed on 8 October 2020).
3. Institute of Medicine. Nutrition-Related Health Concerns, Dietary Intakes, and Eating Behaviors of Children and Adolescents. In *Nutrition Standards for Foods in Schools: Leading the Way Toward Healthier Youth*; The National Academies Press: Washington, DC, USA, 2007. [CrossRef]
4. Story, M.; Holt, K.; Sofka, D. *Bright Futures in Practice*, 2nd ed.; National Center for Education in Maternal and Child Health: Arlington, VA, USA, 2002.
5. Daniels, S.R. The consequences of childhood overweight and obesity. *Future Child* **2006**, *16*, 47–67. [CrossRef]
6. Institute of Medicine. *Preventing Childhood Obesity: Health in the Balance*; The National Academies Press: Washington, DC, USA, 2005.
7. Nasreddine, L.; Naja, F.; Tabet, M.; Habbal, M.-Z.; El-Aily, A.; Haikal, C.; Sidani, S.; Adra, N.; Hwalla, N. Obesity is associated with insulin resistance and components of the metabolic syndrome in Lebanese adolescents. *Ann. Hum. Biol.* **2012**, *39*, 122–128. [CrossRef]
8. Nasreddine, L.; Ouaijan, K.; Mansour, M.; Adra, N.; Sinno, D.; Hwalla, N. Metabolic syndrome and insulin resistance in obese prepubertal children in Lebanon: A primary health concern. *Ann. Nutr. Metab.* **2010**, *57*, 135–142. [CrossRef]
9. Gidding, S.S.; Dennison, B.A.; Birch, L.L.; Daniels, S.R.; Gilman, M.W.; Lichtenstein, A.H.; Rattay, K.T.; Steinberger, J.; Stettler, N.; Van Horn, L. Dietary recommendations for children and adolescents: A guide for practitioners: Consensus statement from the American Heart Association. *Circulation* **2005**, *112*, 2061–2075. [CrossRef]
10. World Health Organization. *Technical paper. Regional strategy on nutrition 2010–2019. Regional Committee for the Eastern Mediterranean. Fifty-Seventh Session. Agenda Item 4 (b)*; WHO: Geneva, Switzerland, 2010.
11. Nasreddine, L.; Naja, F.; Sibai, A.-M.; Helou, K.; Adra, N.; Hwalla, N. Trends in nutritional intakes and nutrition-related cardiovascular disease risk factors in Lebanon: The need for immediate action. *Leb. Med. J.* **2014**, *103*, 1–9. [CrossRef]
12. Popkin, B.M.; Adair, L.S.; Ng, S.W. Global nutrition transition and the pandemic of obesity in developing countries. *Nutr. Rev.* **2012**, *70*, 3–21. [CrossRef]
13. World Health Organization Regional Office for the Eastern Mediterranean. Nutrition. Available online: http://www.emro.who.int/health-topics/nutrition/index.html (accessed on 26 August 2020).
14. Rahim, H.F.A.; Sibai, A.; Khader, Y.; Hwalla, N.; Fadhil, I.; Alsiyabi, H.; Mataria, A.; Mendis, S.; Mokdad, A.H.; Husseini, A. Non-communicable diseases in the Arab world. *Lancet* **2014**, *383*, 356–367. [CrossRef]
15. Moghames, P.; Hammami, N.; Hwalla, N.; Yazbeck, N.; Shoaib, H.; Nasreddine, L.; Naja, F. Validity and reliability of a food frequency questionnaire to estimate dietary intake among Lebanese children. *Nutr. J.* **2015**, *15*, 4. [CrossRef]
16. Bagchi, K. Nutrition in the eastern Mediterranean region of the World Health Organization. *East. Mediterr. Health J.* **2008**, *14*, S107–S113.

17. World Health Organization Regional Office for the Eastern Mediterranean. Countries in the Eastern Mediterranean Region. Available online: http://www.emro.who.int/countries.html (accessed on 15 July 2020).
18. World Health Organization. Global School-Based Student Health Survey (GSHS). Available online: https://www.who.int/ncds/surveillance/gshs/factsheets/en/ (accessed on 11 August 2020).
19. Keats, E.C.; Rappaport, A.I.; Shah, S.; Oh, C.; Jain, R.; Bhutta, Z.A. The dietary intake and practices of adolescent girls in low-and middle-income countries: A systematic review. *Nutrients* **2018**, *10*, 1978. [CrossRef]
20. World Health Organization. *Healthy Diet FACT SHEET N° 394*; WHO: Geneva, Switzerland, 2015.
21. Abbass, M.M.; Mahmoud, S.A.; El Moshy, S.; Rady, D.; AbuBakr, N.; Radwan, I.A.; Ahmed, A.; Abdou, A.; Al Jawaldeh, A. The prevalence of dental caries among Egyptian children and adolescences and its association with age, socioeconomic status, dietary habits and other risk factors. A cross-sectional study. *F1000Research* **2019**, *8*, 1–19. [CrossRef] [PubMed]
22. Hashim, R.; Williams, S.M.; Murray Thomson, W. Diet and caries experience among preschool children in Ajman, United Arab Emirates. *Eur. J. Oral. Sci.* **2009**, *117*, 734–740. [CrossRef] [PubMed]
23. Jaghasi, I.; Hatahet, W.; Dashash, M. Dietary patterns and oral health in schoolchildren from Damascus, Syrian Arab Republic. *East. Mediterr. Health J.* **2012**, *18*, 358–364. [CrossRef]
24. Nasreddine, L.; Naja, F.; Akl, C.; Chamieh, M.C.; Karam, S.; Sibai, A.-M.; Hwalla, N. Dietary, lifestyle, and socio-economic correlates of overweight, obesity and central obesity in Lebanese children and adolescents. *Nutrients* **2014**, *6*, 1038–1062. [CrossRef]
25. Hasanein, M.A.; Jawad, S.H.A. Prevalence of obesity and risk factors among female school-aged children in primary school in Madinah Munawarah. *Life Sci. J.* **2014**, *11*.
26. Kelishadi, R.; Gheisari, A.; Zare, N.; Farajian, S.; Shariatinejad, K. Salt intake and the association with blood pressure in young Iranian children: First report from the middle East and north Africa. *Int. J. Prev. Med.* **2013**, *4*, 475.
27. Khatib, I.; Elmadfa, I. High prevalence rates of anemia, vitamin A deficiency and stunting imperil the health status of Bedouin schoolchildren in North Badia, Jordan. *Ann. Nutr. Metab.* **2009**, *55*, 358–367. [CrossRef]
28. Gharib, N.; Rasheed, P. Energy and macronutrient intake and dietary pattern among school children in Bahrain: A cross-sectional study. *Nutr. J.* **2011**, *10*, 62. [CrossRef]
29. Ali, H.I.; Ng, S.W.; Zaghloul, S.; Harrison, G.G.; Qazaq, H.S.; El Sadig, M.; Yeatts, K. High proportion of 6 to 18-year-old children and adolescents in the United Arab Emirates are not meeting dietary recommendations. *Nutr. Res.* **2013**, *33*, 447–456. [CrossRef]
30. Alsubaie, A.S.R. Intake of fruit, vegetables and milk products and correlates among school boys in Saudi Arabia. *Int. J. Adolesc. Med. Health* **2018**, *1*. [CrossRef]
31. Hassan, A.S.; Al-Dosari, S.N. Breakfast habits and snacks consumed at school among Qatari schoolchildren aged 9–10 years. *Nutr. Food Sci.* **2008**, *38*, 264–270. [CrossRef]
32. Amini, M.; Dadkhah-Piraghaj, M.; Abtahi, M.; Abdollahi, M.; Houshiarrad, A.; Kimiagar, M. Nutritional assessment for primary school children in Tehran: An evaluation of dietary pattern with emphasis on snacks and meals consumption. *Int. J. Prev. Med.* **2014**, *5*, 611. [PubMed]
33. Mirmiran, P.; Ziadlou, M.; Karimi, S.; Hosseini-Esfahani, F.; Azizi, F. The association of dietary patterns and adherence to WHO healthy diet with metabolic syndrome in children and adolescents: Tehran lipid and glucose study. *BMC Public Health* **2019**, *19*, 1457. [CrossRef]
34. Naeeni, M.M.; Jafari, S.; Fouladgar, M.; Heidari, K.; Farajzadegan, Z.; Fakhri, M.; Karami, P.; Omidi, R. Nutritional knowledge, practice, and dietary habits among school children and adolescents. *Int. J. Prev. Med.* **2014**, *5*, S171. [CrossRef]
35. Kelishadi, R.; Ardalan, G.; Gheiratmand, R.; Gouya, M.M.; Razaghi, E.M.; Delavari, A.; Majdzadeh, R.; Heshmat, R.; Motaghian, M.; Barekati, H. Association of physical activity and dietary behaviours in relation to the body mass index in a national sample of Iranian children and adolescents: CASPIAN Study. *Bull. World Health Organ.* **2007**, *85*, 19–26. [CrossRef]
36. Musaiger, A.O.; Al-Mufty, B.A.; Al-Hazzaa, H.M. Eating habits, inactivity, and sedentary behavior among adolescents in Iraq: Sex differences in the hidden risks of noncommunicable diseases. *Food Nutr. Bull.* **2014**, *35*, 12–19. [CrossRef] [PubMed]

37. Mikki, N.; Abdul-Rahim, H.F.; Shi, Z.; Holmboe-Ottesen, G. Dietary habits of Palestinian adolescents and associated sociodemographic characteristics in Ramallah, Nablus and Hebron governorates. *Public Health Nutr.* **2010**, *13*, 1419–1429. [CrossRef]
38. Nabhani-Zeidan, M.; Naja, F.; Nasreddine, L. Dietary intake and nutrition-related knowledge in a sample of Lebanese adolescents of contrasting socioeconomic status. *Food Nutr. Bull.* **2011**, *32*, 75–83. [CrossRef]
39. Waly, I.; Zayed, K.; Al Haddabi, B. Obesity, eating habits and sedentary behaviour of Omani young adolescents: A cross-sectional study. *EC Nutr.* **2017**, *7*, 3–10.
40. Makansi, N.; Allison, P.; Awad, M.; Bedos, C. Fruit and vegetable intake among Emirati adolescents: A mixed methods study. *East. Mediterr. Health J.* **2018**, *24*. [CrossRef]
41. Hejazi, N.; Mazloom, Z. Socioeconomic status, youth's eating patterns and meals consumed away from home. *Pak. J. Biol. Sci.* **2009**, *12*, 730. [PubMed]
42. Abdel-Hady, D.; El-Gilany, A.-H.; Sarraf, B. Dietary habits of adolescent students in Mansoura, Egypt. *Int. J. Collab. Res. Intern. Med. Public Health* **2014**, *6*, 132.
43. El Achhab, Y.; Marfa, A.; Echarbaoui, I.; Chater, R.; El-Haidani, A.; Filali-Zegzouti, Y. Physical inactivity, sedentary behaviors and dietary habits among Moroccan adolescents in secondary school. *Sci. Sport* **2018**, *33*, 58–62. [CrossRef]
44. Hamrani, A.; Mehdad, S.; El Kari, K.; El Hamdouchi, A.; El Menchawy, I.; Belghiti, H.; El Mzibri, M.; Musaiger, A.O.; Al-Hazzaa, H.M.; Hills, A.P. Physical activity and dietary habits among Moroccan adolescents. *Public Health Nutr.* **2015**, *18*, 1793–1800. [CrossRef] [PubMed]
45. Shokrvash, B.; Salehi, L.; Akbari, M.H.; Mamagani, M.E.; Nedjat, S.; Asghari, M.; Majlessi, F.; Montazeri, A. Social support and dairy products intake among adolescents: A study from Iran. *BMC Public Health* **2015**, *15*, 1078. [CrossRef]
46. Nasreddine, L.; Mehio-Sibai, A.; Mrayati, M.; Adra, N.; Hwalla, N. Adolescent obesity in Syria: Prevalence and associated factors. *Child Care Health Dev.* **2010**, *36*, 404–413. [CrossRef]
47. Mahfouz, A.A.; Shatoor, A.S.; Hassanein, M.A.; Mohamed, A.; Farheen, A. Gender differences in cardiovascular risk factors among adolescents in Aseer Region, southwestern Saudi Arabia. *J. Saudi Heart Assoc.* **2012**, *24*, 61–67. [CrossRef]
48. Montazerifar, F.; Karajibani, M.; Dashipour, A.R. Evaluation of dietary intake and food patterns of adolescent girls in Sistan and Baluchistan Province, Iran. *Funct. Foods Health Dis.* **2012**, *2*, 62–71. [CrossRef]
49. Sachithananthan, V.; Gad, N. A Study on the Frequency of Food Consumption and Its Relationship to BMI in School Children and Adolescents in Abha City, KSA. *Cur. Res. Nutr. Food Sci.* **2016**, *4*, 203. [CrossRef]
50. Moukhyer, M.E.; van Eijk, J.T.; De Vries, N.K.; Bosma, H. Health-related behaviors of Sudanese adolescents. *Educ. Health* **2008**, *21*, 184.
51. Musaiger, A.O.; Nabag, F.O.; Al-Mannai, M. Obesity, dietary habits, and sedentary behaviors among adolescents in Sudan: Alarming risk factors for chronic diseases in a poor country. *Food Nutr. Bull.* **2016**, *37*, 65–72. [CrossRef] [PubMed]
52. Musaiger, A.; Bader, Z.; Al-Roomi, K.; D'Souza, R. Dietary and lifestyle habits amongst adolescents in Bahrain. *Food Nutr. Res.* **2011**, *55*, 7122. [CrossRef]
53. Abudayya, A.H.; Stigum, H.; Shi, Z.; Abed, Y.; Holmboe-Ottesen, G. Sociodemographic correlates of food habits among school adolescents (12–15 year) in North Gaza Strip. *BMC Public Health* **2009**, *9*, 185. [CrossRef]
54. Dalky, H.F.; Al Momani, M.H.; Al-Drabaah, T.K.; Jarrah, S. Eating habits and associated factors among adolescent students in Jordan. *Clin. Nurs. Res.* **2017**, *26*, 538–552. [CrossRef]
55. Mahfouz, A.A.; Abdelmoneim, I.; Khan, M.Y.; Daffalla, A.A.; Diab, M.M.; Al-Gelban, K.S.; Moussa, H. Obesity and related behaviors among adolescent school boys in Abha City, Southwestern Saudi Arabia. *J. Trop. Pediatr.* **2008**, *54*, 120–124. [CrossRef] [PubMed]
56. Musaiger, A.O.; Kalam, F. Dietary habits and lifestyle among adolescents in Damascus, Syria. *Ann. Agric. Environ. Med.* **2014**, *21*. [CrossRef] [PubMed]
57. Allafi, A.; Al-Haifi, A.R.; Al-Fayez, M.A.; Al-Athari, B.I.; Al-Ajmi, F.A.; Al-Hazzaa, H.M.; Musaiger, A.O.; Ahmed, F. Physical activity, sedentary behaviours and dietary habits among Kuwaiti adolescents: Gender differences. *Public Health Nutr.* **2014**, *17*, 2045–2052. [CrossRef]
58. Honkala, S.; Honkala, E.; Al-Sahli, N. Consumption of sugar products and associated life-and school-satisfaction and self-esteem factors among schoolchildren in Kuwait. *Acta Odontol. Scand.* **2006**, *64*, 79–88. [CrossRef]

59. Al Muammar, M.; El Shafie, M. Association between dietary habits and body mass index of adolescent females in intermediate schools in Riyadh, Saudi Arabia. *East. Mediterr. Health J.* **2014**, *20*, 39–45. [CrossRef]
60. Bello, L.; Al-Hammad, N. Pattern of fluid consumption in a sample of Saudi Arabian adolescents aged 12–13 years. *Int. J. Paediatr. Dent.* **2006**, *16*, 168–173. [CrossRef]
61. Subih, H.S.; Abu-Shquier, Y.; Bawadi, H.; Al-Bayyari, N. Assessment of body weight, maternal dietary knowledge and lifestyle practices among children and adolescents in north Jordan. *Public Health Nutr.* **2018**, *21*, 2803–2810. [CrossRef]
62. Institute of Medicine; Food and Nutrition Board. Dietary Reference Intakes for Water, Potassium, Sodium, Chloride, and Sulfate. Available online: https://www.nal.usda.gov/sites/default/files/fnic_uploads/water_full_report.pdf (accessed on 10 September 2020).
63. Jomaa, L.; Hwalla, N.; Constant, F.; Naja, F.; Nasreddine, L. Water and beverage consumption among children aged 4–13 years in Lebanon: Findings from a National Cross-Sectional Study. *Nutrients* **2016**, *8*, 554. [CrossRef]
64. Ali, H.I.; Al Dhaheri, A.S.; Elmi, F.; Ng, S.W.; Zaghloul, S.; Ohuma, E.O.; Qazaq, H.S. Water and Beverage Consumption among a Nationally Representative Sample of Children and Adolescents in the United Arab Emirates. *Nutrients* **2019**, *11*, 2110. [CrossRef] [PubMed]
65. Al Sabbah, H.; Vereecken, C.; Kolsteren, P.; Abdeen, Z.; Maes, L. Food habits and physical activity patterns among Palestinian adolescents: Findings from the national study of Palestinian schoolchildren (HBSC-WBG2004). *Public Health Nutr.* **2007**, *10*, 739–746. [CrossRef]
66. Kerkadi, A.; Sadig, A.H.; Bawadi, H.; Al Thani, A.A.M.; Al Chetachi, W.; Akram, H.; Al-Hazzaa, H.M.; Musaiger, A.O. The relationship between lifestyle factors and obesity indices among adolescents in Qatar. *Int. J. Environ. Res. Public Health* **2019**, *16*, 4428. [CrossRef]
67. Al-Hazzaa, H.M.; Abahussain, N.A.; Al-Sobayel, H.I.; Qahwaji, D.M.; Musaiger, A.O. Physical activity, sedentary behaviors and dietary habits among Saudi adolescents relative to age, gender and region. *Int. J. Behav. Nutr. Phys. Act.* **2011**, *8*, 140. [CrossRef]
68. Nazik, M.; Malde, M.; Ahmed, M.; Trovik, T. Correlation between caries experience in Sudanese school children and dietary habits, according to a food frequency questionnaire and a modified 24-hr recall method. *Afr. J. Food Agric. Nutr. Dev.* **2013**, *13*.
69. FAO and FHI 360. *Minimum Dietary Diversity for Women: A Guide for Measurement*; Food and Agriculture Organization of the United Nations: Rome, Italy, 2016.
70. Friel, S.; Hattersley, L.; Snowdon, W.; Thow, A.M.; Lobstein, T.; Sanders, D.; Barquera, S.; Mohan, S.; Hawkes, C.; Kelly, B. Monitoring the impacts of trade agreements on food environments. *Obes. Rev.* **2013**, *14*, 120–134. [CrossRef] [PubMed]
71. El-Gazzar, H.H.; Saleh, S.M.; Khairy, S.A.; Marei, A.S.; ElKelany, K.; Al Soda, M.F. Relationship between dietary intake and obesity among a group of primary school-aged children in Cairo Governorate. *J. Med. Sci. Res.* **2019**, *2*, 42.
72. Khatib, I.; Hijazi, S.S. Micronutrient deficiencies among children may be endemic in underprivileged areas in Jordan. *Jordan Med. J.* **2009**, *43*, 324–332.
73. Al-Rewashdeh, A. Assessment of the nutritional status for preschool children in Jordan. *Bull. Fac. Agric. Cairo Univ.* **2009**, *60*, 423–432.
74. Institute of Medicine; Food and Nutrition Board. Dietary Reference Intakes for Energy, Carbohydrate, Fiber, Fat, Fatty Acids, Cholesterol, Protein and Amino Acids. Available online: https://www.nap.edu/catalog/10490/dietary-reference-intakes-for-energy-carbohydrate-fiber-fat-fatty-acids-cholesterol-protein-and-amino-acids-macronutrients (accessed on 30 April 2017).
75. Jabre, P.; Sikias, P.; Khater-Menassa, B.; Baddoura, R.; Awada, H. Overweight children in Beirut: Prevalence estimates and characteristics. *Child Care Health Dev.* **2005**, *31*, 159–165. [CrossRef]
76. Akl, C. *Prevalence and Determinants of Overweight and Obesity in a Nationally Representative Sample of Lebanese Children 5 to 12 Years Old*; American University of Beirut: Beirut, Lebanon, 2012.
77. Alredaisy, M.; Ibrahim, S. Assessment of nutritional status of children less than 10 years old in rural western Kordafan. *IIOABJ* **2011**, *2*, 40–49.
78. Ng, S.W.; Zaghloul, S.; Ali, H.; Harrison, G.; Yeatts, K.; El Sadig, M.; Popkin, B.M. Nutrition transition in the United Arab Emirates. *Eur. J. Clin. Nutr.* **2011**, *65*, 1328–1337. [CrossRef] [PubMed]

79. Kilani, H.; Al-Hazzaa, H.; Waly, M.I.; Musaiger, A. Lifestyle Habits: Diet, physical activity and sleep duration among Omani adolescents. *Sultan Qaboos Univ. Med. J.* **2013**, *13*, 510. [CrossRef] [PubMed]
80. Bazhan, M.; Kalantari, N.; Houhiar-Rad, A.; Alavi-Majd, H.; Kalantari, S. Dietary habits and nutrient intake in adolescent girls living in Northern Iran. *Arch. Adv. Biosci.* **2013**, *4*.
81. ALFaris, N.A.; Al-Tamimi, J.Z.; Al-Jobair, M.O.; Al-Shwaiyat, N.M. Trends of fast food consumption among adolescent and young adult Saudi girls living in Riyadh. *Food Nutr. Res.* **2015**, *59*, 26488. [CrossRef] [PubMed]
82. Washi, S.A.; Ageib, M.B. Poor diet quality and food habits are related to impaired nutritional status in 13-to 18-year-old adolescents in Jeddah. *Nutr. Res.* **2010**, *30*, 527–534. [CrossRef]
83. Department of Health. Dietary Reference Values for Food Energy, Nutrients for the United Kingdom. In *Report of the Panel on Dietary Values of the Committee on Medical Aspects of Food Policy*, 8th ed.; HMSO: London, UK, 1996.
84. Zaghloul, S.; Al-Hooti, S.N.; Al-Hamad, N.; Al-Zenki, S.; Alomirah, H.; Alayan, I.; Al-Attar, H.; Al-Othman, A.; Al-Shami, E.; Al-Somaie, M. Evidence for nutrition transition in Kuwait: Over-consumption of macronutrients and obesity. *Public Health Nutr.* **2013**, *16*, 596–607. [CrossRef]
85. Jildeh, C.; Papandreou, C.; Mourad, T.A.; Hatzis, C.; Kafatos, A.; Qasrawi, R.; Philalithis, A.; Abdeen, Z. Assessing the nutritional status of Palestinian adolescents from East Jerusalem: A school-based study 2002–03. *J. Trop. Pediatr.* **2011**, *57*, 51–58. [CrossRef]
86. Ahmed, N.M.K.; Onsa, Z.O. Nutritional Assessment of the Adolescents in the Northern State of Sudan. *Pak. J. Nutr.* **2014**, *13*, 79. [CrossRef]
87. Mohseni-Takalloo, S.; Mirmiran, P.; Hosseini-Esfahani, F.; Azizi, F. Dietary fat intake and its relationship with serum lipid profiles in tehranian adolescents. *J. Food Nutr. Res.* **2014**, *2*, 330–334. [CrossRef]
88. World Health Organization. Interim summary of conclusions and dietary recommendations on total fat & fatty acids. In *From the Joint FAO/WHO Expert Consultation on Fats and Fatty Acids in Human Nutrition*; World Health Organization: Geneva, Switzerland, 2008.
89. Nasreddine, L.; Chamieh, M.C.; Ayoub, J.; Hwalla, N.; Sibai, A.-M.; Naja, F. Sex disparities in dietary intake across the lifespan: The case of Lebanon. *Nutr. J.* **2020**, *19*, 1–18. [CrossRef] [PubMed]
90. World Health Organization. Diet, Nutrition and the Prevention of Chronic Diseases. Joint WHO/FAO Expert Consultation. WHO Technical Report Series no. 916. Available online: https://apps.who.int/iris/bitstream/handle/10665/42665/WHO_TRS_916.pdf?sequence=1 (accessed on 1 September 2020).
91. Aounallah-Skhiri, H.; Traissac, P.; El Ati, J.; Eymard-Duvernay, S.; Landais, E.; Achour, N.; Delpeuch, F.; Romdhane, H.B.; Maire, B. Nutrition transition among adolescents of a south-Mediterranean country: Dietary patterns, association with socio-economic factors, overweight and blood pressure. A cross-sectional study in Tunisia. *Nutr. J.* **2011**, *10*, 38. [CrossRef]
92. Huew, R.; Maguire, A.; Waterhouse, P.; Moynihan, P. Nutrient intake and dietary patterns of relevance to dental health of 12-year-old Libyan children. *Public Health Nutr.* **2014**, *17*, 1107–1113. [CrossRef]
93. Montero, P.; Mora Urda, A.; Cherkaoui, M.; Anzid, K. Transition nutritionnelle au Maroc: Étude comparative de l'état nutritionnel des adolescents entre 1991 et 2007. *Bull Séances.* **2009**, *60*, 433–450.
94. Montero, M.D.P.; Mora-Urda, A.I.; Anzid, K.; Cherkaoui, M.; Marrodan, M.D. Diet quality of Moroccan adolescents living in Morocco and in Spain. *J. Biosoc. Sci.* **2017**, *49*, 173. [CrossRef] [PubMed]
95. Anderson, J.W.; Baird, P.; Davis, R.H.; Ferreri, S.; Knudtson, M.; Koraym, A.; Waters, V.; Williams, C.L. Health benefits of dietary fiber. *Nutr. Rev.* **2009**, *67*, 188–205. [CrossRef]
96. Collison, K.S.; Zaidi, M.Z.; Subhani, S.N.; Al-Rubeaan, K.; Shoukri, M.; Al-Mohanna, F.A. Sugar-sweetened carbonated beverage consumption correlates with BMI, waist circumference, and poor dietary choices in school children. *BMC Public Health* **2010**, *10*, 234. [CrossRef]
97. Tayel, D.I.; El-Sayed, N.A.; El-Sayed, N.A. Dietary pattern and blood pressure levels of adolescents in Sohag, Egypt. *J. Egypt Public Health Assoc.* **2013**, *88*, 97–103. [CrossRef]
98. Al-Ansari, J.M.; Al-Jairan, L.Y.; Gillespie, G.M. Dietary habits of the primary to secondary school population and implications for oral health. *J. Allied Health* **2006**, *35*, 75–80. [PubMed]
99. Rifat-uz-Zaman, Z.I.; Ali, U. Dietary Intakes of Urban Adolescents of Sialkot, Pakistan Do Not Meet the Standards of Adequacy. *Pak. J. Nutr.* **2013**, *12*, 460–467. [CrossRef]
100. Aziz, S.; Hosain, K. Carbohydrate (CHO), protein and fat intake of healthy Pakistani school children in a 24 hour period. *J. Pak. Med. Assoc.* **2014**, *64*, 1255–1259.

101. Abuzaid, O.I. *Eating Patterns and Physical Activity Characteristics among Urban and Rural Students in Saudi Arabia*; Nutrition and Health Sciences Department, University of Nebraska-Lincoln: Lincoln, NE, USA, 2012.
102. Institute of Medicine; Food and Nutrition Board. Dietary Reference Intakes: RDA and AI for Vitamins and Elements. Available online: http://www.nationalacademies.org/hmd/~{}/media/Files/Activity%20Files/Nutrition/DRI-Tables/2_%20RDA%20and%20AI%20Values_Vitamin%20and%20Elements.pdf?la=en (accessed on 30 April 2017).
103. Khatib, I. High prevalence of subclinical vitamin A deficiency in Jordan: A forgotten risk. *Food Nutr. Bull.* **2002**, *23*, 228–236. [CrossRef] [PubMed]
104. Salamoun, M.; Kizirian, A.; Tannous, R.; Nabulsi, M.; Choucair, M.; Deeb, M.; Fuleihan, G.E.-H. Low calcium and vitamin D intake in healthy children and adolescents and their correlates. *Eur. J. Clin. Nutr.* **2005**, *59*, 177–184. [CrossRef] [PubMed]
105. Al-Musharaf, S.; Al-Othman, A.; Al-Daghri, N.M.; Krishnaswamy, S.; Yusuf, D.S.; Alkharfy, K.M.; Al-Saleh, Y.; Al-Attas, O.S.; Alokail, M.S.; Moharram, O. Vitamin D deficiency and calcium intake in reference to increased body mass index in children and adolescents. *Eur. J. Pediatr.* **2012**, *171*, 1081–1086. [CrossRef]
106. Saeid, N.; Elmzibri, M.; Hamrani, A.; Latifa, Q.; Belghiti, H.; El Berri, H.; Benjeddou, K.; Bouziani, A.; Benkirane, H.; Taboz, Y. Assessment of sodium and potassium intakes in children aged 6 to 18 years by 24 h urinary excretion in city of rabat, Morocco. *J. Nutr. Metab.* **2018**, *2018*. [CrossRef]
107. Al-Daghri, N.M.; Al-Othman, A.; Alkharfy, K.M.; Alokail, M.S.; Khan, N.; Alfawaz, H.A.; Aiswaidan, I.A.; Chrousos, G.P. Assessment of selected nutrients intake and adipocytokines profile among Saudi children and adults. *Endocrine J.* **2012**, EJ12-0167. [CrossRef]
108. Nasreddine, L.M.; Kassis, A.N.; Ayoub, J.J.; Naja, F.A.; Hwalla, N.C. Nutritional status and dietary intakes of children amid the nutrition transition: The case of the Eastern Mediterranean Region. *Nutr. Res.* **2018**, *57*, 12–27. [CrossRef]
109. Nasreddine, L.; Ayoub, J.J.; Al Jawaldeh, A. Review of the nutrition situation in the Eastern Mediterranean Region. *East. Mediterr. Health J.* **2018**, *24*, 77–91. [CrossRef]
110. Kelishadi, R.; Ardalan, G.; Gheiratmand, R.; Majdzadeh, R.; Hosseini, M.; Gouya, M.; Razaghi, E.; Delavari, A.; Motaghian, M.; Barekati, H. Thinness, overweight and obesity in a national sample of Iranian children and adolescents: CASPIAN Study. *Child Care Health Dev.* **2008**, *34*, 44–54. [CrossRef] [PubMed]
111. Mirmohammadi, S.-J.; Hafezi, R.; Mehrparvar, A.H.; Rezaeian, B.; Akbari, H. Prevalence of overweight and obesity among Iranian school children in different ethnicities. *Iran J. Pediatr.* **2011**, *21*, 514. [PubMed]
112. Nasreddine, L.; Naja, F.; Chamieh, M.C.; Adra, N.; Sibai, A.-M.; Hwalla, N. Trends in overweight and obesity in Lebanon: Evidence from two national cross-sectional surveys (1997 and 2009). *BMC Public Health* **2012**, *12*, 798. [CrossRef] [PubMed]
113. Bener, A.; Kamal, A.A. Growth patterns of Qatari school children and adolescents aged 6–18 years. *J. Health Popul. Nutr.* **2005**, *23*, 250–258.
114. Rootwelt, C.; Fosse, K.B.; Tuffaha, A.; Said, H.; Sandridge, A.; Janahi, I.; Greer, W.; Hedin, L. Qatar s Youth Is Putting on Weight: The Increase in Obesity Between 2003 and 2009. In Proceedings of the Qatar Foundation Annual Research Conference Proceedings, Doha, Qatar, November 2014; Volume 2014, p. HBSP1130.
115. El-Hazmi, M.A.; Warsy, A.S. A comparative study of prevalence of overweight and obesity in children in different provinces of Saudi Arabia. *J. Trop. Pediatr.* **2002**, *48*, 172–177. [CrossRef]
116. Al-Almaie, S.M. Prevalence of obesity and overweight among Saudi adolescents in Eastern Saudi Arabia. *Saudi Med. J.* **2005**, *26*, 607.
117. Al-Nuaim, A.A.; Al-Nakeeb, Y.; Lyons, M.; Al-Hazzaa, H.M.; Nevill, A.; Collins, P.; Duncan, M.J. The prevalence of physical activity and sedentary behaviours relative to obesity among adolescents from Al-Ahsa, Saudi Arabia: Rural versus urban variations. *J. Nutr. Metab.* **2012**, *2012*. [CrossRef]
118. Aounallah-Skhiri, H.; El Ati, J.; Traissac, P.; Romdhane, H.B.; Eymard-Duvernay, S.; Delpeuch, F.; Achour, N.; Maire, B. Blood pressure and associated factors in a North African adolescent population. a national cross-sectional study in Tunisia. *BMC Public Health* **2012**, *12*, 98. [CrossRef]
119. Musaiger, A.O. The state of nutrition in Bahrain. *Nutr. Health* **2000**, *14*, 63–74. [CrossRef]
120. Musaiger, A.O. Overweight and obesity in eastern mediterranean region: Prevalence and possible causes. *J. Obes.* **2011**, *2011*. [CrossRef]

121. Black, R.E.; Victora, C.G.; Walker, S.P.; Bhutta, Z.A.; Christian, P.; De Onis, M.; Ezzati, M.; Grantham-McGregor, S.; Katz, J.; Martorell, R. Maternal and child undernutrition and overweight in low-income and middle-income countries. *Lancet* **2013**, *382*, 427–451. [CrossRef]
122. Itoh, H.; Kanayama, N. Nutritional conditions in early life and risk of non-communicable diseases (NCDs) from the perspective of preemptive medicine in perinatal care. *Hypertens. Res. Pregnancy* **2015**, *3*, 1–12. [CrossRef]
123. Weiss, R.; Dziura, J.; Burgert, T.S.; Tamborlane, W.V.; Taksali, S.E.; Yeckel, C.W.; Allen, K.; Lopes, M.; Savoye, M.; Morrison, J. Obesity and the metabolic syndrome in children and adolescents. *N. Engl. J. Med.* **2004**, *350*, 2362–2374. [CrossRef] [PubMed]
124. Khader, Y.; Batieha, A.; Jaddou, H.; El-Khateeb, M.; Ajlouni, K. Metabolic syndrome and its individual components among Jordanian children and adolescents. *Int. J. Pediatr. Endocrinol.* **2010**, *2010*, 316170. [CrossRef] [PubMed]
125. Taha, D.; Ahmed, O.; Sadiq, B.B. The prevalence of metabolic syndrome and cardiovascular risk factors in a group of obese Saudi children and adolescents: A hospital-based study. *Ann. Saudi Med.* **2009**, *29*, 357–360. [CrossRef] [PubMed]
126. Eapen, V.; Mabrouk, A.; Yousef, S. Metabolic syndrome among the young obese in the United Arab Emirates. *J. Trop. Pediatr.* **2010**, *56*, 325–328. [CrossRef]
127. Ho, K.K.; Ferruzzi, M.G.; Wightman, J.D. Potential health benefits of (poly) phenols derived from fruit and 100% fruit juice. *Nutr. Rev.* **2020**, *78*, 145–174. [CrossRef]
128. Tetens, I.; Alinia, S. The role of fruit consumption in the prevention of obesity. *J. Hortic. Sci. Biotech.* **2009**, *84*, 47–51. [CrossRef]
129. Ello-Martin, J.A.; Roe, L.S.; Ledikwe, J.H.; Beach, A.M.; Rolls, B.J. Dietary energy density in the treatment of obesity: A year-long trial comparing 2 weight-loss diets. *Am. J. Clin. Nutr.* **2007**, *85*, 1465–1477. [CrossRef]
130. Malik, V.S.; Schulze, M.B.; Hu, F.B. Intake of sugar-sweetened beverages and weight gain: A systematic review¯. *Am. J. Clin. Nutr.* **2006**, *84*, 274–288. [CrossRef]
131. Malik, V.S.; Pan, A.; Willett, W.C.; Hu, F.B. Sugar-sweetened beverages and weight gain in children and adults: A systematic review and meta-analysis. *Am. J. Clin. Nutr.* **2013**, *98*, 1084–1102. [CrossRef] [PubMed]
132. Teff, K.L.; Grudziak, J.; Townsend, R.R.; Dunn, T.N.; Grant, R.W.; Adams, S.H.; Keim, N.L.; Cummings, B.P.; Stanhope, K.L.; Havel, P.J. Endocrine and metabolic effects of consuming fructose-and glucose-sweetened beverages with meals in obese men and women: Influence of insulin resistance on plasma triglyceride responses. *J. Clin. Endocrinol. Metab.* **2009**, *94*, 1562–1569. [CrossRef]
133. Stanhope, K.L.; Schwarz, J.M.; Keim, N.L.; Griffen, S.C.; Bremer, A.A.; Graham, J.L.; Hatcher, B.; Cox, C.L.; Dyachenko, A.; Zhang, W. Consuming fructose-sweetened, not glucose-sweetened, beverages increases visceral adiposity and lipids and decreases insulin sensitivity in overweight/obese humans. *J. Clin. Investig.* **2009**, *119*, 1322–1334. [CrossRef]
134. Stanhope, K.L.; Griffen, S.C.; Bair, B.R.; Swarbrick, M.M.; Keim, N.L.; Havel, P.J. Twenty-four-hour endocrine and metabolic profiles following consumption of high-fructose corn syrup-, sucrose-, fructose-, and glucose-sweetened beverages with meals. *Am. J. Clin. Nutr.* **2008**, *87*, 1194–1203. [CrossRef] [PubMed]
135. Stanhope, K.L.; Havel, P.J. Endocrine and metabolic effects of consuming beverages sweetened with fructose, glucose, sucrose, or high-fructose corn syrup. *Am. J. Clin. Nutr.* **2008**, *88*, 1733S–1737S. [CrossRef]
136. Muth, N.D.; Dietz, W.H.; Magge, S.N.; Johnson, R.K.; Pediatrics, A.A.O.; Association, A.H. Public policies to reduce sugary drink consumption in children and adolescents. *Pediatrics* **2019**, *143*. [CrossRef]
137. Engin, A. Fat cell and fatty acid turnover in obesity. In *Obes Lipotoxicity*; Springer: Berlin/Heidelberg, Germany, 2017; pp. 135–160.
138. Liberali, R.; Kupek, E.; Assis, M.A.A.d. Dietary Patterns and Childhood Obesity Risk: A Systematic Review. *Child Obes.* **2020**, *16*, 70–85. [CrossRef] [PubMed]
139. Eyles, H.; Bhana, N.; Lee, S.E.; Grimes, C.; McLean, R.; Nowson, C.; Wall, C. Measuring Children's Sodium and Potassium Intakes in NZ: A Pilot Study. *Nutrients* **2018**, *10*, 1198. [CrossRef]
140. UNICEF-GAIN. Food Systems for Children and Adolescents. In *Working Together to Secure Nutritious Diets*; UNICEF Office of Research: Rome, Italy, 2018.
141. Al-Isa, A. Nutritional Knowledge among High School Male Students in Kuwait. *J. Community Med. Health Educ.* **2018**, *8*. [CrossRef]

142. Al-Yateem, N.; Rossiter, R. Nutritional knowledge and habits of adolescents aged 9 to 13 years in Sharjah, United Arab Emirates: A crosssectional study. *East. Mediterr. Health J.* **2017**, *23*, 551–558. [CrossRef]
143. McClain, A.D.; Chappuis, C.; Nguyen-Rodriguez, S.T.; Yaroch, A.L.; Spruijt-Metz, D. Psychosocial correlates of eating behavior in children and adolescents: A review. *Int. J. Behav. Nutr. Phys. Act.* **2009**, *6*, 54. [CrossRef] [PubMed]
144. Banna, J.C.; Buchthal, O.V.; Delormier, T.; Creed-Kanashiro, H.M.; Penny, M.E. Influences on eating: A qualitative study of adolescents in a periurban area in Lima, Peru. *BMC Public Health* **2015**, *16*, 40. [CrossRef] [PubMed]
145. Becker, A.E.; Burwell, R.A.; Herzog, D.B.; Hamburg, P.; Gilman, S.E. Eating behaviours and attitudes following prolonged exposure to television among ethnic Fijian adolescent girls. *Br. J. Psychiatry* **2002**, *180*, 509–514. [CrossRef]
146. Karimi-Shahanjarini, A.; Omidvar, N.; Bazargan, M.; Rashidian, A.; Majdzadeh, R.; Shojaeizadeh, D. Iranian female adolescent's views on unhealthy snacks consumption: A qualitative study. *Iran J. Public Health* **2010**, *39*, 92. [PubMed]
147. Anthrologica-World Food Programme (WFP). *Bridging the Gap: Engaging Adolescents for Nutrition, Health and Sustainable Development*; World Food Programme: Rome, Italy, 2018.
148. Pachón, H.; Simondon, K.B.; Fall, S.T.; Menon, P.; Ruel, M.T.; Hotz, C.; Creed-Kanashiro, H.; Arce, B.; Domínguez, M.R.L.; Frongillo, E.A. Constraints on the delivery of animal-source foods to infants and young children: Case studies from five countries. *Food Nutr. Bull.* **2007**, *28*, 215–229. [CrossRef]
149. Armar-Klemesu, M.; Osei-Menya, S.; Zakariah-Akoto, S.; Tumilowicz, A.; Lee, J.; Hotz, C. Using ethnography to identify barriers and facilitators to optimal Infant and Young Child Feeding in rural Ghana: Implications for programs. *Food Nutr. Bull.* **2018**, *39*, 231–245. [CrossRef]
150. Burns, J.; Emerson, J.A.; Amundson, K.; Doocy, S.; Caulfield, L.E.; Klemm, R.D. A qualitative analysis of barriers and facilitators to optimal breastfeeding and complementary feeding practices in South Kivu, Democratic Republic of Congo. *Food Nutr. Bull.* **2016**, *37*, 119–131. [CrossRef]
151. Darmon, N.; Drewnowski, A. Contribution of food prices and diet cost to socioeconomic disparities in diet quality and health: A systematic review and analysis. *Nutr. Rev.* **2015**, *73*, 643–660. [CrossRef]
152. Kelly, B.; Halford, J.C.; Boyland, E.J.; Chapman, K.; Bautista-Castaño, I.; Berg, C.; Caroli, M.; Cook, B.; Coutinho, J.G.; Effertz, T. Television food advertising to children: A global perspective. *Am. J. Public Health* **2010**, *100*, 1730–1736. [CrossRef]
153. Nasreddine, L.; Taktouk, M.; Dabbous, M.; Melki, J. The extent, nature, and nutritional quality of foods advertised to children in Lebanon: The first study to use the WHO nutrient profile model for the Eastern Mediterranean Region. *Food Nutr. Res.* **2019**, *63*. [CrossRef]
154. Amini, M.; Omidvar, N.; Yeatman, H.; Shariat-Jafari, S.; Eslami-Amirabadi, M.; Zahedirad, M. Content analysis of food advertising in Iranian children's television programs. *Int. J. Prev. Med.* **2014**, *5*, 1337. [PubMed]
155. World Health Organization. Nutrition-Friendly Schools Initiative (NFSI). Available online: https://www.who.int/nutrition/topics/nutrition_friendly_schools_initiative/en/ (accessed on 8 October 2020).
156. World Health Organization. *Global Accelerated Action for the Health of Adolescents (AA-HA!): Guidance to Support Country Implementation*; World Health Organization: Geneva, Switzerland, 2017.
157. World Health Organization Regional Office for the Eastern Mediterranean. *Implementing the WHO Recommendations on the Marketing of Food and Nonalcoholic Beverages to Children in the Eastern Mediterranean Region*; 9290222247; World Health Organization: Cairo, Egypt, 2018.
158. World Health Organization Regional Office for the Eastern Mediterranean. *Strategy on Nutrition for the Eastern Mediterranean Region 2020–2030*; World Health Organization: Cairo, Egypt, 2019.
159. World Health Organization Regional Office for the Eastern Mediterranean. *Regional Framework for Action on Obesity Prevention 2019–2023*; World Health Organization: Cairo, Egypt, 2019.
160. World Health Organization. *Policy Statement and Recommended Actions for Lowering Sugar Intake and Reducing Prevalence of Type 2 Diabetes and Obesity in the Eastern Mediterranean Region*; World Health Organization: Cairo, Egypt, 2016.
161. World Health Organization. *Policy Statement and Recommended Actions for Reducing Fat Intake and Lowering Heart Attack Rates in the Eastern Mediterranean Region*; World Health Organization: Cairo, Egypt, 2014.

162. World Health Organization. *Policy Statement and Recommended Actions to Lower National Salt Intakes and Lower Death Rates from High Blood Pressure and Strokes in the Eastern Mediterranean Region*; World Health Organization: Cairo, Egypt, 2014.
163. HLPE. Nutrition and food systems. In *A Report by the High Level Panel of Experts on Food Security and Nutrition of the Committee on World Food Security*; High Level Panel of Experts: Rome, Italy, 2017.
164. UNICEF. The Faces of Malnutrition. Available online: https://www.unicef.org/nutrition/index_faces-of-malnutrition.html (accessed on 30 September 2020).

Publisher's Note: MDPI stays neutral with regard to jurisdictional claims in published maps and institutional affiliations.

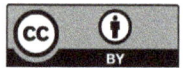

© 2020 by the authors. Licensee MDPI, Basel, Switzerland. This article is an open access article distributed under the terms and conditions of the Creative Commons Attribution (CC BY) license (http://creativecommons.org/licenses/by/4.0/).

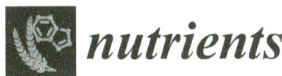

Article

Salt Reduction Strategies in Portuguese School Meals, from Pre-School to Secondary Education—The Eat Mediterranean Program

Ana Isabel Rito [1,2,*], Sofia Mendes [2,3], Mariana Santos [1,3], Francisco Goiana-da-Silva [4], Francesco Paolo Cappuccio [5], Stephen Whiting [6], Ana Dinis [7], Carla Rascôa [7], Isabel Castanheira [1], Ara Darzi [4] and João Breda [6]

1. WHO Collaborating Centre on Nutrition and Childhood Obesity—National Institute of Health Dr. Ricardo Jorge (INSA, IP), 1649-016 Lisbon, Portugal; Mariana.Coelho@insa.min-saude.pt (M.S.); isabel.castanheira@insa.min-saude.pt (I.C.)
2. Centre for Studies and Research in Social Dynamics and Health (CEIDSS), 1649-016 Lisbon, Portugal; sofiamendes@ceidss.com
3. National School of Public Health, NOVA University of Lisbon, 1600-560 Lisbon, Portugal
4. Centre for Health Policy, Institute of Global Health Innovation, Imperial College London, London SW7 2AZ, UK; franciscogoianasilva@gmail.com (F.G.-d.-S.); a.darzi@imperial.ac.uk (A.D.)
5. University of Warwick, WHO Collaborating Centre for Nutrition, Warwick Medical School, Coventry CV2 2DX, UK; f.p.cappuccio@warwick.ac.uk
6. WHO European Office for the Prevention and Control of Noncommunicable Diseases, 125009 Moscow, Russia; whitings@who.int (S.W.); rodriguesdasilvabred@who.int (J.B.)
7. Regional Health Administration of Lisbon and Tagus Valley (ARSLVT), 1700-179 Lisbon, Portugal; ana.dinis@arslvt.min-saude.pt (A.D.); carla.rascoa@arslvt.min-saude.pt (C.R.)
* Correspondence: ana.rito@insa.min-saude.pt; Tel.: +351-217-519-200

Received: 23 June 2020; Accepted: 16 July 2020; Published: 24 July 2020

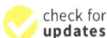

Abstract: High sodium (salt) consumption is associated with an increased risk of developing non-communicable diseases. However, in most European countries, Portugal included, sodium intake is still high. This study aimed to assess the sodium content of school meals before and after the Eat Mediterranean (EM) intervention—a community-based program to identify and correct nutritional deviations through the implementation of new school menus and through schools' food handlers training. EM (2015–2017) was developed in 25 schools (pre to secondary education) of two Portuguese Municipalities, reaching students aged 3–21 years old. Samples of the complete meals (soup + main course + bread) from all schools were collected, and nutritional quality and laboratory analysis were performed to determine their nutritional composition, including sodium content. Overall, there was a significant decrease (−23%) in the mean sodium content of the complete school meals, which was mainly achieved by the significant reduction of 34% of sodium content per serving portion of soup. In conclusion, EM had a positive effect on the improvement of the school meals' sodium content, among the participant schools. Furthermore, school setting might be ideal for nutrition literacy interventions among children, for flavors shaping, and for educating towards less salty food acceptance.

Keywords: community-based program; childhood obesity; school meals; salt intake; sodium consumption

---

1. Introduction

Given the well-established evidence that excessive sodium consumption (1 g of sodium per 100 g represents 2.5 g of salt per 100 g) is linked to an increased risk of developing non-communicable diseases (NCD) [1], a reduction in population's sodium consumption has been a key focus of both the international and national policy agendas. Reducing salt intake in the general population is not only a practical action that can prevent adverse health outcomes—such as increased blood pressure—but it is also a feasible and cost-effective strategy to reduce the growing burden of NCDs and reduce health-care costs for governments and individuals [2].

The World Health Organization (WHO) recommends a population reduction in salt intake as one of the 'best buys' or cost-effective actions that should be prioritized to tackle the global burden of NCDs [3–5]. Targets of a daily salt intake lower than 5 g for adults and 2 g for children have been recommended [6]. In addition, WHO Member States have agreed to work towards the global target of a 30% relative reduction in mean population intake of salt by 2025 relative to 2010 levels. It is crucial that this target is met in order to achieve the overall goal of a 25% reduction in premature mortality from NCDs by 2025 [2].

The overall number of countries implementing a national salt reduction strategy more than doubled from 2010 to 2015. However, despite the remarkable efforts and actions that have since been taken, more needs to be done. Data from 2013 revealed that population salt consumption in most European countries ranged from around 7 g/day (Bulgaria, Cyprus, Germany, and Latvia) to 13 g/day (Czech Republic) [7,8].

Among all dietary habits, excessive salt intake has the most adverse outcomes. The average daily intake of salt per capita among the Portuguese population is 10.7 g [9], which is double the level recommended by WHO (<5 g) [6]. Portugal ranks the highest among European countries regarding salt intake, with excessive intake reported in 63.2% of women and 88.9% of men [10]. The problem also affects younger groups, as research shows that most children and adolescents exceed daily recommendations [11–13].

Excessive salt intake is associated with an increased risk of obesity—partially due to poor diets that are high in both energy and salt, such as regular consumption of breakfast cereals [14] and highly processed foods [10]. Another reason for this association may be that consumption of salty foods stimulates thirst and increases fluid intake, thereby increasing the consumption of sugar-sweetened beverages, which can further fuel obesity [15]. This scenario is of particular interest in Portugal, where the prevalence of childhood overweight has been among the highest in Europe, affecting around one in three children [16]. It is, therefore, urgent to tackle this issue, as even small reductions in salt consumption can bring great health benefits to children by reducing the risk of developing cardiovascular diseases—the leading cause of death and disability in Portugal and worldwide [17,18].

The Portuguese "National Program for the Promotion of Healthy Eating" [19], in line with internationally recommended interventions [20], strongly advocates for the implementation of strategies to reduce dietary salt intake in children by providing information and education on healthy eating as well as the strengthening of consumer protections, particularly by reducing the salt content of school meals.

Several attempts have been made to reach children in schools to encourage healthier eating habits and improve the nutritional quality of the food served to them. These interventions can potentially impact all children of school age, irrespective of their ethnicity or socioeconomic group [21–25]. Primary and secondary schools serve at least one meal every day and can also determine the types of food and beverages that are available or served at schools (i.e., schools' cafeterias and vending machines). Schools can positively impact eating behaviors and promote healthier eating [26–28], for example, by deploying nutrition education classes.

School is a key setting to deliver health education to children, promote healthy lifestyles and social equality, and to ensure access to nutritionally balanced meals, regardless of the family's socioeconomic status [29]. In Portugal, municipalities are responsible for providing school meals (lunch) for pre-school and primary schools as well as for the management [30] of the menu. During secondary education, the supply of school meals is supported by the Directorate General of Education Institutions (DGEstE) [31], except for schools with their own cooking facilities. In Portugal, a set of guidelines for the school food supply has been established, which includes limits on the salt content of the school meal's components—bread, soup, and the main dish [31].

Assuming that lunch represents 30% of the total energy value [32] and considering the WHO recommendation [6], 1.5 g of salt should be the maximum level in this meal. In Portugal, little is known about the nutritional composition of the complete school meal. The amount of different nutrients in food samples can be measured through laboratory analyses, using standardized techniques recommended by international organizations [33]. In the few studies that have been conducted to estimate sodium content of school meals in Portugal, mean salt content has ranged from 2.83 and 3.82 g [34–36], which clearly should be reduced.

Eat Mediterranean—A Program for Eliminating Dietary Inequalities in Schools (EM) [37], was a European Economic Area (EEA) Grant funded project developed as a Portuguese community-based intervention (2015 to 2017) through a multi-sectorial approach involving health, education, and political stakeholders. The program's goal was to reduce nutritional inequalities among school-aged children through the promotion of the Mediterranean diet. The program comprised a comprehensive approach both at the individual level (child and family) and at the group/community level (nutritional education sessions at schools and improvement of school food environments). One of the objectives and key priority areas in the implementation of EM at the community level was to evaluate and improve the nutritional quality of food available in school meals. Within the school food environment, the EM program proposed a qualitative and quantitative (laboratory) analysis and evaluation of the nutritional adequacy of school meals. The aim was to identify nutritional deviations, according to international/national recommendations [29,31,38,39] and correct them by modifying the food composition of school meals through both training of the schools' food handlers and through the development and implementation of new menus.

2. Materials and Methods

2.1. Program and Participant Schools

The EM program was implemented over two school years (2015/2016 (Y1) to 2016/2017 (Y2)) in two Portuguese municipalities: Santarém and Alpiarça. In total, 25 individual public schools and 5773 students (3–21 years old), from pre-school to secondary education, participated in EM.

The entities responsible for the supply of school meals in both pre-schools and primary schools were Santarém Municipality (17 schools) and Alpiarça Municipality (three schools). For secondary schools, DGEstE supplied meals to four schools, while one had their own cooking service.

The specific evaluation and intervention on nutritional adequacy of served school meals (lunch) were organized in three phases:

- Evaluation (Y1): 386 school menus were analyzed qualitatively. Thirty-nine school meal samples were collected from 10 kitchens that served all 25 Schools for analysis during the period between March and June 2016. A report on qualitative and quantitative nutritional adequacy of school meals was presented to school communities.
- Intervention (Y1/Y2): From July 2016 to March 2017, a working group was established to discuss the results of the report from the evaluation phase and to develop a new proposal for school menus. The working group included public health professionals, nutritionists, a municipal food engineer, school cooks, teachers, and parents. The new school menus were developed according to the WHO recommendations [29,38] and national guidelines [32,40], and these were implemented in all participant schools. Additionally, training was provided for the schools' food handlers in order to implement the new changes. During the intervention period, nutritionists from the working group closely followed and guided every step of the process, including food preparation, cooking and serving of the meals while, at the same time, providing training to the food handlers. The training covered topics, such as food safety, cooking methods, and portion guidance (for example, to estimate the amount of salt that could be added to food, a standard measuring spoon or cup was introduced for all food handlers to use). Additionally, technical

sheets of the new menus were developed, and their implementation was conducted under the supervision of members of the working group.
- Post-intervention (Y2): A new set of 39 school meal samples was collected from the same kitchens from April to June 2017, and a qualitative and quantitative evaluation of the changes was performed.

Ethical approval was granted by Lisbon and Tagus Valley Regional Health Administration Ethical Committee (089.CES/INV/2015).

2.2. Food Samples and Sample Preparation

Food samples were collected from all 10 kitchens that served meals to the 25 schools. Of the 10 kitchens, nine served meals at their own schools, so samples were collected at the moment of serving. One school was served by transporting meals from a central kitchen outside the city. In this case, food samples were collected at the school immediately prior to serving.

The samples consisted of the food portions that were served to children at lunchtime. Each food sample consisted of three main items: bread, soup, and the main course (including salad or cooked vegetables and one piece of fruit). These were collected during both evaluation and post-intervention phases in a total of 39 samples in each phase. In one of the schools (school B), it was not possible to analyze the bread samples, as they were not sent to the laboratory. The meal items were weighed on a Mettler-Toledo PB3002-S/FACT (Mettler-Toledo, Inc., Columbus, OH) laboratory scale, with an accuracy of 0.01 g. Samples were collected using latex gloves, placed in sterile polythene bags, and alphabetically coded to maintain confidentiality. The samples were transported to the laboratory, refrigerated, homogenized, and milled using a high-speed grinder, a knife mill Grindomix GM 200; Retsch, Haan, Germany equipped with titanium knives to prevent contamination. The prepared samples were stored in vacuum bags at the freezing temperature ($-20\ °C$) until processing.

2.3. Laboratory Analysis and Interpretation

The analysis was performed in accordance with the methodology recommended by the Official Methods of Analysis of AOAC International [33], under quality assurance conditions complying with the requirements described in standard EN ISO/IEC 17025: 2005 [41]. For sodium determination, the samples were analyzed in triplicate using an inductively-coupled plasma optical emission spectrometer, ICP OES, model iCAP 6000, Thermo Fisher Scientific, Madison, WI, USA for the determination of sodium (Na) content. There are several common sources of sodium in food, including from salt added during preparation or during processing, as well as from the sodium in seasoning (e.g., sodium phosphate, sodium bicarbonate, MSG mono-glutamate, etc.). However, this study assumed that all sodium in food was in the form of sodium chloride and equivalents, so all results were expressed in terms of "salt".

The salt content in g/100 g of food was calculated by the formula: salt (g) = sodium (g) × 2.5 [41]. Considering a school meal (lunch) makes up 30% of the daily total energy intake [32], 1.5 g of salt was the reference value used in the present study (according to the WHO recommendation of salt intake [6]: $0.30 \times 5 = 1.5$ g).

2.4. Statistical Analysis

Data sets were produced using Microsoft Excel® spreadsheets, and statistical analyses were performed using IBM SPSS® statistics for Windows, version 22.0, Armonk, NY, USA [42]. Results were reported as mean (+ standard deviation). Non-parametric tests for comparing means were carried out for paired samples. A significance level of $\alpha = 0.05$ was considered statistically significant.

3. Results

The quantitative analysis of the school menus found that the standardized serving portions collected during the evaluation phase and the post-intervention phase were similar. Regarding the reduction in sodium and salt equivalent of the individual meal components, there was a 34% reduction per serving portion of soup. There were no significant changes in sodium and salt equivalent per serving portion of bread or per serving portion of the main course. In the complete meal, including the three components, there was a 23% reduction in sodium and salt equivalent per serving portion (Table 1).

Table 1. Sodium and salt content of school meals components (soup, main course, and bread) and of the complete meal (all components) analyzed at the evaluation and the post-intervention phases of the eat Mediterranean program.

	n	Serving Portion (g) [a]		Sodium (g/Serving Portion)			Salt (g/Serving Portion) [b]		
		Evaluation	Post-Intervention	Evaluation	Post-Intervention	p-Value	Evaluation	Post-Intervention	p-Value
Soup	10	227.10 ± 30.24	220.30 ± 37.08	0.59 ± 0.12	0.39 ± 0.24	0.017 Change 0.20~34%	1.48 ± 0.29	0.98 ± 0.59	0.017 Change 0.49~34%
Main course	10	262.30 ± 51.71	269.80 ± 61.28	0.68 ± 0.21	0.60 ± 0.25	0.169	1.70 ± 0.54	1.50 ± 0.63	0.169
Bread	9	46.00 ± 14.80	46.56 ± 16.08	0.19 ± 0.09	0.18 ± 0.11	0.441	0.48 ± 0.21	0.45 ± 0.27	0.514
Complete meal	10	-	-	1.50 ± 0.30	1.16 ± 0.45	0.028 Change 0.34~23%	3.75 ± 0.40	2.90 ± 1.12	0.047 Change 0.85~23%

[a] There were no statistically significant differences between serving portions (g) ($p > 0.05$); [b] The salt content was calculated by the formula: salt (g) = sodium (g) × 2.5 [35].

Changes in the mean salt content of the complete school meal in grams (g) at evaluation and at the post-intervention phase are shown, for individual schools and for all schools combined, in Figure 1. For all schools except for two (B and J), there was a decrease in salt content between the two time-points.

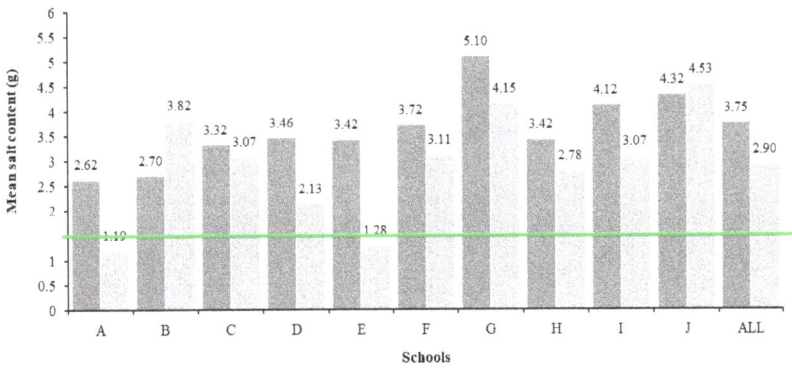

Figure 1. Mean salt content (g) of the complete school meals analyzed at the evaluation phase and the post-intervention phase of the eat Mediterranean program and its adequacy regarding the reference value (maximum 1.5 g of salt/meal), by the school.

4. Discussion

While community-based programs designed to improve the nutritional quality of school meals have been shown to be effective previously [43,44], EM was one of the first programs in Portugal to address qualitative and nutritional laboratory analysis together. Through a multidisciplinary approach targeting the school food environment, a key objective of the program was to improve the nutritional composition of school meals served to young people during lunchtime. In Portugal, addressing the quality of school meals is an important way to promote healthy diets as at least one meal is offered every day, and at pre- and primary education levels, almost every child has lunch at school [45].

The qualitative assessment of the 386 school menus has been presented elsewhere [46]. As part of evaluating EM, this study focused on identifying the nutritional deviations of sodium and salt equivalent content of school meals from international and national recommendations [29,31,38,39] and aimed to correct them by modifying the nutritional composition of school meals. This was done through training of the schools' food handlers and the development and implementation of new menus. The results showed that EM had a positive effect on the improvement of the school meals' salt content among the participating schools, achieving an overall reduction of 23% of the salt content of school meals served at lunchtime.

At the beginning of the EM program, the mean salt content of school meals was 3.75 g of salt per meal. These findings were similar to those reported in previous Portuguese studies [34–36], as well as in studies from other countries that assessed the salt content in school meals served in canteens [47]. Interventions as part of the EM program led to a significant reduction ($p < 0.05$) of salt content (from 3.75 g to 2.90 g of salt per meal, i.e., ~23%); however, it was still far from the reference value of lunch salt content (1.5 g of salt), and it was estimated that it would need to be met to achieve recommended salt consumption levels.

Looking separately at each component of the meal, the main dish was the component with the highest contribution to the salt content of the whole meal. This was also found in the study conducted by Barbosa et al. 2018 [48] in Portuguese University Canteens, in which it was suggested that one possible explanation for this result was the presence of intrinsic sodium in foods, such as meat and fish, which is higher than the sodium intrinsically present in vegetables used for soups [49]. However, we found a significant reduction in the salt content of soup from 1.48 g per serving portion before the intervention to 0.98 g per serving portion after the intervention (~34% reduction).

The values for lunch salt content, after EM intervention, are yet slightly higher than those reported by other Portuguese studies [50,51]. According to the Portuguese 2018 guidelines for menus and school canteens [31], the maximum value that can be added to soups and main dishes during the cooking process is 0.2 g of iodized salt. In addition, it is recommended that salt be replaced by glasswort or aromatic herbs. Regarding the serving of bread included in the school meals, according to the recommendations for Portuguese school meals [31], it should be one small piece of bread of 25 g for pre-school and primary school and 45 g for elementary and secondary school, with a maximum salt composition of 1%, meaning 0.25 g and 0.45 g of salt per serving of bread, respectively. As there was no intervention targeted at reducing bread provided during school meals, this study observed that, despite the level of education, the mean serving of bread was around 45 g, and the salt content of bread per serving, both before and after the intervention, was above the guidelines (0.46 g–0.49 g). In Portugal, there is a culture of always serving bread at mealtime, which is reflected in the official guidelines [31]. It could be suggested that if there was a non-mandatory offer of bread at school meals, at least for young children, and if carbohydrate intake recommendations were met through foods with less salt, a further reduction on overall salt intake could have been observed through this action alone.

There were several challenges in the implementation of the EM program. One of these was to reduce the amount of salt added by cooks while preparing the meals, as while the technical guidance clearly requires that the amount of salt added during meal preparation be accurately measured, several cooks still opted to measure by "hand". This was also described by Gonçalves et al. [52], who found that the amount of added salt was influenced by the taste of the cook, even though many food handlers acknowledged that they did not taste the food before adding salt. That study also pointed out that food handlers were aware of the health problems associated with excessive salt intake as well as the recommended salt intake values, but they mentioned that the greatest difficulty in salt reduction was the opinion and acceptance of the consumers toward less salt in foods [52]. Such limitations reinforce the importance of educating both consumers and food handlers so that programs aiming at reducing the salt content in school meals and other settings can be more effective.

Action to reduce salt consumption is urgent, including among younger populations, in order to reduce the risk of developing cardiovascular diseases. The offer of high sodium meals in a school environment can contribute to individuals acquiring long-term poor eating habits, including increased consumption of processed food, which is already a pattern in Portuguese children [10]. Additionally, emerging evidence suggests dietary sodium intake may be associated with obesity, both through pathophysiological mechanisms and through the induction of thirst and increased consumption of high energy drinks [53–57], enhancing the need to address and tackle this public health issue.

The improvement of the menus introduced by the EM program has shown that it is possible to successfully reduce the salt content of school lunches through existing mechanisms. To ensure school meals are nutritionally adequate, it is essential that trained cooking staff and all responsible parties strictly comply with the technical sheets provided. It is also crucial to continue the education of students, parents, educators, teachers, as well as the monitoring of all stages of preparing and serving meals by the cooking staff. The integrated and concerted work among health departments, research institutions, municipalities, and educational communities was a strong part of the success of the EM program.

Among the common challenges educators face when trying to reduce the amount of added salt to meals is rejection by consumers due to "lack of flavor" [52]. However, the adaptive capacity of the flavors-linked neurological system to small reductions in salt in meals has been well described [57]. Thus, school settings may be ideal not only for nutrition literacy interventions among children but also for flavors, shaping and educating towards less salty food acceptance.

One of the pitfalls of this study was the limited time frame of the intervention to carry out all the activities projected in this comprehensive program without including a post-intervention longer monitoring period. This would have been important to continuously assess the adaptation to the changes implemented in the context of the new school food environment, in particular, the acceptance/preference of less salty meals by the children.

Nonetheless, recognizing the relevance of consumer acceptance in order to obtain long-lasting changes, EM paved the way for further work towards providing healthier meals in the participating schools, including a monitoring system to assess students' acceptance of school meals changes and also regarding food waste. The training, capacity building, and nutritional education offered during the EM intervention to all school community (teachers, parents, children, food handlers, and others) would hopefully contribute to the sustainability of the progress achieved in improvements and support continuous improvements.

5. Conclusions

This study demonstrated the success of the EM program in reducing the salt content of lunch meals served in schools. School meals must be nutritious, and reinforcement of this through regular monitoring and evaluation is a key factor to ensure school food quality. In order for school meals to be nutritionally adequate, trained cooking staff and all responsible parties would need to strictly comply with the provided technical sheets. It is crucial that the health literacy of students, parents, educators, and teachers is developed through continuous education, and the monitoring process at all stages of preparing and serving meals by school food handlers is strengthened. This comprehensive program was built through a collaboration between different stakeholders (health departments and units, research institutions, municipalities, and educational communities), which was both key to its success and ensured a holistic approach towards promoting healthier behaviors.

Author Contributions: The authors' contributions are as follows: A.I.R., was part of the coordinating team of eat Mediterranean and worked in all stages of the research, such as project design, methodology, analysis and interpretation of the data, and conceptualization, preparation and writing of the original manuscript; S.M. worked on the analysis and interpretation of the data; M.S. contributed to the laboratory analysis; A.D. (Ana Dinis) and C.R. coordinated and implemented the eat Mediterranean program, worked on the project design, data collection, and interpretation of the data. A.I.R.; S.M.; M.S.; F.G.-d.-S.; F.P.C.; S.W.; A.D. (Ana Dinis); C.R.; I.C.; A.D. (Ara Darzi); J.B. contributed to the writing, review and editing. All authors have read and agreed to the published version of the manuscript.

Funding: The eat Mediterranean program (2015–2017) was coordinated by ARSLVT, Portugal, co-funded by the Public Health Initiatives Program (PT06) of the EEA Grants (grant application 171 NU2).

Acknowledgments: The authors wish to acknowledge all the nutritionists, psychologists, and other health professionals, children, parents, educators, teachers, school cooking staff, and municipality technicians for their contribution on the fieldwork, as well as the following Institutions for their partnership and support: Agrupamentos de Escolas Ginestal Machado, Sá da Bandeira e de José Relvas; Hospital Distrital de Santarém; CEIDSS—Centre for Studies and Research in Social Dynamics and Health; ISCTEIUL—Instituto Universitário de Lisboa; Municipalities of Alpiarça and Santarém and Instituto Nacional de Saúde Doutor Ricardo Jorge.

Conflicts of Interest: The authors declare no conflict of interest. The writing group takes sole responsibility for the content of this article, and the content of this article reflects the views of the authors only. S.W. and J.B. are staff members of the WHO. The WHO is not liable for any use that may be made of the information contained therein.

References

1. World Health Organization. *Global Status Report on Noncommunicable Diseases 2014*; World Health Organization: Geneva, Switzerland, 2014.
2. World Health Organization. *Global Action Plan for the Prevention and Control of Noncommunicable Diseases 2013-2020*; World Health Organization: Geneva, Switzerland, 2013.
3. Beaglehole, R.; Bonita, R.; Horton, R.; Adams, C.; Alleyne, G.; Asaria, P.; Baugh, V.; Bekedam, H.; Billo, N.E.; Casswell, S.; et al. Priority actions for the non-communicable disease crisis. *Lancet* **2011**, *6736*, 1438–1447. [CrossRef]
4. World Health Organization. *Noncommunicable Diseases Progress Monitor, 2017*; World Health Organization: Geneva, Switzerland, 2017; Available online: http://apps.who.int/iris/bitstream/10665/258940/1/9789241513029-eng.pdf?ua=1 (accessed on 23 September 2019).
5. World Health Organization. *Tackling NCDs: 'Best Buys' and Other Recommended Interventions for the Prevention and Control of Noncommunicable Diseases*; World Health Organization: Geneva, Switzerland, 2017; Available online: https://apps.who.int/iris/handle/10665/259232 (accessed on 23 September 2019).
6. World Health Organization. *Guideline: Sodium Intake for Adults and Children*; World Health Organization: Geneva, Switzerland, 2012; Available online: https://www.who.int/publications/i/item/9789241504836 (accessed on 23 September 2019).
7. European Commission. *Survey on Member Sates' Implementation of the EU Salt Reduction Framework*; Publications Office of the European Union: Luxembourg, 2013; Available online: https://op.europa.eu/en/publication-detail/-/publication/df7ef17e-d643-4593-94b3-84bacfa7a76a (accessed on 23 September 2019).
8. World Health Organization. *Mapping Salt Reduction Initiatives in the WHO European Region*; World Health Organization: Copenhagen, Denmark, 2013; Available online: http://www.euro.who.int/en/publications/abstracts/mapping-salt-reduction-initiatives-in-the-who-european-region (accessed on 23 September 2019).
9. Polonia, J.; Martins, L.; Pinto, F.; Nazare, J. Prevalence, awareness, treatment and control of hypertension and salt intake in Portugal: Changes over a decade the PHYSA study. *J. Hypertens.* **2014**, *32*, 1211–1221. [CrossRef]
10. Lopes, C.; Torres, D.; Oliveira, A.; Severo, M.; Alarcao, V.; Guiomar, S.; Mota, J.; Teixeira, P.J.; Rodrigues, S.; Lobato, L.; et al. Inquérito Alimentar Nacional e de Atividade Física, IAN-AF 2015-2016: Relatório de resultados. Universidade do Porto, 2017. Available online: https://ian-af.up.pt/publicacoes (accessed on 26 September 2019).
11. Goncalves, C.; Abreu, S.; Padrao, P.; Pinho, O.; Graca, P.; Breda, J.; Santos, R.; Moreira, P. Sodium and potassium urinary excretion and dietary intake: A cross-sectional analysis in adolescents. *Food Nutr. Res.* **2016**, *60*. [CrossRef] [PubMed]
12. Correiacosta, L.; Cosme, D.; Nogueirasilva, L.; Morato, M.; Sousa, T.; Moura, C.; Mota, C.; Guerra, A.; Albinoteixeira, A.; Areias, J.C.; et al. Gender and obesity modify the impact of salt intake on blood pressure in children. *Pediatric Nephrol.* **2016**, *31*, 279–288. [CrossRef]
13. Sardinha, L.B.; Santos, D.A.; Silva, A.M.; Coelhoesilva, M.J.; Raimundo, A.; Moreira, H.; Santos, R.; Vale, S.; Baptista, F.; Mota, J. Prevalence of overweight, obesity, and abdominal obesity in a representative sample of Portuguese adults. *PLoS ONE* **2012**, *7*, e47883. [CrossRef] [PubMed]

14. Rito, A.I.; Dinis, A.; Rascoa, C.; Maia, A.; Martins, I.D.; Santos, M.; Lima, J.; Mendes, S.; Padrao, J.; Steinnovais, C. Improving breakfast patterns of portuguese children-an evaluation of ready-to-eat cereals according to the European nutrient profile model. *Eur. J. Clin. Nutr.* **2019**, *73*, 465–473. [CrossRef] [PubMed]
15. Ma, Y.; He, F.; MacGregor, G. High Salt Intake—Independent Risk Factor for Obesity? *Hypertension* **2015**, *66*, 843–849. [CrossRef] [PubMed]
16. Rito, A.I.; Cruz de Sousa, R.; Mendes, S.; Graça, P. *Childhood Obesity Surveillance Initiative: COSI Portugal 2016*; Instituto Nacional de Saúde Dr. Ricardo Jorge (INSA, IP): Lisbon, Portugal, 2017; Available online: http://hdl.handle.net/10400.18/4857 (accessed on 26 September 2019).
17. Programa Nacional para a Promoção da Alimentação Saudável. *Portugal Alimentação Saudável em Números 2015*; Direção-Geral da Saúde: Lisbon, Portugal, 2016; Available online: http://nutrimento.pt/activeapp/wp-content/uploads/2016/03/Relatório-Portugal-Alimentação-Saudável-em-números-2015.pdf (accessed on 27 September 2019).
18. Li, X.; Jan, S.; Yan, L.L.; Hayes, A.J.; Chu, Y.; Wang, H.; Feng, X.; Niu, W.; He, F.J.; Ma, J.; et al. Cost and cost-effectiveness of a school-based education program to reduce salt intake in children and their families in China. *PLoS ONE* **2017**, *12*. [CrossRef]
19. Ministério da Saúde, Direção Geral da Saúde. *Programa Nacional para a Promoção da Alimentação Saudável Orientações Programáticas*; Direção-Geral da Saúde: Lisbon, Portugal, 2012; Available online: http://www.dgs.pt/programas-de-saude-prioritarios.aspx (accessed on 10 October 2019).
20. World Health Organization. *The SHAKE Technical Package for Salt Reduction*; World Health Organization: Geneva, Switzerland, 2016; Available online: https://apps.who.int/iris/rest/bitstreams/1061141/retrieve (accessed on 6 January 2020).
21. Lytle, L.A.; Kubik, M.Y. Nutritional issues for adolescents. *Best Pract. Res. Clin. Endocrinol. Metab.* **2003**, *17*, 177–189. [CrossRef]
22. World Health Organization. *Diet, Nutrition and the Prevention of Chronic Diseases: Report of a Joint WHO/FAO Expert Consultation—Technical Report Series no. 916*; World Health Organization: Geneva, Switzerland, 2003; Available online: https://apps.who.int/iris/bitstream/handle/10665/42665/WHO_TRS_916.pdf;jsessionid=EBC44FFF46A59BECE4352FE155FC349C?sequence=1 (accessed on 25 October 2019).
23. French, S.A.; Stables, G. Environmental interventions to promote vegetable and fruit consumption among youth in school settings. *Prev. Med.* **2003**, *37*, 593–610. [CrossRef]
24. Flodmark, C.E.; Marcus, C.; Britton, M. Interventions to prevent obesity in children and adolescents: A systematic literature review. *Int. J. Obes.* **2006**, *30*, 579–589. [CrossRef]
25. Sharma, M. International school-based interventions for preventing obesity in children. *Obes. Rev.* **2006**, *8*, 155–167. [CrossRef]
26. Centers for Disease Control and Prevention. Guidelines for school health programs to promote lifelong healthy eating. *J. Sch. Health* **1997**, *67*, 9–26. [CrossRef] [PubMed]
27. Branca, F.; Nikogosian, H.; Lobstein, T. *The challenge of obesity in the WHO European Region and the Strategies for Response*; World Health Organization: Copenhagen, Denmark, 2007; Available online: http://www.euro.who.int/en/publications/abstracts/challenge-of-obesity-in-the-who-european-region-and-the-strategies-for-response-the (accessed on 25 October 2019).
28. Commission of the European Communities. *Green Paper—Promoting Healthy Diets and Physical Activity: A European Dimension for The Prevention of Overweight, Obesity and Chronic Diseases*; European Commission: Brussels, Belgium, 2005; Available online: https://eur-lex.europa.eu/legal-content/EN/TXT/PDF/?uri=CELEX:52005DC0637&from=EN26 (accessed on 25 October 2019).
29. World Health Organization. *Report of the Commission on Ending Childhood Obesity*; World Health Organization: Geneva, Switzerland, 2016; Available online: https://www.who.int/end-childhood-obesity/final-report/en/ (accessed on 25 October 2019).
30. Ministério da Educação e da Ciência (2015) Parte C Despacho n°8452-a/2015. Available online: https://www.dgeste.mec.pt/wp-content/uploads/2014/01/Despacho8452A2015ASE.pdf (accessed on 25 October 2019).
31. Lima, R.M. Orientações sobre ementas e refeitórios escolares. *Ministério da Educação—Direção-Geral da Educação*. 2018. Available online: http://www.dge.mec.pt/sites/default/files/Esaude/oere.pdf (accessed on 13 November 2019).
32. Institute of Medicine (US) Committee on Nutrition Standards for National School Lunch and Breakfast Programs. *School Meals: Building Blocks for Healthy Children*; National Academies Press: Washington, DC, USA, 2010.

33. Association of Official Analytical Chemists (AOAC). *International Official Methods of Analysis of AOAC International*; AOAC International: Rockville, MD, USA, 2000.
34. Paiva, I.; Pinto, C.; Queiros, L.; Meister, M.C.; Saraiva, M.; Bruno, P.; Antunes, D.; Afonso, M. Baixo valor calórico e elevado teor de sal. *Acta Médica Portuguesa* **2011**, *24*, 215–222. [PubMed]
35. Viegas, C.; Torgal, J.; Graça, P.; Martins, M. Evaluation of salt content in school meals. *Rev. Nutr.* **2015**, *28*, 165–174. [CrossRef]
36. Fontes, T.; Bento, A.; Matias, F.; Mota, C.; Nascimento, A.; Santiago, S.; Santos, M. O valor nutricional das refeições escolares. In *Boletim Epidemiológico*; INSA, IP Nº especial _ Alimentação e Nutrição: Lisboa, Portugal, 2015.
37. Eat Mediterranean Program. Available online: http://www.ceidss.com/eat-mediterranean/ (accessed on 10 December 2019).
38. World Health Organization. *School Policy Framework: Implementation of the WHO Global Strategy on Diet, Physical Activity and Health*; World Health Organization: Geneva, Switzerland, 2008; Available online: http://www.who.int/dietphysicalactivity/SPF-En.pdf (accessed on 13 November 2019).
39. SPARE—Sistema de Planeamento e Avaliação de Refeições Escolares—Elaboração, Verificação e Monitorização na ótica do Utilizador. Available online: http://www.plataformacontraaobesidade.dgs.pt:8080/SPARE2/index.php (accessed on 15 December 2019).
40. International Organization for Standardization. *General Requirements for the Competence of Testing and Calibration Laboratories*, 2nd ed.; ISO/IEC 17025:2005 (International Standard); International Organization for Standardization: Geneva, Switzerland, 2005.
41. *Regulation (EU) No 1169/2011 of the European Parliament and of the Council of 25 October 2011 on the Provision of Food Information to Consumers*; The Publications Office of the European Union: Luxembourg, 2011.
42. IBM Corp. *IBM SPSS Statistics for Windows*; Version 22.0; IBM Corp: Armonk, NY, USA, 2016.
43. Rocha, A.; Afonso, C.; Santos, M.C.; Morais, C.; Franchini, B.; Chilro, R. System of planning and evaluation of school meals. *Public Health Nutr.* **2014**, *17*, 1264–1270. [CrossRef]
44. Sancho, T.; Candeias, A.; Mendes, C.; Rego, M.; Cartaxo, L. Promoção da qualidade nutricional de refeições em estabelecimentos de educação do Algarve análise comparativa 2004/2005–2006/2007. *Rev. Nutrícias* **2008**, *8*, 1–3.
45. Rocha, A.; Ávila, H.; Barbosa, M. Caracterização da Prestação do Serviço de Refeições Escolares pelos Municípios Portugueses. *Rev. Nutrícias* **2012**, *13*, 3–8.
46. Rito, A.; Dinis, A.; Rascôa, C.; Rodrigues, S.; Stein-Novais, C.; Mendes, S.; Maia, A.; Luís, S.; Luciano, R. Nutrition Qualitative Evaluation and Improvement of School Meals in Portugal—Eat Mediterranean Program. *Acta Port. Nutr.* **2018**, *12*, 6–12. [CrossRef]
47. Ahn, S.; Park, S.; Kim, J.N.; Han, S.N.; Jeong, S.B.; Kim, H.K. Salt content of school meals and comparison of perception related to sodium intake in elementary, middle, and high schools. *Nutr. Res. Pract.* **2013**, *7*, 59–65. [CrossRef]
48. Barbosa, M.; Fernandes, A.; Gonçalves, C.; Pena, M.; Padrão, P.; Pinho, O.; Moreira, P. Sodium and Potassium Content of Meals Served in University Canteens. *Port. J. Public Health* **2018**, *35*, 27–33. [CrossRef]
49. Martins, I.; Porto, A.; Oliveira, L. Tabela de Composição de Alimentos. In *Departamento de Alimentação e Nutrição*; Instituto Nacional de Saúde Doutor Ricardo Jorge: Lisbon, Portugal, 2007.
50. Gonçalves, C.; Silva, G.; Pinho, O.; Camelo, S.; Amaro, L.; Teixeira, V.; Padrão, P.; Moreira, P. Sodium content in vegetable soups prepared outside the home: Identifying the problem. In *International Symposium on Occupational Safety and Hygiene: Book of Abstracts*; Sociedade Portuguesa de Segurança e Higiene Ocupacionais: Guimarães, Portugal, 2012.
51. Goncalves, C.; Monteiro, S.; Padrao, P.; Rocha, A.; Abreu, S.; Pinho, O.; Moreira, P. Salt reduction in vegetable soup does not affect saltiness intensity and liking in the elderly and children. *Food Nutr. Res.* **2014**, *58*, 24825. [CrossRef] [PubMed]
52. Gonçalves, C.; Pinho, O.; Padrão, P.; Santos, C.; Abreu, S.; Moreira, P. Knowledge and practices related to added salt in meals by food handlers. *Rev. Nutrícias* **2014**, *21*, 14–17.
53. Libuda, L.; Kersting, M.; Alexy, U. Consumption of dietary salt measured by urinary sodium excretion and its associated with body weight status in healthy children and adolescents. *Public Health Nutr.* **2012**, *15*, 433–441. [CrossRef] [PubMed]

54. Yoon, Y.S.; Oh, S.W. Sodium density and obesity; the Korea National Health and Nutrition Examination Survey 2007–2010. *Eur. J. Clin. Nutr.* **2013**, *67*, 141–146. [CrossRef] [PubMed]
55. Zhu, H.; Pollock, N.K.; Kotak, I.; Gutin, B.; Wang, X.; Bhagatwala, J.; Parikh, S.; Harshfield, G.A.; Dong, Y. Dietary sodium, adiposity, and inflammation in healthy adolescents. *Pediatrics* **2014**, *133*, e635–e642. [CrossRef]
56. Grimes, A.; Bolhuis, D.; He, F.; Nowson, C. Dietary sodium intake and overweight and obesity in children and adults: A protocol for a systematic review and meta-analysis. *Syst. Rev.* **2016**, *5*, 7. [CrossRef]
57. Cappuccio, F.P.; Capewell, S. Facts, issues and controversies in salt reduction for the prevention of cardiovascular disease. *Funct. Food Rev.* **2015**, *7*, 41–61. [CrossRef]

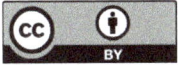

© 2020 by the authors. Licensee MDPI, Basel, Switzerland. This article is an open access article distributed under the terms and conditions of the Creative Commons Attribution (CC BY) license (http://creativecommons.org/licenses/by/4.0/).

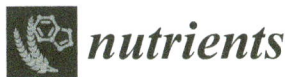

Article

Is the Perceived Fruit Accessibility Related to Fruit Intakes and Prevalence of Overweight in Disadvantaged Youth: A Cross-Sectional Study

Narae Yang and Kirang Kim *

Department of Food Science and Nutrition, College of Natural Sciences, Dankook University, Dandae-ro, Dongnam-gu, Cheonan-si, Chungnam 31116, Korea; skfo2581@daum.net
* Correspondence: kirangkim@dankook.ac.kr; Tel.: +82-41-529-6373

Received: 23 September 2020; Accepted: 19 October 2020; Published: 29 October 2020

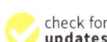

Abstract: Background: Few investigations have studied the relationship between home and school food environments, fruit intakes, and prevalence of overweight in children and adolescents from disadvantaged backgrounds. This study aimed to determine whether food environments for fruit intake at household and school levels affect fruit intakes and risk of overweight among children and adolescents with low household income. Methods: Students (n = 3148) in Seoul, Korea completed questionnaires pertaining to select aspects of their food environments, frequency of fruit intakes, and weight status. Chi-square tests and logistic regressions evaluated associations between the aforementioned variables. Results: Participants consumed fruit an average of 0.77 times per day, though its frequency increased when fruit accessibility was perceived positively. The percentage of overweight participants was 23.5% for boys and 22.8% for girls. Generally, fruit intake frequency was linked to a lower prevalence of overweight. Regular provision of fruit in school lunches was associated with a reduced risk of overweight among elementary school girls (odds ratio (OR): 0.52, 95% confidence interval (CI): 0.30–0.92), and having someone at home to prepare fruit was associated with a reduced risk of overweight in elementary school boys (OR: 0.64, 95% CI: 0.43–0.94) and girls (OR: 0.63, 95% CI: 0.43–0.93). Conclusions: The frequency of fruit intake was low among disadvantaged youth. Increasing access to fruit in their food environments appears to enhance consumption and lower the risk of overweight, especially for elementary school girls.

Keywords: food environment; fruit; children; adolescents; obesity; overweight; home; school

1. Introduction

The epidemic of pediatric overweight and obesity has expanded steadily over the past few decades, currently reaching more than 370 million children worldwide [1]. Consequences of early excess adiposity include a heightened risk of psychological problems such as depression, low self-esteem, and disordered eating in the immediate term, as well as cardiovascular disease and various cancers upon adulthood [2–5]. Adult obesity, implemented in child obesity, makes it difficult to lose weight [6]. Therefore, it is important to prevent obesity in childhood [6]. The prevalence of obesity among children and adolescents has increased in Asia [7]. Although the rising trends of body mass index (BMI) have flattened in high-income countries, the prevalence of obesity is still high in worldwide [7].

Obesity has been explained with reduced intakes of healthy foods and unhealthy eating behaviors [8–11]. Especially fruit, which are rich in water and fiber, to enhance satiety, and low in energy density [12], have been known to prevent obesity, coronary heart disease, stroke, cardiovascular disease, total cancer, and all-cause mortality [13–16]. Obesity prevention interventions that take into account healthy food intake, such as fruit, are needed. For effective obesity intervention, it is important to identify the relationship between eating healthy foods and obesity and to find the main determinants that affect obesity. Previous intervention methods for eating healthy foods to prevent obesity have focused on individual behavior changes. However, individual level interventions fundamentally could not change the obesogenic environment, which have been reported to have little effect on long-term improvement [17,18]. In recent years, the ecological model has been applied to promote health in the public health sector. The multilevel interventions that take an account for both individual and environmental factors have been paid attention for effective behavior change. Among environmental factors, food environments include political, economic, social, physical, and natural environment factors which affect accessibility, availability, and affordability of foods [19,20]. The food environments have been known as an important factor related to food choice and dietary intakes [19,20]. For children and adolescents, the household is the first physical and social environment to learn about food intake [21], and the school is responsible for their lunches and another setting to make them eat healthy food [21]. Thus, for effective intervention, factors at household and school levels that affect the availability and accessibility of foods as well as at the individual level should be included [22].

It has been reported that the food environment has a greater effect on health and nutritional status in the vulnerable group than in the general group [23], but most of the studies have been conducted on the general group [24], and there is a dearth of research exploring how food environments at home and school affect fruit intakes and risk of overweight among disadvantaged children and adolescents. Therefore, research is needed to determine how the food environments of vulnerable children is related to healthy food intake and obesity. For this study, we surveyed low socioeconomic status youth to determine how select aspects of their food environments associate with consumption of fruit and weight status. Therefore, the objective of this study was to investigate whether food environments at household and school levels affect fruit intakes and risk of overweight among disadvantaged children and adolescents.

2. Methods

2.1. Study Population

Participants were recruited in 2015 from the Community Childcare Center, located in Seoul, Korea. They provide welfare services (e.g., protection, education, and meals) after school to youth from disadvantaged backgrounds (e.g., beneficiaries of national basic livelihood or single-parent families, etc.) [25]. During this time, the Community Childcare Center participated in the Healthy Fruit Basket Program, which aims to prevent the development of chronic diseases by providing access to fresh fruits [25,26]. In total, 4154 students (mean age; elementary school: 10.4 y, middle and high school: 14.3 y) were recruited; however, only 3148 were included in the final analyses because they supplied information for all the variables of interest and were of an eligible weight status (i.e., normal and overweight) [27,28]. The Institutional Review Board approved this study, and all participants gave written informed consent and assent (DKU 2015-10-016).

2.2. Weight Status

Height and weight were measured by a trained measurer at the public health centers or the Community Childcare Centers using a nationally certified weight and height scale. BMI was calculated as weight (kg) divided by height squared (m^2). According to the 2007 Korean National Growth Charts for children and adolescents [29], classification of normal weight was defined as having a body weight between the fifth and eighty-fourth percentiles, based on one's gender and age; classification of overweight was defined as having a body weight in the eighty-fifth percentile or above, or BMI 25 kg/m^2 or greater, based on one's gender and age.

2.3. Fruit Intakes

Fruit frequency questionnaires examined fruit intakes from the month preceding study enrollment. Scoring ranged from 0 (never) to 9 (3+ times per day). All responses were converted into times per day and collapsed into two categories (<0.5 times per day vs. ≥0.5 times per day) to determine the association with overweight.

2.4. Food Environments

Participants were asked five questions about their food environments, adapted from those employed in a previous investigation [30]. Here, three dimensions of the physical environment were evaluated: (1) Availability of fruit at home, (2) accessibility of fruit at home (i.e., is there someone who prepares fruit for children to eat?), and (3) accessibility of fruit at school (i.e., does the school provide fruit twice a week?). For the social environment, questions inquired about the habit of frequently eating fruit among parents and friends. Responses for the questions ranged from 1 (strongly disagree) to 5 (strongly agree), and all were collapsed into categories of disagree (strongly disagree, disagree), neutral, and agree (agree, strongly agree).

2.5. Statistical Analysis

Chi-square tests assessed the distribution of participants' general characteristics, the food environment, and weight status according to the frequency of fruit intakes and aspects of the food environment. T-tests evaluated differences in the frequency of fruit intakes by sex and grade level. An analysis of variance and Scheffe's post-hoc test determined differences between the food environments. Logistic regressions analyzed the effects of fruit intakes and food environments on weight status, showing odds ratios (ORs), 95% confidence intervals (95% CI). All analyses were performed by SPSS Statistics (v. 23.0); $p \leq 0.05$ was considered statistically significant.

3. Results

General characteristics of the participants are shown in Table 1. Overall, 49.0% were boys and 71.5% were in elementary school. The percentage of overweight for boys and girls was 23.5% and 22.8%, respectively. The percentage of overweight for elementary school, and middle and high school students was 24.3% and 20.4%, respectively. There was a significant difference of weight status between grades, and the percentage of overweight was high in elementary school students.

Table 1. General characteristics of subjects [1].

	All (n = 3148)	Normal Weight (n = 2419)	Overweight (n = 729)	p [2]
Sex				
Boys	1542 (49.0)	1179 (76.5)	363 (23.5)	0.617
Girls	1606 (51.0)	1240 (77.2)	366 (22.8)	
Grade				
Elementary school	2251 (71.5)	1705 (75.7)	546 (24.3)	0.021
Middle and high school	897 (28.5)	714 (79.6)	183 (20.4)	
Sex, grade				
Boys				
Elementary school	1061 (68.8)	797 (75.1)	264 (24.9)	0.065
Middle and high school	481 (31.2)	382 (79.4)	99 (20.6)	
Girls				
Elementary school	1190 (74.1)	908 (76.3)	282 (23.7)	0.142
Middle and high school	416 (25.9)	332 (79.8)	84 (20.2)	

[1] Qualitative variables are presented as n (%). [2] p-values for differences between the weight statuses were obtained by a chi-square test.

Table 2 details aspects of the participants' food environments. Overall, 59.5% to 63.2% of participants responded positively (i.e., affirmed the availability of fruit at home, a regular provision of fruit in school lunches, having someone at home to prepare fruit for them, and a family habit of frequently eating fruit). Between the sexes, girls perceived their food environments more positively than boys ($p < 0.001$). Between the grade levels, elementary school students perceived their food environments more positively than middle and high school students ($p < 0.001$).

Table 2. Select aspects of participants' food environments [1].

	All	Sex		Grade	
		Boys	Girls	Elementary School	Middle and High School
Availability of fruit at home					
Disagree	458 (14.5)	238 (15.4)	220 (13.7)	313 (13.9)	145 (16.2)
Neutral	816 (25.9)	441 (28.6)	375 (23.3)	557 (24.7)	259 (28.9)
Agree	1874 (59.5)	863 (56.0)	1011 (63.0)	1381 (61.4)	493 (55.0)
p [2]		<0.001		0.004	
Regular provision of fruit in school lunches					
Disagree	259 (8.2)	155 (10.1)	104 (6.5)	145 (6.4)	114 (12.7)
Neutral	959 (30.5)	504 (32.7)	455 (28.3)	624 (27.7)	335 (37.3)
Agree	1930 (61.3)	883 (57.3)	1047 (65.2)	1482 (65.8)	448 (49.9)
p [2]		<0.001		<0.001	
Having someone at home to prepare fruit					
Disagree	439 (13.9)	226 (14.7)	213 (13.3)	295 (13.1)	144 (16.1)
Neutral	718 (22.8)	393 (25.5)	325 (20.2)	471 (20.9)	247 (27.5)
Agree	1991 (63.2)	923 (59.9)	1068 (66.5)	1485 (66.0)	506 (56.4)
p [2]		<0.001		<0.001	
Family habit of eating fruit frequently					
Disagree	282 (9.0)	143 (9.3)	139 (8.7)	193 (8.6)	89 (9.9)
Neutral	954 (30.3)	518 (33.6)	436 (27.1)	618 (27.5)	336 (37.5)
Agree	1912 (60.7)	881 (57.1)	1031 (64.2)	1440 (64.0)	472 (52.6)
p [2]		<0.001		<0.001	
Friends' habit of eating fruit frequently					
Disagree	544 (17.3)	299 (19.4)	245 (15.3)	364 (16.2)	180 (20.1)
Neutral	1378 (43.8)	710 (46.0)	668 (41.6)	936 (41.6)	442 (49.3)
Agree	1226 (38.9)	533 (34.6)	693 (43.2)	951 (42.2)	275 (30.7)
p [2]		<0.001		<0.001	

[1] Values are presented as absolute numbers and percentages. [2] p-values for differences between sexes or grade levels, obtained by a chi-square test.

Table 3 shows the relationship between aspects of participants' food environments and frequency of fruit intakes. Regardless of sex or grade level, fruit intakes differed according to how one's food environment was perceived. Here, the group who perceived their food environments positively was found to consume fruit 0.87 to 0.95 times per day, whereas the group who perceived their food environments negatively was found to consume fruit 0.42 to 0.67 times per day ($p < 0.001$). Interestingly, there were no differences in fruit intakes between sexes when they shared the same perception about their food environments. However, when both grade levels responded positively about their food environments, consumption of fruit was found to be higher among elementary school students. For groups displaying a negative or neutral perception, frequency of fruit intakes was comparable.

Table 3. Relationship between aspects of participants' food environments and frequency of fruit intakes [1].

	All	Sex		Grade	
		Boys	Girls	Elementary School	Middle and High School
All	0.77 ± 0.17	0.74 ± 0.02 [a]	0.80 ± 0.02 [b]	0.85 ± 0.02 [a]	0.59 ± 0.02 [b]
p^2		0.036		<0.001	
		Availability of fruit at home			
Disagree	0.47 ± 0.03 [a]	0.46 ± 0.04 [a]	0.49 ± 0.04 [a]	0.51 ± 0.04 [a]	0.39 ± 0.03 [a]
Neutral	0.55 ± 0.02 [a]	0.54 ± 0.03 [a]	0.55 ± 0.03 [a]	0.60 ± 0.03 [ab]	0.44 ± 0.03 [a]
Agree	0.95 ± 0.02 [b]	0.92 ± 0.03 [b]	0.96 ± 0.03 [b]	1.03 ± 0.03 [c]	0.71 ± 0.03 [b]
p^2	<0.001	<0.001		<0.001	
		Regular provision of fruit in school lunches			
Disagree	0.65 ± 0.05 [a]	0.62 ± 0.06 [a]	0.69 ± 0.08 [ab]	0.64 ± 0.07 [acd]	0.66 ± 0.06 [ad]
Neutral	0.62 ± 0.02 [a]	0.62 ± 0.03 [a]	0.63 ± 0.03 [a]	0.70 ± 0.03 [a]	0.47 ± 0.03 [cd]
Agree	0.87 ± 0.02 [b]	0.83 ± 0.03 [b]	0.89 ± 0.03 [b]	0.93 ± 0.02 [b]	0.64 ± 0.03 [ad]
p^2	<0.001	<0.001		<0.001	
		Having someone at home to prepare fruit			
Disagree	0.60 ± 0.04 [a]	0.55 ± 0.05 [a]	0.64 ± 0.05 [a]	0.67 ± 0.05 [ae]	0.43 ± 0.03 [ad]
Neutral	0.53 ± 0.02 [a]	0.52 ± 0.03 [a]	0.55 ± 0.04 [a]	0.58 ± 0.03 [ac]	0.44 ± 0.03 [cd]
Agree	0.90 ± 0.02 [b]	0.88 ± 0.03 [b]	0.91 ± 0.03 [b]	0.97 ± 0.02 [b]	0.70 ± 0.03 [e]
p^2	<0.001	<0.001		<0.001	
		Family habit of eating fruit frequently			
Disagree	0.42 ± 0.04 [a]	0.42 ± 0.05 [a]	0.43 ± 0.05 [a]	0.46 ± 0.05 [ab]	0.33 ± 0.03 [ab]
Neutral	0.54 ± 0.02 [a]	0.55 ± 0.03 [a]	0.53 ± 0.03 [a]	0.59 ± 0.03 [bc]	0.45 ± 0.03 [ab]
Agree	0.94 ± 0.02 [b]	0.91 ± 0.03 [b]	0.97 ± 0.03 [b]	1.01 ± 0.02 [d]	0.72 ± 0.03 [c]
p^2	<0.001	<0.001		<0.001	
		Friends' habit of eating fruit frequently			
Disagree	0.67 ± 0.03 [a]	0.63 ± 0.04 [a]	0.71 ± 0.05 [ab]	0.75 ± 0.04 [a]	0.49 ± 0.03 [bd]
Neutral	0.67 ± 0.02 [a]	0.68 ± 0.03 [a]	0.67 ± 0.03 [a]	0.73 ± 0.03 [a]	0.56 ± 0.03 [bd]
Agree	0.93 ± 0.03 [b]	0.89 ± 0.04 [bc]	0.96 ± 0.04 [c]	1.00 ± 0.03 [c]	0.69 ± 0.04 [ad]
p^2	<0.001	<0.001		<0.001	

[1] Values are fruit intake per day, presenting as means ± standard errors. [2] p-values for differences between sexes or grade levels, obtained by ANOVA; letters ([a,b,c,d,e]) indicate significant differences between groups (Scheffe's post-hoc test, $p < 0.05$).

Table 4 shows the relationship between aspects of participants' food environments, frequency of fruit intakes, and weight status. The fruit intake frequency was not related to weight status in total subjects but as classified by grade; the lower intake frequency was shown in overweight groups of elementary school students. In terms of fruit environments and overweight, regular provision of fruit in school lunches and having a person at home to prepare fruit were negatively correlated to an overweight status for all participants. A low frequency of fruit intakes was associated with an overweight status among elementary school students. The proportion of overweight students was lower among those who perceived their food environment at school positively compared to those who did not ($p = 0.044$), especially for girls ($p = 0.047$) and elementary school students ($p = 0.005$). In addition, the proportion of overweight students was lower among those who had someone at home to prepare fruit compared to those who did not ($p < 0.001$), notably again for girls ($p = 0.007$) and elementary school students ($p = 0.001$).

Table 4. Relationship between aspects of participants' food environments, frequency of fruit intakes, and weight status [1].

	All		Sex				Grade			
			Boys		Girls		Elementary School		Middle and High School	
	Normal Weight	Over Weight	Normal Weight	Over Weight	Normal Weight	Over Weight	Normal Weight	Over Weight	Normal Weight	Over Weight
Fruits intakes per day										
<0.5	1194 (49.4)	378 (51.9)	610 (51.7)	191 (52.6)	584 (47.1)	187 (51.1)	771 (45.2)	274 (50.2)	423 (59.2)	104 (56.8)
≥0.5	1225 (50.6)	351 (48.1)	569 (48.3)	172 (47.4)	656 (52.9)	179 (48.9)	934 (54.8)	272 (49.8)	291 (40.8)	79 (43.2)
p^2	0.238		0.770		0.179		0.043		0.554	
Food environments										
Availability of fruit at home										
Disagree	348 (14.4)	110 (15.1)	181 (15.4)	57 (15.7)	167 (13.5)	53 (14.5)	232 (13.6)	81 (14.8)	116 (16.2)	29 (15.8)
Neutral	629 (26.0)	187 (25.7)	335 (28.4)	106 (29.2)	294 (23.7)	81 (22.1)	420 (24.6)	137 (25.1)	209 (29.3)	50 (27.3)
Agree	1442 (59.6)	432 (59.3)	663 (56.2)	200 (55.1)	779 (62.8)	232 (63.4)	1053 (61.8)	328 (60.1)	389 (54.5)	104 (56.8)
p^2	0.892		0.929		0.768		0.713		0.838	
Regular provision of fruit in school lunches										
Disagree	187 (7.7)	72 (9.9)	115 (9.8)	40 (11.0)	72 (5.8)	32 (8.7)	99 (5.8)	46 (8.4)	88 (12.3)	26 (14.2)
Neutral	723 (29.9)	236 (32.4)	380 (32.2)	124 (34.2)	343 (27.7)	112 (30.6)	454 (26.6)	170 (31.1)	269 (37.7)	66 (36.1)
Agree	1509 (62.4)	421 (57.8)	684 (58.0)	199 (54.8)	825 (66.5)	222 (60.7)	1152 (67.6)	330 (60.4)	357 (50.0)	91 (49.7)
p^2	0.044		0.535		0.047		0.005		0.775	
Having someone at home to prepare fruit										
Disagree	310 (12.8)	129 (17.7)	160 (13.6)	66 (18.2)	150 (12.1)	63 (17.2)	204 (12.0)	91 (16.7)	106 (14.8)	38 (20.8)
Neutral	539 (22.3)	179 (24.6)	297 (25.2)	96 (26.4)	242 (19.5)	83 (22.7)	342 (20.1)	129 (23.6)	197 (27.6)	50 (27.3)
Agree	1570 (64.9)	421 (57.8)	722 (61.2)	201 (55.4)	848 (68.4)	220 (60.1)	1159 (68.0)	326 (59.7)	411 (57.6)	95 (51.9)
p^2	<0.001		0.055		0.007		0.001		0.135	
Family habit of eating fruit frequently										
Disagree	211 (8.7)	71 (9.7)	107 (9.1)	36 (9.9)	104 (8.4)	35 (9.6)	141 (8.3)	52 (9.5)	70 (9.8)	19 (10.4)
Neutral	730 (30.2)	224 (30.7)	393 (33.3)	125 (34.4)	337 (27.2)	99 (27.0)	454 (26.6)	164 (30.0)	276 (38.7)	60 (32.8)
Agree	1478 (61.1)	434 (59.5)	679 (57.6)	202 (55.6)	799 (64.4)	232 (63.4)	1110 (65.1)	330 (60.4)	368 (51.5)	104 (56.8)
p^2	0.629		0.780		0.778		0.141		0.339	
Friends' habit of eating fruit frequently										
Disagree	421 (17.4)	123 (16.9)	233 (19.8)	66 (18.2)	188 (15.2)	57 (15.6)	275 (16.1)	89 (16.3)	146 (20.4)	34 (18.6)
Neutral	1051 (43.4)	327 (44.9)	541 (45.9)	169 (46.6)	510 (41.1)	158 (43.2)	697 (40.9)	239 (43.8)	354 (49.6)	88 (48.1)
Agree	947 (39.1)	279 (38.3)	405 (34.4)	128 (35.3)	542 (43.7)	151 (41.3)	733 (43.0)	218 (39.9)	214 (30.0)	61 (33.3)
p^2	0.796		0.798		0.702		0.415		0.652	

[1] Values are presented as absolute numbers and percentages. [2] p-values for differences between sexes and grade levels, obtained by a chi-square test.

Table 5. Relationship between aspects of participants' food environments and odds of being overweight.

	Boys						Girls					
	Elementary School		Middle and High School				Elementary School				Middle and High School	
	OR [1] (95% CI)	Adjusted OR [2] (A95% CI)	OR (95% CI)	Adjusted OR (A95% CI)			OR (95% CI)	Adjusted OR (A95% CI)			OR (95% CI)	Adjusted OR (A95% CI)
Availability of fruit at home												
Disagree	1.00	1.00	1.00	1.00			1.00	1.00			1.00	1.00
Neutral	0.87 (0.56–1.35)	0.87 (0.56–1.34)	1.41 (0.69–2.90)	1.41 (0.69–2.88)			1 (0.63–1.60)	1.02 (0.64–1.62)			0.61 (0.29–1.29)	0.61 (0.29–1.27)
Agree	0.8 (0.54–1.19)	0.79 (0.53–1.18)	1.44 (0.74–2.80)	1.41 (0.72–2.77)			1 (0.67–1.50)	1.08 (0.72–1.63)			0.77 (0.40–1.48)	0.7 (0.36–1.37)
p-trend [3]	0.278	0.246	0.342	0.392			0.988	0.652			0.701	0.464
Regular provision of fruit in school lunches												
Disagree	1.00	1.00	1.00	1.00			1.00	1.00			1.00	1.00
Neutral	0.87 (0.52–1.47)	0.87 (0.52–1.47)	0.98 (0.49–1.96)	1 (0.50–1.99)			0.72 (0.39–1.30)	0.72 (0.40–1.31)			0.66 (0.30–1.44)	0.71 (0.32–1.55)
Agree	0.71 (0.43–1.16)	0.7 (0.43–1.15)	1.01 (0.52–1.98)	1.01 (0.52–1.98)			0.52 (0.30–0.92)	0.54 (0.31–0.95)			0.7 (0.34–1.46)	0.71 (0.34–1.49)
p-trend [3]	0.081	0.075	0.939	0.963			0.005	0.01			0.527	0.492
Having someone at home to prepare fruit												
Disagree	1.00	1.00	1.00	1.00			1.00	1.00			1.00	1.00
Neutral	0.76 (0.49–1.19)	0.76 (0.49–1.19)	0.85 (0.44–1.64)	0.85 (0.45–1.64)			0.95 (0.60–1.50)	0.93 (0.59–1.47)			0.56 (0.27–1.16)	0.55 (0.27–1.14)
Agree	0.64 (0.43–0.94)	0.63 (0.42–0.93)	0.72 (0.40–1.32)	0.7 (0.38–1.29)			0.63 (0.43–0.93)	0.65 (0.44–0.96)			0.57 (0.30–1.05)	0.51 (0.27–0.96)
p-trend [3]	0.023	0.019	0.275	0.223			0.004	0.009			0.122	0.06
Family habit of eating fruit frequently												
Disagree	1.00	1.00	1.00	1.00			1.00	1.00			1.00	1.00
Neutral	1.16 (0.69–1.93)	1.15 (0.68–1.92)	0.63 (0.29–1.36)	0.63 (0.29–1.36)			0.81 (0.48–1.37)	0.82 (0.49–1.38)			1.08 (0.45–2.58)	1.03 (0.43–2.46)
Agree	0.83 (0.51–1.36)	0.81 (0.49–1.33)	1.01 (0.48–2.12)	1.00 (0.47–2.13)			0.78 (0.49–1.25)	0.84 (0.52–1.36)			1.09 (0.47–2.50)	0.96 (0.41–2.25)
p-trend [3]	0.097	0.081	0.301	0.346			0.357	0.649			0.879	0.835
Friends' habit of eating fruit frequently												
Disagree	1.00	1.00	1.00	1.00			1.00	1.00			1.00	1.00
Neutral	1.06 (0.72–1.56)	1.06 (0.72–1.56)	1.26 (0.69–2.31)	1.25 (0.69–2.29)			1.06 (0.70–1.59)	1.04 (0.69–1.58)			0.86 (0.45–1.65)	0.85 (0.44–1.63)
Agree	1.02 (0.69–1.52)	1.02 (0.69–1.51)	1.31 (0.67–2.57)	1.29 (0.65–2.54)			0.84 (0.56–1.27)	0.86 (0.57–1.31)			1.13 (0.59–2.17)	1.07 (0.55–2.08)
p-trend [3]	0.962	0.977	0.459	0.496			0.204	0.302			0.586	0.699

[1] Odds ratios (ORs) were derived from logistic regression models. [2] Adjusted ORs adjusted for fruit intake frequency and were derived from logistic regression models. [3] p-values for trends.

Table 5 shows the relationship between aspects of participants' food environments and odds of being overweight, unadjusted and adjusted for fruit intake frequency. For boys, those who had someone at home to prepare fruit were unlikely to be overweight (OR = 0.64, 95% CI = 0.43–0.94, p-trend = 0.023), and these results remained significant after adjusting for frequency of fruit intakes (OR = 0.63, 95% CI = 0.420.93, p-trend = 0.019). For elementary school girls, regular provision of fruit in school lunches (OR = 0.52, 95% CI = 0.30–0.92, p-trend = 0.005) and having someone at home to prepare fruit for them (OR = 0.63, 95% CI = 0.43–0.93, p-trend = 0.004) were negatively related to an overweight status, even after adjusting for frequency of fruit intakes (OR = 0.54, 95% CI = 0.31–0.95, p-trend = 0.01 for regular provision of fruit in school lunches; OR = 0.65, 95% CI = 0.44–0.96, p-trend = 0.009 for having someone at home to prepare fruit). Among middle and high school girls, having someone at home to prepare fruit was significantly associated with a lower risk of being overweight after adjusting for frequency of fruit intakes (OR = 0.51, 95% CI = 0.27–0.96, p-trend = 0.06).

4. Discussion

Because of the prominent influence that food environments exert on an individual's tendency toward obesity, we explored the relationship between aspects of the home and school food environments, fruit intakes, and overweight status among disadvantaged children and adolescents. We found that the frequency of fruit intakes increased when participants perceived their food environments positively, and this was associated with a reduced prevalence of overweight. In particular, regular provision of fruit in school lunches and having someone at home to prepare fruit was associated with a healthier body weight among elementary school students and girls.

Fruit was consumed an average of 0.77 times per day by our participants, which was below the recommended level of the Dietary Reference Intake for Koreans of at least twice per day [31]. According to the Korea National Health and Nutrition Examination Survey [32], low-income families consume less fruit than medium-income families (100.1 vs. 135.2 g/day). In this study, frequency of fruit intake varied according to a participant's perception of their food environment, with higher rates of consumption among those who responded positively. These results provide evidence that food environments to increase fruit intakes would play an important role in fruit consumption.

Previously, review papers and meta-analyses have shown that increasing the availability and accessibility of fruits and vegetables for children at school is effective at preventing obesity [33,34]. In this study, regular provision of fruit in school lunches was positively related to fruit intakes among elementary school students, but not middle and high school students. These findings do not align with those from a related investigation in the United States, wherein high school students who received fruits and vegetables from The Fresh Fruit and Vegetable Program were likely to eat fruit more often than those who did not (59.1% vs. 40.9%) [35]. Given that middle and high school students appear to have more established eating habits, it may be necessary to provide fruit at a higher frequency in order to enhance intakes [35,36]. The school lunch service in Korea could provide fruits as a dessert within the school budget, but the current frequency of provision of fruit at school lunch would not be enough to meet the consumption of fruit for the disadvantaged middle and high school students in Korea. Therefore, additional funding for more frequent provision of fruit at school lunch should be needed to increase their fruit consumption.

Regarding the food environment at home, having someone to prepare fruit for students was found to relate favorably to fruit intakes and weight status. This result was consistent with those from other studies reporting that social support for healthy food intakes aides in the prevention of obesity among vulnerable children [37,38]. A few reasons might explain this. First, caregivers give children fruit in a form that allows them to eat it easily. Several studies have shown that providing fruit in a ready-to-eat form or making it visible to children promotes fruit intakes [39,40]. Because the process of washing, cutting, and peeling fruit has been described as an impediment to consumption, providing or storing it in an accessible form may help children eat fruit more frequently [40,41]. Indeed, analyses from the Healthy Habits randomized trial [42] revealed that the frequency of fruit provision from a parent positively impacted their children's fruit intakes after 12 months. Second, caregivers could promote fruit intakes simply by encouraging their children [43]. Considering that participants in our study hailed from disadvantaged backgrounds, it is unlikely that their caregivers purchase much fruit for them or monitor their intakes at home. Thus, incorporating the Healthy Fruit Basket Program into all Community Childcare Centers and related institutions nationwide may help these individuals increase fruit intakes and attenuate risk of overweight or obesity [25,26].

It is well established that availability of food in the home is a key determinant of consumption among children and adolescents [44–46], and our analyses confirmed this phenomenon for fruit, in particular. Additionally, we observed that a family's habit of eating fruit frequently was connected to high fruit intakes across all participants, similar to findings from other publications [39,42,43].

Interestingly, this investigation detected no difference in fruit intakes between sexes sharing the same perception about their food environments. However, with respect to the grade levels, elementary school students were found to consume fruit more frequently than middle or high school students when their food environment was perceived positively. Childhood is a period of social modeling, as individuals learn how to interact with their environments and behave appropriately [11,47,48]. Hence, the benefits of food environments on fruit intakes may apply more strongly to children than adolescents. For another explanation, a recent study of adults with low socioeconomic position found that self-efficacy on fruit and vegetable consumption was more strongly associated with fruit and vegetable consumption than perceived food environments, which implies the importance of capacity building to partially overcome the poor food environment [49]. As several studies have shown the positive effect of nutritional education on fruit and vegetable intakes [50–52], nutritional education intervention should be included for adolescents with negative perception of food environment who especially have low self-efficacy to increase their fruit and vegetable intakes.

When we examined the relationship between fruit intakes and weight status, a high frequency (>0.5 times per day) was tied to a lower prevalence of overweight in girls. According to systematic reviews, consumption of fruit as a means to prevent pediatric obesity did not always produce consistent results in terms of gender or amount (38,39). For example, one investigation noted that eating fruit more than twice a day was only protective against obesity in boys [53], and another showed that excessive fruit intakes actually engendered obesity [54]. Heeding our results and those from earlier studies, consumption of fruit alone may not be adequate to prevent obesity. Specifically, our investigation found that the effects of some aspects of the food environment on the prevalence of obesity remained significant after adjusting for fruit intake frequency, and a related study observed a positive link between parental concern for their children's diet and fitness practices ($r = 0.552$, $p < 0.001$) [55]. It could suggest that the home environment supporting children to eat fruits could also support other behaviors that can prevent obesity in children, such as encouraging exercise. Further research exploring caretakers' interest in their children's health will provide a more holistic understanding of how environments moderate their risk of obesity.

The present study had several limitations and strengths. Concerning limitations, this was a cross-sectional study, so any causal associations between food environments, fruit intakes, and overweight status have yet to be determined. In addition, the questionnaire evaluating fruit availability and accessibility in the home and school food environments was not validated, although it had been employed in a previous study [30]. Moreover, we did not collect information pertaining to other confounders of overweight, which could offer deeper insight into factors underlying the present findings [25,26]. Granted, this was a highly homogenous cohort since all participants were recruited from the Community Childcare Center, so it is unlikely they possessed any remarkable characteristics that would alter our results. Nonetheless, future studies examining a more diverse population are needed to confirm the relationship between the food environment and risk of obesity by adjusting the confounding factor. Despite limitations, these results provide evidence that food environments play an important role in overweight prevention as well as fruit consumption among underprivileged Asian children and adolescents, using a relatively large sample size.

5. Conclusions

This study found that the frequency of fruit intakes was generally low among children and adolescents from disadvantaged backgrounds; however, those who perceived their food environments positively consumed more fruit and were less likely to be overweight than those who perceived them negatively. Noteworthily, regular provision of fruit in school lunches and having someone at home to prepare fruit were predictive of a high frequency of fruit intakes and lower prevalence of overweight, and these discoveries were most apparent among elementary school students and girls. On the whole, our findings demonstrate that augmenting access to fruit within any realm of the food environment is associated with increased consumption and healthier body weights for low-income youth. Going forward, the school lunch service in Korea could consider increasing fruit servings since current provisions are not sufficient for enabling disadvantaged middle and high school students to meet the dietary guidelines. In addition, a nation-wide program to increase fruit consumption at the Community Childcare Center where they usually spend time would be essential to improve their health.

Author Contributions: K.K. conceived and designed the study; N.Y. analyzed the data and wrote the first draft of the paper; K.K. supervised the data analysis and revised the draft paper. All authors have read and agreed to the published version of the manuscript.

Funding: This research was funded by the National Research Foundation (NRF) of Korea (2019R1A2C1084372).

Conflicts of Interest: All authors declare no conflict of interest.

References

1. Di Cesare, M.; Sorić, M.; Bovet, P.; Miranda, J.J.; Bhutta, Z.; Stevens, G.A.; Laxmaiah, A.; Kengne, A.P.; Bentham, J. The epidemiological burden of obesity in childhood: A worldwide epidemic requiring urgent action. *BMC Med.* **2019**, *17*, 1–20. [CrossRef]
2. Rankin, J.; Matthews, L.; Cobley, S.; Han, A.; Sanders, R.; Wiltshire, H.D.; Baker, J.S. Psychological consequences of childhood obesity: Psychiatric comorbidity and prevention. *Adolesc. Health Med. Ther.* **2016**, *7*, 125–146. [CrossRef]
3. Sagar, R.; Gupta, T. Psychological Aspects of Obesity in Children and Adolescents. *Indian J. Pediatr.* **2018**, *85*, 554–559. [CrossRef]
4. Anthropometric Measures during Infancy and Childhood and the Risk of Developing Cardiovascular Disease or Diabetes Mellitus Type 2 in Later Life: A Systematic Review 2015. Available online: https://www.who.int/maternal_child_adolescent/documents/singh-anthropometry-ncd-infants-children-2015.pdf?ua=1 (accessed on 27 August 2020).
5. Preventing and Managing the Global Epidemic—WHO Technical Report Series. Available online: https://www.who.int/nutrition/publications/obesity/WHO_TRS_894/en/ (accessed on 27 August 2020).
6. Dehghan, M.; Akhtar-Danesh, N.; Merchant, A.T. Childhood obesity, prevalence and prevention. *Nutr. J.* **2005**, *4*, 1–8. [CrossRef]
7. Bentham, J.; Di Cesare, M.; Bilano, V.; Bixby, H.; Zhou, B.; Stevens, G.A.; Riley, L.M.; Taddei, C.; Hajifathalian, K.; Lu, Y.; et al. Worldwide trends in body-mass index, underweight, overweight, and obesity from 1975 to 2016: A pooled analysis of 2416 population-based measurement studies in 128·9 million children, adolescents, and adults. *Lancet* **2017**, *390*, 2627–2642. [CrossRef]
8. Poti, J.; Braga, B.; Quin, B. Ultra-processed food intake and obesity: What really matters for health—Processing or nutrient content? *Curr. Obes. Rep.* **2018**, *6*, 420–431. [CrossRef]
9. Huang, J.-Y.; Qi, S.-J. Childhood obesity and food intake. *World J. Pediatr.* **2015**, *11*, 101–107. [CrossRef]
10. Epstein, L.H.; Paluch, R.A.; Beecher, M.D.; Roemmich, J.N. Increasing healthy eating vs. reducing high energy-dense foods to treat pediatric obesity. *Obesity* **2008**, *16*, 318–326. [CrossRef]
11. Ricotti, R.; Caputo, M.; Prodam, F. Chapter 9—Mediterranean diet, nutrition transition, and cardiovascular risk factor in children and adolescents. In *The Mediterranean Diet: An Evidence-Based Approach*, 2nd ed.; Preedy, V.R., Watson, R.R., Eds.; Academic Press: Cambridge, MA, USA, 2020; pp. 89–95, ISBN 978-0-12-818649-7.

12. Rolls, B.J.; Ello-Martin, J.A.; Tohill, B.C. What Can Intervention Studies Tell Us about the Relationship between Fruit and Vegetable Consumption and Weight Management? *Nutr. Rev.* **2004**, *62*, 1–17. [CrossRef]
13. Aune, D.; Giovannucci, E.; Boffetta, P.; Fadnes, L.T.; Keum, N.N.; Norat, T.; Greenwood, D.C.; Riboli, E.; Vatten, L.J.; Tonstad, S. Fruit and vegetable intake and the risk of cardiovascular disease, total cancer and all-cause mortality-A systematic review and dose-response meta-analysis of prospective studies. *Int. J. Epidemiol.* **2017**, *46*, 1029–1056. [CrossRef]
14. Hebden, L.; O'Leary, F.; Rangan, A.; Singgih Lie, E.; Hirani, V.; Allman-Farinelli, M. Fruit consumption and adiposity status in adults: A systematic review of current evidence. *Crit. Rev. Food Sci. Nutr.* **2017**, *57*, 2526–2540. [CrossRef]
15. Stamler, J.; Dolecek, T. Chapter 13. Relation of food and nutrient intakes to body mass in the special intervention and usual care groups in the Multiple Risk Factor Intervention Trial. *Am. J. Clin. Nutr.* **1997**, *65*, 366S–373S. [CrossRef]
16. Buijsse, B.; Feskens, E.J.M.; Schulze, M.B.; Forouhi, N.G.; Wareham, N.J.; Sharp, S.; Palli, D.; Tognon, G.; Halkjaer, J.; Tjønneland, A.; et al. Fruit and vegetable intakes and subsequent changes in body weight in European populations: Results from the project on Diet, Obesity, and Genes (DiOGenes). *Am. J. Clin. Nutr.* **2009**, *90*, 202–209. [CrossRef]
17. Kamath, C.C.; Vickers, K.S.; Ehrlich, A.; McGovern, L.; Johnson, J.; Singhal, V.; Paulo, R.; Hettinger, A.; Erwin, P.J.; Montori, V.M. Behavioral interventions to prevent childhood obesity: A systematic review and metaanalyses of randomized trials. *J. Clin. Endocrinol. Metab.* **2008**, *93*, 4606–4615. [CrossRef]
18. Swinburn, B.; Egger, G.; Raza, F. The Development and Application of a Framework for Identifying and Prioritizing Environmental Interventions for Obesity. *Dissecting Obesog. Environ.* **1999**, *29*, 563–570.
19. Rideout, K.; Mah, C.; Minaker, L. *Food Environments: An Introduction for Public Health Practice*; National Collaborating Centre for Environmental Health British Columbia Centre for Disease Control: Vancouver, BC, Canada, 2015.
20. Rosenkranz, R.R.; Dzewaltowski, D.A. Model of the home food environment pertaining to childhood obesity. *Nutr. Rev.* **2008**, *66*, 123–140. [CrossRef]
21. Chan, K.; Prendergast, G.; Grønhøj, A.; Bech-Larsen, T. The role of socializing agents in communicating healthy eating to adolescents: A cross-cultural study. *J. Int. Consum. Mark.* **2011**, *23*, 59–74. [CrossRef]
22. Food and Health in Europe: A New Basis for Action. Available online: https://www.who.int/nutrition/publications/Food_and_health_Europe%20_newbasis_for_%20action.pdf (accessed on 27 August 2020).
23. Lytle, L.A. Measuring the Food Environment. State of the Science. *Am. J. Prev. Med.* **2009**, *36*, 1–18. [CrossRef]
24. Micha, R.; Karageorgou, D.; Bakogianni, I.; Trichia, E.; Whitsel, L.P.; Story, M.; Peñalvo, J.L.; Mozaffarian, D. Effectiveness of school food environment policies on children's dietary behaviors: A systematic review and meta-analysis. *PLoS ONE* **2018**, *13*, 1–27. [CrossRef]
25. Ministry of Health and Welfare. *2015 Community Child Centers Support Program Manual*; Ministry of Health and Welfare: Sejong, Korea, 2015; p. 19.
26. Ministry of Health and Welfare; Korea Health Promotion Institute. *Healthy Fruit Basket Program Manual*; Korea Health Promotion Institute: Sejong, Seoul, 2013; p. 9.
27. Aarestrup, J.; Gamborg, M.; Ulrich, L.G.; Sørensen, T.I.A.; Baker, J.L. Childhood body mass index and height and risk of histologic subtypes of endometrial cancer. *Int. J. Obes.* **2016**, *40*, 1096–1102. [CrossRef]
28. Nogueira, L.; Stolzenberg-Solomon, R.; Gamborg, M.; Sørensen, T.I.; Baker, J.L. Childhood Body Mass Index and Risk of Adult Pancreatic Cancer. *Curr. Dev. Nutr.* **2017**, *1*, e001362. [CrossRef]
29. Korea Centers for Disease Control and Prevention; Committee for the Development of Growth Standard for Korean Children and Adolescents; Korean Pediatric Society. *2007 Korean Children and Adolescents Growth Standard (Commentary for the Development of 2007 Growth Chart)*; Korea Centers for Disease Control and Prevention: Cheongju, Korea, 2007; pp. 93–104.
30. Story, M.; Kaphingst, K.M.; Robinson-O'Brien, R.; Glanz, K. Creating Healthy Food and Eating Environments: Policy and Environmental Approaches. *Annu. Rev. Public Health* **2008**, *29*, 253–272. [CrossRef]
31. The Ministry of Health and Welfare; The Korean Nutrition Society. *Dietary Reference Intakes for Koreans 2015*; The Korean Nutrition Society: Sejong, Korea, 2015; pp. 958–959.

32. The Ministry of Health and Welfare; Korea Centers for Disease Control and Prevention. *Korea Health Statistics 2018: Korea National Health and Nutrition Examination Survey (KNHANES VII-3)*; Korea Centers for Disease Control and Prevention: Sejong, Korea, 2020.
33. Pineda, E.; Swinburn, B.; Sassi, F. Effective school food environment interventions for the prevention of childhood obesity: Systematic review and meta-analysis. *Lancet* **2019**, *394*, S77. [CrossRef]
34. Bere, E.; Klepp, K.I.; Øverby, N.C. Free school fruit: Can an extra piece of fruit every school day contribute to the prevention of future weight gain? A cluster randomized trial. *Food Nutr. Res.* **2014**, *58*, 1–5. [CrossRef]
35. Davis, E.M.; Cullen, K.W.; Watson, K.B.; Konarik, M.; Radcliffe, J. A Fresh Fruit and Vegetable Program Improves High School Students' Consumption of Fresh Produce. *J. Am. Diet. Assoc.* **2009**, *109*, 1227–1231. [CrossRef]
36. Ridberg, R.A.; Bell, J.F.; Merritt, K.E.; Harris, D.M.; Young, H.M.; Tancredi, D.J. Effect of a fruit and vegetable prescription program on children's fruit and vegetable consumption. *Prev. Chronic Dis.* **2019**, *16*, 1–13. [CrossRef]
37. Story, M. School-based approaches for preventing and treating obesity. *Int. J. Obes.* **1999**, *23*, S43–S51. [CrossRef]
38. Heredia, N.I.; Ranjit, N.; Warren, J.L.; Evans, A.E. Association of parental social support with energy balance-related behaviors in low-income and ethnically diverse children: A cross-sectional study. *BMC Public Health* **2016**, *16*, 1–12. [CrossRef]
39. Ray, C.; Roos, E.; Brug, J.; Behrendt, I.; Ehrenblad, B.; Yngve, A.; Te Velde, S.J. Role of free school lunch in the associations between family-environmental factors and children's fruit and vegetable intake in four European countries. *Public Health Nutr.* **2013**, *16*, 1109–1117. [CrossRef]
40. Wyse, R.; Campbell, E.; Nathan, N.; Wolfenden, L. Associations between characteristics of the home food environment and fruit and vegetable intake in preschool children: A cross-sectional study. *BMC Public Health* **2011**, *11*, 938. [CrossRef]
41. McMorrow, L.; Ludbrook, A.; Macdiarmid, J.I.; Olajide, D. Perceived barriers towards healthy eating and their association with fruit and vegetable consumption. *J. Public Health* **2017**, *39*, 330–338. [CrossRef]
42. Wyse, R.; Wolfenden, L.; Bisquera, A. Characteristics of the home food environment that mediate immediate and sustained increases in child fruit and vegetable consumption: Mediation analysis from the Healthy Habits cluster randomised controlled trial. *Int. J. Behav. Nutr. Phys. Act.* **2015**, *12*, 1–9. [CrossRef]
43. Pearson, N.; Biddle, S.J.H.; Gorely, T. Family correlates of fruit and vegetable consumption in children and adolescents: A systematic review. *Public Health Nutr.* **2009**, *12*, 267–283. [CrossRef]
44. Yee, A.Z.H.; Lwin, M.O.; Ho, S.S. The influence of parental practices on child promotive and preventive food consumption behaviors: A systematic review and meta-analysis. *Int. J. Behav. Nutr. Phys. Act.* **2017**, *14*, 1–14. [CrossRef]
45. Befort, C.; Kaur, H.; Nollen, N.; Sullivan, D.K.; Nazir, N.; Choi, W.S.; Hornberger, L.; Ahluwalia, J.S. Fruit, vegetable, and fat intake among non-hispanic black and non-hispanic white adolescents: Associations with home availability and food consumption settings. *J. Am. Diet. Assoc.* **2006**, *106*, 367–373. [CrossRef]
46. Spurrier, N.J.; Magarey, A.A.; Golley, R.; Curnow, F.; Sawyer, M.G. Relationships between the home environment and physical activity and dietary patterns of preschool children: A cross-sectional study. *Int. J. Behav. Nutr. Phys. Act.* **2008**, *5*, 1–12. [CrossRef]
47. Goslin, D.A. *Handbook of Socialization Theory and Research*, 4th ed.; Rand McNally: Chicago, IL, USA, 1969; pp. 213–262, ISBN 0528686801.
48. Schmitt, R. The Stages of Moral Development: A Basis for an Educational Concept? *Int. Rev. Educ.* **1980**, *26*, 207–216.
49. de Menezes, M.C.; Diez Roux, A.V.; Souza Lopes, A.C. Fruit and vegetable intake: Influence of perceived food environment and self-efficacy. *Appetite* **2018**, *127*, 249–256. [CrossRef]
50. Wagner, M.G.; Rhee, Y.; Honrath, K.; Blodgett Salafia, E.H.; Terbizan, D. Nutrition education effective in increasing fruit and vegetable consumption among overweight and obese adults. *Appetite* **2016**, *100*, 94–101. [CrossRef]
51. Honrath, K.; Wagner, M.G.; Rhee, Y. Does Nutrition Education with Fruit and Vegetable Supplementation Increase Fruit and Vegetable Intake and Improve Anthropometrics of Overweight or Obese People of Varying Socioeconomic Status? *Ecol. Food Nutr.* **2018**, *57*, 32–49. [CrossRef]

52. Clark, R.L.; Famodu, O.A.; Holásková, I.; Infante, A.M.; Murray, P.J.; Olfert, I.M.; McFadden, J.W.; Downes, M.T.; Chantler, P.D.; Duespohl, M.W.; et al. Educational intervention improves fruit and vegetable intake in young adults with metabolic syndrome components. *Nutr. Res.* **2019**, *62*, 89–100. [CrossRef]
53. Santiago, S.; Zazpe, I.; Martí, A.; Cuervo, M.; Martínez, J.A. Gender differences in lifestyle determinants of overweight prevalence in a sample of Southern European children. *Obes. Res. Clin. Pract.* **2013**, *7*, e391–e400. [CrossRef]
54. Field, A.E.; Gillman, M.W.; Rosner, B.; Rockett, H.R.; Colditz, G.A. Association between fruit and vegetable intake and change in body mass index among a large sample of children and adolescents in the United States. *Int. J. Obes.* **2003**, *27*, 821–826. [CrossRef]
55. Attorp, A.; Scott, J.E.; Yew, A.C.; Rhodes, R.E.; Barr, S.I.; Naylor, P.J. Associations between socioeconomic, parental and home environment factors and fruit and vegetable consumption of children in grades five and six in British Columbia, Canada. *BMC Public Health* **2014**, *14*, 1–9. [CrossRef]

Publisher's Note: MDPI stays neutral with regard to jurisdictional claims in published maps and institutional affiliations.

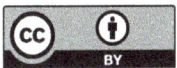 © 2020 by the authors. Licensee MDPI, Basel, Switzerland. This article is an open access article distributed under the terms and conditions of the Creative Commons Attribution (CC BY) license (http://creativecommons.org/licenses/by/4.0/).

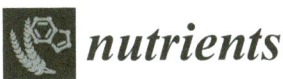

Article

How Minority Parents Could Help Children Develop Healthy Eating Behaviors: Parent and Child Perspectives

Chishinga Callender [1], Denisse Velazquez [1], Meheret Adera [1], Jayna M. Dave [1], Norma Olvera [2], Tzu-An Chen [3], Shana Alford [4] and Debbe Thompson [1,*]

1. USDA/ARS Children's Nutrition Research Center, Department of Pediatrics, Baylor College of Medicine, 1100 Bates Street, Houston, TX 77030, USA; Chishinga.Callender@bcm.edu (C.C.); himedenisse@gmail.com (D.V.); msa8@rice.edu (M.A.); jmdave@bcm.edu (J.M.D.)
2. Psychological, Health, and Learning Sciences Department, University of Houston, 3657 Cullen Boulevard Room 491, Houston, TX 77204, USA; nolvera@central.uh.edu
3. HEALTH Research Institute, University of Houston, 4849 Calhoun Road, Houston, TX 77204, USA; ann0516@gmail.com
4. Common Threads, 222 W. Merchandise Mart Plaza, Suite 1212, Chicago, IL 60654, USA; salford@commonthreads.org
* Correspondence: dit@bcm.edu; Tel.: +1-713-798-7076

Received: 22 October 2020; Accepted: 15 December 2020; Published: 18 December 2020

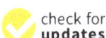

Abstract: Minority children and children living in under-resourced households are at the greatest risk for obesity and diet-related disparities. Identifying effective strategies to reduce these risks is an important step in child obesity prevention. Parents influence the home environment and play a critical role in child obesity prevention. Eighteen parent–child dyads living in under-resourced Houston area communities participated in a mixed methods study (online surveys, telephone interviews). The purpose of the research reported here was to conduct a secondary analysis of the qualitative data to explore Black/African American and Hispanic parent and child perspectives of the ways in which parents could help their children make healthy food choices. Descriptive statistics were calculated for parent and child demographic characteristics; hybrid thematic analysis was used to code and analyze the interview transcripts. Frequencies were calculated for children's interview responses to rating scales and the grade they gave their eating habits. Mothers' responses were grouped into two broad categories: facilitators (modeling, availability, and teaching) as ways parents could help their child eat healthy, and barriers (lack of time, cost of healthy foods, and lack of knowledge) to helping their child eat healthy. Alternatively, child responses focused on ways in which parents could provide support: environmental support (home availability, home cooking, and introducing new foods) and personal support (providing child choice, teaching, and encouragement). Most children reported that eating healthy was easy, and most rated their personal eating habits as an A or B. These findings suggest that understanding the perspectives of Black/African American and Hispanic parent–child dyads can provide insight into the development of culturally and economically relevant healthy eating strategies and interventions for families living in under-resourced communities.

Keywords: minority; parents; children; obesity; prevention; diet; nutrition promotion; Black/African American; Hispanic; qualitative

1. Introduction

The high prevalence of child obesity in the United States is a significant public health issue [1], with the highest prevalence among Black/African American and Hispanic children [2,3] and children living in low-income households [4]. Identifying effective strategies to reduce the risk of child obesity and related disparities is an important step in child obesity prevention [5].

Several factors influence child obesity risk, including diet, physical activity, and sedentary behavior [6,7]. Through excessive caloric intake, diet plays a significant role in obesity risk [6,7]. Several factors influence dietary intake, including the home food environment [8], parenting styles [9], family meals [9], personal food preferences [10], and household income [11]. Furthermore, the diet quality of children in the United States falls below the national dietary recommendations [12].

Similar to obesity-related disparities, diet-related disparities exist, and it is imperative to address them as well. Racial and ethnic minorities (i.e., Black/African American, Hispanic) experience diet-related disparities and tend to have poorer diet quality compared to their white counterparts [13]. In addition, these disparities exist in low-income populations, as poor diet quality is associated with socioeconomic status [14]. For example, a study found that lower-income individuals ate lower-quality foods than their higher-income counterparts [14]. Families living in under-resourced communities are more likely to be exposed to advertising of less healthy foods and beverages [15], have more access to fast food restaurants [16], and less access to stores with affordable healthy foods [17]. Thus, minority, under-resourced families may be at the greatest risk for experiencing diet-related disparities. Understanding how these factors influence child dietary behaviors is essential in developing effective interventions to reduce poor diet quality for children.

Parents exert a strong influence on the home food environment [9,18]. Therefore, they play an important role in child obesity prevention. It is critical for parents to encourage children to engage in healthy dietary behaviors at an early age to reduce children's risk of obesity and related diseases and to help them develop and maintain a healthy lifestyle into adulthood. Previous research identifies the challenges that families living in under-resourced communities experience accessing healthy foods [11,19]. In addition, previous studies have identified parents' perspectives on strategies to promote healthy eating behaviors [20–23]. However, few studies have explored perspectives of racial and ethnic minority parent–child dyads regarding ways parents can help their children practice healthy eating behaviors. The perspectives of parents and children in minority and under-resourced communities are essential for developing effective, culturally appropriate, and acceptable obesity prevention and nutrition promotion interventions. Thus, the purpose of this research was to expand the voices of minority families in the literature by investigating both parent and child perspectives of the ways in which parents can help their children make healthy food choices.

2. Materials and Methods

This is a secondary data analysis of data from a larger, mixed methods study designed to identify thoughts, expectations, and preferences of parents and children toward cooking and nutrition education programs promoting healthy eating. This paper was guided by the following research question: From the perspectives of both parents and children, how can parents help their children make healthy food choices?

2.1. Design

This study re-examined qualitative data from a larger mixed-methods study. The protocol was approved by the institutional review board at Baylor College of Medicine (H-44683).

2.2. Study Participants

Inclusionary criteria for the families included: child 8–13 years old; parent/guardian of a child 8–13 years old; both parent and child fluent in English or Spanish; child receives and/or is eligible for free or reduced price meals at school; healthy (i.e., no physical, health, or medical condition that would affect diet or participation in a telephone interview or focus group); parent and child living in the same household; the parent has primary responsibility for family food shopping/acquisition and/or meals; transportation to focus group (focus group participation only); families also needed to be willing to provide contact information, to participate in study activities, and have focus group/telephone interview audio recorded. Exclusionary criteria included unwillingness to have the telephone interview or focus group recorded and to take photos for the study.

2.3. Recruitment

Families living in under-resourced communities in the Greater Houston, TX metropolitan area were recruited for this study. A more detailed description of the recruitment procedures is reported elsewhere [24]. Briefly, recruitment started in early May 2019 and ended in mid-August 2019. Recruitment methods included contacting potential families from the volunteer database at the USDA/ARS Children's Nutrition Research Center (CNRC) and referrals from recruited families. All families provided written informed consent prior to participation. During the consent process, parents had the option for their family to participate in either separate telephone interviews or focus groups in their preferred language (English or Spanish). All families chose to participate in telephone interviews.

2.4. Data Collection

Data collection for the larger study began in June 2019 and ended in October 2019. In that study, parents and children completed online surveys, took photographs of situations that made it easy or hard to make healthy food choices, and completed telephone interviews. Surveys were available in English and Spanish, and telephone interviews were conducted in participants' preferred language (English or Spanish). Trained research coordinators conducted semi-structured telephone interviews [25]. Interviews were scripted and contained open-ended, non-leading questions; probes and prompts were used to clarify, expand, and understand responses. Separate scripts guided parent and child interviews. This paper reports demographic data, as well as parent and child responses to the following interview questions: "How can parents help their children to eat healthy?" (parents); "How could your parents help you make healthy food choices at home?" (child). To explore children's perspectives related to their personal eating habits, child responses to the following interview questions are also reported: (1) "On a scale of 1 (hard), 2 (not hard or easy), 3 (easy), how easy or hard is it to eat healthy?" (2) "What grade would you give your eating habits (i.e., A, B, C, D, F like in school grades)?" Each interview was digitally recorded, transcribed, and reviewed for accuracy prior to analysis.

2.5. Data Analysis

2.5.1. Surveys

A single dataset was created by combining the English and Spanish language surveys. Parent and child data were analyzed separately. Descriptive statistics (frequencies, percentages) were calculated for demographic and household characteristics.

2.5.2. Interviews

Two independent coders used hybrid thematic analysis to code and analyze verbatim transcripts [26]. Transcripts were reviewed for accuracy prior to analysis. To provide structure to the coding process, transcripts were initially coded using a priori codes guided by the research question. Emergent codes were generated as transcripts that were reviewed and coded to provide flexibility to the coding process and ensure that parent and child perspectives were fully captured. After coding was complete, the codes were reviewed for relevance to the research question. During this process, some codes were dropped, and others were grouped into categories based on their similarities. Then, categories were reviewed and grouped into higher-order categories as appropriate. Analysis was conducted on English language transcripts (i.e., English language transcripts and translated Spanish language transcripts). Separate parent and child codebooks were maintained and routinely updated to reflect new emergent codes, definitions, and key decisions. Frequencies were calculated for children's responses to rating scales and the grade they gave their eating habits. Their reasons for selecting a rating or grade were used to expand the findings and provide additional insight.

Verbatim quotes, used to support qualitative findings, were labeled as follows: P = Parent; C = child; A = Black/African American; H = Hispanic. To help differentiate the quotes, a number (from 1–18) was assigned to each parent/child dyad.

3. Results

3.1. Family Characteristics

Eighteen parent–child dyads enrolled in the study. All participating parents were mothers (100%), mostly 40–49 years old (61%), Black/African American (56%), Hispanic (44%), and married/living with significant other (61%). Over half of the children were female (56%) and Black/African American (56%). Half of the children's ethnicity (50%) was reported as Hispanic by the mothers. The ages of children participating included 8–10 years old (22%) and 11–13 years old (78%).

The highest level of household education varied, with 33% of families having less than a college education, 33% having some college coursework, 22% having a college degree, and 11% having a postgraduate degree. Annual household income for the majority of families (66%) was below $41,000. To add context, 39% of mothers reported two adults in the household, and 50% reported having two children under the age of 18 living in the household. Although the majority of mothers reported high/marginal food security (89%), more than half reported using one to three food assistance programs (67%). The majority of families (61%) spoke mostly English at home. All families recruited for the study met the inclusionary criteria.

3.2. Interview Findings

Interviews ranged from an average of 43 min (children) to 56 min (mothers). As previously stated, the a priori codes were generated from the research question prior to coding. Then, emergent codes were added throughout coding based on parents and children responses. After coding all transcripts, the emergent codes were reviewed, collapsed, and grouped into categories. Parents' responses were grouped into two categories: facilitators (what made it easy to help their child make healthy food choices) and barriers (what made it difficult to help their child make healthy food choices). Children's responses were also grouped into two categories: environmental support (how parents create healthy eating choices at home) and personal support (how parents actively influence the child to eat healthy). The categories are presented in Figure 1 (parent) and Figure 2 (child).

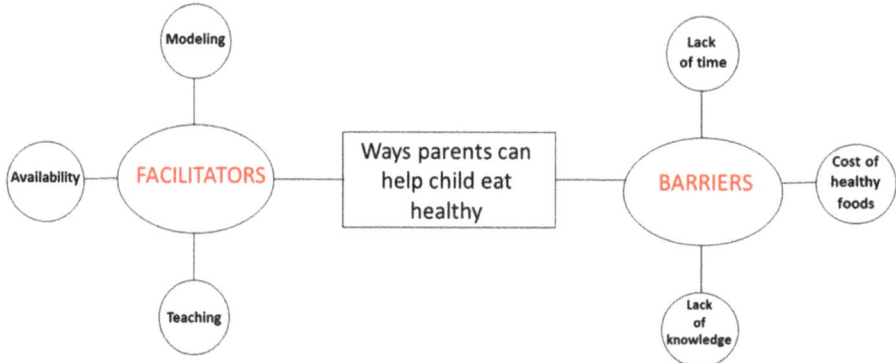

Figure 1. Visual representation of mothers' perspectives on ways parents can help their children eat healthy. (Note: Red font indicates the categories. Bold black font indicates the supporting categories that emerged.)

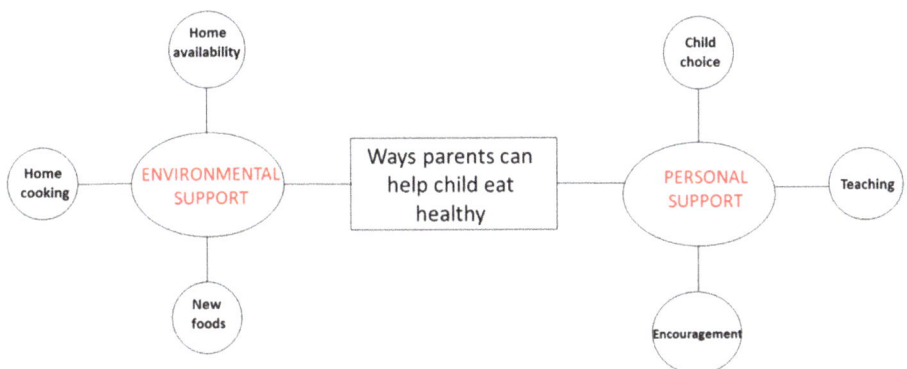

Figure 2. Visual representation of children's perspectives on ways parents can help their children eat healthy. (Note: Red font indicates the categories. Bold black font indicates the supporting categories that emerged.)

3.2.1. Parents

When parents were asked, "How can parents help their child eat healthy?" two main categories emerged: facilitators and barriers to helping their child eat healthy (Figure 1). Each is described in more detail below in order of prevalence and presented in Table 1.

Table 1. Categories and subcategories from qualitative data analysis of interviews with parents on ways parents can help their children eat healthy.

Categories	Subcategories	Definitions
Facilitators	• Modeling • Availability • Teaching	• Modeling healthy eating behaviors • Having healthy foods easily available • Teaching healthy eating behaviors
Barriers	• Lack of time • Cost of healthy foods • Lack of knowledge	• Lack of time to prepare or serve healthy foods • High cost of healthy foods • Lack of knowledge about healthy eating and cooking

Facilitators. Three ways parents could help their children make healthy food choices were mentioned: (1) modeling healthy eating behaviors, (2) having healthy foods easily available for the child (availability), and (3) teaching the child about healthy eating. Several mothers shared that modeling healthy eating is beneficial to a child: *"By eating healthy themselves. Kids follow what we do. And if they see a parent eating healthy, they are more likely to follow in their parent's footsteps"* (P.15A). Mothers shared examples of ways to make healthy foods easily available for their children. One mother mentioned, *"I think that ... the healthy way depends on what kind of food. Because I try to use those tricks in the soup so that they eat it. So that they can eat healthier. And with fruit, I try to keep as many containers full of fruit as possible, so that they don't have to wash them, so that they can see it [as] appetizing there, in the refrigerator"* (P.6H). A few mothers shared their perspective about teaching healthy eating habits to their children. For example, one mother taught her children about the benefits of healthy eating: *"By explaining to them that our food is our medicine, and our medicine has to be our food, because we are what we eat. By showing them the effects that diseases caused by unhealthy food have on different people"* (P.17H). Another mother shared teaching children about preparing healthy foods: *"I think that as a parent, we help them package up food portions, be it in Ziploc bags or in Tupperware, teaching them how to divide up food and have it prepared for when they come back from school, or some sport, grab it and eat"* (P.18H).

Barriers. Parents mentioned three types of barriers to helping children eat healthy: (1) lack of time, (2) cost of healthy foods, and (3) parent's lack of knowledge about healthy eating and cooking. Lack of time to prepare or serve healthy foods was noted as a barrier by several mothers. For example, one mother shared how time affects working mothers: *"Sometimes, you know, when the mother works or both parents work, especially the mother, there is no time to prepare, like, maybe healthy food. So, maybe, you know, 'cause you need to cook or to grill or whatever. So the things that are not healthy in a can or fast food that you buy, you know, it's easier, so the family ends up eating unhealthy because their mother would be tired and all that. But I think time really plays a role, especially if the mother is working"* (P.2A). However, stay-at-home mothers did not see lack of time as a barrier: *"Time? No, not right now because the children are on vacation. I'm here with them, I don't work. So, of course I can go to the store to buy the ingredients or whatever I need. No, time is no obstacle"* (P.12H).

The high cost of healthy foods was also seen as a barrier for some mothers: *"Economics. If a parent feels as though they don't have the money for the healthy food, they're likely to buy what's cheap"* (P.15A). One mother shared her personal experience with household finances impacting eating choices for her family: *"Yes, one of the first obstacles is that sometimes... The day you don't eat healthy at home is for lack of... it's because our budget is really low. But, we try to do the best we can"* (P.3H).

Knowledge also emerged as a barrier to helping children make healthy food choices. For example, one mother shared how lack of knowledge of *" ... how to cook [or] prepare ... food"* was a barrier to helping children eat healthy (P.11A). Another shared how some parents are not knowledgeable about healthy ingredient substitutions for meals they enjoy cooking: *"And they may not know that you can cook the foods you love but you don't have to use—you can use different ingredients to get the flavor and the taste you want"* (P.1A).

3.2.2. Children

When children were asked, "How could your parents help you make healthy food choices at home?" two main categories emerged: environmental and personal support by parents (Figure 2). Each is described in more detail below in order of prevalence and presented in Table 2.

Table 2. Categories and subcategories from coding of interviews with children on ways parents can help their children eat healthy.

Categories	Subcategories	Definitions
Environmental Support	• Home availability • Home cooking • New foods	• Healthy foods easily available at home • Cooking foods at home • Introduction to new or different foods
Personal Support	• Child choice • Teaching • Encouragement	• Giving child the opportunity to choose foods, preparation methods, and meals • Teaching healthy eating behaviors • Encouraging child to practice healthy eating behaviors

Environmental support. Three ways parents could encourage a child's healthy eating choices in the home environment were mentioned by children: (1) home availability (i.e., healthy foods easily available at home), (2) home cooking, and (3) introducing new foods. Several children suggested that their parents could make healthy foods more available. For example, one child shared, *"Maybe by like buying more healthier food like more fruits and vegetables"* (C.15A). Another child shared how their mother makes healthy foods available at home: *"Well, she would help me by like at home, we would find things in the house that would be healthy. Like, fruit in yogurt and stuff. Sometimes, we'll make, like, smoothies, like, but they would have, like, lots of vegetables. Well, like, vegetables and things inside. Plus, we have a lot of vegetable things we cook with"* (C.16A).

For home cooking, children also noted that preparing foods in a healthy way would be helpful: *"Or maybe when we cook not putting as much grease and butter and unhealthy foods like that"* (C.15A). Some children also suggested including more vegetables in meals. For example, one child shared, *" . . . my mom and my dad could help me in the kitchen with different types of vegetables and different types of protein, things that I need"* (C.8A).

Introduction to new or different foods was also suggested by children: *"And—but I think to help us more she could, like, start influencing us by giving us more creative things and different foods that sometimes we've never tried. Because if you keep eating the same thing over and over, even though it's healthy, it might get boring and you don't want to eat it anymore"* (C.10H). Children shared examples of how their parents introduced new foods, including through sharing new recipes, watching their mothers cook, and cooking foods from different cultures. For example, one child shared her experience with cultural foods: *"Mainly, my mom influences me to try new food because since she's, like, from . . . she's from Mexico, she, like, influenced me to try a lot of new foods from other places"* (C.10H). It is worth noting that a majority of children identified their mothers as an influence to try new foods.

Personal support. Children mentioned three types of personal support parents could use to help children eat healthy: (1) giving the child choice, (2) teaching, and (3) providing encouragement. Giving the child choice (i.e., opportunities to choose foods, preparation methods, and meals) was recommended by a few children. For example, one child shared how parents could ask questions about making healthy food choices: *"I think if they asked more about what type of food we want to eat that is healthy"* (C.2H). A few children expressed interest in making choices at the grocery store: *"Going with her to the grocery store to pick out the vegetables and fruits I want"* (C.7H).

For teaching, a child was interested in her mother teaching her to cook healthy: *"My mom could teach me how to cook healthier meals so that way when I [get] hungry I could just cook that and I would be able to eat healthy"* (C.13A). A few children shared that their mothers taught them about cooking through showing them: *"Mom teaches us how she does things. And then my mom does it"* (C.12H). For encouragement, one child shared how his mother encouraged him to make healthy snack choices: *"Well, sometimes . . . because most of the time, I like to walk to the store and buy chips, but my mom told me that I shouldn't be walking to the store and getting chips because chips are unhealthy, so she just doesn't give me the money. She says if you go to the store you better come back with some fruit cups or something."* A child also shared how her mother encouraged her to make healthy choices at restaurants: *"So when we go places, like, for example Chick-fil-A and all that stuff that has a lot of grease, she encourages me to try, like, salads and stuff"* (C.16A). Simple words of encouragement with reasoning were also noted as helping a child with eating healthy: *"She says you won't know if you won't taste it"* (C.11A).

3.2.3. Children's Perspectives on Making Healthy Dietary Choices

Ease and Difficulty of Healthy Eating

When children were asked, "on a scale of 1 (hard), 2 (not hard or easy), 3 (easy), how easy or hard is it to eat healthy," the following ratings were reported: rating of 1 ($n = 3$), rating of 2 ($n = 5$), and rating of 3 ($n = 10$). Reasons for choosing the ratings varied. For example, one child who gave a rating of 1 noted eating habits as a reason healthy eating was difficult for the general population: *"Well, I think it's hard to eat healthy because some people might be so used to eating unhealthy that they'll just like they're are going to keep eating unhealthy. But they might eat something healthy not very often, but they'll probably eat it every once in a while"* (C.1A). Children shared a variety of reasons for choosing a rating of 2. A child mentioned how temptation can influence eating healthy: *"Because it's not hard to eat healthy, but it's not also easy to eat healthy. Because if it's easy to eat healthy but if you see stuff that's unhealthy and it looks good or smells good, you might want it"* (C.9A). Another shared how types of foods can influence eating choices: *"I chose two because it can be easy sometimes but not always is, but it's not hard either. It depends on the food I'm eating and the taste"* (C.14H).

Children also shared a variety of reasons for choosing a rating of 3. A few children noted parental and/or family influences on their eating choices. For example, one child shared how the entire family encourages healthy eating: *"Because in my household, my family, like my sisters, especially my older sister, my dad, my mom, they really, like, encourage us to eat foods that don't contain things that are bad for your body and healthy things"* (C.10H). Another child shared that her mother *"buys fruits and vegetables"* (C.4A). Some children also noted their eating habits as a reason for choosing a rating of 3: *"Because I like eating lots of apples and salads so it's much easier to do that"* (C.11A) and *"Because I normally eat healthy"* (C.13A). The benefits of healthy eating were also mentioned as a reason: *"Three cause it doesn't really matter really what you eat, you have to have a lot of—I mean, not a lot, less calories and you have to have a lot of vegetables and stuff like lettuce, carrots, tomatoes, a lot of things that will help your body"* (C.16A).

Personal Eating Habits Assessment

When children were asked, "What grade would you give your eating habits?" they reported the following grades: A ($n = 3$), B ($n = 10$), C ($n = 2$), and D ($n = 2$). Reasons varied for choosing the grades. For example, a child who reported an A for their eating habits mentioned his mother's cooking: *"'Cause most of the things I eat, my mom cooks and she cooks a lot with a lot of vegetables and stuff so to help be healthy"* (C.16A). Similarly, a child with an "A" grade mentioned eating healthy foods at home and school: *"At school, the food is very healthy. They give us balanced meals, but sometimes the taste just isn't so great. Sometimes it's a bit hard to eat. And at home it's an A, because most of the time, almost all the time it's very healthy and the taste is good so it's easier to eat"* (C.14H). Another described their favorite types of foods, while also noting fruit purchases made by his mother as the reason for reporting an A.

Several children who reported a "B" or "C" grade for their eating habits mentioned mixed eating habits (i.e., eating healthy and unhealthy foods) as a reason. One child shared the following: *"Because I don't, like, all the time it won't always be healthy food but sometimes it's healthy food. And then sometimes I do have sweets now and then"* (C.8A). One child noted differences in foods eaten in the home and school environment as a reason for a "B" grade: *"Because I eat great at home, but at school not that well"* (C.17H). Interestingly, one child compared their eating habits to their friends as the reason for a "B" grade: *" . . . because I'm not that healthy that I over overpass everything. But I do consider myself eating healthier than a lot of my friends"* (C.10H). Both children who reported a "D" grade shared a lack of vegetable consumption as the reason.

4. Discussion

The purpose of this research was to investigate the perspectives of minority parents and children on the ways in which parents could help their children make healthy eating choices. Although a few studies [27,28] have presented interview findings from parent–child dyads regarding healthy eating, this study is unique in that it highlights both parent and child perspectives of the ways parents could help their children eat healthy. This study is also distinctive as it presents interview findings from children about the ease and difficulty of eating healthy and an assessment of their personal eating habits.

For mothers in this sample, modeling, availability, and teaching served as the main facilitators for parents to help children practice healthy eating behaviors. Similar to our research, parental roles of modeling healthy eating behaviors [29,30], making healthy foods available [8,29], and teaching about healthy eating [29] have been reported by parents in other studies. Previous studies have also found that availability of healthy foods [8,31] in the home and modeling [31] have been associated with child's diet quality. Contrary to previous research, child's weight was not mentioned as a motivation to encourage healthy eating behaviors in children [27]. These findings suggest that interventions promoting healthy eating behaviors for minority children living in under-resourced communities should promote strategies such as modeling, making healthy foods available at home, and teaching children how to eat and cook healthy, while avoiding an emphasis on child's body weight.

For mothers in this sample, lack of time, cost of healthy foods, and lack of knowledge were highlighted as barriers to helping children practice healthy eating behaviors. Lack of time to prepare healthy meals [27,30,32–34] is consistently reported by parents as a barrier to healthy eating. This could be due to parents from under-resourced families working long hours and/or having multiple jobs [32]. However, a few mothers in our study did not report a lack of time as a barrier due to their role as stay-at-home mothers. Similar to mothers in our study, parents from previous studies, including those with limited income, also identified the cost of healthy foods as a barrier and also believed that healthy eating is expensive [21,27,30,32–34]. Lack of knowledge was also reported as a barrier by parents with limited income [32] and minority families [27]. These findings highlight the need for developing parent-focused interventions for minority and under-resourced communities with a focus on teaching time management strategies for preparing healthy meals, providing affordable options for purchasing healthy foods (e.g., purchasing fresh fruits and vegetables in season), and promoting nutrition and cooking skills knowledge.

Children reported that home availability, home cooking, and new foods were environmental support factors to be practiced by parents to help children eat healthy. Home availability [35], home cooking [36], and willingness to try new foods [37] were reported by children in other studies as ways in which parents helped them make healthy eating choices. In our study, both mothers and children reported that home availability of healthy foods can support the creation of a healthy home food environment. The availability of healthy foods is consistently supported in the literature as an agent for changing children's dietary behaviors [9,29]. In addition to availability, it is imperative that nutrition education/promotion interventions are inclusive of strategies on home cooking (e.g., healthful preparation methods, cooking with the child) and how to introduce new foods.

Children also reported that giving the child choice, teaching, and encouragement were personal support factors to helping children eat healthy. These factors were found to be similar to concepts in previous research, including instrumental and emotional social support for healthful eating from the parent's perspective [38] and positive parental parenting (i.e., feeding practices) [39]. Comparable to our study, middle school aged children in the northeastern United States noted that their food choices were influenced by their parent's guidance [40]. Interestingly, child choice was seen differently by children in Spain, as they did not have a choice in how the foods were prepared, but they were given an option for the amount and type of foods eaten [37]. Similar to our study, children noted that parents shared advice on fruit and vegetable consumption and encouraged them to eat foods prepared at home instead of foods prepared outside of the home [36].

Furthermore, similar to our study, teaching and encouragement were identified as active guidance in five research studies, and a positive relationship was found with vegetable consumption in one study [29]. In our study, the environmental and personal support factors were primarily influenced by mothers. The literature consistently supports mothers influencing the eating behaviors of their children [9]. It is important to note that both children and mothers mentioned teaching as a way parents can help their children eat healthy. Future research should explore the role of fathers in the environmental and personal support factors for children's dietary behaviors. Based on the above findings, intervention programs should include strategies for parents on ways to offer choices in healthy foods, teaching about them (e.g., types of healthy foods, benefits of healthy eating), and encouraging their child to eat them.

Our study highlighted another contribution to the literature: children's perspectives on the ease and difficulty of eating healthy. A variety of reasons (i.e., eating habits, benefits of healthy eating, and temptations) were mentioned in considering healthy eating choices. It is critical to note that a few of the children's responses reflected parental influences (i.e., maternal encouragement and purchasing of fruits and vegetables). Children's perspectives on their personal eating habits also contribute to the literature. A majority of the children rated their eating habits highly, while only a few rated their eating habits below a B. Similar to reasons for the ease and difficulty of eating healthy, children noted parental influences (i.e., home cooking, mother purchasing fruits) attributing to their eating choices. Comparable to our study, children in England shared parental influences on their eating choices [41]. Food choices at school, mixed eating habits, and a lack of vegetable consumption were also mentioned as reasons for the personal eating habits grade. Further investigation is needed into children's perspectives on their personal eating habits. Although parents believed that they needed to make ample effort to help their children eat healthy, children simply wanted environmental modifications (e.g., having healthy foods available, home cooked meals, introduction of new foods) and personal support from parents (e.g., the freedom to make their own food choices, lessons on healthy eating, healthy eating encouragement). This suggests that future interventions to encourage healthy eating among minority children and children living in under-resourced communities should focus on encouraging these types of changes.

The strengths of this study included semi-structured interviews and interviewers trained in qualitative methods. One limitation included the differences in mothers' responses to the interview question; there was a lack of clarity in whether mothers were speaking of their personal experiences or their beliefs about the experiences of other parents. A second limitation included children's responses to the interview questions on the ease and difficulty of healthy eating; the data did not lend itself to hybrid thematic analysis. Despite the limitations, the findings provide an opportunity to identify parent and child perspectives of the ways in which parents can help their children make healthy dietary choices.

5. Conclusions

Insights from minority parents and children are critical to the development of effective child obesity prevention and nutrition education programs for families living in under-resourced communities.

Strategies centered on environmental and personal support are needed for parents to help their children develop and practice healthy eating behaviors. It is important that child nutrition promotion strategies tailor to the perspectives of families with the priority of reducing diet-related disparities among racial/ethnic minorities and under-resourced communities.

Author Contributions: Conceptualization, C.C. and D.T.; methodology, D.T., J.M.D., N.O., and C.C.; validation, C.C. and D.T.; formal analysis, T.-A.C., C.C., and D.T.; investigation, C.C., D.V., and M.A.; data curation, C.C.; writing—original draft preparation, C.C.; writing—review and editing, C.C., D.T., M.A., D.V., J.M.D., N.O., T.-A.C., and S.A.; visualization, C.C.; supervision, D.T.; project administration, S.A.; funding acquisition, D.T. All authors have read and agreed to the published version of the manuscript.

Funding: This project was supported by funding from Common Threads (to Thompson). This work is also a publication of the United States Department of Agriculture, Agricultural Research Service (USDA/ARS), Children's Nutrition Research Center, Department of Pediatrics, Baylor College of Medicine, Houston, Texas, and funded in part with federal funds from the USDA/ARS under Cooperative Agreement No. 58-3092-5-001. The contents of this publication do not necessarily reflect the views or policies of the USDA, nor does mention of trade names, commercial products, or organizations imply endorsement from the U.S. government.

Acknowledgments: We would like to thank the families who participated in this research.

Conflicts of Interest: The authors declare no conflict of interest.

References

1. Fryar, C.D.; Carroll, M.D.; Ogden, C.L. Prevalence of Overweight, Obesity, and Severe Obesity among Children and Adolescents Aged 2–19 Years: United States, 1963–1965 through 2015. Available online: https://www.cdc.gov/nchs/data/hestat/obesity_child_15_16/obesity_child_15_16.htm (accessed on 29 June 2020).
2. Mejia de Grubb, M.C.; Levine, R.S.; Zoorob, R.J. Diet and obesity issues in the underserved. *Prim. Care* **2017**, *44*, 127–140. [CrossRef] [PubMed]
3. Hales, C.M.; Carroll, M.D.; Fryar, C.D.; Ogden, C.L. Prevalence of obesity among adults and youth: United States 2011–2014. *NCHS Data Brief.* **2017**, *2017*, 1–8.
4. Ogden, C.L.; Carroll, M.D.; Fakhouri, T.H.; Hales, C.M.; Fryar, C.D.; Li, X.; Freedman, D.S. Prevalence of obesity among youths by household income and education level of head of household—United States 2011–2014. *MMWR Morb. Mortal. Wkly. Rep.* **2018**, *67*, 186–189. [CrossRef] [PubMed]

5. U.S. Department of Health and Human Services. Healthy People. Available online: https://www.healthypeople.gov/ (accessed on 29 June 2020).
6. Wilfley, D.E.; Saelens, B. Epidemiology and causes of obesity in children. In *Eating Disorders and Obesity: A Comprehensive Handbook*, 2nd ed.; Fairburn, C.G., Brownell, K.D., Eds.; The Guildford Press: New York, NY, USA, 2002; pp. 429–432.
7. Kumar, S.; Kaufman, T. Childhood obesity. *Panminerva Med.* **2018**, *60*, 200–212. [CrossRef] [PubMed]
8. Santiago-Torres, M.; Adams, A.K.; Carrel, A.L.; LaRowe, T.L.; Schoeller, D.A. Home food availability, parental dietary intake, and familial eating habits influence the diet quality of urban Hispanic children. *Child. Obes.* **2014**, *10*, 408–415. [CrossRef] [PubMed]
9. Scaglioni, S.; De Cosmi, V.; Ciappolino, V.; Parazzini, F.; Brambilla, P.; Agostoni, C. Factors influencing children's eating behaviours. *Nutrients* **2018**, *10*, 706. [CrossRef] [PubMed]
10. Beckerman, J.P.; Alike, Q.; Lovin, E.; Tamez, M.; Mattei, J. The development and public health implications of food preferences in children. *Front. Nutr.* **2017**, *4*, 66. [CrossRef]
11. French, S.A.; Tangney, C.C.; Crane, M.M.; Wang, Y.; Appelhans, B.M. Nutrition quality of food purchases varies by household income: The SHoPPER study. *BMC Public Health* **2019**, *19*, 231. [CrossRef]
12. Banfield, E.C.; Liu, Y.; Davis, J.S.; Chang, S.; Frazier-Wood, A.C. Poor adherence to US dietary guidelines for children and adolescents in the National Health and Nutrition Examination Survey population. *J. Acad Nutr. Diet.* **2016**, *116*, 21–27. [CrossRef]
13. Satia, J.A. Diet-related disparities: Understanding the problem and accelerating solutions. *J. Am. Diet. Assoc.* **2009**, *109*, 610–615. [CrossRef]
14. Block, J.P.; Subramanian, S.V. Moving beyond "food deserts": Reorienting United States policies to reduce disparities in diet quality. *PLoS Med.* **2015**, *12*, e1001914. [CrossRef] [PubMed]
15. Lucan, S.C.; Maroko, A.R.; Sanon, O.C.; Schechter, C.B. Unhealthful food-and-beverage advertising in subway stations: Targeted marketing, vulnerable groups, dietary intake, and poor health. *J. Urban. Health* **2017**, *94*, 220–232. [CrossRef] [PubMed]
16. Fleischhacker, S.E.; Evenson, K.R.; Rodriguez, D.A.; Ammerman, A.S. A systematic review of fast food access studies. *Obes. Rev.* **2011**, *12*, e460–e471. [CrossRef] [PubMed]
17. Hager, E.R.; Cockerham, A.; O'Reilly, N.; Harrington, D.; Harding, J.; Hurley, K.M.; Black, M.M. Food swamps and food deserts in Baltimore City, MD, USA: Associations with dietary behaviours among urban adolescent girls. *Public Health Nutr.* **2017**, *20*, 2598–2607. [CrossRef]
18. Gruber, K.J.; Haldeman, L.A. Using the family to combat childhood and adult obesity. *Prev. Chronic Dis.* **2009**, *6*, A106.
19. Laraia, B.A.; Leak, T.M.; Tester, J.M.; Leung, C.W. Biobehavioral factors that shape nutrition in low-income populations: A narrative review. *Am. J. Prev. Med.* **2017**, *52*, S118–S126. [CrossRef]
20. Evans, A.; Chow, S.; Jennings, R.; Dave, J.; Scoblick, K.; Sterba, K.R.; Loyo, J. Traditional foods and practices of Spanish-speaking Latina mothers influence the home food environment: Implications for future interventions. *J. Am. Diet. Assoc.* **2011**, *111*, 1031–1038. [CrossRef]
21. Nepper, M.J.; Chai, W. Parents' barriers and strategies to promote healthy eating among school-age children. *Appetite* **2016**, *103*, 15–64. [CrossRef]
22. Parks, E.P.; Kazak, A.; Kumanyika, S.; Lewis, L.; Barg, F.K. Perspectives on stress, parenting, and children's obesity-related behaviors in Black families. *Health Educ. Behav.* **2016**, *43*, 632–640. [CrossRef]
23. Taverno Ross, S.E.; Macia, L.; Documét, P.I.; Escribano, C.; Kazemi Naderi, T.; Smith-Tapia, I. Latino parents' perceptions of physical activity and healthy eating: At the intersection of culture, family, and health. *J. Nutr. Educ. Behav.* **2018**, *50*, 968–976. [CrossRef]
24. Thompson, D.; Callender, C.; Velazquez, D.; Gonzalez, A.; Adera, M.; Li, P.; Mackey, G.; Dave, J.M.; Olvera, N.; Chen, T.A.; et al. *Common Threads Grant—Final Report*; Baylor College of Medicine: Houston, TX, USA, 2020; unpublished work.
25. Jamshed, S. Qualitative research method-interviewing and observation. *J. Basic Clin. Pharm.* **2014**, *5*, 87–88. [CrossRef] [PubMed]
26. Fereday, J.; Muir-Cochrane, E. Demonstrating rigor using thematic analysis: A hybrid approach of inductive and deductive coding and theme development. *Int. J. Qual. Methods* **2006**, *5*, 80–92. [CrossRef]
27. Lilo, E.A.; Muñoz, M.; Cruz, T.H. Perceptions of healthy eating among Hispanic parent-child dyads. *Health Promot. Pract.* **2019**, *20*, 231–238. [CrossRef] [PubMed]

28. Danford, C.A.; Martyn, K.K. Exploring eating and activity behaviors with parent-child dyads using event history calendars. *J. Fam. Nurs.* **2013**, *19*, 375–398. [CrossRef] [PubMed]
29. Yee, A.Z.; Lwin, M.O.; Ho, S.S. The influence of parental practices on child promotive and preventive food consumption behaviors: A systematic review and meta-analysis. *Int. J. Behav. Nutr. Phys. Act.* **2017**, *14*, 47. [CrossRef] [PubMed]
30. van der Velde, L.A.; Schuilenburg, L.A.; Thrivikraman, J.K.; Numans, M.E.; Kiefte-de Jong, J.C. Needs and perceptions regarding healthy eating among people at risk of food insecurity: A qualitative analysis. *Int. J. Equity Health* **2019**, *18*, 184. [CrossRef]
31. Couch, S.C.; Glanz, K.; Zhou, C.; Sallis, J.F.; Saelens, B.E. Home food environment in relation to children's diet quality and weight status. *J. Acad. Nutr. Diet.* **2014**, *114*, 1569–1579.e1. [CrossRef]
32. Dave, J.M.; Thompson, D.I.; Svendsen-Sanchez, A.; Cullen, K.W. Perspectives on barriers to eating healthy among food pantry clients. *Health Equity* **2017**, *1*, 28–34. [CrossRef]
33. Oates, G.R.; Phillips, J.M.; Bateman, L.B.; Baskin, M.L.; Fouad, M.N.; Scarinci, I.C. Determinants of obesity in two urban communities: Perceptions and community-driven solutions. *Ethn. Dis.* **2018**, *28*, 33–42. [CrossRef]
34. Callender, C.; Thompson, D. Text messaging based obesity prevention program for parents of pre-adolescent African American girls. *Children* **2017**, *4*, 105. [CrossRef]
35. St. George, S.M.; Wilson, D.K. A qualitative study for understanding family and peer influences on obesity-related health behaviors in low-income African-American adolescents. *Child. Obes.* **2012**, *8*, 466–476. [CrossRef] [PubMed]
36. Banna, J.C.; Buchthal, O.V.; Delormier, T.; Creed-Kanashiro, H.M.; Penny, M.E. Influences on eating: A qualitative study of adolescents in a periurban area in Lima, Peru. *BMC Public Health* **2016**, *16*, 40. [CrossRef] [PubMed]
37. Lopez-Dicastillo, O.; Grande, G.; Callery, P. School children's own views, roles and contribution to choices regarding diet and activity in Spain. *Child. Care Health Dev.* **2013**, *39*, 109–117. [CrossRef] [PubMed]
38. Dave, J.M.; Evans, A.E.; Condrasky, M.D.; Williams, J.E. Parent-reported social support for child's fruit and vegetable intake: Validity of measures. *J. Nutr. Educ. Behav.* **2012**, *44*, 132–139. [CrossRef] [PubMed]
39. Haines, J.; Haycraft, E.; Lytle, L.M.; Nicklaus, S.; Kok, F.; Merdji, M.; Fisberg, M.; Moreno, L.A.; Goulet, O.J.; Hughes, S.O. Nurturing children's healthy eating: Position statement. *Appetite* **2019**, *137*, 124–133. [CrossRef] [PubMed]
40. Holsten, J.E.; Deatrick, J.A.; Kumanyika, S.; Pinto-Martin, J.; Compher, C.W. Children's food choice process in the home environment. A qualitative descriptive study. *Appetite* **2012**, *58*, 64–73. [CrossRef]
41. Pearce, A.; Kirk, C.; Cummins, S.; Collins, M.; Elliman, D.; Connolly, A.; Law, C. Gaining children's perspectives: A multiple method approach to explore environmental influences on healthy eating and physical activity. *Health Place* **2009**, *15*, 614–621. [CrossRef]

Publisher's Note: MDPI stays neutral with regard to jurisdictional claims in published maps and institutional affiliations.

© 2020 by the authors. Licensee MDPI, Basel, Switzerland. This article is an open access article distributed under the terms and conditions of the Creative Commons Attribution (CC BY) license (http://creativecommons.org/licenses/by/4.0/).

Article

Development of RisObIn.Com, a Screening Tool for Risk of Childhood Obesity in the Community

Ana Catarina Moreira [1,2,*], Patrícia Almeida Oliveira [1,3], Rute Borrego [1], Telma Nogueira [4,5], Raquel Ferreira [1,6] and Daniel Virella [7]

1. Escola Superior de Tecnologia da Saúde de Lisboa, Instituto Politécnico de Lisboa, 1990-096 Lisboa, Portugal; patricia.aao@gmail.com (P.A.O.); rute.borrego@estesl.ipl.pt (R.B.); raquel.ferreira@cm-sintra.pt (R.F.)
2. H &TRC—Health & Technology Research Center, 1990-096 Lisboa, Portugal
3. Faculdade de Medicina, Universidade de Lisboa, 1649-004 Lisboa, Portugal
4. Laboratório de Nutrição, Faculdade de Medicina, Universidade de Lisboa, 1649-028 Lisboa, Portugal; telmanogueira@medicina.ulisboa.pt
5. Instituto de Saúde Ambiental, Faculdade de Medicina, Universidade de Lisboa, 1649-028 Lisboa, Portugal
6. Núcleo de Educação e Qualidade Alimentar, Câmara Municipal de Sintra, 2710-307 Sintra, Portugal
7. Research Unit, Centro Hospitalar Universitário Lisboa Central, 1150-199 Lisboa, Portugal; danielvirella@chlc.min-saude.pt
* Correspondence: ana.moreira@estesl.ipl.pt

Received: 28 September 2020; Accepted: 23 October 2020; Published: 27 October 2020

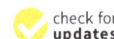

Abstract: The prevalence of childhood overweight has increased considerably in the past three decades and there is evidence that childhood obesity can persist into adulthood. A simple tool to identify relevant risk factors may alert families and prevent overweight and obesity. This study aims to develop a pre-school screening tool to assess the risk of childhood obesity. Child anthropometric measurements and several risk factors for childhood obesity factors were obtained. The effect of the variables on the outcome of obesity (defined as increased anthropometry-estimated adiposity) was assessed by binary logistic regression analyses. The identified variables were submitted for expert panel validation and combined for the tool development. A total of 304 children were included. Eight items were included in the tool. A higher score of the tool indicates a greater risk for obesity in childhood with the cutoff point set at 0. The tool sensitivity for obesity was 95%, specificity was 74.4%, the positive predictive value was 37.3%, and negative predictive value was 98.9%. The Risk of childhood Obesity In the Community (RisObIn.Com) tool is proposed to be a comprehensive tool to identify children at high risk for late childhood obesity at admission to primary school. Further studies are needed to assess the performance of the tool.

Keywords: childhood overweight; children; risk; community; screening; tool

1. Introduction

The prevalence of childhood overweight and obesity has increased considerably in the past decades, mostly in high-income countries but recently also rising in low- and middle-income countries. Although in high-income countries, a recent decrease has been observed [1], prevalence remains very high [2,3]. Obesity is defined as an abnormal fat accumulation that impairs health [4] but it has been shown that obesity defined by Body Mass Index (BMI) alone is a remarkably heterogeneous condition with varying cardiovascular and metabolic manifestations across individuals, which may differ according to age and gender [5]. This is a chronic disease that increases heavily the burden on citizens, health care systems, productivity, cities, and society and should be considered a top priority and main target to combat the increasing non-communicable diseases epidemic [6]. There is evidence that childhood obesity can persist into adulthood [7], lead to physical obesity-related complications, and affect psychological health and social and emotional well-being [8]. This emphasizes the importance of early intervention to prevent the onset of obesity in childhood. A comprehensive and proactive strategy to deal with the challenges imposed by the obesity epidemic is needed and requires the development and implementation of programs for prevention, early diagnosis, and treatment, especially in children [6]. However, interventions to reduce childhood obesity show limited effectiveness, particularly for weight-related outcomes [9].

Therefore, sustainable and effective interventions to prevent childhood obesity should target higher-risk children [10]. Obesity development involves a complex interplay between physiological, environmental, psychological, social, and behavioral exposures [11,12]. There is evidence of epigenetic processes in utero that contribute to infant obesity, including DNA methylation, and gut microbiome alterations [13]. Breastfeeding is also associated with obesity protection [14,15]. Additional life course exposures include socio-economic status, food production and marketing, food insecurity, and obesogenic environments, that can promote unhealthy lifestyles. In this environment, some individuals are genetically more susceptible to develop obesity [16].

A simple tool to identify relevant obesity risk factors early in life may alert families and caretakers into positive changes, improving a child's weight trajectory and preventing overweight and obesity. Tools to identify children at risk for obesity have been published [17–19]. To our best knowledge, none of these include a large diversity of parameters known to affect weight gain trajectory; the broad variables related to obesity require a more comprehensive tool.

This study aims to develop a pre-school screening tool to assess the risk for childhood obesity based on a broad spectrum of risk factors considering peri-natal, anthropometric, sociodemographic, past eating habits, current eating habits, subjective anthropometry perception, subjective eating habits perception and physical activity, and sleeping habits, at a multivariable level.

2. Materials and Methods

Data from the community-based participatory research Sintra Grows Healthy (SGH) [20] was used for independent analysis, as a cross-sectional with nested case-control study. The study sample comprises schoolchildren aged 6–12 years attending the first to fourth grades of six public primary schools in Sintra municipality, Portugal. Anthropometric measurements of children were assessed and a wide set of data was obtained by the application of a questionnaire to the children's legal guardian, mainly their parents. For the purpose of the present study, an additional set of questions relevant for the study of obesity risk factors was collected by applying a second questionnaire to the children's legal guardian. Only children for whom both these questionnaires were filled, were selected for this study. Data were collected between 2017 and 2018. Written informed consent was obtained and the safety and confidentiality of all the collected and archived data were ensured. Approval was obtained from the National Commission of Data Protection and the Ethics Commission of Lisbon Academic Medical Center.

Anthropometric measurements were obtained directly by trained members of the SGH research team, using standardized anthropometric procedures [21]. Children were barefoot and wearing minimal clothing to assess height and weight. Height was assessed using a portable stadiometer to the nearest 0.1 cm (SECA 213®) in the vertical position, with feet together and the head in the Frankfort plane. Weight was assessed through a portable calibrated scale (SECA Robusta 813®, SECA Deutschland, Hamburg, Germany), expressed up to 0.1 kg. Body Mass Index (BMI) was calculated as weight (kg) divided by height squared (cm^2). BMI was classified according to age and gender z-scores of the World Health Organization for children aged 5 to 19 years old [22]. Waist circumference was directly measured on the skin to the nearest 0.1 cm according to the World Health Organization method with a non-extensible and flexible tape (SECA 201®, SECA Deutschland, Hamburg, Germany) [23]. Waist-to-Height Ratio (WtHR) was calculated as waist circumference (cm) divided by height (cm) and classified as an indicator for early health risk as ≤0.5 or >0.5 [24].

The set of questions specifically included for the present study were gathered and developed through a literature review regarding childhood obesity [11,12,16]. Children were asked to fill the questionnaire at home with their parents. To assure data confidentiality, each child was assigned a subject identification code. The questionnaires were collected by teachers and sent back to the SGH team. Data entry and revision was conducted through a standardized procedure. The information collected for the present analysis included (a) parental nationality; (b) parental level of education; (c) family type (nuclear/extended two-/one-parented); (d) number and age of siblings; (e) mean monthly income; (f) parental current employment status; (g) present parental weight and height (from which BMI was calculated and categorized into underweight, normal weight, overweight, or obese) and (h) father's and mother's body image perception. The caretakers were asked to recall peri-natal information: (a) maternal weight before and after pregnancy (from which BMI pre-pregnancy and adequacy of weight gain during pregnancy were calculated according to the Institute of Medicine recommendations [25]); (b) maternal tobacco consumption during pregnancy; (c) diagnosis of gestational diabetes and/or pre-eclampsia; (d) information given by the assistant physician during pregnancy on adequateness of the fetus for gestational age; and (e) the gestational age in complete weeks (to determine if the birth was pre-term or term). Information regarding anthropometric data throughout childhood was retrieved from the records in the child health bulletin: (a) birth weight and length [from which BMI was calculated through World Health Organization Anthro software for Windows, version 3.2.2. (World Health Organization—Department of Nutrition, Geneva, Switzerland), and classification into small for gestational age (SGA, < 10th percentile), appropriate for gestational age (10th–89th percentile), and large for gestational age (LGA, > 90th percentile) were obtained]; (b) weight and length at the ages of 12, 18, and 24 months and 3 and 5 years old [from which BMI z-score was calculated through the World Health Organization Anthro software for Windows, version 3.2.2. (World Health Organization—Department of Nutrition, Geneva, Switzerland)]. Overweight (including obesity) was defined according to age and sex z-scores (above 2) of the World Health Organization for children up to 5 years old [26]; since the medical visits from birth to 5-years-old may not have occurred at the exact dates selected to recall anthropometric data, the health record information closer to those ages and respective dates were collected to correctly assess z-scores. To classify anthropometric measurements at each visit, the exact age was calculated by the difference between birth date and the records visit date.

We collected data on child and family feeding patterns at two moments. We asked about breastfeeding (total and exclusive duration) and the introduction of solid foods (age, appetite, and type of meal first introduced). For present feeding pattern, we asked about: child's appetite, the Mediterranean diet pattern index of the child (KIDMED [27]) through adapted questions, and its family (PREDIMED [28]), and one question to both child and caretakers regarding child's intake when worried, irritated, or anxious, extracted from the from Child Eating Behaviour Questionnaire [29]. To assess the child's and caretaker's perception of the quantity of child usual intake, we used images of four meal plates with different portions of food (A to D, ascendingly). According to children's height-for-age, we determined the two images closer to their recommended portion (z-score ≤ 1 corresponded to images A and B; z-score > 1 corresponded to images B and C). Image D represented an excessive food portion for any children of our sample. We compared the adequacy of the caretaker's answers and classified them as adequate, excessive, or lower. Caretakers were asked to select an option regarding the child's nutritional status for age between "low weight," "adequate weight," or "excessive weight" and compared to the child's BMI. This perception was categorized as correct, underestimated, or overestimated.

Children and caretakers identified the child's body figure through body image scales [30]. We compared that perception with the corresponding child's BMI and categorized it as incorrect, relatively correct, or correct to child's BMI, as previously done [31]. The perceptions were additionally categorized as correct, underestimated, or overestimated. Caretakers also identified their own body figures through body image scales [32]. We compared that perception with the corresponding parental

BMI and categorized it as incorrect, relatively correct, or correct to child's BMI, as previously done [33]. The perceptions were additionally categorized as correct, underestimated, or overestimated.

We questioned about the physical activity and sedentary behaviors of the child, the frequency of consumption of meals in front of a screen, and the number of hours of sleep.

Variables were grouped into eight dimensions: peri-natal, anthropometric, sociodemographic, previous eating habits, current eating habits, subjective anthropometry (perception), subjective eating habits (perception), physical activity, and hours of sleep.

2.1. Development of the Risk Index Tool and Scoring

As the BMI, as a single measurement of obesity, does not reflect the whole complexity of the condition [6], the European Association for the Study of Obesity proposed to improve the diagnostic criteria for obesity with the inclusion of other dimensions, including the degree of adiposity [34]. Therefore, to increase the accuracy of the outcome measure, to reflect an adiposity-based condition, a composite variable was created using BMI and WtHr. Thus, the primary outcome measure in this study is increased adiposity, defined as overweight (including obesity) with WtHr > 0.5, while in primary school. To test the effect of the factors under investigation on the primary outcome, binary logistic regression analyses were performed. Exposures were tested within the aforementioned dimensions (dependent variable: overweight (including obesity) with WtHr > 0.5; factors: all risk factors by dimension).

The regression analysis was used to identify factors associated with the primary outcome on each of the eight dimensions. The studied risk factors that showed an association with our primary outcome were presented to an expert pediatric panel (nutrition, education, nursing, pediatrician, and exercise physiology experts) for external construct validation with the purpose of developing the proposed tool: RisObIn.Com (Risk of childhood Obesity In the Community).

The most agreed risk factor variables were then combined to develop the RisObIn.Com tool. At least one item from every considered dimension was included in the score if any of the items revealed significant statistical relevance. The Beta (β) values to a decimal case were used to generate the scoring system as an indicator of the association between each variable, and 0 and 1 scores were assigned to the response option regarding their association with the outcome variable (overweight including obesity with WtHr > 0.5). As an example, on the physical activity item, a score of 0 was assigned to the response option "plays regular and programmed physical activity," and a score of 1 to the response option "doesn't play regular and programmed physical activity." This score was then multiplied by 1.6 to obtain the item's score, as β was 1.642. The final score of the RisObIn.Com tool was obtained by the sum of all item scores and a correction factor was added to obtain zero as the cut-off value.

2.2. Statistical Analysis

All data were checked for entry errors. Statistical analysis was done using IBM SPSS Statistics for Windows, version 26 (IBM Corp, Armonk, NY, USA). OpenEpi Version 3.01 was used to calculate confidence intervals (CI) [35]. Continuous data were checked for normal distribution using the Kolmogorov-Smirnov test and graphically by evaluating histograms and expressed as mean and standard deviation. Non-normally distributed data were expressed as median (Min-Max). Comparisons between the participants studied and those not included were made by using t-tests for normally distributed continuous variables, Mann-Whitney rank-sum tests for non-normally distributed continuous variables, and χ2 tests for categorical variables.

Cutoff point analysis was performed to identify the optimal value that differentiates the risk of obesity from non-risk of obesity in children. The threshold was defined by the largest distance from the diagonal line of the receiver operating characteristic (ROC) curve (sensitivity × (1 − specificity)). Using the cutoff point obtained, both sensitivity and specificity and positive and negative predictive values were calculated, with their 95% CI. All P values reported were based on two-sided hypotheses and compared to a significance level of 5%.

3. Results

3.1. Study Sample Characteristics

Data was collected from 593 subjects. From those, 289 had incomplete data on crucial information to proceed with the analysis (for example, sex information) and therefore were excluded. The remain 304 gathered anthropometric measurements and data regarding our set of questions and therefore were included, despite some were not complete. In the portion of not included subjects, the children's median age was 8.0 (5.8–10.8) years old (missing 162), 7.8 (5.9–10.8) for girls, and 8.1 (5.8–10.4) for boys. The mother's median age was 39.0 (25.0–54.0) years old (missing 62), and father's was 41.0 (25.0–66.0) years old (missing 62). There were no significant differences between the child's age (U = 2371.0, $p = 0.166$), mother's age (U = 41,256.5, $p = 0.153$), child's BMI z-score (U = 23,156.0, $p = 0.204$), mother's (U = 38,080.0, $p = 0.240$) or father's nationality (U = 33,481.5, $p = 0.207$), parental current employment status (U = 30,097.5, $p = 0.308$), mean monthly income (U = 33,703.5, $p = 0.510$), and father's level of education (U = 36,689.0, $p = 0.939$) between the children included in the sample and those not included. The father's age (U = 33,362.5, $p = 0.021$) and the mother's level of education (U = 39,273.0, $p = 0.035$) was significantly different between the children included in the sample and those not included. The sociodemographic characteristics of the sample are presented in Table 1.

Table 1. Sociodemographic characteristics of the study sample.

	Sample Characteristics		n	%	Girls n	Boys n
Child	Age n = 300		Median 8.0 (5.9–10.2) years old			
	Sex n = 304	Girls	148	48.7	n/a	n/a
		Boys	156	51.3	n/a	n/a
	Body Mass Index n = 304	Underweight	4	1.3	1	3
		Normal weight	208	68.4	95	113
		Overweight	63	20.7	38	25
		Obesity	29	9.5	14	15
Caretakers	Mother's age n = 300		Median 38.0 (26.0–52.0)			
	Father's age n = 280		Median 40.0 (26.0–63.0)			
	Mother's Body Mass Index n = 288	Underweight	9	3.1	3	6
		Normal weight	165	57.3	82	83
		Overweight	84	29.2	43	41
		Obesity	30	10.4	14	16
	Father's Body Mass Index n = 275	Underweight	0	0	0	0
		Normal weight	104	37.8	57	47
		Overweight	132	48.0	55	77
		Obesity	39	14.2	22	17
	Mother's nationality n = 290	Portuguese	270	93.1	137	133
		Non-Portuguese	20	6.9	9	11
	Father's nationality n = 277	Portuguese	265	95.7	131	134
		Non-Portuguese	12	4.3	6	6

Table 1. Cont.

	Sample Characteristics		n	%	Girls n	Boys n
Caretakers	Mother's education n = 297	Basic education or lower	62	20.9	32	30
		Higher secondary education or a professional course	119	40.1	68	51
		Graduation or bachelor's degree	99	33.3	44	55
		Master or doctoral degree	17	5.7	3	14
	Father's education n = 280	Basic education or lower	91	32.5	48	43
		Higher secondary education or a professional course	129	46.1	59	70
		Graduation or bachelor's degree	46	16.4	22	24
		Master or doctoral degree	14	5.0	6	8
	Professional situation n = 263	Both parents are employed	209	79.5	108	101
		Only one parent is employed	44	16.7	21	23
		Both parents are jobless	10	3.8	3	7
	Mean monthly household income n = 271	Less than €500	9	3.32	4	5
		€500–€1000	80	29.52	40	40
		€1000–€1500	80	29.52	36	44
		€1500–€2000	52	19.18	28	24
		€2000–€3000	41	15.12	17	24
		Above €3000	9	3.32	3	6

n/a—not applicable.

The overall prevalence estimates of underweight, normal weight, overweight, and obesity, and central adiposity are shown in Table 2. Overall, the prevalence rate was 20.7% for overweight and 9.5% for obesity. Most children (80.8%, n = 244) had WtHr ≤ 0.5. Combining BMI and WtHr, 16.8% [95% CI 13.0–21.4] (n = 51) children were overweight (including obesity) with WtHr > 0.5. Only seven children had a WtHr > 0.5 with a normal weight and four children had a WtHr ≤ 0.5 with obesity.

3.2. Risk Factors for Overweight (Including Obesity) with WtHr > 0.5

Risk estimation models for overweight (including obesity) with WtHr > 0.5 were explored within each dimension of variables. The significant risk factors on each of the eight dimensions are presented in Table 3 and Supplementary Table S1.

3.2.1. Peri-Natal Dimension

The only variable retained in the final peri-natal dimension estimation model was maternal pre-pregnancy BMI; being classified as overweight increases, in mean, 2.6-fold the risk of overweight (including obesity) with WtHr > 0.5, and being classified as obese increases, in mean, 4.1-fold the risk of overweight (including obesity) with WtHr > 0.5.

3.2.2. Anthropometric Dimension

For the anthropometric dimension, the retained variable was the BMI at 5 years old; being classified as overweight increases, in mean, 4.2-fold the risk of overweight (including obesity) with WtHr > 0.5.

Table 2. Characterization of anthropometric measurements and calculated indexes.

		Total				Girls				Boys			
				95% Confidence Interval				95% Confidence Interval				95% Confidence Interval	
		n	%	Lower Level	Upper Level	n	%	Lower Level	Upper Level	n	%	Lower Level	Upper Level
Body Mass Index z-Score							Median 0.36 (−2.77–3.89)							
	Underweight	4	1.3	0.5	3.3	1	0.68	0.1	3.7	3	1.92	0.7	5.5
Body Mass Index Class	Normal Weight	208	68.4	62.9	73.4	95	64.19	56.2	71.5	113	72.44	64.9	78.8
	Overweight	63	20.7	16.6	25.6	38	25.68	19.3	33.3	25	16.02	11.1	22.6
	Obesity	29	9.5	6.7	13.4	14	9.45	5.7	15.3	15	9.62	5.9	15.3
	n Total	304	100.0	-	-	148	100.0	-	-	156	100.0	-	-
Waist Circumference							Median 58.5 (37.5–91.5)							
Waist-to-Height ratio							Median 0.46 (0.34–0.66)							
	≤0.5	244	80.8	75.9	84.8	110	74.8	67.2	81.2	134	86.5	80.2	90.9
	>0.5	58	19.2	15.5	24.4	37	25.2	18.9	32.8	21	13.5	9.0	19.8
	n Total	302	100.0	-	-	147	100.0	-	-	155	100.0	-	-
Overweight (Including Obesity) with Waist-to-Height ratio	>0.5	51	16.8	13.0	21.4	31	20.9	15.3	28.4	20	12.8	8.5	18.9
	n Total	304	-	-	-	148	-	-	-	156	-	-	-

Table 3. Variables retained in the statistical models.

Dimension	Variables		Exp(β) (95% Confidence Interval)	p-Value
Peri-natal	Pre-pregnancy Body Mass Index	Pre-pregnancy Body Mass Index of Overweight	2.591 (1.164–5.766)	0.020
		Pre-pregnancy Body Mass Index of Obesity	4.145 (0.925–8.570)	0.063
	Body Mass Index z-score 5-years-old		4.159 (2.404–8.497)	0.000
	Paternal Body Mass Index	Paternal Body Mass Index of Overweight	0.772 (0.252–2.364)	0.650
		Paternal Body Mass Index of Obesity	4.041 (1.271–12.844)	0.018
	Type of meal introduced in solid food introduction	Soup	0.401 (0.176–0.914)	0.030
Current eating habits	Child's appetite	Would eat only with insistence or frequently would not eat in totality; Would eat all and be satisfied	0.174 (0.050–0.603)	0.006
	Caretaker's perception of child's intake through image		1.489 (0.985–2.249)	0.059
	Family Mediterranean pattern (PREDIMED)	How many vegetable servings do you consume per day?	0.624 (0.389–0.999)	0.050
		How many servings of butter, margarine, or cream do you consume per day?	1.535 (0.976–2.413)	0.063
Subjective anthropometry perception	Adequacy of father's body image perception vs. actual Body Mass Index	Relatively correct	4.902 (1.116–21.536)	0.035
		Correct	2.597 (0.634–10.643)	0.185
	Adequacy of the caretaker's opinion on the child's nutritional status vs. child's Body Mass Index	Relatively correct	3.483 (0.882–13.753)	0.075
		Correct	31.605 (6.055–164.951)	0.000
Subjective eating habits perception	Caretaker's perception regarding child's intake when anxious	No	0.260 (0.056–1.204)	0.085
	Caretaker's perception of the adequacy of the child's food intake for age	Inferior or adequate	0.083 (0.024–0.286)	0.000
Physical activity and hours of sleep	Child's participation in programmed sport activity	Yes	0.194 (0.052–0.724)	0.015

3.2.3. Sociodemographic Dimension

The sociodemographic variable retained in the final estimation model was paternal BMI; paternal BMI reflecting overweight decreases, in mean, 33% the risk of overweight (including obesity) with WtHr > 0.5, and paternal BMI reflecting obesity increases, in mean, 4-fold the risk of overweight (including obesity) with WtHr > 0.5.

3.2.4. Past Eating Habits Dimension

For the past eating habits dimension, the only variable included in the final model was the type of meal used for solid foods introduction; if soup (rather than cereals) was the first solid food introduced, it decreases, in mean, 60% (the risk of overweight (including obesity) with WtHr > 0.5.

3.2.5. Current Eating Habits Dimension

For current eating habits, the variables child's appetite, the caretaker's perception of the child's intake through image, and the PREDIMED questions regarding vegetable daily intake and butter, margarine, and cream daily intake were included in the final model. The child's appetite decreases, in mean, 83% the risk of overweight (including obesity) with WtHr > 0.5. The caretaker's perception of the child's intake through image increases, in mean, 1.5-fold the risk of overweight (including obesity) with WtHr > 0.5. The PREDIMED question regarding vegetable daily intake decreases, in mean, 38% (the risk of overweight (including obesity) with WtHr > 0.5, and the PREDIMED question regarding butter, margarine, and cream daily intake increases, in mean, 1.5-fold the risk of overweight (including obesity) with WtHr > 0.5.

3.2.6. Subjective Anthropometry Perception Dimension

For subjective anthropometry perception, the two variables retained in the final model were (1) the adequacy of father's own body image perception in comparison to his real BMI; and (2) the adequacy of the caretaker's opinion regarding the child's nutritional status in comparison to the child's real BMI. The relatively correct adequacy of father's own body image perception compared to real BMI increases, in mean, 4.9-fold the risk of overweight (including obesity) with WtHr > 0.5, and the correct adequacy of father's own body image perception compared to real BMI increases, in mean, 2.6-fold the risk of overweight (including obesity) with WtHr > 0.5. Regarding the adequacy of the caretaker's opinion regarding the child's nutritional status compared to the child's real BMI, correct adequacy decreases, in mean, 31.6-fold the risk of overweight (including obesity) with WtHr > 0.5.

3.2.7. Subjective Eating Habits Perception Dimension

In the eating habits subjective data, the variables retained in the final estimation model were the caretaker's perception of child's food intake when worried, irritated, or anxious and the caretaker's perception of the adequacy of the child's food intake for age. The caretaker's perception that the child's food intake when worried, irritated, or anxious is not affected decreases, in mean, 74% the risk of overweight (including obesity) with WtHr > 0.5. The caretaker's perception that the child's food intake is inferior or adequate for age decreases, in mean, 92% the risk of overweight (including obesity) with WtHr > 0.5.

3.2.8. Physical Activity and Sleeping Habits Dimension

For physical activity and hours of sleep, the variables included in the final model were the child's participation in programmed sports activity, the number of sedentary hours in a weekday, the number of sedentary hours on a weekend day, and the total number of sedentary hours in a week. The child's participation in programmed sports activity decreases, in mean, 81% the risk of overweight (including obesity) with WtHr > 0.5.

3.3. Scoring and Risk Index

The set of 13 variables identified for the items of the screening tool were submitted to the pediatric expert panel.

The variable father's BMI from the sociodemographic dimension was excluded as two members of the panel did not agree with its inclusion in the tool, for lack of evidence of the variable impact in childhood obesity.

The current eating habits dimension variables for PREDIMED vegetable servings daily intake and butter, margarine, and cream servings daily intake, and the caretaker's perception of the child's intake through image were excluded. One member of the panel did not agree with the inclusion of the butter, margarine, and cream daily intake variable in the tool, for lack of evidence of the variable impact in childhood obesity.

The adequacy of the father's body image perception vs. BMI from the subjective anthropometry perception was excluded as two members of the panel did not agree with its inclusion in the tool, for lack of evidence of the variable impact in childhood obesity.

For the physical activity and sleep hours dimension, only the programmed physical activity practice variable was included. The remaining were excluded due to the observed lack of measurable effect.

Eight items were included in the tool and all dimensions except the sociodemographic were included. The items and respective scores are presented in Table 4.

Table 4. Items included in the Risk of childhood Obesity in the Community (RisObIn.Com) tool, categorization, and scoring.

Dimension	Item	Response Options and Scoring	Scoring
Anthropometric	Body Mass Index at 5 years old	0—Overweight	−2.3 ($p = 0.031$)
		1—Underweight, Normal weight	
Peri-natal	Mother's pre-pregnancy Body Mass Index	0—Obesity	−1.0 ($p = 0.063$)
		1—Underweight, Normal weight, Overweight	
Current eating habits	Child's appetite	0—Would eat only with insistence or frequently would not eat in totality; Would eat all and be satisfied	1.5 ($p = 0.015$)
		1—Would eat more than what is offered	
Previous eating habits	Type of meal introduced in solid food introduction	0—Soup	−0.9 ($p = 0.030$)
		1—Infant cereal	
Subjective eating habits perception	Caretaker's perception of the adequacy of the child's food intake for age	0—Less than adequate; Adequate	2.5 ($p = 0.000$)
		1—More than adequate	
	Caretaker's perception regarding the child's higher intake when worried, irritated, or anxious	0—No	1.4 ($p = 0.085$)
		1—Yes	
Subjective anthropometry perception	Adequacy of the caretaker's opinion on the child's nutritional status vs. child's Body Mass Index	0—Correct	3.4 ($p = 0.000$)
		1—Incorrect	
Physical activity and hours of sleep	Child's participation in programmed sport activity	0—Yes	1.6 ($p = 0.015$)
		1—No	

Applying the tool items to every child who gathered responses to all the tool items ($n = 145$), the sum of the items ranged from −4.20 to 4.60. Higher values of the tool indicated a greater risk of obesity in childhood. The area under the ROC curve was 0.897 [95%CI 0.825-0.968; $p < 0.001$] for girls and 0.779 [95%CI 0.612–0.947; $p = 0.016$]—Figure 1. The uncorrected optimal cutoff point of the RisObIn.Com tool was -1, thus, a correction factor (+1) was applied to obtain a cutoff point value of zero. The tool sensitivity, based on the optimal cutoff point, was 95.0%; that is, 95.0% of children who had overweight (including obesity) with WtHr > 0.5 while on primary school, got a score greater than 0 in the transition from pre-school to primary school had overweight (including obesity) with WtHr > 0.5 while on primary school. The specificity was 74.4%, meaning that 74.4% of children who did not have overweight (including obesity) with WtHr > 0.5 while on primary school, got a score equal or less than 0 in the transition from pre-school to primary school did not have overweight (including obesity) with WtHr > 0.5 while on primary school. The positive predictive value was 37.3%, meaning that among those who had a score greater than 0, the probability of having the condition was 37.3%. The negative predictive value was 98.9%, meaning that among those who had a score equal or less than 0, the probability of not having the condition was 98.9%.

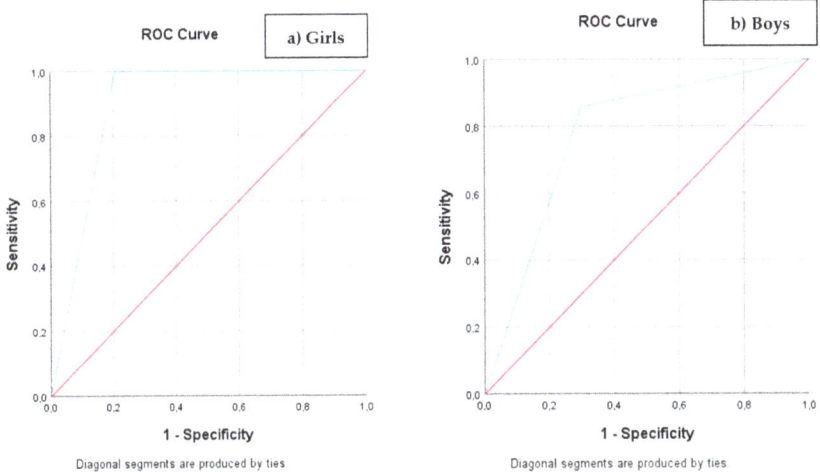

Figure 1. Performance of the proposed screening tool (RisObIn.Com) to identify girls (**a**) and boys (**b**) in the transition from pre-school to primary school that had overweight (including obesity) with WtHr > 0.5 while in primary school. The receiver operating characteristic (ROC) curves were calculated for the cutoff point value of zero. The area under the ROC curve was 0.897 (95%CI 0.825–0.968; $p < 0.001$) for girls; and the area under the ROC curve was 0.779 (95%CI 0.612–0.947; $p = 0.016$) for boys. CI: Confidence Interval; WtHr: Waist-to-Height Ratio.

4. Discussion

Preschool and primary school ages are among the most critical periods for determining obesity later in life [36]. A screening tool applied at this occasion will signal cases that will benefit from general and customized intervention, improving resources to prevent child obesity.

This new proposed tool combines elements that reflect the multifactor nature of obesity: maternal BMI before pregnancy; the child's own BMI at 5 years old; the first solid food introduced for diversification; the caretakers perception of the current appetite of the child; the parental opinion regarding the child's intake adequacy; the child's food intake when worried, irritated, or anxious; the parental perception of the child's nutritional status; and the regular practice of programmed physical activities. Through this weighted combination, RisObIn.Com provides a score that estimates the risk of obesity through school age.

To the best of our knowledge, this is the first screening tool to assess the risk of obesity in children at the entrance of primary school that includes a set of parameters from different dimensions and specific periods, acknowledged to affect weight gain trajectory. The development of this tool contrasts with other existing tools, which selected items through the opinion of experts [17] or literature review [37], focusing only on a specific period of childhood, such as the peri-natal period [18] or the present moment of assessment [19]; others attempted to associate a large number of variables to childhood obesity risk through data mining [38]. The inclusion of all these dimensions can justify the large areas under the ROC curve obtained by RisObIn.Com, larger than other tools [18,19,38]. We observed a difference between boys and girls regarding the ROC findings considering the sex variable, but we consider that it is not possible to infer this difference is maintained when the tool is applied in samples differ in dimension or population characteristics. RisObIn.Com achieves 95% sensitivity and 74.4% specificity despite the tool having been developed using a smaller sample than other studies.

4.1. Peri-Natal Dimension

Maternal pre-pregnancy BMI was the only variable retained in the final estimation model from the peri-natal dimension set. This variable has been shown to be positively associated with infant adiposity, as well as childhood obesity and overweight [12]. A recent meta-analysis identified significantly higher odds for childhood obesity with higher pre-pregnancy maternal BMI, 89% for the offspring of overweight women before pregnancy and 264% for those who were obese before pregnancy [39].

4.2. Anthropometric Dimension

On the anthropometric dimension, the retained variable was the BMI at 5 years of age. The growth patterns of BMI during childhood, particularly during critical periods, are closely related to adult obesity risk [40]. The second physiological rise in BMI occurs, in general, between 3 and 7 years [41]. Pei et al., in 2013, on the German birth cohorts GINIplus—The German Infant Study on the Influence of Nutrition Intervention plus Air pollution and Genetics on Allergy Development, and LISAplus—Influence of Life-style factors on Development of the Immune System and Allergies in East and West Germany plus Air Pollution and Genetics on Allergy Development, also found that BMI at 60–64 months of age was significantly associated with overweight at the age of 10 years [42]. Children with higher BMI at 5 years of age probably have already experienced an adiposity rebound, and early age at adiposity rebound is known to be a risk factor for later obesity [43].

4.3. Previous Eating Habits Dimension

Evidence shows that breastfeeding is a protective factor for obesity [14,15]. However, in this study, regarding previous eating habits, we found that only the type of first complementary solid food introduced was associated with overweight (including obesity) with WtHr > 0.5 while in primary school. Recent data does not support the hypothesis that the quality of complementary foods has a direct effect on the risk for later obesity [44]. Soup can be prepared using many different vegetables as ingredients; the quality and quantity of vegetables and fat used have a strong influence on its nutritional value. By opposition, infant cereals do not allow nutrient composition modifications, thus having a more constant energy value. In countries [45] such as Portugal, the traditional recommendation of the first complementary food to be introduced is infant cereals [46]. One can only speculate that, in infants that present a higher BMI or rapid weight gain [47], health professionals will recommend that the first food to introduce should be soup, since it allows to manipulate the amount of vegetables and fat content, in the attempt to reduce energy intake.

4.4. Current Eating Habits Dimension

In the current eating habits dimension, the parameters retained in the final model were the child's appetite and the caretaker's perception of high, low, or adequate appetite of the child. These measures relate to appetite and reflect self-regulation of energy intake. Biological regulation of appetite is very complex, engaging a number of tissues, organs, hormones, and neural circuits with several feedback pathways between the brain and peripheral tissues [48]. These mechanisms can be influenced and modulated by several factors, beyond the aim of the development of a screening tool. Adequate nutritional status children eat smaller portions at lunch/dinner and may eat more snacks throughout the day; the energy of those snacks is usually greater than the energy of lunch or dinner meals [49].

When parents perceive their child as having increased appetite, they may try to implement restrictive feeding practices. These practices can increase the preoccupation of the child with food and affect eating behaviors, eventually leading to paradoxical weight gain [50]. As both extremes of feeding practices could shape children's relation to food, we cannot exclude that, in the past, parents may have forced their children to eat after they are satisfied, promoting a dysregulation on this equilibrium, once the tendency to encourage children to clear their plate is reported to be associated with obesity [51].

The variables from the PREDIMED index, collected in the SGH study, while explored in the analysis, were excluded, because this Mediterranean diet assessment tool is not yet validated for Portugal; therefore, it may not be adapted to Portuguese food habits. The caretaker's perception of the child's intake through image was also excluded. We presented caretakers a set of four images of a lunch/dinner plate. By presenting an even number of options instead of an odd number, we avoid the tendency for the selection of the central option, improving the reliability of the answer. However, since the need to use images will be a challenge for the application of this tool and the removal of the item had a small effect in the final model, it was removed.

4.5. Subjective Perception of Anthropometry Dimension

Regarding the subjective perception of anthropometry, this study found a high proportion of parents that misclassified the nutritional status of their child. It has been speculated that the high prevalence of overweight and obesity in children in the last decades can influence the misinterpretation of the child's normal weight [52], leading to the perception of "normal" weight despite the BMI indication of overweight. If parents cannot recognize their child as overweight, they will not act to change behaviors and the situation can exacerbate, leading to obesity.

4.6. Subjective Perception of Eating Habits Dimension

Adequate dietary habits are important for health throughout life, but particularly during childhood, considering that the dietary habits during this specific period are potentially perpetuated into adulthood [53]. In the dimension related to the subjective perception of eating habits, the variables retained in the final estimation model were the caretaker's perception of the child's food intake while worried, irritated, or anxious and the caretaker's perception of the adequacy for age of the child's usual food intake. Previous studies have shown psychopathology to be associated with overweight in children [54,55]; validity data indicate that children as young as 4 years old can report on their own anxiety symptoms [56]. In reaction to anxiety, emotional eating acts as a biological response that provides temporary feelings of gratification/satisfaction [57]. The intervention approach for children with anxiety symptoms and emotional eating should be adapted to address the negative emotions underlying eating behaviors as well as teaching healthy coping strategies for these emotions [58]. Parents and their own perception of the child's dietary habits is one of the most important factors for the dietary habits of children [59]. Childhood obesity experts recommend that childhood overweight prevention should focus on parents, according to the growing evidence of the role of parental practices and family environment in promoting effective changes [11,12].

4.7. Physical Activity and Sleeping Habits Dimension

For the dimension concerning physical activity and sleeping habits, the variables included in the final model were the child's participation in programmed sports activity. The levels of physical inactivity are rising in many countries with major implications for general health and the prevalence of non-communicable diseases, such as obesity. The association had already been identified in a similar population living in Portugal's capital (Greater Lisbon) [60]. A recent multinational cross-sectional study demonstrated that low levels of moderate-to-vigorous physical activity or high sedentary levels during weekdays and weekends were associated with higher odds of obesity in 9–11-year-old children in 12 countries [61].

The RisObIn.Com tool seems to be a comprehensive tool to identify, at school entrance, 5-to-6-year-old children at higher risk for late childhood obesity. It was conceived to be applied either by the parents or by teachers or school health professionals, such as a school nurse, school nutritionist, or school social worker, with parental feedback and the child's health bulletin for easier recall of mother pre-pregnancy BMI and anthropometric measures at the age of 5 years. The tool carries a small and simple set of instructions for its effective use. A web-based tool allows a quick, simple, and automated form of application. RisObIn.Com is hosted in Health & Technology Research Center webpage available at https://htrc.estesl.ipl.pt/risobin-com/.

The synergy between the authors of this study and the SGH research team benefited from the logistics associated with data collection and allowed the enhancement and efficiency of resources. The methodology included direct anthropometric measurements, assessment of a set of variables identified as influent in obesity development (from peri-natal to the present moment, including sociodemographic, anthropometric, past and current eating habits, subjective anthropometry, and eating habits perception, and physical activity and hours of sleep) and had the endorsement of an expert panel group composed by skilled professionals from different areas. As a positive asset, the selected outcome measure reflects adiposity by the cumulative outcome of overweight (including obesity) with WtHr > 0.5, which allows both a better characterization of the nutritional status and better accuracy. On the other hand, the mixed design of case-control study nested on a cross-sectional study is a limitation, due to recollection bias, and causal inferences to be made, just epidemiologic and statistic associations. Another source of bias was related to maternal weight before and after pregnancy that was reported and not measured. The local nature of the sample and the differences observed between the children included and not included in the study do not allow immediate generalization of the findings to other populations; therefore, external validation of the screening tool and the study of its performance in different samples is required. Eventual ethnic differences were not explored, due to national ethical and legal restrictions related to data protection. The effective sample size was smaller than expected and it probably affected the ability to identify more exposure variables significantly associated with the study outcome; a larger sample would probably have improved the observed results. Longitudinal data analysis would allow evaluating the tool's ability to predict BMI change over time.

The RisObIn.Com screening tool is proposed to be routinely used by teachers and other school personnel with the participation of parents or caretakers for early identification of children who might benefit from preventive actions, but its use could also be extended to health care professionals such as nurses, family physicians, or pediatricians. The RisObIn.Com screening tool is a simple and inexpensive tool that can provide an evaluation of the risk factors for pediatric obesity and may identify those in need for healthy lifestyle changes.

5. Conclusions

The RisObIn.Com tool is proposed to be a comprehensive tool to identify children at high risk for late childhood obesity at admission to primary school, by the age of 5 to 6 years old. Further studies are needed to assess the external validity and the generalization of the findings, as well as to confirm both the performance of this tool to identify children with obesity risk at admission into primary school and the effect of the subsequent intervention to prevent obesity in children.

Supplementary Materials: The following are available online at http://www.mdpi.com/2072-6643/12/11/3288/s1, Table S1: Variables in the statistical model.

Author Contributions: Conceptualization, A.C.M.; methodology, A.C.M., R.F., T.N., P.A.O., and D.V.; software, D.V., and P.A.O.; formal analysis, D.V.; investigation, A.C.M. and R.B.; resources, R.F. and T.N.; data curation, T.N. and P.A.O.; writing—original draft preparation, P.A.O., A.C.M., and D.V.; writing—review and editing, P.A.O., A.C.M., and D.V.; supervision, A.C.M. All authors agreed on the submitted version of the manuscript.

Funding: This research received no external funding.

Acknowledgments: We would like to acknowledge the members of the experts panel whose contribution was valuable for the development of the present tool (Bandola, L.; Barrigas, C.; Cunha, S.; Neves, C.; Sousa, J.). The present study is part of the MSc thesis in Clinical Nutrition of one of the authors (P.A.O.) (supervisor A.C.M.), from Faculty of Medicine of Lisbon and Lisbon School of Health Technology, Lisbon, Portugal. The authors are grateful to the SGH team and to its coordinator Joana Sousa, to whom we express our recognition. H&TRC authors gratefully acknowledge the FCT/MCTES national support through the UIDB/05608/2020 and UIDP/05608/2020.

Conflicts of Interest: The authors declare no conflict of interest.

References

1. Abarca-Gómez, L.; Abdeen, Z.A.; Hamid, Z.A.; Abu-Rmeileh, N.M.; Acosta-Cazares, B.; Acuin, C.; Adams, R.J.; Aekplakorn, W.; Afsana, K.; Aguilar-Salinas, C.A.; et al. Worldwide trends in body-mass index, underweight, overweight, and obesity from 1975 to 2016: A pooled analysis of 2416 population-based measurement studies in 128·9 million children, adolescents, and adults. *The Lancet* **2017**, *390*, 2627–2642. [CrossRef]
2. Wijnhoven, T.M.A.; Van Raaij, J.M.A.; Sjöberg, A.; Eldin, N.; Yngve, A.; Kunešová, M.; Starc, G.; Rito, A.I.; Duleva, V.; Hassapidou, M.; et al. WHO European childhood obesity surveillance initiative: School nutrition environment and body mass index in primary schools. *Int. J. Environ. Res. Public Health* **2014**, *11*, 11261–11285. [CrossRef]
3. Spinelli, A.; Buoncristiano, M.; Kovacs, V.A.; Yngve, A.; Spiroski, I.; Obreja, G.; Starc, G.; Pérez, N.; Rito, A.I.; Kunešová, M.; et al. Prevalence of Severe Obesity among Primary School Children in 21 European Countries. *Obes. Facts* **2019**, *12*, 244–258. [CrossRef]
4. WHO Consultation on Obesity. Diseases WHOD of N World Health Organization. In Proceedings of the Programme of Nutrition F and, R.H. Obesity: Preventing and Managing the Global Epidemic: Report of a WHO Consultation on Obesity, Geneva, Switzerland, 3–5 June 1997; World Health Organization: Geneva, Switzerland, 1997.
5. Neeland, I.J.; Poirier, P.; Després, J.P. Cardiovascular and Metabolic Heterogeneity of Obesity: Clinical Challenges and Implications for Management. *Circulation* **2018**, *137*, 1391–1406. [CrossRef] [PubMed]
6. Frühbeck, G.; Busetto, L.; Dicker, D.; Yumuk, V.; Goossens, G.H.; Hebebrand, J.; Halford, J.G.C.; Farpour-Lambert, N.J.; Blaak, E.E.; Woodward, E.; et al. The ABCD of obesity: An EASO position statement on a diagnostic term with clinical and scientific implications. *Obes. Facts* **2019**, *12*, 131–136. [CrossRef] [PubMed]
7. Simmonds, M.; Burch, J.; Llewellyn, A.; Griffiths, C.; Yang, H.; Owen, C.; Duffy, S.; Woolacott, N. The use of measures of obesity in childhood for predicting obesity and the development of obesity-related diseases in adulthood: A systematic review and meta-analysis. *Health Technol. Assess.* **2015**, *19*, 1–336. [CrossRef] [PubMed]
8. Bhadoria, A.; Sahoo, K.; Sahoo, B.; Choudhury, A.; Sufi, N.; Kumar, R. Childhood obesity: Causes and consequences. *J. Fam. Med. Prim. Care* **2015**, *4*, 187. [CrossRef]
9. van de Kolk, I.; Gerards, S.M.; Harms, L.S.E.; Kremers, S.P.J.; Gubbels, J.S. The effects of a comprehensive, integrated obesity prevention intervention approach (SuperFIT) on children's physical activity, sedentary behavior, and BMI z-score. *Int. J. Environ. Res. Public Health* **2019**, *16*, 5016. [CrossRef] [PubMed]
10. Lobstein, T.; Jackson-Leach, R.; Moodie, M.L.; Hall, K.D.; Gortmaker, S.L.; Swinburn, B.A.; James, W.P.T.; Wang, Y.; McPherson, K. Child and adolescent obesity: Part of a bigger picture. *Lancet* **2015**, *385*, 2510–2520. [CrossRef]
11. Birch, L.L.; Ventura, A.K. Preventing childhood obesity: What works? *Int. J. Obes.* **2009**, *33*, S74–S81. [CrossRef]
12. Davison, K.K.; Birch, L.L. Childhood overweight: A contextual model and recommendations for future research. *Obes. Rev.* **2001**, *2*, 159–171. [CrossRef] [PubMed]
13. Golab, B.P.; Santos, S.; Voerman, E.; Lawlor, D.A.; Jaddoe, V.W.; Gaillard, R.; Barros, H.; Bergström, A.; Charles, M.A.; Chatzi, L.; et al. Influence of maternal obesity on the association between common pregnancy complications and risk of childhood obesity: An individual participant data meta-analysis. *Lancet Child Adolesc. Health* **2018**, *2*, 812–821. [CrossRef]
14. Rito, A.I.; Buoncristiano, M.; Spinelli, A.; Salanave, B.; Kunešová, M.; Hejgaard, T.; Solano, M.G.; Fijałkowska, A.; Sturua, L.; Hyska, J.; et al. Association between Characteristics at Birth, Breastfeeding and Obesity in 22 Countries: The WHO European Childhood Obesity Surveillance Initiative–COSI 2015/2017. *Obes. Facts* **2019**, *12*, 226–243. [CrossRef] [PubMed]
15. Yan, J.; Liu, L.; Zhu, Y.; Huang, G.; Wang, P.P. The association between breastfeeding and childhood obesity: A meta-analysis. *BMC Public Health* **2014**, *14*, 1267. [CrossRef] [PubMed]
16. Schrempft, S.; Van Jaarsveld, C.H.M.; Fisher, A.; Herle, M.; Smith, A.D.; Fildes, A.; Llewellyn, C.H. Variation in the Heritability of Child Body Mass Index by Obesogenic Home Environment. *JAMA Pediatr.* **2018**, *172*, 1153–1160. [CrossRef]
17. Santos, M.; Cadieux, A.; Gray, J.; Ward, W. Pediatric Obesity in Early Childhood: A Physician Screening Tool. *Clin. Pediatr.* **2016**, *55*, 356–362. [CrossRef]

18. Manios, Y.; Birbilis, M.; Moschonis, G.; Birbilis, G.; Mougios, V.; Lionis, C.; Chrousos, G.P. Childhood Obesity Risk Evaluation based on perinatal factors and family sociodemographic characteristics: CORE Index. *Eur. J. Pediatr.* **2013**, *172*, 551–555. [CrossRef]
19. Simpson, J.R.; Keller, H.; Rysdale, L.; Beyers, J. Nutrition Screening Tool for Every Preschooler (NutriSTEP™): Validation and test-retest reliability of a parent-administered questionnaire assessing nutrition risk of preschoolers. *Eur. J. Clin. Nutr.* **2008**, *62*, 770–780. [CrossRef]
20. Sintra Cresce Saudável. Sintra Cresce Saudável [Internet]. Available online: http://crescesaudavel.sintra.pt/ (accessed on 26 September 2020).
21. World Health Organization. *Physical Status: The Use and Interpretation of Anthropometry*; WHO: Geneva, Switzerland, 1995.
22. de Onis, M.; Lobstein, T. Defining obesity risk status in the general childhood population: Which cut-offs should we use? *Int. J. Pediatr. Obes.* **2010**, *5*, 458–460. [CrossRef]
23. World Health Organization. *The WHO STEPwise Approach to Noncomunicable Disease Risk Factor Surveillance (STEPS)*; WHO: Geneva, Switzerland, 2017.
24. Taylor, R.W.; Williams, S.M.; Grant, A.M.; Taylor, B.J.; Goulding, A. Predictive Ability of Waist-to-Height in Relation to Adiposity in Children Is Not Improved With Age and Sex-Specific Values. *Obesity* **2011**, *19*, 1062–1068. [CrossRef]
25. Rasmussen, K.M.; Yaktine, A.L.; Institute of Medicine (U.S.). Committee to Reexamine IOM Pregnancy Weight Guidelines. In *Weight Gain during Pregnancy: Reexamining the Guidelines*; National Academies Press: Washington, DC, USA, 2009; p. 854.
26. World Health Organization. *Training Course on Child Growth Assessment: Interpreting Growth Indicators*; WHO: Geneva, Switzerland, 2008.
27. Serra-Majem, L.; Ribas, L.; Ngo, J.; Ortega, R.M.; García, A.; Pérez-Rodrigo, C.; Aranceta, J. Food, youth and the Mediterranean diet in Spain. Development of KIDMED, Mediterranean Diet Quality Index in children and adolescents. *Public Health Nutr.* **2004**, *7*, 931–935. [CrossRef] [PubMed]
28. Martínez-González, M.A.; García-Arellano, A.; Toledo, E.; Salas-Salvadó, J.; Buil-Cosiales, P.; Corella, D.; Covas, M.I.; Schröder, H.; Arós, F.; Gómez-Gracia, E.; et al. A 14-item Mediterranean diet assessment tool and obesity indexes among high-risk subjects: The PREDIMED trial. *PLoS ONE* **2012**, *7*, e43134. [CrossRef] [PubMed]
29. Viana, V.; Sinde, S.; Saxton, J. Questionário do Comportamento Alimentar da Criança (CEBQ). In *Instrumentos e Contextos de Avaliação Psicológica*; Almedina: Lisbon, Portugal, 2011.
30. Collins, M.E. Body figure perceptions and preferences among preadolescent children. *Int. J. Eat. Disord.* **1991**, *10*, 199–203. [CrossRef]
31. Daraganova, G. Data and measurement. In *The Longitudinal Study of Australian Children Annual Statistical Report 2013*; Australian Institute of Family Studies: Melbourne, Australia, 2014.
32. Stunkard, A.J.; Sørensen, T.I.A.; Schulsinger, F. Use of the Danish Adoption Register for the study of obesity and thinness. *Res. Publ. Assoc. Res. Nerv. Ment. Dis.* **1983**, *60*, 115–120.
33. Freedman, D.S.; Khan, L.K.; Serdula, M.K.; Dietz, W.H.; Srinivasan, S.R.; Berenson, G.S. Inter-relationships among childhood, B.M.I.; childhood height, and adult obesity: The Bogalusa Heart Study. *Int. J. Obes.* **2004**, *28*, 10–16. [CrossRef]
34. Hebebrand, J.; Holm, J.C.; Woodward, E.; Baker, J.L.; Blaak, E.; Durrer Schutz, D.; Farpour-Lambert, N.J.; Frühbeck, G.; Halford, J.G.C.; Lissner, L.; et al. A Proposal of the European Association for the Study of Obesity to Improve the ICD-11 Diagnostic Criteria for Obesity Based on the Three Dimensions Etiology, Degree of Adiposity and Health Risk. *Obes Facts* **2017**, *10*, 284–307. [CrossRef]
35. Dean, A.; Sullivan, K.; Soe, M. OpenEpi: Open Source Epidemiologic Statistics for Public Health, Version 3.01. Updated 2013/04/06 [Internet]. Available online: www.OpenEpi.com (accessed on 26 September 2020).
36. Toschke, A.M.; Grote, V.; Koletzko, B.; Von Kries, R. Identifying Children at High Risk for Overweight at School Entry by Weight Gain during the First 2 Years. *Arch. Pediatr. Adolesc. Med.* **2004**, *158*, 449–452. [CrossRef]
37. Avis, J.L.S.; Holt, N.L.; Maximova, K.; van Mierlo, T.; Fournier, R.; Padwal, R.; Cave, A.L.; Martz, P.; Ball, G.D.C. The Development and Refinement of an e-Health Screening, Brief Intervention, and Referral to Treatment for Parents to Prevent Childhood Obesity in Primary Care. *Telemed. e-Health* **2016**, *22*, 385–394. [CrossRef]

38. Hammond, R.; Athanasiadou, R.; Curado, S.; Aphinyanaphongs, Y.; Abrams, C.; Messito, M.J.; Gross, R.; Katzow, M.; Jay, M.; Razavian, N.; et al. Predicting childhood obesity using electronic health records and publicly available data. *PLoS ONE* **2019**, *14*, e0215571. [CrossRef]
39. Heslehurst, N.; Vieira, R.; Akhter, Z.; Bailey, H.; Slack, E.; Ngongalah, L.; Pemu, A.; Rankin, J. The association between maternal body mass index and child obesity: A systematic review and meta-analysis. *PLoS Med.* **2019**, *16*, e1002817. [CrossRef]
40. Zhang, T.; Whelton, P.K.; Xi, B.; Krousel-Wood, M.; Bazzano, L.; He, J.; Chen, W.; Li, S. Rate of change in body mass index at different ages during childhood and adult obesity risk. *Pediatr. Obes.* **2019**, *14*, e12513. [CrossRef] [PubMed]
41. Cole, T.J. Children grow and horses race: Is the adiposity rebound a critical period for later obesity? *BMC Pediatr.* **2004**, *4*, 6. [CrossRef]
42. Pei, Z.; Flexeder, C.; Fuertes, E.; Thiering, E.; Koletzko, B.; Cramer, C.; Berdel, D.; Lehmann, I.; Bauer, C.-P.; Heinrich, J.; et al. Early life risk factors of being overweight at 10 years of age: Results of the German birth cohorts GINIplus and LISAplus. *Eur. J. Clin. Nutr.* **2013**, *67*, 855–862. [CrossRef] [PubMed]
43. Williams, S.M.; Goulding, A. Patterns of gowth associated with the timing of adiposity rebound. *Obesity* **2009**, *17*, 335–341. [CrossRef]
44. Grote, V.; Theurich, M.; Koletzko, B. Do complementary feeding practices predict the later risk of obesity? Vol. 15, Current Opinion in Clinical Nutrition and Metabolic Care. *Curr. Opin. Clin. Nutr. Metab. Care* **2012**, *15*, 293–297. [CrossRef] [PubMed]
45. Miles, G.; Siega-Riz, A.M. Trends in food and beverage consumption among infants and toddlers: 2005–2012. *Pediatr. Am. Acad. Pediatr.* **2017**, *139*, e20163290. [CrossRef]
46. Rêgo, C.; Lopes, C.; Durão, C.; Pinto, E.; Mansilha, H.; Pereira da Silva, L.; Nazareth, M.; Graça, P.; Ferreira, R.; Lima, R.M.; et al. *Alimentação Saudável dos 0 aos 6 anos–Linhas De Orientação Para Profissionais E Educadores*; Direção-Geral da Saúde: Lisbon, Portugal, 2019.
47. Zheng, M.; Lamb, K.E.; Grimes, C.; Laws, R.; Bolton, K.; Ong, K.K.; Campbell, K. Rapid weight gain during infancy and subsequent adiposity: A systematic review and meta-analysis of evidence. *Obes. Rev.* **2018**, *19*, 321–332. [CrossRef]
48. MacLean, P.S.; Blundell, J.E.; Mennella, J.A.; Batterham, R.L. Biological control of appetite: A daunting complexity. *Obesity* **2017**, *25* (Suppl. 1), S8–S16. [CrossRef]
49. Santos, T.; Moreira, A.C. Alimentação em contexto pré-escolar: Relação com estado nutricional e local de residência. *Acta Port. Nutr.* **2017**, *8*, 34–37. [CrossRef]
50. Eagleton, S.G.; Brown, C.L.; Moses, M.J.; Skelton, J.A. Restrictive feeding and excessive hunger in young children with obesity: A case series. *Clin. Case Rep.* **2019**, *7*, 1962–1967. [CrossRef]
51. Robinson, E.; Aveyard, P.; Jebb, S.A. Is plate clearing a risk factor for obesity? A cross-sectional study of self-reported data in US adults. *Obesity* **2015**, *23*, 301–304. [CrossRef] [PubMed]
52. Robinson, E. Overweight but unseen: A review of the underestimation of weight status and a visual normalization theory. *Obes. Rev.* **2017**, *18*, 1200–1209. [CrossRef]
53. Klesges, R.C.; Stein, R.J.; Eck, L.H.; Isbell, T.R.; Klesges, L.M. Parental influence on food selection in young children and its relationships to childhood obesity. *Am. J. Clin. Nutr.* **1991**, *53*, 859–864. [CrossRef] [PubMed]
54. Pinto, I.; Wilkinson, S.; Virella, D.; Alves, M.; Calhau, C.; Coelho, R. Anxiety, family functioning and neuroendocrine biomarkers in obese children. *Acta Med. Port.* **2017**, *30*, 273–280. [CrossRef]
55. Pinto, I.; Wilkinson, S.; Virella, D.; Alves, M.; Calhau, C.; Coelho, R. Attachment Strategies and Neuroendocrine Biomarkers in Obese Children. *Acta Med. Port.* **2016**, *29*, 332–339. [CrossRef]
56. Luby, J.L.; Belden, A.; Sullivan, J.; Spitznagel, E. Preschoolers' Contribution to their Diagnosis of Depression and Anxiety: Uses and Limitations of Young Child Self-Report of Symptoms. *Child Psychiatry Hum. Dev.* **2007**, *38*, 321–338. [CrossRef]
57. Fox, C.K.; Gross, A.C.; Rudser, K.D.; Foy, A.M.H.; Kelly, A.S. Depression, Anxiety, and Severity of Obesity in Adolescents. *Clin. Pediatr.* **2016**, *55*, 1120–1125. [CrossRef]
58. Sheinbein, D.H.; Stein, R.I.; Hayes, J.F.; Brown, M.L.; Balantekin, K.N.; Conlon, R.P.K.; Saelens, B.E.; Perri, M.G.; Welch, R.R.; Schechtman, K.B.; et al. Factors associated with depression and anxiety symptoms among children seeking treatment for obesity: A social-ecological approach. *Pediatr. Obes.* **2019**, *14*, e12518. [CrossRef] [PubMed]

59. Rodgers, R.F.; Paxton, S.J.; Massey, R.; Campbell, K.J.; Wertheim, E.H.; Skouteris, H.; Gibbons, K. Maternal feeding practices predict weight gain and obesogenic eating behaviors in young children: A prospective study. *Int. J. Behav. Nutr. Phys. Act.* **2013**, *10*, 24. [CrossRef]
60. Gouveia, C.; Pereira-da-Silva, L.; Silva, P.; Virella, D.; Videira-Amaral, J. [Physical activity and sedentarism in adolescent students in Lisbon] Actividade física e sedentarismo em adolescentes escolarizados do Concelho de Lisboa. *Acta Pediatr. Port.* **2007**, *38*, 7–12.
61. Li, N.; Zhao, P.; Diao, C.; Qiao, Y.; Katzmarzyk, P.T.; Chaput, J.P.; Fogelholm, M.; Kuriyan, R.; Kurpad, A.; Lambert, E.V.; et al. Joint associations between weekday and weekend physical activity or sedentary time and childhood obesity. *Int. J. Obes.* **2019**, *43*, 691–700. [CrossRef] [PubMed]

Publisher's Note: MDPI stays neutral with regard to jurisdictional claims in published maps and institutional affiliations.

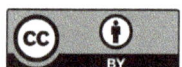

© 2020 by the authors. Licensee MDPI, Basel, Switzerland. This article is an open access article distributed under the terms and conditions of the Creative Commons Attribution (CC BY) license (http://creativecommons.org/licenses/by/4.0/).

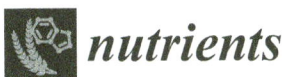 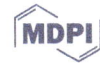

Article

Play with Your Food and Cook It! Tactile Play with Fish as a Way of Promoting Acceptance of Fish in 11- to 13-Year-Old Children in a School Setting—A Qualitative Study

Rikke Højer [1,2,*], Karen Wistoft [3] and Michael Bom Frøst [2]

1. Center for Nutrition and Rehabilitation, Nutrition and Health, University College Absalon, Slagelsevej 70-74, 4180 Sorø, Denmark
2. Department of Food Science, Design and Consumer Behaviour, University of Copenhagen, Rolighedsvej 26, 1958 Frederiksberg, Denmark; mbf@food.ku.dk
3. Department of Educational Sociology Emdrup, Danish School of Education, Tuborgvej 164, Building D, 143, 2400 Copenhagen, Denmark; kawi@edu.au.dk
* Correspondence: rho@pha.dk; Tel.: +45-21448894

Received: 23 August 2020; Accepted: 15 October 2020; Published: 17 October 2020

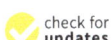

Abstract: Despite a tradition of consuming fish in Denmark and despite the health benefits of eating fish, Danish children consume only one-third of the officially recommended amount of fish. The objective of this study was to explore an experiential and sensory-based exercise in a school setting with focus on tactile play and cooking as a way of promoting 11- to 13-year-old children's acceptance of fish. The design was a qualitative exploratory multiple-case design using participant observation in a school setting. Six classes were recruited from the Eastern part of Denmark ($n = 132$). Based on an exercise with cooking fish and gyotaku (fish print), four meta-themes were identified by applying applied thematic analysis: rejection, acceptance, craftsmanship, and interaction. Rejection and acceptance appeared along a rejection–acceptance continuum related to how the fish was categorised (animal, non-animal, food) in different phases of the experiment. Rejection was promoted by mucus, smell, animalness, and texture, whereas helping each other, tactile play, and craftsmanship promoted acceptance. In conclusion, this study found that tactile play combined with cooking could be a way of promoting acceptance of fish. The findings also support a school setting as a potential gateway in promoting healthy food behaviour.

Keywords: food acceptance; tactile play; cooking; children; fish; health promotion

1. Introduction

1.1. Background

Children aged 11 to 13 years are in the early adolescent life phase [1], a phase defined by a developmental plasticity [2], where lifelong habits can be established [3]. The adolescent life phase is critical when it comes to behavioural changes in, for example, dietary habits [4]. The changes in dietary habits are due to, for example, an increase in autonomy and a decrease in family influence [5,6].

Consumption of fish provides valuable nutrients. Especially fatty fish have a high content of vitamin D, which is important for e.g., calcium (Ca) absorption, bone health, and childhood growth stages [7,8]. Regular consumption of fish, especially those high in n-3 poly unsaturated fatty acids (PUFA), also reduce incidences of, for example, diabetes mellitus, systemic arterial hypertension, central obesity and hyper-lipidemia [9,10], and seem to positively influence intestinal microbiota [11].

Furthermore, the macro nutrient content of fish with regard to protein is 15–20% and fish contains all the essential amino acids [12], which is beneficial for the diet as the sulphur-containing amino acids, cysteine and methionine, are absent in plant protein. Furthermore, proteins from fish have a high degree of digestibility i.e., 85–95% [12,13]. Studies have shown positive health effects as a result of fish protein intake e.g., by decreasing the risk of metabolic syndromes and increasing insulin sensitivity [14–17].

1.1.1. Acceptance and Rejection of Food

This study focuses on fish as part of a healthy diet. According to a national study, Danish children aged 10 to 17 years eat only 105 g of fish per week [18], one-third of the Nordic recommendations of 350 g per week [19]. The intake of fish among Danish early adolescent phase children corresponds with international observations [20–22]. Furthermore, to the authors' knowledge, little research has been conducted in the area of early adolescent phase children's acceptance of fish.

Rozin and Fallon [23,24] have developed a framework in which they have identified three principal motivations within the taxonomy of food acceptance and rejection, which drive food acceptance and rejection: sensory-affective factors (e.g., liking/disliking taste or smell), anticipated consequences (e.g., negative/positive physiological or social), and ideational factors (e.g., knowledge of the nature or origin of a food). These motivations and attributes can lead to either rejection or acceptance: the psychological rejection categories are distaste (the concept distaste includes all sensory characteristics, real or imagined [25,26]), danger, inappropriateness, and disgust, and the acceptance categories are good taste, beneficial, appropriate, and transvalued [25,27]. Furthermore, Rozin and Vollmecke [27] point out that the influence of culture and context are predominant factors influencing acceptance and rejection, and that acquired likes can be promoted by social encounters with people outside the family, especially peers. The framework of rejection and acceptance developed by Rozin and colleagues [23,24,27] has been applied repeatedly in studies investigating food behaviour (e.g., [25,26,28,29]).

Based on the limited research conducted within and around the target group of this study, Prell, Berg, and Jonsson [30] identified a negative attitude towards the smell, the fear of finding bones, the accompaniments, and friends' behaviour as primary barriers to eating fish. In a study focusing on foods in general, Frerichs et al. [31] found that appearance and texture were primary drivers for accepting or rejecting food. Furthermore, Mitterer-Daltoé, Latorres, Treptow, Pastous-Madureiraa, and Queiroz [32] and Latorres, Mitterer-Daltoé, and Queiroz [33] found that young children had a higher acceptance of fish than older children. This might be due to the older children's cognitive maturation, leading to food-related cognitions increasing and becoming more complex [34]. The animal origin of fish could also play a role in rejection, since foods of animal origin tend to promote an attitude of disgust more than those of vegetable origin [24,25,35,36]. Increasing acceptance of food through tactility (the sense of touch by using the hands) or tactile play is a research area that has yet to be explored in greater depth. Five recent studies have been conducted in this research area [37–42], but these studies all fall outside the age-related sample of this study. Nevertheless, the results are interesting and relevant to this study as they point to a positive impact of tactile play on food neophobia and/or food acceptance.

Another way of influencing food behaviour and promoting acceptance of healthy foods has been sought through a hands-on approach and cooking programmes. A review of the effect of cooking programmes by Utter, Fay, and Denny [43] concluded that cooking programmes may have a positive impact on food-related beliefs, knowledge, skills, and behaviours. Of the 20 studies included in the review, only three were on children in the age range of the sample group in the present study. However, none of the studies included in the review focused on foods of animal origin. Furthermore, observations of children's food behaviour and learning processes have been included in studies by, for example, Block et al. [44], Fisher and Birch [45], and Gibbs et al. [46]. The relevance of applying observation as a research method relates to the objective of revealing actual behaviour.

Nelson, Corbin, and Nickols-Richardsson [47] argue that culinary skills education offers a unique opportunity for experiential learning, which they illustrated through the use of the Kolb Cycle of Experiential Learning [48] combined with culinary skills education (Figure 1).

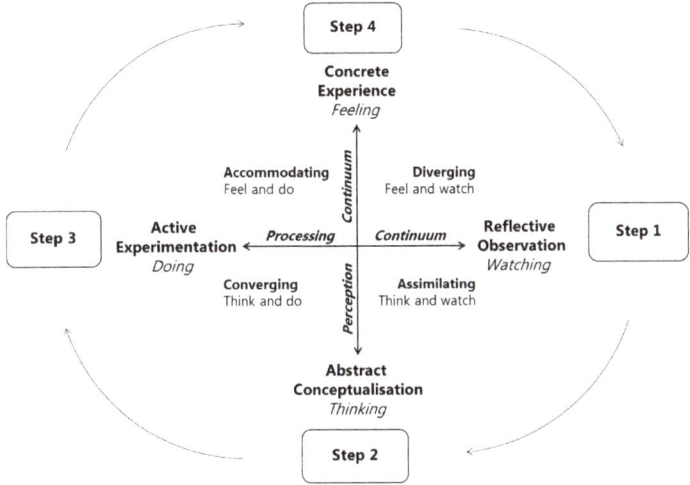

Figure 1. Model of culinary skills education as a process for Kolb's cycle of experiential learning developed by Nelson, Corbin, and Nickols-Richardsson [47]. Figure by first author R. Højer.

According to Nelson et al. [47], culinary skills education promotes knowledge through experience, as illustrated in Figure 1. As students move from observational to experiential learning stages and engage in culinary concepts, a foundation for promoting critical thinking and learning skills and technical proficiencies is laid out, all aimed at promoting healthy food behaviour. Furthermore, Nelson et al. [47] conclude that nutrition knowledge alone, aimed at promoting healthy food behaviour, seems incomplete without the dimension of experiential learning via interactions with food and cooking equipment.

1.1.2. The Subject Food Knowledge

In 2014, the subject Food Knowledge replaced the subject Home Economics as part of a reform of the Danish compulsory primary and lower secondary schools. The subject is mandatory for one year and can be taken in 4th, 5th, or 6th grade. In the subject Food Knowledge, students focus on four areas of competencies: Food and Health, Knowledge of Food, Cooking and Dining, and Food Cultures. The purpose of the reform was to ensure that Food Knowledge provides students with an opportunity to work with senses and experiences. Experimentation, creation, and communication in relation to food and meals are also key elements, as is the development of, for example, new skills and knowledge through motor skills, cognition, and perception [49].

1.1.3. Gyotaku Explained

Gyotaku is a traditional Japanese art form (see Figure 2); gyo is the Japanese for fish and taku for rubbing or printing: fish rubbing or fish printing [50].

Gyotaku was used by Japanese fishermen more than a hundred years ago [51]. To avoid misunderstanding, the fishermen used it to replicate the correct size of the fish, whereby it became a documentation method. During the twentieth century, the practice of gyotaku has been turned into an art form.

As an example of an experiential exercise, gyotaku was adapted to firstly include a tactile art exercise, which was the traditional part of the exercise to be explored in this study. Secondly, after the art part of the exercise in which the fish served as an art medium, the fish would then be included in a cooking exercise. The gyotaku exercise was chosen for its novelty in a Danish context and for its tactile hands on approach to the fish.

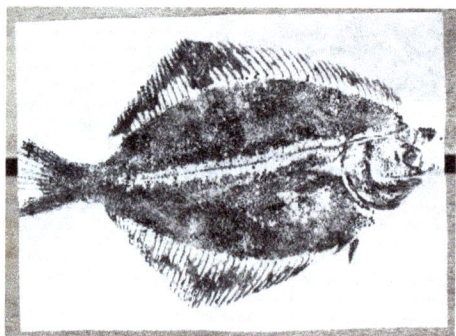

Figure 2. Gyotaku of flounder *(Platichthys flesus)*, artist: R. Højer, photo: Marilyn Koitnurm.

1.2. Study Aim

The aim of this study was to promote children's acceptance of fish. Based on the hypothesis that through hands on experience with fish it is possible to promote acceptance of fish, the objective of this study was, through an intervention, to explore the potential of a sensory-based experiential exercise in a school setting with focus on cooking and tactile play as a way of promoting 11- to 13-year-old children's acceptance of fish. The two main research questions to be answered were: (1) how do children respond to handling, preparing and cooking fresh fish? and (2) how does the process of the sensory-based tactile experiment gyotaku affect children's acceptance of fish?

2. Materials and Methods

2.1. Study Design

This study was an intervention with a multiple-case study design [52]. Six cases in six different classes from six different schools were included in the intervention. All participating classes underwent the experiential gyotaku exercise one class at a time. The qualitative method used to collect data consisted of participant observation [53].

The gyotaku exercise was integrated into the (in Denmark) compulsory subject Food Knowledge (*Danish: Madkundskab*) [49] in the fifth and sixth grades and it meets the official learning goals (for 2017–2018 and 2019) for the subject Food Knowledge set by the Ministry of Children and Education [54].

Ethics Approval

Ethics approval for this study was given by the joint Research Ethics Committee of the Faculty of Science and the Faculty of Health and Medical Sciences, University of Copenhagen, Denmark (reference 504-0005/17-5000).

2.2. Participants

We recruited six classes from fifth and sixth grades (11 to 13 years of age) from six different Danish public schools ($n = 132$). Four classes were from the capital region and two from the region of Zealand (see Table 1 for participant characteristics). Recruitment was geographically limited to the eastern part of Denmark due to convenience. The recruitment was done by sending out information letters via e-mail to schools in the eastern part of Denmark addressed to the school's Food Knowledge teachers. For all participating children, written informed consent was given by the legally appointed caregiver parent or either parent if the parents were married or had joint custody. Children's refusal to touch, handle, and/or taste the fish was respected by the researchers.

Table 1. Participant characteristics.

School	Classes	Grade	n	Sex (♀/♂)	Teachers *
School SA **	1	6th	32	21/11	2
School SB	1	6th	24	14/10	2
School SC	1	5th	18	10/8	2
School MB ***	1	6th	21	13/8	1
School MC	1	5th	18	9/9	1
School MD	1	6th	19	11/8	1
Total	6		132	78/54	9

* Number of teachers present during the gyotaku exercise. ** Schools SA, SB, and SC are schools from workshops during Science Week 2016. *** Schools MB, MC, and MD are schools from the main study 2017.

2.3. Setting and Gyotaku Exercise

School SA, SB, and SC took part in gyotaku workshops in a teaching kitchen at the Department of Food Science at the University of Copenhagen, Frederiksberg, Denmark, in a field trip setting. School MB, MC, and MD were in their natural educational setting, since the gyotaku exercise took place on three different occasions at schools in the ordinary school teaching kitchen. This differentiated setup was due to practical organization as the classes SA, SB and SC participated as part of Science Week 2016, a yearly returning science festival in Denmark, whereas the classes MB, MC, and MD did not participate in Science Week 2016 and data were collected during early spring 2017. All classes carried out the gyotaku exercises based on the same exercise guide.

The sensory-based experiential exercise was a four-phase exercise consisting of a) gyotaku (fish printing), which also gave its name to the complete experiment, b) filleting a fish, c) cooking the fish fillets by a commonly used Danish method, and d) tasting.

Materials for the gyotaku experiment (per group of four children): one fresh whole flatfish with head (either dab (*Limanda limanda*) or flounder (*Platichthys flesus*)), one lemon, squid ink diluted with tap water in a cup, a small sponge, five A4 pieces of paper cut into eight equal parts, paper towels, printing paper, a cutting board, a sharp filleting knife, rye flour, salt, pepper, butter, rye bread, a frying pan, a stove and written experimental instructions.

General organisation: all of the children worked in groups of four. Each group received one fresh fish to be shared during printing, filleting, and cooking (1 fish = 4 fillets).

Phase a: Gyotaku (printing): The printing procedure was the actual gyotaku exercise. The children chose and picked up their group's fish from a box containing fresh fish on ice. The fish was then cleaned by washing it under cold running water while rubbing it with a slice of fresh lemon (this dissolves the fish's natural mucus cover). The fish was then dried with paper towels and placed on a cutting board. Paper squares were placed around the edge of the fish to avoid getting squid ink on the cutting board. Diluted squid ink was applied with a sponge to the surface of the fish until it was covered with ink. The paper squares around the fish were removed, and printing paper was placed on top of the fish. The print was transferred to the paper by stroking the fish on top of the paper. The paper was gently pulled off the fish, and a mirrored print of the fish had been transferred to the paper (see Figure 2).

Phase b: Filleting: If they wanted to, each child in the group filleted their own fish fillet by following the handout picture instructions. After the child had felt the fillet with his/her fingers to ensure that no fish bones were present, the fillet was ready to be cooked.

Phase c: Cooking: The fish fillets were turned in rye flour containing salt and pepper and were then fried in butter on a hot pan. This is the traditional way of cooking fish fillets in Danish cuisine.

Phase d: Tasting: The fried fish fillets were served on a slice of rye bread with butter and a slice of lemon. Tasting/eating was voluntary. This is a common way of serving fish fillets in Danish cuisine.

After the experiment, the children could take the gyotaku home, or the school could use it, for example in an art exhibition.

2.4. Data Collection—Participant Observation

The participant observation was primarily concept-driven [55] and based on the framework of Rozin and Fallon's [23] and Rozin and Vollmecke's [27] taxonomy of food rejection and acceptance. Therefore, a loosely structured observation guide, with room for exploratory inquiry, was constructed based on the main framework of acceptance and rejection with the following themes: (1) the social/group interaction element, (2) the children's interaction with the fish, (3) the process of the exercise, and (4) development/changes in attitude throughout the experiment. Documentation methods used during the participant observation were in the form of written field notes and situational photos to document the setting, various situations, and child–fish interactions. The field note strategy was inscription and transcription [55], in which descriptions of behaviours (inscriptions) and informants' own words and dialogues (transcription) were recorded in an observational journal based on the loosely constructed and pre-thematised observational guide.

The same researcher participated in all gyotaku exercises by observing and interacting with the children through informal conversations based on the observation guide. In all cases except two (school MB and MD), observation assistants were present throughout the gyotaku exercise. At schools SA, SB, SC, three observation assistants were present, and at school MC one observation assistant was present. In all cases, the observation assistants had a semi-participatory role while also documenting the gyotaku exercise through photos. During the participant observations, researchers and assistants interacted with the children through informal conversations based on the situation while the children were working with the fish. Questions were based on "free narrative" [56] to promote situational comfort and to get and keep the conversation flowing. The questions were directed towards the children's perspectives of the situational experiences; for example (to the whole group): "How is it going here?" and "How do you feel about filleting a fish?". Probing [53] was used to follow up on short answers, for example "Can you tell me some more about that?". The focus was on informality and conversations steered by the children and their point of view. If a child asked what had been written down during a conversation, he/she was given the opportunity to read it. After each observation session, observational journals and photos were compared and evaluated. Post-intervention notes were documented by the research group. Furthermore, the field notes in the observational journal were immediately after the observation separated into direct observations of behaviour, dialogues based on children's peer-to-peer dialogues and researcher–child dialogues, and researcher reflections. A pre-coding was conducted based on concept-driven coding [55]; for example based on the framework of acceptance and rejection [25,27], fish handling, sensory aspects, and group work.

2.5. Data Analytical Method

Data analysis was conducted by using Applied Thematic Analysis (ATA) developed by Guest, MacQueen, and Namey [57]. ATA was applied to identify themes and to analyse patterns of meaning in relation to the research questions under study and was chosen for its flexibility with regard to type of texts, for example field notes [57], and its ability to highlight similarities and differences across cases [58].

Through a concept-driven [55] processing of data based on the research questions, four meta-themes were identified by organizing the pre-coded text into a matrix based on the frequency of re-occurrence of documented observed behaviours and dialogues. The identified meta-themes were rejection, acceptance, craftsmanship, and interaction. A thematic map was constructed to create a visual outline of possible sub-themes [57,58]. Finally, themes were re-considered to ensure accurate representation by re-reading the data set [57,58]. (See Figure 3 for presentation of the ATA data processing. This resulted in the appearance of sub-theme clusters as situational events, behaviours, etc. (see Figure 4).

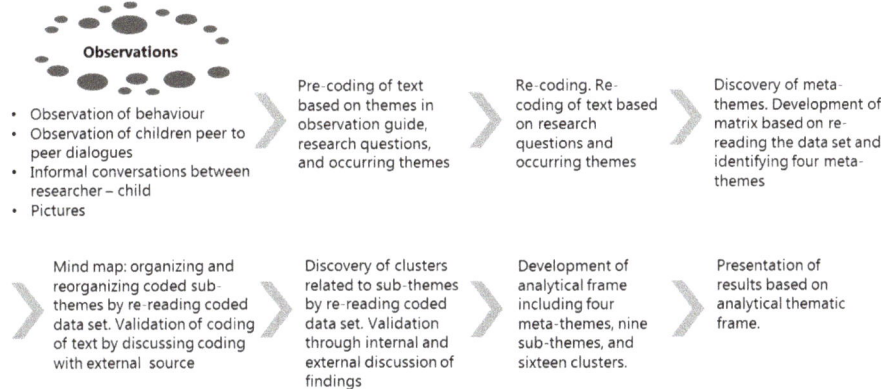

Figure 3. The ATA (Applied Thematic Analysis) data processing.

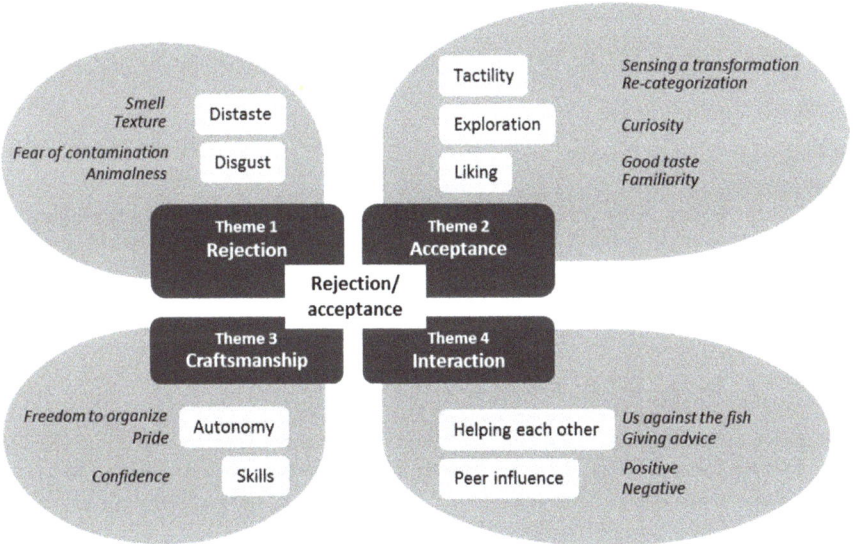

Figure 4. ATA frame for presentation of data: main category, meta-themes, sub-themes, and related clusters.

Data not relevant for the research questions were excluded from the data set and analysis after being re-read to ensure lack of relevance. Furthermore, the ATA frame (analysis, results, and discussion hereof) was read by and discussed with researchers within the research group, but for those who had not been present at the interventions the frame was read by and discussed with an experienced researcher outside of the research group.

The essence of meta-themes and sub-themes are presented in Table 2. Data were not only sorted by meta-theme and sub-theme but also by exercise phase (see Table A1: Data set).

Table 2. Essence of meta-themes and sub-themes.

	Meta-Theme/Sub-Theme	Essence
1.	Rejection: distaste and disgust	The theme 'rejection' concerns children's behaviour and verbal expressions that can be characterised as distaste or disgust as defined by Martins and Pliner [25], Rozin and Fallon [24], and Angyal [35]; distaste is defined as a sensory-driven reaction (e.g., smell, touch, taste, appearance, texture, sound), and disgust as a concern with contamination or being soiled as a result of contact with what is perceived as animal bodily waste products. The latter is defined by observed body language, for example turning away, holding a hand in front of the mouth and/or nose, mimicking nausea and/or vomiting, etc. [24,35]. The theme refers to observed behaviour and verbal expressions motivated by any interaction with the fresh fish, which could promote or is a direct rejection of tasting the cooked fish at the end of the experiment. Rejection could also be a result of a perception of a food [27].
2.	Acceptance: tactility, exploration, and liking	The theme "acceptance" concerns children's behaviour and verbal expressions concerning tactility, limited to include the sense of touch with the hands, exploration driven by curiosity, and liking, which refers to a positive affective response to food. Acceptance is understood as a willingness to taste the food, but it can then be rejected. Acceptance does not depend on liking, since other motives can exist for accepting a food (e.g., for its health benefits) [24,27].
3.	Craftsmanship: autonomy and skills	The theme "craftsmanship" concerns observed behaviour and verbal expressions related to the defined activity of preparation and cooking. Craftsmanship is understood as a physical, bodily practice that leads to a tactile experience and relational understanding [59]. Craftsmanship covers a tacit experience-based set of knowledge and skills within cooking – in this case, the fish. Even though Sennett [59] defines craftsmanship as "the skill of making things well", in this case the effort and attempt matter just as much, and maybe more than the outcome, an approach also supported by Martin [60]. In craftsmanship, Martin [60] underlines the importance of creating an environment in which the child feels independent and thereby learns by making decisions. In this space of autonomy, intrinsic motivation may promote pride in the work, thereby increasing curiosity with regard to tasting the fish.
4.	Interaction: helping each other and peer influence	The theme "interaction" refers to observed behaviour and verbal expressions related to social facilitation either related to the children helping each other or by peer influence. Through behaviour and verbal expressions, the children might influence each other with regard to accepting or rejecting the fish at the end of the experiment [27,61,62].

3. Results

In Figure 4 two main categories, four meta-themes, nine related sub-themes, and sixteen clusters *(italic)* are presented.

Data are presented according to the ATA frame (Figure 4) by including relevant examples from the data set to support the ATA. Abbreviations applied in the analysis: Obs: observation, ic: informal conversation. Phases of the exercise: $^{\#1}$ = Before printing; $^{\#2}$ = During printing; $^{\#3}$ = Between printing and filleting; $^{\#4}$ = During filleting; $^{\#5}$ = Frying; $^{\#6}$ = Tasting.

3.1. Meta-Theme 1: Rejection

3.1.1. Sub-Theme: Distaste

Rejection based on distaste, which includes all sensory characteristics, both real or imagined [25,26], was based on two main sensory characteristics: smell and texture. Rejection based on smell was primarily present in two phases of the experiment. Firstly, at the beginning of the printing phase when the children were presented with the fresh fish:

$^{\#1}$ When the lid is removed from the fish on ice, several children say: *"Ugh, it smells fishy"* [in a bad way] (School all, obs.)

Secondly, smell was a source of rejection based on distaste in the final experiment phase (tasting):

$^{\#6}$ Some children do not want to taste the fish. Int.: *"Why?"* Response: *"It smells of fish. We know we do not like fish because it feels weird in the mouth"*. A girl says: *"That is also why my dad does not like fish"* (School MC, ic).

Furthermore, the texture of the fish in the mouth was a factor in rejecting the fish based on distaste:

$^{\#6}$ A girl nibbles on the fried fish: *"I don't like the fish. It is kind of ... mushy"*. (School MD, obs).

$^{\#6}$ Everyone in the class tastes the fried fish, but three boys spit it out and agree that they do not like to chew it as it is too mushy and soft in the mouth. (School MB, obs).

3.1.2. Sub-Theme: Disgust

Apart from behaviours and verbal expressions promoting rejection based on distaste, rejection was also observed for the affective response of disgust.

Fear of contamination was observed primarily in two situations. Firstly, at the beginning of the experiment (phase a) when children picked up the fresh fish using only the tips of their thumb and index finger as shown in Figure 5. Most often the task of picking up the fish would be done by two children going to the fish box. One would pick up the fish (as illustrated in Figure 5) while the child not picking up the fish would often stand in the background in order to not get too close to the fish, although still leaning forward to have a look.

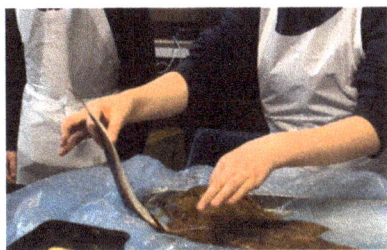

Figure 5. A display of disgust: picking up the fish, photo: R. Højer.

Secondly, in relation to filleting (phase b):

#4 Several children put on latex gloves before starting filleting (School MB, obs.).

Rejections driven by disgust also appeared as a reaction to the idea of "animalness". These reactions were also predominant at the beginning of the experiment (phase a) and during the filleting phase (phase b):

#1 Girl, when fish has been collected: *"Yuck! Look, it has eyes"* [pinches her nose] (School SC, obs).

#4 Int.: *How is it going with filleting the fish?* The girl cutting responds: *"I think that sound when you kind of hit the bone with the knife and that sound it makes . . . ugh"* [shrugs] (School MD, ic).

#4 Girl, during filleting: *"Yuck, it has fish guts inside* [viscera]*"* [she pinches her nose and turns away, holding her hands in front of her mouth] (School MD, obs).

3.2. Meta-Theme 2: Acceptance

3.2.1. Sub-Theme: Tactility

Acceptance through tactility was observed in two forms: "sensing a transformation" and "reduction of animalness" through the sense of touch and a re-categorisation of the fish from animal to non-animal. The former displayed itself at the beginning of the experiment (phase a) after the fish's natural mucus layer had been washed and removed:

#1 Boy group after washing the fish: they stroke it and agree that it is weird because it was so slimy before but now it is soft to the touch (School MD, obs).

When the children started the printing process (phase a), it seemed like the fish had been re-categorised from animal to an art medium. Touching the fish was no longer an issue:

#2 During the printing process, great attention is given to getting the right amount of ink on the eyes, fins, and the mouth to get them onto the paper. This is done by unfolding the fins with their fingers and dabbing the sponge lightly on the eyes, fins, and the mouth (School all, obs.).

#2 Between prints, the fish is gently patted and stroked by several children; it is "tickled" between the eyes and around the mouth (School all, obs).

3.2.2. Sub-Theme: Exploration

Exploration was predominant in two main scenarios: exploring the fish before and after filleting (phase b). There were clear signs of curiosity, as shown in the following example:

#3 A girl is exploring the fish. She opens the fish's mouth and looks into it: *"I just had to look inside. You can see its teeth . . . I just had to touch"*. Another girl in the group: *"Ohh yes, its mouth can get really big"*. The first girl replies: *"Yes, it can eat big fish"* (School MC, ic).

This exploratory scenario is also seen in Figure 6 with children putting their fingers in the fish's mouth to feel its teeth.

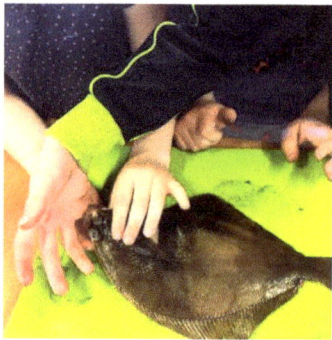

Figure 6. Children exploring the fish, photo: R. Højer.

After filleting, children explored the fish:

#4 Roe in fish: at first the children do not want to touch or even look, but after a while they start to pick at it with the knife tip, and then cut it, mash it, and study the small eggs (School SA, SB, SC, obs.).

Both exploratory scenarios led to a greater child interaction with the fish.

3.2.3. Sub-Theme: Liking

Acceptance due to liking was primarily driven by the sensory characteristic "taste" (the fish tasted good). It also seemed like taste familiarity was a factor in liking it.

#6 A girl is eating her fish fillet: *"Mmm, I love fish fillet"* Int.: *"Why?"* Girl: *"It is kind of a little bit sweet but also just good. We also get it at home"* (School MD, ic).

#6 A girl tastes a little bit of roasted fish roe and says: *"Mmm, it actually tastes like cod roe . . . but it is a little bit grainy and dry in the mouth"* (School MD, obs).

3.3. Meta-Theme 3: Craftsmanship

3.3.1. Sub-Theme: Autonomy

Throughout the experiment, autonomy was a sub-theme, since all of the assignments were carried out through group negotiation and decision-making; there was freedom to organise the work themselves (no teacher involvement), for example, who should pick up the fish, who should fry the fish etc. Pride in their work was especially evident during printing (phase a) and filleting (phase b):

#3 After the printing, children show their self-made print to teachers and other groups (School all, obs).

#4 They want to try to fillet the fish themselves. The experimenter (first author) is not allowed to help too much, only to correct them if they have made a wrong cut (School all, obs).

3.3.2. Sub-Theme: Skills

Skills were developed, particularly in the filleting process (phase b). It was observed that the children initially had difficulties in holding the knife correctly and actually filleting the fish. During the filleting process, they became more confident in using the knife and in how to fillet the fish (School all, obs.). During cooking (phase c), skills were developed when they were trained how to cook a fish for the correct amount of time:

#5 While frying the fish, the children are very preoccupied with cooking it for the right amount of time so it is not raw, but they are also focused on not cooking it for too long. They comment on the colour and use it as a way of telling if it is done (School all, obs).

A clear indication of the acquired skills can be seen in the following extract:

#5 After frying the fish, a girl says: *"Ah, now I know how to make fish fillet. I would like to try it at home if mom will buy a fish"* (School MC, ic).

3.4. Meta-Theme 4: Interaction

3.4.1. Sub-Theme: Helping Each Other

The sub-theme "helping each other" appeared primarily as "us against them/the fish" and giving advice. A concept of "we are in this together" and "us against the fish" appeared, particularly at the beginning of the experiment (phase a), where the children had to pick up the fish and prepare it for printing:

#1 Two girls are washing and drying a dab before printing. They help each other by holding the fish at each end and carrying it together to the printing table (School MC, obs.).

Children also helped each other when washing the fish to remove the fish skin mucus prior to the printing (phase a). For example, one child supported the fish's tail, while another rubbed it with a lemon slice to remove mucus from the fish. Furthermore, helping each other was observed when, for example, applying the ink and giving advice on how to apply ink to the fish during printing, and giving advice on how to make a correct cut with the knife during the filleting phase (phase b):

#4 The girls give advice on how and where to cut: *"You have to start with the moon-shaped cut there"*. The boys correct each other more often (School MB, obs).

3.4.2. Sub-Theme: Peer Influence

Peer influence was observed throughout the exercise and resulted in the other children in the group reacting either positively or negatively to the fish. The following two extracts illustrate peer influence leading to a positive reaction to the fish (the first extract) and a negative reaction to the fish (the second extract):

#3 After printing, two girls in a group of four are touching the fish, while the other two do not want to touch it. After observing the girls touching the fish for a little while, the other two girls change their mind and come over to the fish and try to touch it (School MB, obs.).

#6 Everyone in the class tastes the fried fish, but three boys from the same group spit it out and agree that they do not like to chew it as it is too mushy and soft in the mouth (first one boy spits it out, then the rest of the group) (School MB, obs).

The ATA is summarised visually in Figure 7, which shows meta-themes, sub-themes, and predominant clusters within identified sub-themes related to the different phases in the experiment.

			Phase a: Printing			Phase b: Filleting	Phase c: Cooking	Phase d: Tasting
Theme	**Sub-theme**	**Cluster**	#1 Before printing	#2 During printing	#3 Between print/fillet	#4 Filleting	#5 Frying	#6 tasting
Rejection	Distaste	Smell	+*					+
		Texture						+
	Disgust	Fear of contamination	+			+		
		Animalness	+			+		
Acceptance	Tactility	Sensing a transformation	+	+				
		Re-categorization		+				
	Exploration	Curiosity			+	+		
	Liking	Good taste						+
		Familiarity						+
Craftsmanship	Autonomy	Freedom to organize	+	+	+	+	+	
		Pride		+		+		
	Skills	Confidence				+	+	
Interaction	Helping each other	Us against the fish	+					
		Giving advice		+		+		
	Peer influence	Positive	+			+		+
		Negative	+			+		+

* '+' indicates observations and/or verbal expressions identified related to theme/sub-theme/cluster and experiment phase

Figure 7. Applied thematic analysis (ATA) summary visualised.

4. Discussion

Based on thematic analysis, we propose the following diagram to explain a rejection–acceptance continuum (Figure 8).

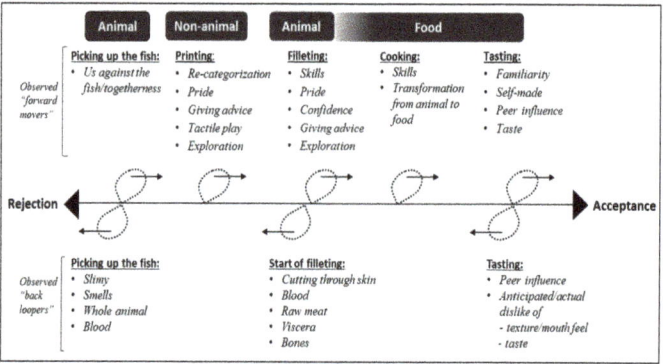

Figure 8. A rejection–acceptance continuum based on fish categorisation with examples of elements driving acceptance forward or backwards. Developed by first author Højer, inspired by and Rozin and Fallon [24].

Figure 8 illustrates elements which drive either rejection or acceptance along the continuum. Our observations on the categorisation and re-categorisation of the fish as animal, non-animal, and food were in line with what Rozin and Fallon [63] and Martins and Pliner [25] refer to as "animalness". This animalness can be reduced in a fish by, for example, removing the head and bones, cutting it up, cooking it, and serving it without it resembling what it is: a fish and an animal [63].

At the beginning of the exercise, the fish was categorised as an animal due to its smell, slimy texture, and visual appearance (whole animal with head, fins, blood, etc.) and thereby promoted rejection. The whole fish represented a high degree of animalness, since it did not resemble what the children would typically eat (a breaded fish fillet). According to the results of a Danish citizen science project on Danes' fish eating habits, the hot fish dish most often eaten by children was breaded fish fillet (39%), and in the form of cold cuts (eaten on rye bread) the favourites were mackerel in tomato sauce (33%) and fish cakes (21%) [64]. According to Fischler [65], this could be categorized as gastro-anomie, because the consumer has problems in identifying food and food origin as a result of processing [65]. Rejection based on animalness was also found in a Norwegian study on adolescents' (16 to 17 years of age) attitudes towards meat from farm animals. Females, in particular, rejected meat due to its association with, for example, blood and animal parts [66]. The study also found that participants in regular contact with farm animals displayed no disgust reaction and had a more relaxed attitude towards meat production [66]. In an empirical study on what motivates food disgust, Martins and Pliner [25] found that animalness was not the complete explanation for a food disgust reaction, as non-animal food products were also capable of promoting disgust. According to Martins and Pliner [25], an explanation could be found in the experienced texture of, for example, slime, as it could be related to decay. Through multidimensional scaling analysis, they were able to identify independent (i.e., unique) dimensions, suggesting that both aversive textural properties and the reminders of animalness are primary variables accounting for perceptions of food disgust [25,67]. Egolf, Siegrist, and Hartmann [28] also found in their study on how people's food disgust sensitivity shapes eating and food behaviour that surface texture of food was capable of promoting disgust.

According to our observations during the printing phase, the fish was re-categorised from animal to non-animal, because it was perceived as an art/play medium and rejection cues were not evident. In this phase, tactility through touching the fish, as part of the assignment of printing, appeared to promote acceptance of the fish. This observation correlates with the findings of Coulthard and Sealy [38], who found that pre-school children tried more fruits and vegetables after participating in a sensory play activity with real fruits and vegetables than children in a non-food sensory play task ($p < 0.001$) and in a visual exposure task ($p < 0.001$). Similar results were also found by Nederkoorn, Theißen, Tummers, and Roefs [41]: tactility increased the acceptance of food with the same texture.

The observed acceptance could also be promoted by the reduction in mucus on the fish after washing, which would reduce the texture-induced disgust as proposed by Martins and Pliner [25]. Nevertheless, this does not account for the following tactile exploration of the fish, where the children, driven by curiosity about something unfamiliar, put their fingers in the fish's mouth, touched the gills, eyes, tongue, etc., with all parts of the fish still covered by or containing mucus (see Figure 6).

At the beginning of the filleting phase of the exercise, the fish was again categorised as an animal, and rejection was promoted. A behavioural example was the observation of the children putting on latex gloves in this phase, although this behaviour could also be a result of peer influence.

Rejection was primarily due to the cutting through of the skin of the fish and cutting close to the bones. Both sound and visual cues reminded them that they were cutting into an animal, thereby increasing the perceived animalness. Later in the filleting phase, the fish were re-categorised from animal to food, because the fish was now fish fillets. The bones, skin, viscera, head, etc. were disposed of. What remained was a form of the fish that was familiar to the children: fish fillets. Applying Lévi-Strauss' [68] concept of nature-culture, we see that, through the filleting process, the fish had gone from a natural form to a more cultivated form, and through the frying of the fish the final step in the cultivating process had been reached.

Furthermore, during the filleting and cooking phase, the children started to learn technical skills, and they clearly took pride in their work, which could be an expression of what Sennett [59] calls the emotional reward for attaining a skill and doing it well, like a craftsman. This finding of promoted self-efficacy, as defined by Bandura [69], is supported by the findings of Cunningham-Sabo and Lohse [70] in an interventional study with fourth-graders. Not only did they find an increase in cooking and food self-efficacy but also an increase in fruit and vegetable preference. Most notable is the finding that non-cookers particularly benefitted from the intervention [70]. An increase in cooking efficacy was also confirmed in a similar study including an experiential approach by Jarpe-Ratner, Folkens, Sharma, Daro, and Edens [71], although no definition of the concept experiential was given.

At the end of the experiment, the fish were fried, and the re-categorisation from animal to food was complete. Observations showed that the majority of children chose to taste and eat the fish fillet on rye bread; the reason given was the good taste, a reason corresponding to the findings of Sick, Højer, and Olsen [29] in a study on children's self-evaluated reasons for accepting and rejecting foods.

Rejection was promoted by, for example, the texture of the cooked fish in the mouth. Rejection of fish based on texture was found by Donadini, Fumi, and Porretta [72], where fish was rejected due to softness, a jelly-like texture, fast melting, and tendency to fall apart easily textures. Texture was also found to be a key rejection characteristic by Sick, Højer, and Olsen [29]. For the children that showed reluctance throughout the experiment and ended up tasting the fish fillet, an "I filleted and cooked it myself" effect could be a possible explanation. A similar effect of "I cooked it myself" was found by Dohle, Rall, and Siegrist [73] and Allirot, da Quinta, Chokupermal, and Urdaneta [74]. Allirot et al. [74] and van der Horst, Ferrage, and Rytz [75] also point to the context or atmosphere in which the food exposure took place and the "cooking together" factor as relevant factors impacting food likes and dislikes and thereby promoting acceptance or rejection. Since the gyotaku experiment took place in a school(-like) setting, the "cooking together" and "helping each other" factors promoted acceptance of fish. According to Lukas and Cunningham-Sabo [76], there is a difference between cooking with friends and classmates. In a qualitative study, they found that classmates were typically associated with rules, structure, and restrictions, while friends are defined by fun and freedom [76]. Yet, when Lukas and Cunningham-Sabo [76] compared data across focus groups, they found that the cooking and tasting group did not make a clear distinction between classmates and friends, and the children in this group seemed to consider their classmates as friends in this "cooking together" context. This was not the case in the two other groups. However, other studies [77,78] have not found a correlation between an experience-based approach and positive change in acceptance, preference or liking of foods.

5. Strengths and Limitations

This section considers the credibility, transferability, dependability, and confirmability [53,79] of the study findings.

Credibility was sought in this study by comparing the findings with those of previous studies that have focused on similar research. Furthermore, to reduce observer bias, observer assistants were present in all but two cases, and after the experiment had ended, dialogues took place between the experimenter and assistant regarding what had been observed. Dependability was sought via a thorough description of the study design and the gyotaku experiment itself in order to ensure that other researchers are able to execute a study in a similar way. Even though true objectivity of the researcher rarely exists, confirmability was sought through a sampling process, whereby the participating classes entered the study according to the rule of "first responders to the information letter" sent out via email (regional) and shared in a Food-Knowledge-specific Facebook group for teachers (national).

Geographically, the data were only collected in the eastern part of Denmark. Therefore, in terms of transferability, it could be said that this case study is not representative of the general population of children in Denmark. Nevertheless, the findings can be seen as indications transferable to similar contexts, since the observations seemed stable and comparable across the cases (schools and classes). Furthermore, even though the experiment varied in terms of setting, the observations across the two settings seemed stable and comparable. Additionally, a research participation effect [80] cannot be completely eliminated as the presence of the research and assistant group in the gyotaku experiment situation is an addition to the typical setting situation. Furthermore, analysis and ATA frame was validated by a researcher not part of the study, but with extensive research experience to reduce bias.

Even though more research in this area is needed, this finding opens up the possibility of transferring the gyotaku exercise and the expected outcome to settings outside the conventional school setting.

We recognise that the present study holds certain limitations investigation-wise that need to be addressed in future research. One such limitation is the aspect of how children categorise and re-categorise fish and how this is connected to the experimental context, the school arena. Furthermore, a more focused investigation of how tactile play might influence children's acceptance of food, especially outside the area of fruit and vegetables, is warranted.

6. Conclusions

With regard to how children responded to handling, preparing, and cooking the fish and how the process of the gyotaku experiment affected the acceptance, we identified that response of rejection and acceptance moved back and forth on a continuum. Rejection was driven by slimy touch, whole animal, smell, cutting through skin, texture of fish meat in the mouth, and taste, and acceptance was promoted by togetherness, helping each other, tactile play, re-categorisation of the fish, exploration, pride, skills, and was self-made. Furthermore, the movement back and forth was determined by how the fish was categorised (as animal, non-animal, or food). The study revealed that autonomy, skills, pride, and helping each other in the groups were important factors in promoting acceptance, whereas the texture of the fish, for example, led to rejection. Furthermore, we found that using the fish as a creative medium for tactile play became an important motivator in promoting acceptance. The findings in this study highlight that cooking combined with tactile play could be a way of promoting acceptance of fish, and as such serve as a potential strategy in promoting healthy food behaviour. The same exercise could be used with other food groups as well, for example with vegetables, fruit, chicken (e.g., print of feet or wings before preparing) etc. where the squid ink is substituted with berry juice or beet root juice. At the same time, our findings support the importance of the school setting and the subject Food Knowledge as a potential experiential learning gateway to promoting healthy food behaviour through focusing on children's food and culinary knowledge and skills, which has also been recommended by Nelson et al. [47].

Author Contributions: Conceptualization and methodology, R.H., K.W. and M.B.F.; data collection and data analyses, R.H., interpretation of data, R.H., K.W. and M.B.F., writing of the manuscript, R.H., review and editing, K.W. and M.B.F., supervision and funding acquisition, M.B.F. All authors have read and agreed to the published version of the manuscript.

Funding: This work is part of the research project Smag for Livet (Taste for Life) and was partly funded by the Nordea Foundation, Denmark, and by University College Absalon, Center for Nutrition and Rehabilitation, Nutrition and Health, Slagelsevej 70-74, 4180 Sorø, Denmark. The funding parties had no involvement in the work.

Acknowledgments: A special thank you to Margit Dall Aaslyng, University College Absalon, Center for Nutrition and Rehabilitation, Nutrition and Health, Sorø, Denmark, for invaluable comments provided in relation to the applied thematic analysis process.

Conflicts of Interest: The authors declare no conflict of interest with regard to authorship, research, funding and/or publication of this article.

Appendix A

Table A1. Data set: Meta-themes, sub-themes, and data extracts from field note journal (obs: observation *, ic: informal conversation **).

Meta-Theme	Sub-Theme	Data Extract
1. Rejection	Distaste	#1. When the lid is removed from the fish on ice, several children say "Ugh, it smells fishy" [in a bad way]. (School MB, MC, MD, SA, SB, SC, obs *).
		#6 Some children do not want to taste the fish.
		Int.: "Why?"
		Response: "It smells of fish", "We know we do not like fish because it feels weird in the mouth". A girl says: "That is also why my dad does not like fish" (School MC, ic**).
		#6 Int.: "Do you like the fish?" (asked to a girl group after frying the fish). Girl, not eating her fish fillet: "I do not like the smell of fish". (School SB, ic).
		#6 After tasting the fried fish fillet, a boy said: "Arhh, that is not for me".
		Int.: "How come?"
		Boy: "It feels mushy in my mouth and tastes fishy". (School SA, ic).
		#6 Two girls absolutely do not want to taste the fried fish, because they know that they do not like fish. (School SB, ic).
		#6 A girl nibbles at the fried fish: "I don't like the fish. It is kind of … mushy". (School MD, obs).
		#6 Three boys did not want to taste the fish: "We do not like the taste and smell of fish". (School SC, ic).
		#6 Everyone in the class tastes the fried fish, but three boys spit it out and agree that they do not like to chew it as it is too mushy and soft in the mouth. (School MB, obs).
		#1 When the lid is removed from the fresh fish, many children react by turning away from the fish, holding their hands in front of their mouth and/or nose, pinching their nose, mimicking vomiting, making "yuck" noises, closing their eyes, etc. (School MB, MC, MD, SA, SB, SC, obs).
		#1 "Ugh, it is GROSS and sooo slimy …".
		Some children mimic vomiting (School SA, obs **).
		#1 Girl, after fish has been cleaned and is placed on the cutting board: "It is not normal". (School MD, obs).
		#1 Girl, when fish has been collected: "Yuck! Look, it has eyes" [pinches her nose]. (School SC, obs).
		#1 A boy does not want to touch the fish: "It is slimy". [no special facial expression/body language]. (School MD, obs).
		#1 A boy pokes the fish before washing: "Ugh, it is sticky". (School MB, obs).
2.	Disgust	#1 Several children try to pick up the fish from the box using only the tips of their thumb and index finger (School MB, MC, MD, SA, SB, SC, obs).
		#2 A boy says that the fish is really disgusting, makes "yuck" sounds, but at the same time he cannot help himself poking it in the eye followed by big arm swings and screeching. Then he runs over to wash his fingers and goes back and pokes the fish again. (School MD, obs).
		#4 A group of girls purse their lips at the sight of blood from the fish. Some close their eyes and turn away from the fish. (School MD, obs).
		#4 Int.: How is it going with filleting the fish? (Question to a girl group). The girl cutting responds: "I think that sound when you kind of hit the bone with the knife and that sound it makes…. ugh" [shrugs] (School MD, ic).
		#4 During filleting. Girl: "Yuck, it has fish guts inside [visceral]". [she pinches her nose and turns away while holding her hands in front of her mouth]. (School MD, obs).
		#4 Several children put on latex gloves before starting filleting. (School MB, obs).
		#5 When the fillets have to be turned in breadcrumbs, they are moved/lifted by holding the fillet in the tail end with the tip of the thumb and index finger (to touch as little meat as possible). (School MB, MC, MD, SA, SB, SC, obs).

Table A1. *Cont.*

Meta-Theme	Sub-Theme	Data Extract
	Tactility	#1 After washing the fish. Girl, stroking the fish: *"It is kind of rough but now it is soft"*. (School MB, obs).
		#1 Boy group after washing the fish: they stroke it and agree that it is weird because it was so slimy before but is now soft to the touch (School MD, obs).
		#1 Int.: *"What was it like to touch the fish?"* Girl: *"It was fun because when you stroke it in the opposite direction, it was ... kind of rough"*. (School MC, ic).
		#2 During the printing process, great attention is given to getting the right amount of ink on the eyes, fins and the mouth to get them onto the paper. This is done by unfolding the fins with the fingers and dabbing the sponge lightly on the eyes, fins and the mouth (the girls are more aware of this than the boys). (School SA, SB, SC, MB, MC, and MD, obs).
		#2 Girl: *"Use your fingers, it's much easier"*. The group quickly shifts from using a spoon to using their fingers to ensure that the paper absorbs ink during the printing [stroking the fish on top of the paper]. (School MD, obs).
		#2 Between prints, the fish is gently patted and stroked by several children; it is 'tickled' between the eyes and around the mouth. (School MB, MC, MD, SA, SB, SC, obs).
		#3 A girl group are stroking their fish and give it a name (School SA, obs).
		#3 A girl group are gently stroking their fish, and a girl says: *"I can't eat it now"* (School SB, obs).
		#4 After the filleting process, they use their fingers to check for small bones in the fillets (School SA, SB, SC, MB, MC, and MD, obs).
		#2 A boy turns the fish to its white side and asks: *"Why is it white underneath?"* Int.: [gives an explanation]. Boy: *"Ohh, that is smart"*. (School MC, ic).
		#3 A girl is exploring the fish. She opens the fish's mouth and looks into it: *"I just had to look inside. You can see its teeth ... I just had to touch"*. Another girl in the group: *"Ohh yes, its mouth can get really big"*. The first girl replies: *"Yes, it can eat big fish"*. (School MC, ic).
2. Acceptance	Exploration	#3 The children open the mouth of the fish and feel inside with their fingers. Feeling the teeth, in particular, makes them more curious, and they keep exploring, also by touching the tongue. (School SA, SB, SC, MB, MC, and MD, obs).
		#3 Girl: *"Can you eat the squid ink?"* Int. *"Yes, you can. Do you want to taste it?"* More children gather around the table, and several of them taste the ink. *"Ugh, it is very salty"*. (School MC, ic).
		#3 After printing, a boy asks: *"Can you eat the eyes ... and may I?"* (School MB, obs).
		#3 Int.: *"Have you ever tried to open the mouth of a fish?"* Boy group: *"Nooo ... "*. Int.: *"Try it"*. A boy holds the fish, while another boy opens the mouth. All: *"Whoa!"*. (School MB, ic).
		#4 A girl says: *"The viscera are not disgusting but mysterious"*. (School MD, obs).
		#4 Boys start to explore the viscera of the fish. They ask what parts they are and whether they can be eaten. (School MB, MC, MD, SA, SB, SC, obs).
		#4 Boys start to pull out the intestines in their full length. (School SA, SC, obs).
		#4 Girls cutting roe out from the fish. Int.: *"Do you know what that is?"* Girl: *"No ... "*

115

Table A1. Cont.

Meta-Theme	Sub-Theme	Data Extract
		Other girl in group: "I do . . . it is roe. Can you eat it?"
		Int.: "Yes"
		Girl: "Let's try and fry it and taste it". (School SC, ic)
		#4 Roe in fish: first the children do not want to touch or even look, but after a while they start to pick at it with the knife tip and then cut it, mash it and study the small eggs. (School SA, SB, SC, obs).
		#1 Girl: "It smells good and bad at the same time" (School MD, obs).
		#1 Girl, when the lid is removed from the fish: "It smells fresh . . . of the sea and salt". (School MB, obs).
	Liking	#6 A girl who says that she does not like fish chooses to taste it anyway: "Ohh, but it tastes like chicken". (School MB, obs).
		#6 A girl eats fried roe: "Ohh, it tastes OK—just like the rest of the fish". (School SB, ic)
		#6 A boy fries the liver: "It tastes like chicken—not bad . . . like chicken and a little bit of blood". (School SB, obs)
		#6 A girl tastes a little bit of roasted fish roe and says: "Mmm, it actually tastes like cod roe . . . but it is a little bit grainy and dry in the mouth". (School MD, obs)
		#6. After the fish has been fried, a group of boys are talking about the taste of the fish. Boy: "It actually tastes good". Another boy replies: "Yes, much better than the ones I get at home". (School MC, ic)
		#6 Four boys taste the fried fish: "Yes, it is good". The other boys agree by nodding their heads. (School MD, obs).
		#6 A girl is eating her fish fillet: "Mmm, I love fish fillet"
		Int.: "Why?"
		Girl: "It is kind of a little bit sweet but also just good. We also get it at home". (School MD, ic)
		#6 Most children choose to taste the fried fish. Only a few do not eat all of it (School SA, SB, SC, obs).
		#all All assignments are carried out through group decision making and negotiation in the group (no teacher involvement), for example, who should pick up the fish, or who should fry the fish. (School MB, MC, MD, SA, SB, SC, obs).
	Autonomy	#2 A teacher wants to help a group with the printing, but the group says that they want to do it themselves. (School MC, obs).
		#3 After the printing, children show their self-made print to teachers and other groups. (School MB, MC, MD, SA, SB, SC, obs).
		#4 They want to try to fillet the fish themselves. I (the experimenter) am not allowed to help too much, only to correct them if they have made a wrong cut. (School MB, MC, MD, SA, SB, SC, obs).
		#4 A group asks for help with the filleting process, but the child holding the knife does not want to let it go (School MD, obs).
		#4 All of the children who filleted their own fish take great pride in their work; they show me their fillet and want me to praise them (prior to the filleting I made it clear that it was difficult and nobody can do it perfectly the first time they try it). (School MB, MC, MD, SA, SB, SC, obs).
3. Craftsman-ship		#1 Before printing, groups evaluate the freshness of the fish based on what they remember from the theme course material (they remember the video material better than that from the booklet). They evaluate the freshness by smelling and agree that the fish should smell of salt and seaweed. (School MC, obs).
	Skills	#2 During the printing process, great attention is given to applying the right amount of ink on all parts of the fish—this is more pronounced among the girls than the boys, who are more concerned with getting it done; a lot of them call me to show me their work. (School MB, MC, MD, SA, SB, SC, obs).
		#4 While filleting, several children refer to the You Tube video on filleting flatfish (a part of the theme course material): "You just have to let the knife do the work for you" becomes a phrase they repeat in the groups. (School MB, MC, MD, obs).
		#4 It is evident that the children are not used to filleting fresh fish; one class has been on a cooking camp where they worked with fish, but they did not try to fillet their own fish. (School MB, MC, MD, SA, SB, SC, obs/ic)

116

Table A1. Cont.

Meta-Theme	Sub-Theme	Data Extract
4. Child interaction	Helping each other	#4 When the children start to fillet, they have great difficulty in holding the filleting knife correctly. However, when they try to fillet their own fish, they become more confident in using the knife and hold it more correctly. (School MB, MC, MD, SA, SB, SC, obs).
		#5 When frying the fish, the children are very preoccupied with cooking it for the right amount of time, so it is not raw, but they are also focused on not cooking it for too long. They comment on the colour and use that as a way of telling if it is done. (School MB, MC, MD, SA, SB, SC, obs).
		#5 After frying the fish, a girl says: "*Ahh, now I know how to make fish fillet. I would like to try it at home if mom will buy a fish*". (School MC, ic).
		#all Groups are very preoccupied with justice; that all group members get to make a print, fillet and get to taste an equal amount of fish. (School MB, MC, MD, SA, SB, SC, obs).
		#1 Two girls are washing and drying a dab before printing. They help each other by holding the fish at each end and carrying it together to the printing table (School MC, obs).
		#1 Two boys are collecting the fish from the box. They end up picking it up together and carry it to the sink. (School SA, obs).
		#1 A boy and a girl are helping each other, holding the fish and washing it under running water; one of them holds the fish, while the other rubs it with lemon. (School SB, obs).
		#2 During printing, the group members give advice to the child applying the ink, for example in order to get ink on the eyes, mouth and fins. Advice is also given to avoid large ink blobs on the finished print. (School MB, MC, MD, SA, SB, SC, obs).
		#2 During printing, they help each other apply the ink correctly on the fish; they also help each other rub the paper and lift the fish print. (School MB, MC, MD, SA, SB, SC, obs).
		#2 The boys seem to correct each other, whereas the girls support each other (School MC, obs).
		#4 During the filleting, the group members give advice to the child filleting, for example, on how and where to cut. (School MB, MC, MD, SA, SB, SC, obs).
		#4 The girls give advice on how and where to cut: "*You have to start with the moon-shaped cut there*". However, the boys correct each other more often. (School MB, obs).
		#6 Before eating, the children help arrange the fish fillets on small platters, so it looks like a small dish, while others set the table. They all sit down and eat at two tables laid with cutlery, glasses, water jugs and napkins. (School MD, obs).
		#1 When the lid is removed from the box containing fish, the disgust behaviour spreads in small groups—if one person in the group reacts, the others react too. (School MB, MC, MD, SA, SB, SC, obs).
		#3 After printing, two girls in a group of four touch the fish, while the other two do not want to touch it. After observing the girls touching the fish for a little while, the other two girls change their mind and come over to the fish and try to touch it (School MB, obs).
	Peer influence	#4 While a group of boys explore the viscera and eyes of the fish, they challenge each other to touch the eye (School MC, obs).
		#4 During the filleting process, when children find viscera and roe in the fish, they start to react to it in the group. If one person reacts by holding a hand in front of the mouth, other group members react in a similar way. (School MB, MC, MD, SA, SB, SC, obs).
		#4 A girl does not want to fillet a fish, but after observing the other girls in her group, she ends up doing it (and even eating it after it has been fried). (School MB, obs).
		#6 Everyone in the class tastes the fried fish, but three boys from the same group spit it out and agree that they do not like to chew it as it is too mushy and soft in the mouth (first one boy spits it out, then the rest of the group). (School MB, obs).

Phase in the experiment: #1 = Before printing; #2 = During printing; #3 = Between printing and filleting; #4 = During filleting; #5 = Frying; #6 = Tasting; #all = All phases of the experiment. obs: observation *, ic: informal conversation **.

References

1. World Health Organization (WHO); South-East Asia Regional Office (SEARO). *Strategic Guidance on Acelerating Actions for Adolescent Health (2018–2022)*; WHO: Geneva, Switzerland, 2018; ISBN 9789290226475.
2. Hochberg, Z. Developmental plasticity in child growth and maturation. *Front. Endocrinol. Lausanne* **2011**, *2*, 41. [CrossRef] [PubMed]
3. Todd, A.S.; Street, S.J.; Ziviani, J.; Byrne, N.M.; Hills, A.P. Overweight and obese adolescent girls: The importance of promoting sensible eating and activity behaviors from the start of the adolescent period. *Int. J. Environ. Res. Public Health* **2015**, *12*, 2306. [CrossRef] [PubMed]
4. Alberga, A.S.; Sigal, R.J.; Goldfield, G.; Prud Homme, D.; Kenny, G.P. Overweight and obese teenagers: Why is adolescence a critical period? *Pediatr. Obes.* **2012**, *7*, 261–273. [CrossRef] [PubMed]
5. Birch, L.L.; Fisher, J.O. Development of eating behaviour among children. *Pediatrics* **1998**, *101*, 539–549.
6. Demory-Luce, D.; Morales, M.; Nicklas, T.; Baranowski, T.; Zakeri, I.; Berenson, G. Changes in food group consumption patterns from childhood to young adulthood: The Bogalusa Heart Study. *J. Am. Diet. Assoc.* **2004**, *104*, 1684–1691. [CrossRef] [PubMed]
7. Braegger, C.; Campoy, C.; Colomb, V.; Decsi, T.; Domellof, M.; Fewtrell, M.; Hojsak, I.; Mihatsch, W.; Molgaard, C.; Shamir, R.; et al. Vitamin d in the healthy European paediatric population. *J. Pediatr. Gastroenterol. Nutr.* **2013**, *56*, 692–701. [CrossRef] [PubMed]
8. Petersen, R.A.; Damsgaard, C.T.; Dalskov, S.M.; Sørensen, L.B.; Hjorth, M.F.; Ritz, C.; Kjølbæk, L.; Andersen, R.; Tetens, I.; Krarup, H.; et al. Vitamin D status and its determinants during autumn in children at northern latitudes: A cross-sectional analysis from the optimal well-being, development and health for Danish children through a healthy New Nordic Diet (OPUS) School Meal Study. *Br. J. Nutr.* **2016**, *115*, 239–250. [CrossRef] [PubMed]
9. Kelli, H.M.; Kassas, I. Cardio Metabolic Syndrome: A Global Epidemic. *J. Diabetes Metab.* **2016**, *6*. [CrossRef]
10. Mouritsen, O.G.; Bagatolli, L.A. *Life—As a Matter of Fat. Lipids in a Membrane Biophysics Perspective*; Springer International Publishing: New York, NY, USA, 2016; ISBN 978-3-319-22614-9.
11. Rondanelli, M.; Rigon, C.; Perna, S.; Gasparri, C.; Iannello, G.; Akber, R.; Alalwan, T.A.; Freije, A.M. Novel insights on intake of fish and prevention of sarcopenia: All reasons for an adequate consumption. *Nutrients* **2020**, *12*, 307. [CrossRef]
12. Balami, S.; Sharma, A.; Karn, R. Significance of Nutritional Value of Fish for Human Health. *Malays. J. Halal Res.* **2020**, *2*, 32–34. [CrossRef]
13. Khalili Tilami, S.; Sampels, S. Nutritional Value of Fish: Lipids, Proteins, Vitamins, and Minerals. *Rev. Fish. Sci. Aquac.* **2018**, *26*, 243–253. [CrossRef]
14. Dort, J.; Sirois, A.; Leblanc, N.; Côté, C.H.; Jacques, H. Beneficial effects of cod protein on skeletal muscle repair following injury. *Appl. Physiol. Nutr. Metab.* **2012**, *37*, 489–498. [CrossRef] [PubMed]
15. Aadland, E.K.; Lavigne, C.; Graff, I.E.; Eng, Ø.; Paquette, M.; Holthe, A.; Mellgren, G.; Jacques, H.; Liaset, B. Lean-seafood intake reduces cardiovascular lipid risk factors in healthy subjects: Results from a randomized controlled trial with a crossover design 1,2. *Am. J. Clin. Nutr.* **2015**, *102*, 582–592. [CrossRef]
16. Tørris, C.; Molin, M.; Cvancarova, M.S. Lean fish consumption is associated with lower risk of metabolic syndrome: A Norwegian cross sectional study. *BMC Public Health* **2016**, *16*, 347. [CrossRef] [PubMed]
17. Aadland, E.K.; Graff, I.E.; Lavigne, C.; Eng, Ø.; Paquette, M.; Holthe, A.; Mellgren, G.; Madsen, L.; Jacques, H.; Liaset, B. Lean Seafood Intake Reduces Postprandial C-peptide and Lactate Concentrations in Healthy Adults in a Randomized Controlled Trial with a Crossover Design. *J. Nutr.* **2016**, *146*, 1027–1034. [CrossRef] [PubMed]
18. Pedersen, A.N.; Christensen, T.; Matthiessen, J.; Knudsen, V.K.; Rosenlund-Sørensen, M.; Biltoft-Jensen, A.; Hinsch, H.; Ygil, K.H.; Kørup, K.; Saxholt, E.; et al. *Danskernes Kostvaner*, 1st ed.; DTU Fødevareinstituttet: Kongens Lyngby, Denmark, 2015; ISBN 9788793109391.
19. Nordic Council of Ministers. *Nordic Nutrition Recommendations 2012: Integrating Nutrition and Physical Activity*; Nordic Council of Ministers: Copenhagen, Denmark, 2014.
20. Commonwealth Scientific Industrial Research Organisation (CSIRO) Preventative Health National Research Flagship, USA. *2007 Australian National Children's Nutrition and Physical Activity Survey: Main Findings*; CSIRO: Canberra, Australia, 2008; ISBN 1741867568.

21. Kranz, S.; Jones, N.R.V.; Monsivais, P. Intake levels of fish in the UK paediatric population. *Nutrients* **2017**, *9*, 392. [CrossRef]
22. Madrigal, C.; Soto-Méndez, M.J.; Hernández-Ruiz, Á.; Valero, T.; Ávila, J.M.; Ruiz, E.; Villoslada, F.L.; Leis, R.; de Victoria, E.M.; Moreno, J.M.; et al. Energy intake, macronutrient profile and food sources of spanish children aged one to <10 years—Results from the esnupi study. *Nutrients* **2020**, *12*, 893. [CrossRef]
23. Rozin, P.; Fallon, A. The psychological categorization of foods and non-foods: A preliminary taxonomy of food rejections. *Appetite* **1980**, *1*, 193–201. [CrossRef]
24. Rozin, P.; Fallon, A.E. A perspective on disgust. *Psychol. Rev.* **1987**, *94*, 23–41. [CrossRef]
25. Martins, Y.; Pliner, P. "Ugh! That's disgusting!": Identification of the characteristics of foods underlying rejections based on disgust. *Appetite* **2006**, *46*, 75–85. [CrossRef]
26. Brown, S.D.; Harris, G. Disliked food acting as a contaminant during infancy. A disgust based motivation for rejection. *Appetite* **2012**, *58*, 535–538. [CrossRef]
27. Rozin, P.; Vollmecke, T.A. Food Likes and Dislikes. *Annu. Rev. Nutr.* **1986**, *6*, 433–456. [CrossRef] [PubMed]
28. Egolf, A.; Siegrist, M.; Hartmann, C. How people's food disgust sensitivity shapes their eating and food behaviour. *Appetite* **2018**, *127*, 28–36. [CrossRef] [PubMed]
29. Sick, J.; Højer, R.; Olsen, A. Children's self-reported reasons for accepting and rejecting foods. *Nutrients* **2019**, *11*, 2455. [CrossRef] [PubMed]
30. Prell, H.; Berg, C.; Jonsson, L. Why don't adolescents eat fish? Factors influencing fish consumption in school. *Scand. J. Nutr.* **2002**, *46*, 184–191. [CrossRef]
31. Frerichs, L.; Intolubbe-Chmil, L.; Brittin, J.; Teitelbaum, K.; Trowbridge, M.; Huang, T.T.K. Children's Discourse of Liked, Healthy, and Unhealthy Foods. *J. Acad. Nutr. Diet.* **2016**, *116*, 1323–1331. [CrossRef]
32. Mitterer-Daltoé, M.; Latorres, J.; Treptow, R.; Pastous-Madureira, L.; Queiroz, M. Acceptance of breaded fish (Engraulis anchoita) in school meals in extreme southern Brazil. *Acta Aliment.* **2013**, *42*, 275–282. [CrossRef]
33. Latorres, J.M.; Mitterer-Daltoé, M.L.; Queiroz, M.I. Hedonic and Word Association Techniques Confirm a Successful Way of Introducing Fish into Public School Meals. *J. Sens. Stud.* **2016**, *31*, 206–212. [CrossRef]
34. Zeinstra, G.G.; Koelen, M.A.; Kok, F.J.; de Graaf, C. Cognitive development and children's perceptions of fruit and vegetables; A qualitative study. *Int. J. Behav. Nutr. Phys. Act.* **2007**, *4*, 30. [CrossRef]
35. Angyal, A. Disgust and related aversions. *J. Abnorm. Soc. Psychol.* **1941**, *36*, 393–412. [CrossRef]
36. Pliner, P.; Pelchat, M.L. Neophobia in humans and the special status of foods of animal origin. *Appetite* **1991**, *16*, 205–218. [CrossRef]
37. Coulthard, H.; Williamson, I.; Palfreyman, Z.; Lyttle, S. Evaluation of a pilot sensory play intervention to increase fruit acceptance in preschool children. *Appetite* **2018**, *120*, 609–615. [CrossRef]
38. Coulthard, H.; Sealy, A. Play with your food! Sensory play is associated with tasting of fruits and vegetables in preschool children. *Appetite* **2017**, *113*, 84–90. [CrossRef] [PubMed]
39. Coulthard, H.; Thakker, D. Enjoyment of Tactile Play Is Associated with Lower Food Neophobia in Preschool Children. *J. Acad. Nutr. Diet.* **2015**, *115*, 1134–1140. [CrossRef] [PubMed]
40. Nederkoorn, C.; Jansen, A.; Havermans, R.C. Feel your food. The influence of tactile sensitivity on picky eating in children. *Appetite* **2015**, *84*, 7–10. [CrossRef]
41. Nederkoorn, C.; Theißen, J.; Tummers, M.; Roefs, A. Taste the feeling or feel the tasting: Tactile exposure to food texture promotes food acceptance. *Appetite* **2018**, *120*, 297–301. [CrossRef] [PubMed]
42. Dazeley, P.; Houston-Price, C. Exposure to foods' non-taste sensory properties. A nursery intervention to increase children's willingness to try fruit and vegetables. *Appetite* **2015**. [CrossRef]
43. Utter, J.; Fay, A.P.; Denny, S. Child and Youth Cooking Programs: More Than Good Nutrition? *J. Hunger Environ. Nutr.* **2017**, *12*, 554–580. [CrossRef]
44. Block, K.; Gibbs, L.; Staiger, P.K.; Gold, L.; Johnson, B.; Macfarlane, S.; Long, C.; Townsend, M. Growing Community: The Impact of the Stephanie Alexander Kitchen Garden Program on the Social and Learning Environment in Primary Schools. *Health Educ. Behav.* **2012**, *39*, 419–432. [CrossRef]
45. Fisher, J.O.; Birch, L.L. Restricting access to palatable foods affects children's behavioral response, food selection, and intake. *Am. J. Clin. Nutr.* **1999**, *69*, 1264–1272. [CrossRef]
46. Gibbs, L.; Staiger, P.K.; Johnson, B.; Block, K.; Macfarlane, S.; Gold, L.; Kulas, J.; Townsend, M.; Long, C.; Ukoumunne, O. Expanding Children's Food Experiences: The Impact of a School-Based Kitchen Garden Program. *J. Nutr. Educ. Behav.* **2013**, *45*, 137–146. [CrossRef]

47. Nelson, S.A.; Corbin, M.A.; Nickols-Richardson, S.M. A call for culinary skills education in childhood obesity-prevention interventions: Current status and peer influences. *J. Acad. Nutr. Diet.* **2013**, *113*, 1031–1036. [CrossRef]
48. Kolb, D.A. *Experiential Learning: Experience as The Source of Learning and Development*; Prentice-Hall Inc.: Upper Saddle River, NJ, USA, 1984; pp. 20–38. [CrossRef]
49. Wistoft, K.; Christensen, J. Taste as a didactic approach: Enabling students to achieve learning goals. *Int. J. Home Econ.* **2016**, *9*, 20.
50. Baggett, P.; Shaw, E. The Art and Science of Gyotaku: There's Somethin' Fishy Goin' On Here . . . . *Sci. Act. Cl. Proj. Curric. Ideas* **2008**, *45*, 3–8. [CrossRef]
51. Stokes, N.C. The fin art of science. *Sci. Teach.* **2001**, *68*, 22–26.
52. Yin, R.K. *Case Study Research Design and Methods*, 4th ed.; SAGE Publications: Thousand Oaks, CA, USA, 2009; ISBN 9781412960991.
53. Bryman, A. *Social Research Methods*; Oxford University Press: Oxford, UK, 2016; ISBN 978-0-19-968945-3.
54. Ministry of Children and Education. Madkundskab Fælles Mål. 2019. Available online: https://emu.dk/sites/default/files/2019-08/GSK---F\T1\aellesMål---Madkundskab.pdf (accessed on 2 February 2020).
55. Gibbs, G. *Analyzing Qualitative Data (Qualitative Research Kit)*; Flick, U., Ed.; Sage Publications Ltd.: Thousand Oaks, CA, USA, 2008; ISBN 0761949801.
56. Fargas-Malet, M.; McSherry, D.; Larkin, E.; Robinson, C. Research with children: Methodological issues and innovative techniques. *J. Early Child. Res.* **2010**, *8*, 175–192. [CrossRef]
57. Guest, G.; MacQueen, K.; Namey, E. *Applied Thematic Analysis*; SAGE Publications: Thousand Oaks, CA, USA, 2014.
58. Braun, V.; Clarke, V. Using thematic analysis in psychology Using thematic analysis in psychology. *Qual. Res. Psychol.* **2006**, *3*, 77–101. [CrossRef]
59. Sennett, R. *The Craftsman*; Yale University Press: London, UK, 2008; ISBN 9780300119091.
60. Martin, R.J. Craftsmanship and Schooling. *J. Thought* **1978**, *13*, 187–195.
61. Birch, L.L. Effects of Peer Models' Food Choices and Eating Behaviors on Preschoolers' Food Preferences. *Child Dev.* **1980**. [CrossRef]
62. Lafraire, J.; Rioux, C.; Giboreau, A.; Picard, D. Food rejections in children: Cognitive and social/environmental factors involved in food neophobia and picky/fussy eating behavior. *Appetite* **2015**. [CrossRef]
63. Rozin, P.; Fallon, A. *The Acquisition of Likes and Dislikes for Foods*; National Academies Press: Washington, DC, USA, 1986.
64. Vuholm, S.; Damsgaard, C. Kan citizen science give os ny viden om danskernes fiskeindtag? *Diætisten* **2019**, *157*, 7–11.
65. Fischler, C. Food habits, social change and the nature/culture dilemma. *Soc. Sci. Inf.* **1980**, *19*, 937–953. [CrossRef]
66. Kubberød, E.; Ueland, Ø.; Tronstad, Å.; Risvik, E. Attitudes towards meat and meat-eating among adolescents in Norway: A qualitative study. *Appetite* **2002**. [CrossRef]
67. Martins, Y.; Pliner, P. Human food choices: An examination of the factors underlying acceptance/rejection of novel and familiar animal and nonanimal foods. *Appetite* **2005**, *45*, 214–224. [CrossRef] [PubMed]
68. Lévi-Strauss, C. *The Raw and the Cooked. Mythologiques Vol. 1*; The University of Chicago: Chicago, IL, USA, 1983; ISBN 13:9780226474878.
69. Bandura, A. Self-efficacy mechanism in human agency. *Am. Psychol.* **1982**, *37*, 122–147. [CrossRef]
70. Cunningham-Sabo, L.; Lohse, B. Cooking with kids positively affects fourth graders' vegetable preferences and attitudes and self-efficacy for food and cooking. *Child. Obes.* **2013**, *9*, 549–556. [CrossRef] [PubMed]
71. Jarpe-Ratner, E.; Folkens, S.; Sharma, S.; Daro, D.; Edens, N.K. An Experiential Cooking and Nutrition Education Program Increases Cooking Self-Efficacy and Vegetable Consumption in Children in Grades 3–8. *J. Nutr. Educ. Behav.* **2016**, *48*, 697–705. [CrossRef] [PubMed]
72. Donadini, G.; Fumi, M.D.; Porretta, S. Hedonic response to fish in preschoolers. *J. Sens. Stud.* **2013**, *28*, 282–296. [CrossRef]
73. Dohle, S.; Rall, S.; Siegrist, M. I cooked it myself: Preparing food increases liking and consumption. *Food Qual. Prefer.* **2014**. [CrossRef]

74. Allirot, X.; da Quinta, N.; Chokupermal, K.; Urdaneta, E. Involving children in cooking activities: A potential strategy for directing food choices toward novel foods containing vegetables. *Appetite* **2016**, *103*, 275–285. [CrossRef]
75. Van der Horst, K.; Ferrage, A.; Rytz, A. Involving children in meal preparation. Effects on food intake. *Appetite* **2014**, *79*, 18–24. [CrossRef]
76. Lukas, C.V.; Cunningham-Sabo, L. Qualitative investigation of the cooking with kids program: Focus group interviews with fourth-grade students, teachers, and food educators. *J. Nutr. Educ. Behav.* **2011**, *43*, 517–524. [CrossRef]
77. Davis, J.N.; Martinez, L.C.; Spruijt-Metz, D.; Gatto, N.M. LA Sprouts: A 12-Week Gardening, Nutrition, and Cooking Randomized Control Trial Improves Determinants of Dietary Behaviors. *J. Nutr. Educ. Behav.* **2016**. [CrossRef] [PubMed]
78. Mustonen, S.; Rantanen, R.; Tuorila, H. Effect of sensory education on school children's food perception: A 2-year follow-up study. *Food Qual. Prefer.* **2009**. [CrossRef]
79. Morrow, S.L. Quality and trustworthiness in qualitative research in counseling psychology. *J. Couns. Psychol.* **2005**, *52*, 250–260. [CrossRef]
80. McCambridge, J.; Witton, J.; Elbourne, D.R. Systematic review of the Hawthorne effect: New concepts are needed to study research participation effects. *J. Clin. Epidemiol.* **2014**, *67*, 267–277. [CrossRef]

Publisher's Note: MDPI stays neutral with regard to jurisdictional claims in published maps and institutional affiliations.

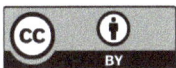

© 2020 by the authors. Licensee MDPI, Basel, Switzerland. This article is an open access article distributed under the terms and conditions of the Creative Commons Attribution (CC BY) license (http://creativecommons.org/licenses/by/4.0/).

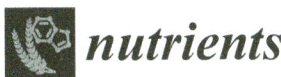

Review

Promoting Healthy Eating among Young People—A Review of the Evidence of the Impact of School-Based Interventions

Abina Chaudhary [1], František Sudzina [2,3,*] and Bent Egberg Mikkelsen [4]

1. Independent Researcher, Kastrupvej 79, 2300 Copenhagen, Denmark; abinachaudhary@yahoo.com
2. Department of Materials and Production, Faculty of Engineering and Science, Aalborg University, A. C. Meyers Vænge 15, 2450 Copenhagen, Denmark
3. Department of Systems Analysis, Faculty of Informatics and Statistics, University of Economics, nám. W. Churchilla 1938/4, 130 67 Prague, Czech Republic
4. Department of Geosciences and Natural Resource Management, Faculty of Science, University of Copenhagen, Rolighedsvej 23, 1958 Frederiksberg C, Denmark; bemi@ign.ku.dk
* Correspondence: sudzina@business.aau.dk or frantisek.sudzina@vse.cz

Received: 1 July 2020; Accepted: 3 September 2020; Published: 22 September 2020

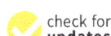

Abstract: Intro: Globally, the prevalence of overweight and obesity is increasing among children and younger adults and is associated with unhealthy dietary habits and lack of physical activity. School food is increasingly brought forward as a policy to address the unhealthy eating patterns among young people. Aim: This study investigated the evidence for the effectiveness of school-based food and nutrition interventions on health outcomes by reviewing scientific evidence-based intervention studies amongst children at the international level. Methods: This study was based on a systematic review using the PRISMA guidelines. Three electronic databases were systematically searched, reference lists were screened for studies evaluating school-based food and nutrition interventions that promoted children's dietary behaviour and health aiming changes in the body composition among children. Articles dating from 2014 to 2019 were selected and reported effects on anthropometry, dietary behaviour, nutritional knowledge, and attitude. Results: The review showed that school-based interventions in general were able to affect attitudes, knowledge, behaviour and anthropometry, but that the design of the intervention affects the size of the effect. In general, food focused interventions taking an environmental approach seemed to be most effective. Conclusions: School-based interventions (including multicomponent interventions) can be an effective and promising means for promoting healthy eating, improving dietary behaviour, attitude and anthropometry among young children. Thus, schools as a system have the potential to make lasting improvements, ensuring healthy school environment around the globe for the betterment of children's short- and long-term health.

Keywords: school children; food and nutrition; intervention; healthy eating

1. Introduction

Childhood is one of the critical periods for good health and development in human life [1,2]. During this age, the physiological need for nutrients increases and the consumption of a diet high in nutritional quality is particularly important. Evidence suggests that lifestyle, behaviour patterns and eating habits adopted during this age persist throughout adulthood and can have a significant influence on health and wellbeing in later life [3,4]. Furthermore, the transition from childhood into adolescence is often associated with unhealthy dietary changes. Thus, it is important to establish healthful eating behaviours early in life and specially focus on the childhood transition period. A healthy diet during the primary age of children reduces the risk of immediate nutrition-related health problems of primary concern to school children, namely, obesity, dental caries and lack of physical activity [5–7].

Furthermore, young people adopting these healthy habits during childhood are more likely to maintain their health and thus be at reduced risk of chronic ailments in later life [7–9]. Thus, healthy behaviours learnt at a young age might be instrumental in reaching the goals of good health and wellbeing of the 2030 Sustainability Agenda which has implications at the global level.

Globally, the prevalence of overweight and obesity rose by 47.1% for children and 27.5% for adults between 1980 and 2013 [10]. A recent WHO (World Health Organization) Commission report [10] stated that if these same trends were to continue, then by 2025, 70 million children are predicted to be affected [11]. Hence, the increased prevalence might negatively affect child and adult morbidity and mortality around the world [12,13]. Worldwide the dietary recommendations for healthy diets recommend the consumption of at least five portions of fruits and vegetables a day, reduced intake of saturated fat and salt and increased consumption of complex carbohydrates and fibres [14]. However, studies show that most children and adolescent do not meet these guidelines [15,16] and, thus, as a result, childhood and adolescent obesity are alarming nearly everywhere [17]. Recent figures show that the prevalence has tripled in many countries, making it the major public health issue in the 21st century [18–21]. According to WHO [4], 1 in 3 children aged 6–9 were overweight and obese in 2010, up from 1 in 4 children of the same age in 2008.

The increased prevalence of overweight and obesity has fuelled efforts to counteract the development, as seen for instance in the action plan on childhood obesity [17]. Increasingly policy makers have been turning their interest to the school setting as a well-suited arena for the promotion of healthier environments [18]. As a result, schools have been the target of increased attention from the research community to develop interventions and to examine the school environment to promote healthful behaviours including healthy eating habits.

Globally, interventions in the school environment to promote healthier nutrition among young people have received considerable attention from researchers over the past years. But there is far from a consensus on what are the most effective ways to make the most out of schools' potential to contribute to better health through food-based actions. Is it the environment that makes a difference? Is it the education or is it the overall attention given to food and eating that plays the biggest role? School food and nutrition intervention strategies have witnessed a gradual change from knowledge orientation to behavioural orientation [22] and from a focus on the individual to the food environment. Research evidence has shown that adequate nutrition knowledge and positive attitudes towards nutrition do not necessarily translate to good dietary practices. Similarly, research has shown that the food environment plays a far bigger role in behaviour than originally believed [23,24].

School-based interventions can a priori be considered as an effective method for promoting better eating at the population level. Schools reach a large number of participants across diverse ethnic groups. It not only reaches children, but school staffs, family members as well as community members [8,25]. Schools can be considered a protected place where certain rules apply and where policies of public priority can be deployed relatively easily. In addition, schools are professional spaces in which learning and formation is at the heart of activities and guided by a skilled and professional staff. Schools, as such, represent a powerful social environment that hold the potential to promote and provide healthy nutrition and education. Besides the potential to create health and healthy behaviours, good nutrition at school has, according to more studies, the potential to add to educational outcomes and academic performance [26–28].

However, taking the growth in research studies and papers in the field into account, it is difficult for both the research community and for policy makers to stay up to date on how successful school-based interventions have been in improving dietary behaviours, nutritional knowledge and anthropometry among children. Also, the knowledge and insights into how it is possible to intervene in the different corners of the school food environment has developed which obviously has influenced over recent decades how programs and interventions can be designed. It has also become clear that food at school is more than just the food taken but includes curricular and school policy components. The findings from school-based studies on the relationship between school, family as well as community-based interventions and health impact suggest that health impacts are dependent on the context in which they have been carried out as well as the methodology. Thus, an updated overview as well as a more detailed analysis of initiatives is needed in order to develop our understanding of the nature of the mechanisms through which the school can contribute to the shaping of healthier dietary behaviour among children and adolescents before more precise policy instruments can be developed. Our study attempted to fill the need for better insight into which of the many intervention components works best. It attempted to look at school food and nutrition interventions reported in the literature that have been looking at healthy eating programmes, projects, interventions or initiatives.

School-based interventions in the Western world are traditionally targeted at addressing obesity and over-nutrition, but school food interventions are also addressing under nutrition and, as such, their role in a double burden of disease perspective should not be underestimated. Many studies have reported on micronutrient malnutrition among school-aged children in developing countries (for instance [29–31]) but it has also been reported in the context of developed countries [32]. Against this backdrop, the aim of this study was to provide an analysis of the evidence of the effectiveness of school-based food interventions by reviewing recent scientific, evidence-based intervention studies on healthy eating promotion at school. The specific objectives of the study were to identify which interventions had an effect on primary outcomes, such as BMI, or on secondary outcomes such as dietary behaviour, nutritional knowledge and attitude.

2. Materials and Methods

The functional unit of the review were healthy eating programmes, projects or initiatives that have been performed using the school as a setting. We included only programmes, projects or initiatives that were studied in a research context, in the sense that they were planned by researchers, carried out under controlled settings using a research protocol, and reported in the literature. School-based programmes, projects, interventions or initiatives are, per definition, cluster samples where a number of schools first were chosen for intervention followed by performing an outcome measurement before and after the intervention and, in most cases, also in one or more control schools. The outcome measurement in the studies reviewed was performed on a sample of students that was drawn from each school (cluster).For this, the systematic review and meta-analysis (PRISMA) guidelines and the standardised quality assessment tool "effective public health practice project (EPHPP) quality assessment tool for quantitative studies" were used for analysing the quality assessment of the included studies [33]. This EPHPP instrument can be used to assess the quality of quantitative studies with a variety of study designs.

2.1. Literature Search

The literature review involved searches in PubMed, Web of Science and Cochrane Library database. The search strategy was designed to be inclusive and focused on three key elements: population (e.g., children); intervention (e.g., school-based); outcome (e.g., diet and nutrition, knowledge, attitude and anthropometrics). The search terms used in PubMed database were: "effectiveness of school food AND nutrition AND primary school children", "effectiveness of school food AND nutrition AND interventions OR programs AND among primary school children AND increase healthy consumption", "primary school children and education and food interventions", "Effectiveness of school-based food interventions among primary school", "effectiveness of school-based nutrition and food interventions", "primary school interventions and its effectiveness", and "obesity prevention intervention among Primary schools". Search terms such as: "effectiveness of school-based food interventions among primary school", "effectiveness of school based food and nutrition interventions", "primary school interventions and its effectiveness" and "obesity prevention interventions", were used in the Web of Science database. Lastly, search terms such as: "nutrition interventions in primary schools" and "Nutrition education interventions in school" were used in the Cochrane Library database to find the articles. In addition, reference lists of all retrieved articles and review articles [34] were screened for potentially eligible articles. The search strategy was initially developed in PubMed and adapted for use in other databases. In addition, snowballing of the reference list of the selected articles was conducted.

2.2. Inclusion Criteria

Studies selected for the inclusion were studies which investigated the effectiveness of a school-based interventions targeting food and nutrition behaviour, healthy eating and nutrition education as a primary focus during the intervention. Also, to be included in this review, only articles from 2014 to 2019 were selected and of those inclusion criteria included articles targeting primary school children aged between 5 and 14 years. Participants included both boys and girls without considering their socio-economic background. Study design included randomized controlled trial "RCT", cluster randomized controlled trial "RCCT", controlled trial "CT", pre-test/post-test with and without control "PP", experimental design "Quasi". Studies which did not meet the intervention components/exposures, such as information and teaching (mostly for the target group and parents were additional), family focus on social support and food focus (which mainly focuses on the availability of free foods including food availability from school gardening), were excluded. Systematic review papers and studies written in different language except for English were excluded as well. Studies which met the intervention criteria but had after school programs were excluded.

2.3. Age Range

Since the review covers a broad range of different countries and since school systems are quite different, the sampling principle had to include some simplification and standardisation. The goal of the review was to cover elementary (primary) and secondary education and, as a result, the age range of 5–14 was chosen to be the best fit, although it should be noted that secondary education in some countries also covers those 15–18 years of age. In most countries, elementary education/primary education is the first—and normally obligatory—phase of formal education. It begins at approximately age 5 to 7 and ends at about age 11 to 13 and in some countries 14. In the United Kingdom and some other countries, the term primary is used instead of elementary. In the United States the term primary refers to only the first three years of elementary education, i.e., grades 1 to 3. Elementary education is, in most countries, preceded by some kind of kindergarten/preschool for children aged 3 to 5 or 6 and normally followed by secondary education.

2.4. Assessment of Study Eligibility

For the selection of the relevant studies, all the titles and abstracts generated from the searches were examined. The articles were rejected on initial screening if the title and abstract did not meet the inclusion criteria or met the exclusion criteria. If abstracts did not provide enough exclusion information or were not available, then the full text was obtained for evaluation. The evaluation of full text was done to refine the results using the aforementioned inclusion and exclusion criteria. Thus, those studies that met predefined inclusion criteria were selected for this study.

2.5. Analytical Approach

The first step of data collection was aimed at organizing all studies with their key information. In the second step, we created coded columns. A coded column served as a basis for being able to do further statistical analysis. In other words, in a coded column we added a new construct not originally found in the papers as a kind of dummy variable that standardized otherwise non-standardized information, allowing us to treat otherwise un-calculable data statistically. For the impact columns, we used the following approach to construct codes where impacts where put on a 1–4-point Likert scale with 1 being "ineffective", 2 "partially effective", 3 "effective" and 4 "very effective".

For the design column, the following approach was adopted as illustrated in the Table 1. Quasi experimental/pre–post studies were labelled QED and were considered to always include a baseline and follow-up outcome measurement. As the simplest design with no comparison but just a pre/post study of the same group, we constructed a power column and assigned 1 to this for a QED design. For the controlled trial (CT), we assigned the power 2. A controlled trial is the same as QED but with a comparison/control in which no interventions are made and with no randomization. We considered a study to be of that kind if some kind of controls were made which could be, for instance, matching. All CTs in our study included 2 types of comparisons: pre and post (baseline and follow-up) as well as a comparison between intervention/no intervention. For the RCT/RCCT—a trial that is controlled through the randomization—we assigned the power 3. This "top of hierarchy" design includes the case (intervention) and a control (no intervention) and normally two types of comparisons (pre and post) as well as an intervention/no intervention. For the context of this study, we did not differentiate between RCTs and RCCTs. The latter is sometimes used to stress the fact that the school (or the class) is the sampling unit from which the subjects are recruited. But since in the context of schools RCCT is simply a variation of RCT, we coded them in the same class of power. We simply assumed that when authors spoke about an RCT, they in fact meant an RCCT since they could not have been sampling subjects without using the school as the unit.

Table 1. Coding table for study designs. The table shows the types of studies examined in the review and the power assigned to them.

Code	Design	Power
PP	Pre-Test/Post-Test	1
OBS	Observational	1
CT	Controlled Trial	2
RCT	Randomized Controlled Trial	3
RCCT	Randomized Controlled Cluster Trial	3

Codes and categorization were used to standardize the information found in the papers for our statistical analysis. Categorisation of the age/class level, such as EA—Early age, EML—Early middle late, EL—Early late, was used.

For the intervention components ("what was done") we translated all studies into three columns: information and teaching, family and social support and environmental components, food provision and availability. The latter was further expanded into three columns labelled as: focus on and provisioning of F & V; free food availability through school gardening and availability of food and healthier food environment. Our inclusion criteria were that studies should contain at least one of these components. For the environmental component—food provision and availability intervention components—we identified 2 distinct types: either a broad healthier eating focus or a narrow and more targeted fruit and vegetable focus. After the coding, we started to ask questions about the data. Most importantly, we were interested in knowing whether there existed a relationship between "what was done" and "what was the impact". In other words, we were interested in knowing more whether there was a pattern in the way the studies intervened and the outcomes.

2.6. Queries Made

We performed queries for each intervention component (the independent variable in columns K, L and M) for each single outcome measure.

Is there a relationship between age and outcome? We used the coded column (EA, EML, etc.) to study that relationship.

In addition, we made queries regarding the relationship among study designs. For instance, would the duration of studies influence whether an effect could be found or not? Would more powerful designs result in more impact?

Furthermore, we made queries on the relationship between one intervention and a multi-interventional component and their effect on the outcome measure. Also, the queries on target groups were made. Codes such as S and NS (refer Table 4) in the column were used to study the relationship. In our analysis a distinction was made between "standard" and "extreme" (special cases). From the reviewed papers, it was clear that some studies put little emphasis on the school selected. We classified those as standard (S). However, a few papers used a stratification approach and case/cluster selection that can be classified as an "extreme" or non-standard case. We coded these as non-standard (NS). For instance, studies could be targeted to include only refugees or subjects of low socio-economic status. It can be speculated that being a "special case" or extreme case could have an influence. As a result, we reserved a code for these cases, although it became clear that they represented only a minority.

In our study, availability plays a central role, since it is used in many food-at-school intervention studies. Availability signals that food is "pushed" as opposed to being used in the "pull" mode, where individuals are expected to request food in the sense that is the behaviour of the individual that becomes the driving force rather than the "out thereness". Availability is in most studies used in combination with the idea of a food environment. The literature shows that availability can be of two types. One is when food is made available for the individual to take where visibility, salience, product placement, etc., are used as factors. The other type of availability is when it is made free and the individual as a result does not have to pay. Free availability has been studied extensively in intervention studies but for obvious reason it is difficult to implement "post-study" since there needs to be a permanent financing present. The only exceptions to this are the collective meal models found in countries such as Sweden, Finland, Estonia and Brazil as well as in the EU scheme where the EU subsidizes the fruit.

Study design and other characteristics are provided in Table 2, and their findings are provided in Table 3.

Table 2. The review sample: study design/characteristics. The table shows the 43 studies of the review illustrating study design and study characteristics of the included studies.

Author	Year	Title/Reference	Main Aim (from Abstract)	Main Aim in Brief	Program Name (Acronym)	Location & Country	Study Design (Column I)	Study Design Coded (RCT, PP, CT, RCCT, Quasi)	Power	Intervention Components			
										Information and Teaching	Food Focus		Family/Social Support
											Environmental/Food Focus on Healthy Meal Availability	Environmental/Food Focus through School Gardening	
Harake et al. [ ]	2018	Impact of pilot school-based nutrition intervention on dietary knowledge, attitudes, behaviours and nutritional status of Syrian refugee children in the Bekaa, Lebanon	This study aimed to evaluate the impact of a six-month pilot school-based nutrition intervention on changes in dietary knowledge, attitude, and behavior of Syrian refugee children enrolled in informal primary schools located in the rural region of the Bekaa in Lebanon. A secondary objective of the study was to explore the effect of the intervention on the dietary intake and nutritional status of children.	Nutritional knowledge, attitude, HE & FV	GHATA	Bekaa Lebanon	Quasi experimental	QED	1	x		x	
Adab P. et al. [ ]	2018	Effectiveness of a childhood obesity prevention programme delivered through schools, targeting 6 (more than 6 years) and 7 years old cluster randomised controlled trial (WAVES study)	To assess the effectiveness of a school and family based healthy lifestyle programme (WAVES intervention) compare with usual practice, in preventing childhood obesity.	Anthropometry, HE & FV	WAVES	UK primary schools from the West Midlands within 35 miles of the study centre	Randomized Controlled Cluster Trials	RCCT	3	x			
Harley A. et al. [ ]	2018	Youth Chef Academy: Pilot Results From a Plant-Based Culinary and Nutrition Literacy Program for Sixth and Seventh Graders	The study aim was to examine the effectiveness of Youth Chef Academy (YCA), a classroom-based experiential culinary and nutrition literacy intervention for sixth and seventh graders (11- to 13-year-old) designed to impact healthy eating.	HE & FV, Nutritional knowledge	YCA	US (exact location is missing)	Controlled Trial (CT)	CT	2	x			
Hermans R.C.J. et al. [ ]	2018	Feed the Alien! The Effects of a Nutrition Instruction Game on Children's Nutritional Knowledge and Food Intake	The aim of this study was to test the short-term effectiveness of the Alien Health Game, a videogame designed to teach elementary school children about nutrition and healthy food choices.	HE & FV, Nutritional knowledge	AHG	Dutch, Netherland	Pre-test post-test, experimental study design	QED	1	x			

129

Table 2. Cont.

Author	Year	Title/Reference	Main Aim (from Abstract)	Main Aim in Brief	Program Name Acronym	Location & Country	Study Design	Study Design Coded RCT, PP, CT, RCCT, Quasi	Power	Intervention Components				
										Information and Teaching	Environmental/Food Focus on Healthy Meal Availability	Food Focus Environmental/Food Focus through School Gardening		Family/Social Support
Piana N., et al. [30]	2017	An innovative school-based intervention to promote healthy lifestyles	To describe an innovative school-based intervention to promote healthy lifestyles. To evaluate its effects on children's food habits and to highlight the key components which contribute most to the beneficial effects obtained from children's, teachers' and parents' perspectives.	HE & FV, Nutritional knowledge, Physical activity	Kidmed test	Spoleto, Umbria	Pre-test post-test	PP	1	x				x
Battjes-Fries M.C.E, et al. [31]	2017	Effectiveness of Taste Lessons with and without additional experiential learning activities on children's willingness to taste vegetables	The aim of this study was to assess the effect of Taste Lessons with and without extra experiential learning activities on children's willingness to taste unfamiliar vegetables, food neophobia, and vegetable consumption.	HE & FV, attitude	TLVM	Dutch province of Gelderland	Quasi experimental design	QED	1	x				
Bogart L.M., et al. [32]	2014	A Randomized Controlled Trial of Students for Nutrition and eXercise (SNaX): A Community-Based Participatory Research Study	To conduct a randomized controlled trial of Students for Nutrition and eXercise (SNaX), a 5-week middle-school-based obesity-prevention intervention combining school-wide environmental changes, multimedia, encouragement to eat healthy school cafeteria foods, and peer-led education.	HE & FV, Nutritional knowledge	SNaX	Los Angeles Unified School District	Randomized Controlled Trial	RCT	3	x				
Shriqui V.K., et al. [33]	2016	Effects of a School-Based comprehensive intervention on Nutritional Knowledge and Habits of Low-Socioeconomic School Children in Israel: A Cluster Randomized Controlled Trial	Examining the effect of a school-based comprehensive intervention on nutrition knowledge, eating habits, and behaviours among low socioeconomic status (LSES) school-aged children was performed	Anthropometry, HE & FV, Nutritional knowledge	NRI & PA	Beer Sheva, a big metropolis in southern Israel	Randomized Controlled Cluster Trial	RCCT	3	x				x

Table 2. Cont.

Author	Year	Title/Reference	Main Aim (from Abstract)	Main Aim in Brief	Program Name Acronym	Location & Country	Study Design Column 1	Study Design Coded RCT, PP, CT, RCCT, Quasi	Power	Information and Teaching	Environmental/Food Focus on Healthy Meal Availability	Environmental/Food Focus	Environmental/Food Focus through School Gardening	Family/Social Support
Sharma S.V. et al.	2016	Evaluating a school-based fruit and vegetable co-op in low-income children: A quasi-experimental study	The purpose of this study was to evaluate the effectiveness of a new school-based food co-op program, Brighter Bites (BB), to increase fruit and vegetable intake, and home nutrition environment among low-income 1st graders and their parents.	HE & FV, Nutritional knowledge	BB	Houston, Texas	Quasi-experimental non-randomized controlled study	QED	1	x		x		x
Lawlor A.D. et al.	2016	The Active for Life Year 5 (AFLY5) school-based cluster randomised controlled trial: effect on potential mediators	To determine the effect of the intervention on potential mediators	Anthropometry, HE & FV	AFLY5	South East of England	Cluster RCT	RCCT	3	x				x
Steyn P.N. et al.	2016	Did Health kick, a randomised controlled trial primary school nutrition intervention improve dietary quality of children in low-income settings in South Africa?	To promote healthy eating habits and regular physical activity in learners, parents and educators by means of an action planning process	HE & FV, PA	HK	Western Cape (WC) Province	Cluster RCT	RCCT	3	x				
Jones M. et al.	2017	Association between Food for Life, a Whole Setting Healthy and Sustainable Food Programme, and Primary School Children's Consumption of Fruit and Vegetables: A cross Sectional Study in England	The aim of the study was to examine the association between primary school engagement in the Food for Life programme and the consumption of fruit and vegetables by children aged 8–10 years.	HE & FV, Nutritional knowledge	FLP	England	Cross sectional school matched comparison approach	Cross-sectional study design	1	x		x		
Larsen L.A. et al.	2015	RE-AIM analysis of a randomized school-based nutrition intervention among fourth-grade classrooms in California	To promote healthy eating behaviours and attitudes in children	HE & FV, Nutritional knowledge, Attitude	NPP	California	RCT with pre-, post-, and follow-up assessments	RCT	3	x				x

Table 2. Cont.

Author	Year	Title/Reference	Main Aim (from Abstract)	Main Aim in Brief	Program Name Acronym	Location & Country	Study Design Column I	Study Design Coded RCT, PP, CT, RCCT, Quasi	Power	Intervention Components				
										Information and Teaching	Food Focus			Family/Social Support
											Environmental/Food Focus on Healthy Meal Availability	Environmental/Food Focus through School Gardening		
Shen, Hu and Sun []	2015	Assessment of School-Based Quasi-Experimental Nutrition and Food Safety Health Education for Primary School Students in Two Poverty-Stricken Counties of West China	Aimed to assess the reliability of the knowledge, attitude and behaviour of nutrition and food safety questionnaire for primary school students (Grade 4 to 6) in poverty-stricken counties of China, and evaluate the effectiveness of health education through a quasi experiment, in order to promote policy establishment for child and adolescent health in the future	HE & FV, Nutritional knowledge, Attitude	NPSE	West China (Shaanxi and Yunnan provinces)	Quasi-experimental design	QED	1	x				
Gallotta C.M. et al. []	2016	Effects of combined physical education and nutritional programs on schoolchildren's healthy habits	To evaluate the efficacy of three 5-month combined physical education (PE) and nutritional interventions on body composition, physical activity (PA) level, sedentary time and eating habits of schoolchildren	Anthropometry, HE & FV, Nutritional knowledge, PA	ESPS	Rome (Italy)	Randomised Controlled Cluster Trial	RCCT	3	x				x
Fairclough J.S. et al. []	2013	Promoting healthy weight in primary school children through physical activity and nutrition education: a pragmatic evaluation of the CHANGE! randomised intervention study	To assess the effectiveness of the CHANGE! intervention on measures of body size, PA and food intake	Anthropometry, HE & FV, PA	CHANGE	Wigan Borough in northwest England, UK	Cluster randomised intervention	RCCT	3	x				
Cunha B.D. et al. []	2013	Effectiveness of a randomized school-based intervention involving families and teachers to prevent excessive weight gain among Adolescents in Brazil	To evaluate the effectiveness of a school-based intervention involving the families and teachers that aimed to promote healthy eating habits in adolescents; the ultimate aim of the intervention was to reduce the increase in body mass index (BMI) of the students	Anthropometry, HE & FV, PA	PAPPAS	Duque de Caxias, Rio de Janeiro, Brazil	Paired cluster randomized school-based trial	RCCT	3	x				

Table 2. Cont.

Author	Year	Title/Reference	Main Aim (from Abstract)	Main Aim in Brief	Program Name Acronym	Location & Country	Study Design	Study Design Coded RCT, PP, CT, RCCT, Quasi	Power	Information and Teaching	Environmental/Food Focus on Healthy Meal Availability	Environmental/Food Focus	Environmental/Food Focus through School Gardening	Family/Social Support
Aviles O.A. et al. [ ]	2017	A school-based intervention improved dietary intake outcomes and reduced waist circumference in adolescents: a cluster randomized controlled trial	The program aimed at improving the nutritional value of dietary intake, physical activity (primary outcomes), body mass index, waist circumference and blood pressure (secondary outcomes)	Anthropometry, HE & FV, PA	ACTIVITAL	Urban area of Cuenca, Ecuador	Pair-matched cluster randomized controlled trial	RCCT	3					x
Muros J.J. et al. [ ]	2013	Results of a seven-week school-based physical activity and nutrition pilot program on health-related parameters in primary school children in Southern Spain	To determine the effect of nutrition education combined with sessions of vigorous extracurricular physical activity (VEPA) on the improvement of health-related parameters in children in primary education	Anthropometry, HE & FV, PA	VEPA	Southern Spain	Pilot study, PP	QED	1	x				
Moss A et al. [ ]	2013	Farm to School and Nutrition Education: Positively Affecting Elementary School-Aged Children's Nutrition Knowledge and Consumption Behavior	To introduce the CATCH nutrition curriculum and Farm to School program to assess nutrition knowledge of 3rd grade students, and increase their fruit and vegetable consumption behavior	HE & FV, Nutritional knowledge	CATCH	Southern Illinois	Quasi-experimental design	QED	1	x				
Zota D. et al. [ ]	2016	Promotion of healthy nutrition among students participating in a school food aid program: a randomized trial	To evaluate the potential benefits on students' eating habits, of incorporating healthy nutrition education as part of a school food aid program	Anthropometry, HE & FV	DIATROFI	Greece	Randomised Controlled Trial with the aspects of pre and post intervention questionnaire	RCT	3	x		x		x
Gold A. et al. [ ]	2017	Classroom Nutrition Education Combined With Fruit and Vegetable Taste Testing Improves Children's Dietary Intake	To test the classroom curriculum, go wild with fruits & veggies! (GWWFV) effectiveness to increase FV intake of third graders in rural and urban communities in North Dakota	HE & VF	GWWFV	North Dakota	Intervention study with RCT aspects (the schools were randomized to control and intervention school)	RCT, Intervention study	3	x				
Mbhatsani H.V., et al. [ ]	2017	Development and Implementation of Nutrition Education on Dietary Diversification for Primary School Children	To ensure that people consume a variety of foods that, together, provide adequate quantities of all the essential micronutrients necessary for health	HE & FV, Nutritional knowledge	NET & HBoIF	Vhembe District of Limpopo Province in South Africa	Quasi-experimental, with a one-group pre-test/post-test intervention	QED	1	x				

Table 2. Cont.

Author	Year	Title/Reference	Main Aim (from Abstract)	Main Aim in Brief	Program Name	Location & Country	Study Design	Study Design Coded	Power	Information and Teaching	Environmental/Food Focus on Healthy Meal Availability	Environmental/Food Focus on Healthy Food Focus	Environmental/Food Focus through School Gardening	Family/Social Support
					Acronym		Column I	RCT, PP, CT, RCCT, Quasi						
Hutchinson J. et al.	2015	Evaluation of the impact of school gardening interventions on children's knowledge of and attitudes towards fruit and vegetables. A cluster randomised controlled trial	To evaluate whether ongoing gardening advice and gardening involvement from the Royal Horticultural Society (RHS) gardening specialists was associated with better fruit and vegetable outcomes in children than those at teacherled schools that obtained standard advice from the RHS Campaign for School Gardening	Nutritional knowledge, Attitude	CFSG	London boroughs, Wandsworth, Tower Hamlets, Greenwich and Sutton	Randomised Controlled Cluster Trial	RCCT	3	x			x	
Viggiamo A et al.	2018	Healthy lifestyle promotion in primary schools through the board game Kaledo: a pilot cluster randomized trial	The board game Kaledo seems to improve knowledge in nutrition and helps to promote a healthy lifestyle in children attending middle and high schools. So, this study was conducted to investigate whether similar effects of Kaledo could be found in younger children in primary school.	Anthropometry, HE & FV, Nutritional knowledge	Kaledo	Campania, Italy	Pilot cluster randomized trial	RCCT	3	x				
Waters E. et al.	2017	Cluster randomised trial of a school-community child health promotion and obesity prevention intervention: findings from the evaluation of fun 'n healthy in Moreland!	Fun 'n healthy in Moreland! aimed to improve child adiposity, school policies and environments, parent engagement, health behaviours and child wellbeing.	Anthropometry, HE & FV	FHM	Victoria, Australia	Randomised Controlled Cluster Trial	RCCT	3	x				
Xu F et al.	2015	Effectiveness of a Randomized Controlled Lifestyle Intervention to Prevent Obesity among Chinese Primary School Students: CLICK-Obesity Study	To evaluate whether the lifestyle intervention was able to reduce obesity risk and increase healthy behaviors and knowledge	Anthropometry, Nutritional knowledge	CLICK-Obesity	Mainland China	Randomised Controlled Cluster Trial	RCCT	3	x				x
Jung et al.	2018	Influence of school-based nutrition education program on healthy eating literacy and healthy food choice among primary school children	To examine the effectiveness of a school-based healthy eating intervention program, the Healthy Highway Program, for improving healthy eating knowledge and healthy food choice behavior among elementary school students	Nutritional knowledge, HE & FV	Healthy highway program	Oswego County, New York State	Pre/post-test	QED	1	x				

Table 2. Cont.

Author	Year	Title/Reference	Main Aim (from Abstract)	Main Aim in Brief	Program Name Acronym	Location & Country	Study Design	Study Design Coded RCT, PP, CT, RCCT, Quasi	Power	Intervention Components			
										Information and Teaching	Food Focus Environmental/Food Focus on Healthy Meal Availability	Food Focus Environmental/Food Focus through School Gardening	Family/Social Support
Jhou W et al. [-]	2014	Effectiveness of a school-based nutrition and food safety education program among primary and junior high school students in Chongqing, China	To examine the effectiveness of a school-based nutrition and food safety education program among primary and junior high school students in China	Nutritional knowledge, attitude	school-based nutrition and food safety education	Chongqing, China	Pre/post-test	QED	1	x			
Anderson EL, et al. [-]	2016	Long-term effects of the Active for Life Year 5 (AFLY5) school-based cluster-randomised controlled trial	To investigate the long-term effectiveness of a school-based intervention to improve physical activity and diet in children.	HE & FV, PA	AFLY5	Southwest of England	Randomised Controlled Cluster Trial	RCCT	3	x			
Griffin TL et al. [-]	2015	A Brief Educational Intervention Increases Knowledge of the Sugar Content of Foods and Drinks but Does Not Decrease Intakes in Scottish Children Aged 10–12 Years	To assess the effectiveness of an educational intervention to improve children's knowledge of the sugar content of food and beverages	Nutritional knowledge, attitude	NEMS	Aberdeen, Scotland	Randomised Controlled Cluster Trial	RCCT	3	x			
Kipping R.R. et al. [-]	2014	Effect of intervention aimed at increasing physical activity, reducing sedentary behaviour, and increasing fruit and vegetable consumption in children: Active for Life Year 5 (AFLY5) school-based cluster randomised controlled trial	To investigate the effectiveness of a school-based intervention to increase physical activity, reduce sedentary behaviour, and increase fruit and vegetable consumption in children	HE & FV, PA	AFLY5	South west of England	Randomised Controlled Cluster Trial	RCCT	3	x			
Caar V.M. et al. [-]	2014	Effects of an intervention aimed at reducing the intake of sugar-sweetened beverages in primary school children: a controlled trial	Aimed at reducing children's SSB consumption by promoting the intake of water	Nutritional knowledge, attitude	Water campaign	Rotterdam, Netherland	Controlled trial	CT	2	x			
Moore GF et al. [-]	2014	Impacts of the Primary School Free Breakfast Initiative on socio-economic inequalities in breakfast consumption among 9–11-year-old schoolchildren in Wales	To examine the impacts of the Primary School Free Breakfast Initiative in Wales on inequalities in children's dietary behaviours and cognitive functioning	HE & FV	PSM	Wales, UK	Randomised Controlled Cluster Trial	RCCT	3			x	

135

Table 2. Cont.

Author	Year	Title/Reference	Main Aim (from Abstract)	Main Aim in Brief	Program Name Acronym	Location & Country	Study Design	Study Design Coded RCT, PP, CT, RCCT, Quasi	Power	Intervention Components Information and Teaching	Food Focus Environmental/Food Focus on Healthy Meal Availability	Environmental/Food Focus through School Gardening	Family/Social Support
Nyberg, G. et al. [68]	2016	Effectiveness of a universal parental support programme to promote health behaviours and prevent overweight and obesity in 6-year-old children in disadvantaged areas, the Healthy School Start Study II, a cluster-randomised controlled trial	To develop and evaluate the effectiveness of a parental support programme to promote healthy dietary and physical activity habits and to prevent overweight and obesity in six-year-old children in disadvantaged areas	Anthropometry, HE & FV	A Healthy School Start	Stockholm, Sweden	Randomised Controlled Cluster Trial	RCCT	3	x			
Mittmann S., Austel A., and Ellrott T. [69]	2016	Behavioural effects of a short school-based fruit and vegetable promotion programme: 5-a-Day for kids	To evaluate the acceptance of the scheme as well as the short- and intermediate-term effects of the German "5-a-day for kids" project	HE & FV	5-a-day for kids	Hannover, Germany	Pre/post-test	PP	1	x			
Huys N. et al. [70]	2019	Effect and process evaluation of a real-world school garden program on vegetable consumption and its determinants in primary schoolchildren	To investigate the effectiveness of a school garden program on children's vegetable consumption and determinants and to gain insight into the process of the program	HE & FV, Nutritional knowledge	Taste Garden	Ghent, Belgium	Non-equivalent pre-test. Post-test control group design	PP	1	x	x		
Weber K.S. et al. [71]	2017	Positive effects of promoting physical activity and balanced diet in a primary school setting with a high proportion of migrant school children	To evaluate the effects of a school-based intervention offering additional hours of supervised physical activity and dietary education for 3rd and 4th graders in primary schools	HE & FV, Nutritional knowledge	'Be smart. Join in. Be fit.'	Düsseldorf, Germany	Controlled trial	CT	2	x			
Llargue's E. et al. [72]	2016	Four-year outcomes of an educational intervention in healthy habits in schoolchildren: the Avall 3 Trial	To investigate the impact of the intervention on physical activity, BMI and prevalence of overweight and obesity after 4 years	Anthropometry	The Avall project	Granollers, Spain	Randomised Controlled Cluster Trial	RCCT	3	x			
Martins M.L. et al. [73]	2015	Strategies to reduce plate waste in primary schools—experimental evaluation	To determine and compare the effect of two interventions in reducing the plate waste of school lunches	Nutritional Knowledge	Reduce plate waste	City of Porto, Portugal	Controlled trial	CT	2	x		x	

Table 2. *Cont.*

Author	Year	Title/Reference	Main Aim (from Abstract)	Main Aim in Brief	Program Name Acronym	Location & Country	Study Design	Study Design Coded RCT, PP, CT, RCCT, Quasi	Power	Intervention Components				
										Information and Teaching	Environmental/Food Focus on Healthy Meal Availability	Food Focus	Environmental/Food Focus through School Gardening	Family/Social Support
Rosario R. et al. [ ]	2016	Impact of a school-based intervention to promote fruit intake: a cluster randomized controlled trial	To examine the effects of a six-month dietary education programme, delivered and taught by trained teachers, on the consumption of fruit as a dessert in children aged 6–12 years	HE & FV	Dietary education intervention programme	City in north of Portugal	Randomised Controlled Cluster Trial	RCCT	3	x				
Zafiropulos V. et al. [ ]	2015	Preliminary results of a dietary intervention among primary school children	To evaluate the effectiveness of the dietary intervention by measuring body composition and dietary behaviour of children prior to and after the intervention	Anthropometry, HE & FV	WBDI	central/eastern Crete Greece	RCT with the aspects of pre and post intervention	RCT	3	x				

Table 3. The review sample-findings. The table shows the findings from the 43 studies of the review.

Author	Year	Age	Age Coded			Sample Size, n	Time Duration/Month	Outcome Measures				Effectiveness Among Children				Target Group	Target Group Coded	
		Years	EA	EMI	EL			Anthropometry	HE/FV	Nutritional Knowledge	Attitude	Anthropometry	HE/FV	Nutritional Knowledge	Attitude		S	NS
Harake et al. [ ]	2018	6–14 years	x	x	x	183	6	x	x	x	x	3	3	4	2	Syrian refugee children in grade 4 to 6 from three informal primary schools (2 intervention and one control)		x
Adab P, et al [ ]	2018	6–7 years	x			1392	12		x	x		1	1			UK primary schools	x	
Harley A, et al. [ ]	2018	11–13 years		x		248	1 and half	x	x	x		3	4	4		8 public kindergarten		x
Hermans R.C.J. et al. [ ]	2018	10–13 years		x	x	108	N.A.	x	x	x			1	1		Dutch children (elementary school children)—3 primary school in the souther part of Netherland	x	
Pana N., et al. [ ]	2017	7–9 years	x	x		190	4		x	x			4	4		11 primary school classes in five schools	x	
Batjies-Fries M.C.E, et al. [ ]	2017	10–11 years		x	x	1010	3		x		x		1		1	children of 34 elementary school grade 6 and 7	x	
Bogart L.M, et al. [ ]	2014	N.A.				2997	41		x	x			4	4		10 schools	x	
Shriqui V.K., et al. [ ]	2016	4–7 years	x			240	10	x	x	x		2	4	4		Children attending LSES school classes	x	

Table 3. *Cont.*

Author	Year	Age	Age Coded			Sample Size, n	Time Duration/Month	Outcome Measures				Effectiveness Among Children				Target Group	Target Group Coded	
		Years	EA	EMl	El			Anthropometry	HF/FV	Nutritional Knowledge	Attitude	Anthropometry	HF/FV	Nutritional Knowledge	Attitude		S	NS
Sharma S.V. et al. [43]	2016	N.A. (first grade students)	x			172	24						3	3		Public or charter schools 1st grade students and their family members		x
Lawlor A.D. et al. [44]	2016	9–10 years			x	2221 (valid data for the 10 mediators were available for 87% to 96% of participants)	36	x	x	x		1	1			primary school children	x	
Steyn P.N. et al. [45]	2016	Mean age 9.9 years	x			500 intervention and 498 control	36		x				1			primary school children from low income settings	x	
Jones M. et al. [46]	2017	8–10 years		x		2411	24		x	x			4	4		schools engaged with the Food for Life programme	x	
Larsen L.A. et al. [47]	2015	(fourth grade students) average 9 years	x			1713	2		x	x	x		4	4	3	47 fourth-grade California classrooms	x	
Shen, Hu and Sun [48]	2015	10.80 ± 1.14			x	478	8		x	x	x		4	4	1	Twelve primary schools in west China	x	
Gallotta C.M. et al. [21]	2016	8–11 years	x		x	230	5	x	x	x		3	4	3		three primary schools in the rural area in the north of the city of Rome (Italy)	x	
Fairclough J.S. et al. [49]	2013	10–11 years	x		x	318	6	x	x			3	1			12 primary schools	x	
Cunha B.D. et al. [50]	2013	10–11 years	x		x	574	9	x		x		1		3		20 schools with fifth grade classes	x	
Aviles O.A. et al. [51]	2017	12–14 years			x	1430	28	x	x			2	3			20 schools	x	
Muros J.J. et al. [52]	2013	10–11 years	x		x	54	2	x	x			2	2			2 schools from rular environment with same socio economic status	x	
Moss A et al. [?]	2013	N.A. 3rd grade students				65	1		x	x			3	4		3rd grade students	x	
Zota D. et al. [54]	2016	4–11 years	x	x	x	21261	12	x	x	x		3	4	3		students attending both elementary and secondary schools in areas of low socioeconomic status (SES)	x	

Table 3. *Cont.*

Author	Year	Age	Age Coded			Sample Size, n	Time Duration/Month	Outcome Measures				Effectiveness Among Children				Target Group	Target Group Coded	
		Years	EA	EMI	EL			Anthropometry	HE/FV	Nutritional Knowledge	Attitude	Anthropometry	HE/FV	Nutritional Knowledge	Attitude		S	NS
Gold A. et al. [ ]	2017	8–9 years		x		662	12		x				4			3rd grade children from 26 schools	x	
Mbhatsani H.V., et al. [ ]	2017	9–14 years		x	x	172	6		x	x			3	3		2 rural primary schools with similar socioeconomic backgrounds	x	
Hutchinson J. et al. [ ]	2015	7–10 years	x	x		1256	12		x	x	x		3	3	2	21 London schools	x	
Viggiano A et al. [ ]	2018	7–11 years	x	x	x	1313	2.5	x	x	x		2	3	3		10 primary schools	x	
Waters E. et al. [ ]	2017	5–12 years	x	x	x	2965	42	x	x	x		1	3	3		24 schools of Moreland municipality	x	
Xu F et al. [ ]	2015	Mean age 10.2		x		1182	10			x		2		3		4th grade students from 8 schools of Nanjing, China	x	
Jung et al. [ ]	2018	NA (elementry school-kindergarden, 2nd, 3rd, 4th, 5th and 6th graders)	x	x		646	12		x	x	x		2	3	2	2 elementary schools	x	

The information from abstracts were organized in a table with the following information:

Column A: Authors. The column lists the researchers/authors conducting the study.

Column B: Year. The column shows the year of the publication of the article.

Column C: Title/Reference. The column lists the title of the article.

Column D: Main aim. The column lists the main aim presented by authors in the abstract of each article.

Column E: Main aim in brief. This column is a constructed variable that refers to the main aim of each study. The idea was to give in brief the study idea and which outcome measures was focused on in the study.

Column F: Program name. The column gives the name of the project, program or intervention reported in in the article.

Column G: Location and Country. The column lists the specific place or location where the study was performed.

Column H: Study design. The column shows research design of the study according to authors.

Column I: Study design coded. This column is a constructed variable to capture the research design of the study and used to make an analysis of power possible, see Column J.

Column J: Power. The column was constructed to express the strength of the design. It is a dummy variable that was assigned a numerical value that allowed for a quantitative analytical approach.

Column K, L and M: Intervention components. The column shows which intervention components that was used in the study. We used a model that categorizes components into three different mechanisms of influence: cognitive (K), environmental (L, M, N) and social (O).

The environmental component includes actions where availability of meals—or fruit and vegetable (F & V)—were increased. Either through passive provision (F & V and meals) or through active participation such as gardening. The social category included actions where families and/or peers were actively influencing the participants. The cognitive category included teaching and learning.

Column L: Environmental/food focus on F & V. In this column, interventions which were targeted towards fruits and vegetables were flagged. This includes interventions whose focus was providing cooking lessons and maintaining healthy cafeterias during the intervention periods. Also, maintaining healthy cafeteria here refers to school canteens providing healthy options to its menu where children's while buying food have healthier options to choose.

Column M: Environmental/food focus on increasing availability through school gardening. In this column, interventions which provided free foods among participants through gardening within the school were listed.

Column N: Environmental/food interventions focused on healthy meal availability. Interventions which provided healthy meals, breakfast, snacks during the school hours and distributed fresh fruits among the participants were listed in this column.

Column O: Family/social support. In this column interventions that included social components were flagged. These interventions included peer and family influence mechanisms.

Column P: Age. The column lists the age of the targeted groups of the intervention expressed in years according to the primary article data provided by authors.

Column Q: Age construct EA. This column shows a constructed variable for the age categorization based on the primary data given by authors. The constructed code was made to make statistical analyses possible. The construct Early Age (EA) was assigned if intervention were carried out in early school.

Column R: Age construct EML. This column shows a constructed variable for the age categorization based on the primary data given by authors. The code Early Middle Late (EML) was assigned if intervention was targeted all age groups.

Column S: Age construct EL. This column shows a constructed variable for the age categorization based on the primary data given by authors. The code EL refers to Early late and was assigned if the intervention was targeted early and early and late school.

Column T: Sample size. The number of young people enrolled in the intervention was listed in this column.

Column U: Time duration. This column shows the length of the intervention expressed in months. It is a constructed variable based on the primary data given by authors and was made to standardize duration and make it ready for cross study analysis.

Columns V, W, X, Y: Outcome measures. In Columns T, U, V, W, the outcome measures named as Anthropometry, HE/FV (healthy eating fruits and vegetables), Nutritional knowledge, and Attitude, respectively, were listed according to our outcome model shown in Figure 1. Only a few include all outcome measures, but all studies included at least one of them.

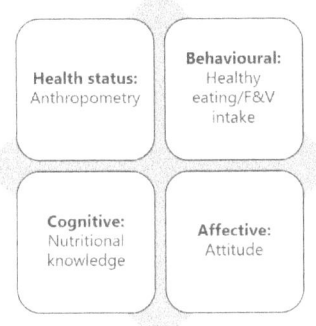

Figure 1. Outcome measures model. The figure illustrates the four types of outcome measures found in the interventions.

Columns X, AA, AB, AC: Effectiveness. The effectiveness as measured by the outcomes measured are listed in this column. Each outcome measure was rated using a Likert scale from 0–4. The effectiveness of outcome measures among participants as measured by the measures in our model (Figure 1): attitude, anthropometry, HE/FV, nutritional knowledge and attitude were listed in the Columns X, Y, Z, AA, respectively.

Column AD: Target group. This column provides information on the target group of interventions such as information on grades of subjects and municipalities.

Columns AE, AF: Target group. This column is a constructed variable created to capture if the intervention had a special ethnic or socio-economic focus. Columns AC and AD consisted of coded target group named as Standard (S) and Non-Standard (NS). The "NS" here represents the target group either from refugees or immigrants or lower socio-economic classes.

Column AG: Keywords. This column lists the keywords found in the interventions.

Ordinary least squares regression was applied in this study; specifically, we used the linear regression function in IBM SPSS 22. We opted for a multi-variate approach; i.e., multiple linear regression was used. Anthropometry, behaviour (healthy eating and food focus), attitude and nutritional knowledge were used as dependent variables. In order to better account for control variables, such as sample size and study length, a dummy variable was introduced for study length of one year and more; and a logarithm of the sample size was used instead of the actual sample size to eliminate scaling effects. We grouped countries by continents (while splitting Europe into North and South as there were enough studies and no countries in between) and introduced related dummy variables. The remaining variables were used as independent variables without any additional manipulations.

Since the aim was to create models consisting only of independent variables that significantly influence the dependent variables, we used the backwards function. Because there were too many independent variables for the backwards function for the attitude model (with only eight observations), the stepwise function was used instead.

Information and teaching was present in all but one study. Free food was found only in two studies and focus on fruit and vegetables in three studies. Therefore, it is not surprising that neither of the three variables were found to be significant in any of the models.

2.7. Study Sample

The search strategy resulted in 1826 titles which were screened for duplicates and potential relevance. After this initial screening, 345 titles and abstracts were assessed against the inclusion and exclusion criteria. Articles that studied school interventions after school hours were excluded. In addition, articles which studied interventions among children in out of school context such as at community level were excluded. The justification is that both "after school" and "out of school" since can be regarded as non-typical school environments. We aimed to study the "school" as an artefact that can be considered as a "standard" across countries despite some national differences. For both "after school" and "out of school", we argue that there are considerable differences among countries and that an inclusion of such studies would negatively influence our analytical approach. In total, 42 articles were identified as relevant and full papers were obtained as the final sample. Figure 2 below illustrates the search terms and selection process of articles.

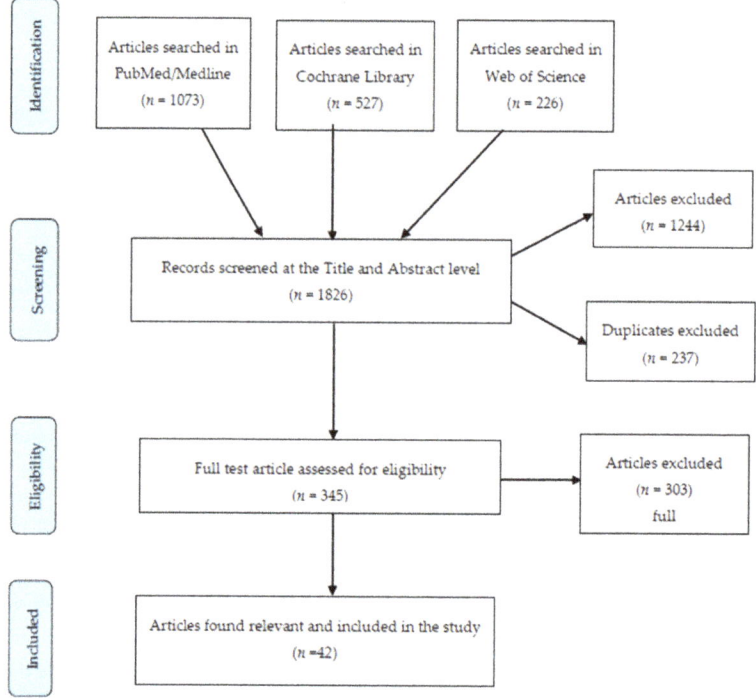

Figure 2. Review flow chart. The figure shows the progress of the literature review process following the PRISMA 2009 approach.

2.8. Intervention Study Characteristics

For all 43 items in our sample, Table 2 provides the information about the study, intervention methodologies, characteristics strategies, etc. In our extract of studies, the sample size ranged from 65-2997 subjects/participants, and the intervention duration ranged from 1 and half month to 36 months. The systematic review locations identified by the author were: 26 from Europe [21,36,38–40,44,46,49,52,54,57,58,63–75], six from Asia [35,42,48,59,60,62], 10 from America [37,41,43,45,47,50,51,53,55,61] and one from Africa [56]. We categorized all interventions according to their intervention components. To this end, we had constructed three classes: Information and Teaching, Food Focus and Family/Social support as illustrated. The interventions characteristics of each included study are shown in Table 2.

Of the total study sample, the majority of studies ($n = 41$) involved "Information and Teaching" components consisting mainly of classroom-based activities (e.g., an adapted curriculum and distribution of educational materials, health and nutrition education program). Another 12 studies along with "Information and Teaching" involved a food focus and availability component. These food and availability components which consisted mainly of supervised school gardening, environmental modifications to stimulate a more healthful diet, such as increased availability and accessibility of healthy foods, distributions free food programmes, school provided free breakfast, school lunch modifications and incentives. Only two studies combined all the three intervention components of this study. Family/social support intervention was clearly focused on in nine study. In other studies, even though their interventions were not primarily or secondarily focused on family/social support component, they indirectly acknowledged the importance of parents and included them in their studies.

All of the reviewed studies included intervention components that were delivered in school settings and within school hours. Our sample showed that consumption of fruit and vegetables was the most used intervention component and was include in more than half of the interventions. Most studies were designed and carried in a way where a research assistant was trained by senior researchers/co-authors to ensure that each members of the research team followed same procedures for data collection. Since all studies were "in situ" studies included a close researcher/school staff cooperation component. In most of the listed studies, teachers being the responsible person to implement the interventions were trained beforehand.

2.9. Types of Interventions

Table 2 shows an overview of the programmes and their intervention components. From the table, it can be seen that studies differed according to how broadly they intervened. Some studies have included a narrow intervention (i.e., only one intervention components which targeted behavioural components), whereas others included multicomponent approaches where all three intervention components were used in the study.

3. Results

Finding the right approach to intervening for healthier eating at school is a major challenge. In other words, which interventions create which impacts and how should the public best invest in new policies, strategies, and practices at school if long term health is the intended end point?

The purpose of this review was to compile the evidence regarding the effectiveness of successful school-based interventions in improving dietary behaviours, nutritional knowledge, attitudes and anthropometry among children. The analysis of the data showed a number of relationships between outcome effect and a number of other characteristics of the intervention (i.e., age, location/region, intervention type, duration). Descriptive statistics are provided in Table 4.

Table 4. Descriptive statistics.

	N	Minimum	Maximum	Mean	Standard Deviation
Power	42	1.00	3.00	2.2619	0.91223
InfoAndTeach	42	0.00	1.00	0.9762	0.15430
FandV	42	0.00	1.00	0.0714	0.26066
FreeFood	42	0.00	1.00	0.0476	0.21554
AvailFood	42	0.00	1.00	0.1667	0.37720
FamilySocialSupport	42	0.00	1.00	0.2143	0.41530
EA—early age	42	0.00	1.00	0.3810	0.49151
EML—early middle late age	42	0.00	1.00	0.7381	0.44500
EL—early late age	42	0.00	1.00	0.5476	0.50376
SampleSize	42	54.00	21261.00	1464.2619	3277.18184
log10SampleSize	42	1.73	4.33	2.7904	0.54986
Months	41	1.00	112.00	14.6585	19.00245
YearOrMore01	41	0.00	1.00	0.4390	0.50243
AnthropometryScale	18	0.00	4.00	2.0000	1.13759
HEFVScale	36	1.00	4.00	2.5556	1.27491
NutritionalKnowledgeScale	26	1.00	4.00	3.1923	0.89529
AttitudeScale	9	1.00	3.00	1.7778	0.66667

The linear regression models carried out for each intervention component is added in the text and the tables have been referred to each associated result. Out of 42 studies, 36 studies reported the outcome on HE/FV behaviour scale while anthropometry and attitude impacts were observed in 18 and six studies, respectively. The item one of the results in this article presents the most general finding from the literature review, item two describes the variable found significant in two cases, while the remaining variables were significant in once case each. Additionally, item four, five and six are related "design" phenomena effects in the sense that they are not related to intervention components but to the study was designed your study. The rest is related to (intervention components rather than designs. In Table 5, the outcome measures for which an effect could be seen has been listed. The linear regression model describing what influences the attitude is provided in Table 6.

Table 5. Linear regression model for attitude.

Model	Unstandardized Coefficients		Standardized Coefficients	t	Significance
	B	SE	Beta		
(Constant)	1.250	0.177		7.071	0.000
FamilySocialSupport	1.000	0.395	0.500	2.530	0.045
EA—early age	0.750	0.250	0.593	3.000	0.024

Table 6. Linear regression model for anthropometry.

Model	Unstandardized Coefficients		Standardized Coefficients	t	Significance
	B	SE	Beta		
(Constant)	4.140	1.008		4.109	0.001
Power	1.511	0.468	0.859	3.231	0.007
AvailFood	3.432	0.804	0.976	4.267	0.001
YearOrMore	0.870	0.403	0.384	2.161	0.050
log10SampleSize	−2.437	0.503	−1.267	−4.846	0.000

With regards to the explanatory power of the model, $R^2 = 0.789$, R^2 adj. $= 0.719$, and significance $= 0.009$. The linear regression model describing what influences the anthropometry is provided in Table 6. With regards to the explanatory power of the model, $R^2 = 0.683$, R^2 adj. $= 0.586$, and significance $= 0.003$. The linear regression model describing what influences the behaviour is provided in Table 7.

Table 7. Linear regression model for behaviour.

Model	Unstandardized Coefficients		Standardized Coefficients	t	Significance
	B	SE	Beta		
(Constant)	2.321	0.229		10.131	0.000
FamilySocialSupport	1.054	0.486	0.348	2.168	0.037

With regards to the explanatory power of the model, $R^2 = 0.121$, R^2 adj. $= 0.096$, and significance = 0.037.

An alternative linear regression model describing what influences the behaviour is provided in Table 8.

Table 8. Alternative linear regression model for behaviour.

Model	Unstandardized Coefficients		Standardized Coefficients	t	Significance
	B	SE	Beta		
(Constant)	3.227	0.205		15.761	0.000
Neurope	−1.727	0.328	−0.670	−5.260	0.000

With regards to the explanatory power of the model, $R^2 = 0.449$, R^2 adj. $= 0.432$, and significance < 0.001.

3.1. School-Based Interventions in General Create Impact

Looking across the whole study sample, it can be seen that in general the interventions created an impact in one or more ways either on knowledge, intentions, eating habits and/or anthropometry. In other words, it was hard to find studies that created no impact. This finding adds to the body of evidence that suggests that food-based interventions are a well-suited and effective policy tool when it comes to promoting healthier eating among young people.

3.2. Family Support Affects Healthier Eating Behaviour and Attitude

Out of all the included studies, nine studies focused on family support as an intervention component. But out of those, our analysis showed that the family involvement was impactful among participants when it comes to promoting healthier food choices. Parents being influencers and role models in the family in these studies seemed to help to influence children's dietary habits. Studies which involved participants' parents in the intervention and provided them with nutritional knowledge and healthy cooking skills (i.e., knowledge about the importance of healthy food and nutrition during the early age of their children), seemed to be able to help young people prepare more healthy and nutritious food at home. As studies showed, this seemed to increase children's intentions towards eating more fruits and vegetables and eventually resulted in consumption of more healthy foods. However, this did not seem to be the case for all ages. Intention to eat more fruits and vegetables was seen among early age participants (EA) either alone or with family support. It should be noted that the regression models did not include interactions, since the number of analysed studies was only ~40. It was not possible to include age as a continuous variable in the models because (as it can be seen in Table 5) age was a range, and sometimes even a wide range, e.g., 8–11 or 4–11. Family support increases the outcome measure by approximately 1 in both cases. Please refer to Tables 5 and 7 for detailed linear regression model used for attitude and behaviour.

3.3. Interventions Done in Northern Europe (7 Studies) Had a Smaller Impact on Behaviour than the Studies Conducted in the Rest of the World (22 Studies)

The results from the models which was created to measure the efficiency of HE/FV highlighted the fact that HE/FV scale depends only on region where the intervention was done. The behaviour outcome for Northern Europe was on average 1.5 while the average for the rest was 3.2 (please refer to Table 8).

3.4. Effect of Anthropometry Measures Increases with Study Power

The results suggested that the design of the study plays a role when it comes to be able to show impact of interventions. From the findings, it was clear that the anthropometry measured among the participants were increasing with the power of the study. That is, the stronger the design the greater the likelihood of being able to measure impact on anthropometric outcomes—a unit increase in the design power is associated with an outcome increase of approximately 1.5 (please refer to Table 6). To examine the influence of study design we used the score that was constructed for the purpose (please refer to Table 1). This score assigns a higher power to randomized designs than non-randomized ones.

3.5. Study Duration Impacts Anthropometric Outcomes

It was also clear that the intervention duration does have impact on the outcome, i.e., the longer the duration better the anthropometric results among the children. Interventions that lasted a year or more, had the outcome measure on average almost one unit higher than shorter studies (please refer to Table 6).

3.6. Larger Samples Impacts Anthropometry Measures

Results showed that anthropometric outcome decreased within the sample size. Increasing the sample size by a factor of 10, from approximately 100 to 1000, decreased the outcome measure by almost 2.5 (please refer to Table 6). Thus, bigger the sample size a reverse effect on outcome was obtained. The studies whose intervention was done for long period of time (i.e., couple of months or year and among small participants) were found to be effective in the outcome. It might be the case that it was hard to administer the same thing to large sample size post intervention and thus could have decreased the anthropometry outcome among the participants.

3.7. Food Availability Interventions Influence Anthropometric Outcomes

Our analyses showed that a food focus, specifically healthy meal availability had an impact on the children's anthropometric outcomes—increasing it by almost 3.5 on average (please refer to Table 6).

3.8. Interventions among Younger Students Influence Attitude Among Participants

Results showed that the younger the study subjects were, the more influence interventions had on attitudes (the outcome was on average 0.75 higher than for other age groups). Thus, the result suggests that the participants' attitude increases when they are in their early age (EA) i.e., 4–7 years old. Furthermore, results suggest that increased family support associated with participants' attitude towards healthy eating helps in changing the behaviour among them. Early age (EA) and family support seemed to impact positively both alone and together. Meaning that the intervention had positive impacts on participants (i.e., EA participants) attitudes towards healthy eating either with the involvement of their family support or without the involvement of family support. Please refer to Table 5 for detail linear regression model for attitude.

3.9. No Effect of School Based Interventions on Nutritional Knowledge

Findings showed that nutritional knowledge among participants (i.e., of all age group) does not depend on school-based interventions. Thus, none of the collected variables have influences on nutritional knowledge.

4. Discussion

4.1. Discussion of Results of This Review in Relation to Others

In the discussion we aim to relate our findings with what has been found in previous studies, discuss our methodological approach and reflect on what are the policy implications. Since the discussion on how to counteract the unhealthy eating pattern and the worrying increase in nutrition related disorders among young people is attracting much attention and since the discussion on how the school could contribute we aim to give policy makers and practitioners an up to date insight into the potentials of the school to act as a hub for promotion of healthier eating and provide inspiration for the development of new types of school-based interventions and strategies.

The huge interest in using the infrastructure of the school to initiate and promote healthier eating among young people has resulted in a large number of interventions studies over the past decades. This research interest per definition as the same time creates a need for syntheses of the findings in order to make them feed into the public health and school policy cycle and to "send the results to work". Taken the huge investment that better food at school strategies at school will cost for states it is worth appreciating that the Evidence-Informs-Policy pathway seems to be working. At the same time the conceptual approaches and the understanding of what intervention components might work better than others, which age groups might benefit the most etc. as developed considerably which again adds to the rationale for synthesis of intervention study findings. Most recent reviews by Julie et al. [76], Noguera el al. [77], Evans et al. [78], Cauwenberghe et al. [34] and Brown et al. [79] has created a time gap of almost five years. Covering the last five years of research our review makes a needed contribution and in addition we argue it makes a needed contribution to a standardization and conceptualization of both sampling and intervention design methodologies.

Overall, the findings from this review suggest that school-based interventions that include intervention components such as information and teaching, food focus and family support are effective in improving the HE/FV, anthropometric measurements and attitude towards healthy dietary behaviour among the participants. On the other hand, nutritional knowledge among participants did not seem to be influenced much by any of the intervention components used.

Impacts on HE/FV behaviours were observed, but mostly among early age children revealing a distinct age pattern in the findings. Thus, age was seen as a significant factor in determining effectiveness in several study [35,37,39,42]. Impact was greater on young children in the 4–7 year old age range, suggesting that dietary influences may vary with age.

Multicomponent approaches that includes good quality instruction and programs, a supportive social environment both at school and home, family support has been effective in addressing childhood related diseases through focusing on diet and physical activity. Most of the studies in this review implemented with combination of school staff and intervention specialists provide evidence for the effectiveness of the program. Thus, evidence supports that family involvement and nutrition education curriculum delivered by the teacher under supervision of intervention specialists can alter the intake of fruit and vegetables while impacting positively on anthropometric measurements. Teacher led interventions have been effective and can be the most sustainable approach for long term impact of the program. The same conclusion was found in a review done in investigating the effectiveness of school-based interventions in Europe which provided the effectiveness of multicomponent intervention promoting a healthy diet in school aged children in Europe [34].Studies with a food focus in their intervention approaches showed significant improvements in BMI [35,54,58]. Significant improvements in BMI here refers to the studies whose probability value was less or equal to 0.05. This means that the interventions in that case showed reduction in body mass of participants. We looked at studies whose aim was to focus on interventions of obesity prevention or reduction among primary school children's. Thus, search term such as: "obesity prevention intervention among primary schools", was used as explained in the methods section. When performing the search for school-based interventions we did not encounter any studies that were focusing on underweight. Making the options for healthy choices of food in the school cafeterias and having the option of free food from the school gardens decreases the sugar sweetened beverages and junk options among the children's and thus resulting in improvements in BMI. This review evidence further highlights that duration of the intervention, i.e., a year or more has an impact on anthropometric measurements. This is in contrast to reviews of Julie et al. [76] and Cauwenberghe et al. [34] review that found that making the better options of food choices and duration of the studies were effective in reducing the sedentary behaviour and noting improvements in BMI. This study also found that larger sample sizes reverse the outcome of anthropometric measurements (i.e., sample size negatively influences the outcome). This might be the case because it might be harder to administer the same thing to more individual. Thus, more studies are needed to examine the effects of bigger sample sizes.

Our study is far from being the first to create overview of the large number of studies that are studying interventions that can promote healthier eating habits and that can counteract the worrying increase in obesity and overweight among young people the general. The huge interest is reflected in the number of studies trying to assess the impact and effectiveness of school-based interventions as well as in the number of reviews aiming to synthesize the findings from the growing body of evidence of the effect of school-based food interventions into actionable school food policies. Our study adds to this body of knowledge and fills a gap since our study looks at the most recent studies.

Comparing our review with others we find that the majority of the studies on school food-based interventions have been conducted in high income countries. This is also the case in our study and this fact is important to keep in mind since it introduces a bias in the insight created from school food effectiveness reviews. It is also important to keep in mind that studies—and as a result also reviews-covers different types of school food cultures. These cultures can roughly be divided in collective, semi collective and non-collective types. In the collective type found in countries such as Sweden, Finland, Estonia and Brazil school food provision is an integrated—and mainly free—part of the school day. In semi-collective approaches food is in most cases traditionally a part of what is offered at school, but due to payment. In the non-collective approach found in countries such as Denmark, Norway and the Netherlands there is little infrastructure and tradition for school organized foodservice. In this approach parents organized lunch boxes as well as competitive foods traditionally play a bigger role.

A further important note to make is the distinction between narrow F & V approaches and broader healthier eating intervention approaches. This classification can also be seen in previous studies and in more recent reviews. The first type of interventions that follow the six-a-day tradition that to some extent has been fuelled by the European School Fruit program introduced by the EU in 2009 was reviewed by Noguera et al. [77] and by Evans et al. [78]. In a study by Noguera el al. [77] a meta-analysis on F&V interventions was done but limited to educational interventions in the sense that it only looked at computer-based interventions and covering mostly European research. The study showed that this targeted but narrowed approach was effective in increasing FV consumption but that broader multicomponent types of interventions including free/subsidized FV interventions were not effective. In the review paper from 2012 by Evans et al. [78] examined studies done in United Kingdom, United States, Canada, Denmark, New Zealand, Norway and the Netherlands. Evans and co-workers [78] found that school-based interventions were able to moderately improve fruit intake but that they had only minimal impact on vegetable intake. These reviews and previous ones generally conclude that F&V targeted interventions are able to improve young people's eating patterns towards higher intake of fruit.

In the category of reviews taking a broader approach to healthier lifestyle promotion we find studies and reviews that looks at promotion of healthier eating in general—and that in some cases include physical activity. A review by Julie et al. [76] covered studies from United States, United Kingdom, Australia, Spain and the Netherlands. This review also included physical activity as part of broader school-based obesity prevention interventions. In particular, interventions should focus on extending physical education classes, incorporating activity breaks, and reducing sedentary behaviours to improve anthropometric measures. Julie et al. concluded that interventions taking a broader approach should include employing a combination of school staff and intervention specialists to implement programs; that they should include psychosocial/psychoeducational components; involve peer leaders; use incentives to increase fruit and vegetable consumption and should involve family. In a study by Cauwenberghe et al. [34] intervention studies done in a European union studies were reviewed. This review—as our study do—made an age distinction in the sense that a categorization was done between children and adolescents. Among children the authors found a strong evidence of effect for multicomponent interventions on fruit and vegetable intake. For educational type of interventions Cauwenberghe et al. [34] found limited evidence of effect as found when looking at behaviour and fruit and vegetable intakes. The study found limited evidence on effectiveness of interventions that specifically targeted children from lower socio-economic status groups. For adolescents Cauwenberghe et al. [34] found moderate evidence of effect was found for educational interventions on behaviour and limited evidence of effect for multicomponent programmes on behaviour. In the same way as our review authors distinguished between behaviour and anthropometrics and found that effects on anthropometrics were often not measured in their sample. Therefore, evidence was lacking and resulted in inconclusive evidence. Cauwenberghe et al. [34] concluded that there was evidence was found for the effectiveness of especially multicomponent interventions promoting a healthy diet but that evidence for effectiveness on anthropometrical obesity-related measures was lacking. In a review by Brown et al. [79] studies mostly from Europe but also covering United States, New Zealand, Canada and Chile it was found that intervention components most likely to influence BMI positively included increased physical activity, decreased sugar sweetened beverages intake, and increased fruit intake.

Our review adds to the increasing support for the idea that school should play a role in promoting healthier eating habits among young people. As such the school can be seen as an important actor when it comes to the promotion of human rights. In particular; the right to adequate food, the right to the highest attainable standard of health and right to the education, school plays an integral part which has also been highlighted in the "United Nations System Standing Committee on Nutrition" new statement for school-based and nutrition interventions [25]. Furthermore, Mikkelsen and colleagues [80] in their study have also suggested the fact that the international framework of human rights should invoke its strategies, policies, and regulations in the context of school and that national, regional, and local level actors has important roles to play. Additionally, they have highlighted that ensuring healthy eating in school environment can be a good investment in children short- and long-term health and education achievements. Thus, schools, as a system have the potential to make lasting improvements in students nutrition both in terms of quality and quantity and simultaneously contribute to realization of human rights around the globe [25].

4.2. Discussion of Methods

Strengths and Limitations

All attempts to reduce complexity of research studies in a research field suffers from in built weaknesses. Standardising the work of others in attempts to make generalizations is always difficult. As per definition a review includes attempts to standardize its study material in order to create an overview of "what works" and what "this that works" depends on. For obvious reasons research protocols depends very much on the context of the study: What is doable in one study setting on one country might not work on other settings. Additionally, reporting procedures vary among authors. The aim of a review is to standardize this heterogeneity to something that is homogenous and computable. So, in our case our constructs represent an attempt to make different studies with similar but slightly different approaches and methodologies comparable by making them computable. This has obviously some disadvantages.

Another limitation is that our review restricted itself to cover only published English language articles. Therefore, publication bias cannot be excluded, as it is possible that the inclusion of unpublished articles written in other languages than English will have affected the results of this review. Second, most of the studies included in the present were carried out in countries from Southern and Northern parts of Europe. This raises questions about the generalisability of these results to other countries in Europe, especially because contextual variables were often lacking in the included studies. And the same questions about the generalisability could be raise in other parts of the world i.e., in Latin America, North America, Asia and Africa, as very few studies were reported from this part of the world.

On the other hand, large dropouts were reported in many listed studies and the study follow up were reported in few studies and was for short time period. Among these studies which did follow up, was right after the end of the intervention period and thus this could have affected the effectiveness among this study outcomes. Long-term follows-up post-interventions would help to study the retention of behaviour change and effect on the body composition among the participants. Thus, long terms studies post interventions are needed to draw the conclusion about the sustainability of an intervention. Additionally, in future studies to improve the quality of the evidence of effectiveness in this kind of interventions, studies with high quality, rigorous design, appropriate sample size, post interventions long term follow up, assessment of implementation issues and cost effectiveness of the intervention should be executed.

On the strength side the standardisation approach helps to find patterns and to create overview of a large material within a given field of research. The strength of this study is that it provides a broad up to date overview of what is known about the relationship between school-based intervention and policies and healthy eating outcomes among children and that it contributes to the deeper understanding of the fact that current research findings are quite limited. This is among the very few recent reviews which evaluated the effect of school-based food at nutrition interventions among children only. A systematic review approach of this study attempted efficiently to integrate existing information and provide data for researchers' rationale in the decision making of future research. Furthermore, the applied explicit methods used in this limited bias and, contributed to improved reliability and accuracy of drawn conclusions. Other advantages are that this study looks specifically at the evidence available in Northern and Southern Europe. Statistical analyses of pooled data have facilitated a more through synthesis of the result is one of the biggest strengths of this study.

4.3. Policy Implications

The evidence of the impact of school intervention derived from our review suggests several topics to be dealt with in future research not only in Europe but also the other part of the world. First, this review highlights the need for researchers to recognize the importance of further investigations on the measures of anthropometrics, nutritional knowledge, and attitude. Among these 42 studies carried out in different regions very few looked upon the effects on participants' attitudes and anthropometrics measures. And of those showed positive impact if family support was provided, if started at early age and lastly if food focus was part of the intervention. Additionally, most of the included studies were not aiming to contribute to obesity prevention. Thus, it is highly recommendable that there is urgent need for more studies to be done that includes more measures of efficiency of participants' attitude towards the healthy behaviour and healthy lifestyle and measures for anthropometrics. Second, to increase the comparability between studies and to facilitate the assessment of effectiveness, more agreement is needed for best measures of the diet and questionnaires. Third, more research is needed to be done among specific groups like low socio-economic group, immigrants or minorities. As mention earlier, only few listed studies included this specific group in their studies. Furthermore, evidence suggest that health inequalities such as prevalence of overweight are as a result of dietary habits and ethnicity and socio-economic status are identified as determinants of health eating. Thus, future research should not exclude these specific groups as European countries have become ethnically diverse.

To improve or decrease childhood diseases such as overweight and obesity and other aspects of health, many policy documents have been calling for the development of the effective strategies among children's and adolescents. Even though the limited to moderate impact and evidence was found among these school-based interventions, it should be noted that interventions were not primarily targeting obesity prevention but, in many cases, had a broader scope. Thus, in order to deliver these evidence-based recommendations to policy makers factors such as sustainability of intervention, context and cost effectiveness should be considered. Additionally, the policy makers should ensure school policies and the environment that encourage physical activity and a healthy diet.

5. Conclusions

Findings from this systematised review suggest that applying multicomponent interventions (environmental, educational, and physical strategies) along with parental involvement and of long-term initiatives may be promising for improving dietary habits and other childhood related diseases among primary school children. Despite being challenging to find experimental studies done in related fields, those studies found showed positive trend. Thus, to conclude, evidence of the effect was found among school-based food and nutrition initiatives among primary school children. However, to strengthen the perspectives of this study, further systematic review targeting the more long-term studies assessing the long-term sustainability of the interventions should be considered. Also, studies with goal to increase efficiency of anthropometric measurements in their future school-based interventions could include increasing PA, increasing fruit and vegetable intake and decreasing sedentary behaviour. This study has provided fundamentals background on which further research could be done in this area of school-based food and nutrition interventions. Thus, the findings from this systematic review can be used as guidelines for future interventions in school settings related to food and nutrition. Also, the categorization of intervention components we see as useful for the planning of future interventions.

Author Contributions: Conceptualization, B.E.M. and A.C.; methodology, B.E.M., A.C. and F.S.; validation B.E.M.; formal analysis, F.S.; investigation, A.C.; resources B.E.M. and A.C.; data curation, A.C. and F.S.; writing—original draft preparation, B.E.M., A.C. and F.S.; writing—review and editing, B.E.M., A.C. and F.S.; project administration, B.E.M. All authors have read and agreed to the published version of the manuscript.

Funding: This research received no external funding.

Conflicts of Interest: The authors declare no conflict of interest.

References

1. Micha, R.; Karageorgou, D.; Bakogianni, I.; Trichia, E.; Whitsel, L.P.; Story, M.; Penalvo, J.L.; Mozaffarian, D. Effectiveness of school food environment policies on children's dietary behaviors: A systematic review and meta-analysis. *PLoS ONE* **2018**, *13*, e0194555. [CrossRef]
2. WHO Europe. *Food and Nutrition Policy for Schools Copenhagen, Security PfNaF*; WHO: Geneva, Switzerland, 2006.
3. EU Commission. *EU Action Plan on Childhood Obesity 2014–2020*; EU Commission: Brussels, Belgium, 2014.
4. Lytle, L.A.; Kubik, M.Y. Nutritional issues for adolescents. *Best Pract. Res. Clin. Endocrinol. Metab.* **2003**, *17*, 177–189. [CrossRef]
5. WHO. Obesity and Overweight 2020. Available online: https://www.who.int/news-room/fact-sheets/detail/obesity-and-overweight (accessed on 20 July 2020).
6. WHO. *Diet, Nutrition and The Prevention of Chronic Diseases*; Contract No.: WHO Technical Report Series 916; WHO: Geneva, Switzerland, 2003.

7. Serra-Paya, N.; Ensenyat, A.; Castro-Vinuales, I.; Real, J.; Sinfreu-Bergues, X.; Zapata, A.; Mur, J.M.; Galindo-Ortego, G.; Solé-Mir, E.; Teixido, C. Effectiveness of a Multi-Component Intervention for Overweight and Obese Children (Nereu Program): A Randomized Controlled Trial. *PLoS ONE* **2015**, *10*, e0144502. [CrossRef] [PubMed]
8. Hruby, A.; Hu, F.B. The Epidemiology of Obesity: A Big Picture. *Pharmacoeconomics* **2015**, *33*, 673–689. [CrossRef] [PubMed]
9. WHO. *Interim Report of the Commission on Ending Childhood Obesity*; WHO: Geneva, Switzerland, 2015.
10. Aceves-Martins, M.; Llauradó, E.; Tarro, L.; Moreno-García, C.F.; Trujillo Escobar, T.G.; Sola, R.; Giralt, M. Effectiveness of social marketing strategies to reduce youth obesity in European school-based interventions: A systematic review and meta-analysis. *Nutr. Rev.* **2016**, *74*, 337–351. [CrossRef] [PubMed]
11. Cali, A.M.G.; Caprio, S. Obesity in children and adolescents. *J. Clin. Endocrinol. Metab.* **2008**, *93*, S31–S36. [CrossRef]
12. Abdelaal, M.; le Roux, C.W.; Docherty, N.G. Morbidity and mortality associated with obesity. *Ann. Transl. Med.* **2017**, *5*, 161. [CrossRef] [PubMed]
13. WHO. Child and Adolescent Health Copenhagen: UN City 2019. Available online: http://www.euro.who.int/en/health-topics/Life-stages/child-and-adolescent-health/child-and-adolescent-health (accessed on 20 July 2020).
14. Lynch, C.; Kristjansdottir, A.G.; Te Velde, S.J.; Lien, N.; Roos, E.; Thorsdottir, I.; Krawinkel, M.; de Almeida, M.D.V.; Papadaki, A.; Ribic, C.H.; et al. Fruit and vegetable consumption in a sample of 11-year-old children in ten European countries—The PRO GREENS cross-sectional survey. *Public Health Nutr.* **2014**, *17*, 2436–2444. [CrossRef] [PubMed]
15. Rippin, H.L.; Hutchinson, J.; Jewell, J.; Breda, J.J.; Cade, J.E. Child and adolescent nutrient intakes from current national dietary surveys of European populations. *Nutr. Res. Rev.* **2019**, *32*, 38–69. [CrossRef]
16. EU Science Hub. Childhood Obesity: Local Data Feeds Local Solutions 2018. Available online: https://ec.europa.eu/jrc/en/news/childhood-obesity-local-data-feeds-local-solutions (accessed on 21 July 2020).
17. Stefan, S.G.B.; Joao, B.; Sandra, C.; Michael, N.; Jan, W. School Food and Nutrition in Europe: Policies, Interventions and Their Impact: EU Science Hub. 2019. Available online: https://ec.europa.eu/jrc/en/publication/eur-scientific-and-technical-research-reports/school-food-and-nutrition-europe-policies-interventions-and-their-impact (accessed on 20 July 2020).
18. WHO. Obesity UN City Marmorvej 51 DK-2100 Copenhagen Ø: WHO Regional Office for Europe. 2018. Available online: http://www.euro.who.int/en/health-topics/noncommunicable-diseases/obesity/obesity (accessed on 21 July 2020).
19. ROfE WHO. *WHO European Childhood Obesity Surveillance Initiative (COSI): UN City*; Marmorvej 51 DK-2100; ROfE WHO: Copenhagen, Denmark, 2014; Available online: http://www.euro.who.int/en/health-topics/disease-prevention/nutrition/activities/who-european-childhood-obesity-surveillance-initiative-cosi (accessed on 21 July 2020).
20. Gallotta, M.C.; Iazzoni, S.; Emerenziani, G.P.; Meucci, M.; Migliaccio, S.; Guidetti, L.; Baldari, C. Effects of combined physical education and nutritional programs on schoolchildren's healthy habits. *PeerJ* **2016**, *4*, e1880. [CrossRef]
21. Contento, I.R. Nutrition education: Linking research, theory, and practice. *Asia Pac. J. Clin. Nutr.* **2008**, *17*, 176–179. [PubMed]
22. Glanz, K. Measuring Food Environments: A Historical Perspective. *Am. J. Prev. Med.* **2009**, *36*, S93–S98. [CrossRef] [PubMed]
23. Vereecken, C.; Haerens, L.; De Bourdeaudhuij, I.; Maes, L. The relationship between children's home food environment and dietary patterns in childhood and adolescence. *Public Health Nutr.* **2010**, *13*, 1729–1735. [CrossRef] [PubMed]
24. Nutrition UNSSCo. *Schools as a System to Improve Nutrition*; UNSCN: Geneva, Switzerland, 2017; p. 64.
25. Hollar, D.; Messiah, S.E.; Lopez-Mitnik, G.; Hollar, T.L.; Almon, M.; Agatston, A.S. Effect of a Two-Year Obesity Prevention Intervention on Percentile Changes in Body Mass Index and Academic Performance in Low-Income Elementary School Children. *Am. J. Public Health* **2010**, *100*, 646–653. [CrossRef]
26. Florence, M.D.; Asbridge, M.; Veugelers, P.J. Diet Quality and Academic Performance. *J. Sch. Health* **2008**, *78*, 209–215. [CrossRef]

27. Anderson, M.L.; Gallagher, J.; Ritchie, E.R. School meal quality and academic performance. *J. Public Econ.* **2018**, *168*, 81–93. [CrossRef]
28. Amare, B.; Moges, B.; Fantahun, B.; Tafess, K.; Woldeyohannes, D.; Yismaw, G.; Ayane, T.; Yabutani, T.; Mulu, A.; Ota, F.; et al. Micronutrient levels and nutritional status of school children living in Northwest Ethiopia. *Nutr. J.* **2012**, *11*, 108. [CrossRef]
29. Herrador, Z.; Sordo, L.; Gadisa, E.; Buño, A.; Gómez-Rioja, R.; Iturzaeta, J.M.; Armas, L.F.D.; Benito, A.; Aseffa, A.; Moreno, J.; et al. Micronutrient Deficiencies and Related Factors in School-Aged Children in Ethiopia: A Cross-Sectional Study in Libo Kemkem and Fogera Districts, Amhara Regional State. *PLoS ONE* **2014**, *9*, e112858. [CrossRef]
30. Christian, P.; Murray-Kolb, L.E.; Khatry, S.K.; Katz, J.; Schaefer, B.A.; Cole, P.M.; Leclerq, S.C.; Tielsch, J.M. Prenatal Micronutrient Supplementation and Intellectual and Motor Function in Early School-aged Children in Nepal. *JAMA* **2010**, *304*, 2716–2723. [CrossRef]
31. The NEMO Study Group. Effect of a 12-mo micronutrient intervention on learning and memory in well-nourished and marginally nourished school-aged children: 2 parallel, randomized, placebo-controlled studies in Australia and Indonesia. *Am. J. Clin. Nutr.* **2007**, *86*, 1082–1093. [CrossRef]
32. Effective Public Health Practice Project. Available online: https://merst.ca/ephpp/ (accessed on 21 July 2020).
33. Van Cauwenberghe, E.; Maes, L.; Spittaels, H.; van Lenthe, F.J.; Brug, J.; Oppert, J.M.; De Bourdeaudhuij, I. Effectiveness of school-based interventions in Europe to promote healthy nutrition in children and adolescents: Systematic review of published and 'grey' literature. *Br. J. Nutr.* **2010**, *103*, 781–797. [CrossRef] [PubMed]
34. El Harake, M.D.; Kharroubi, S.; Hamadeh, S.K.; Jomaa, L. Impact of a Pilot School-Based Nutrition Intervention on Dietary Knowledge, Attitudes, Behavior and Nutritional Status of Syrian Refugee Children in the Bekaa, Lebanon. *Nutrients* **2018**, *10*, 913. [CrossRef] [PubMed]
35. Adab, P.; Pallan, M.J.; Lancashire, E.R.; Hemming, K.; Frew, E.; Barrett, T.; Bhopal, R.; Cade, J.E.; Canaway, A.; Clarke, J.L.; et al. Effectiveness of a childhood obesity prevention programme delivered through schools, targeting 6 and 7 year olds: Cluster randomised controlled trial (WAVES study). *BMJ* **2018**, *360*, k211. [CrossRef] [PubMed]
36. Harley, A.; Lemke, M.; Brazauskas, R.; Carnegie, N.B.; Bokowy, L.; Kingery, L. Youth Chef Academy: Pilot Results From a Plant-Based Culinary and Nutrition Literacy Program for Sixth and Seventh Graders. *J. Sch. Health* **2018**, *88*, 893–902. [CrossRef]
37. Hermans, R.C.; van den Broek, N.; Nederkoorn, C.; Otten, R.; Ruiter, E.L.; Johnson-Glenberg, M.C. Feed the Alien! The Effects of a Nutrition Instruction Game on Children's Nutritional Knowledge and Food Intake. *Games Health J.* **2018**, *7*, 164–174. [CrossRef]
38. Piana, N.; Ranucci, C.; Buratta, L.; Foglia, E.; Fabi, M.; Novelli, F.; Casucci, S.; Reginato, E.; Pippi, R.; Aiello, C.; et al. An innovative school-based intervention to promote healthy lifestyles. *Health Educ. J.* **2017**, *76*, 716–729. [CrossRef]
39. Battjes-Fries, M.C.; Haveman-Nies, A.; Zeinstra, G.G.; van Dongen, E.J.; Meester, H.J.; van den Top-Pullen, R.; van't Veer, P.; de Graaf, K. Effectiveness of Taste Lessons with and without additional experiential learning activities on children's willingness to taste vegetables. *Appetite* **2017**, *109*, 201–208. [CrossRef]
40. Bogart, L.M.; Cowgill, B.O.; Elliott, M.N.; Klein, D.J.; Dawson, J.H.; Uyeda, K.; Elijah, J.; Binkle, D.G.; Schuster, M.A. A randomized controlled trial of students for nutrition and eXercise: A community-based participatory research study. *J. Adolesc. Health* **2014**, *55*, 415–422. [CrossRef]
41. Kaufman-Shriqui, V.; Fraser, D.; Friger, M.; Geva, D.; Bilenko, N.; Vardi, H.; Elhadad, N.; Mor, K.; Feine, Z.; Shahar, D.R. Effect of a School-Based Intervention on Nutritional Knowledge and Habits of Low-Socioeconomic School Children in Israel: A Cluster-Randomized Controlled Trial. *Nutrients* **2016**, *8*, 234. [CrossRef]
42. Sharma, S.V.; Markham, C.; Chow, J.; Ranjit, N.; Pomeroy, M.; Raber, M. Evaluating a school-based fruit and vegetable co-op in low-income children: A quasi-experimental study. *Prev. Med.* **2016**, *91*, 8–17. [CrossRef]
43. Lawlor, D.A.; Jago, R.; Noble, S.M.; Chittleborough, C.R.; Campbell, R.; Mytton, J.; Howe, L.D.; Peters, T.J.; Kipping, R.R. The Active for Life Year 5 (AFLY5) school-based cluster randomised controlled trial: Effect on potential mediators. *BMC Public Health* **2016**, *16*, 68. [CrossRef] [PubMed]

44. Steyn, N.P.; Villiers, A.D.; Gwebushe, N.; Draper, C.E.; Hill, J.; Waal, M.D.; Dalais, L.; Abrahams, Z.; Lombard, C.; Lambert, E.V. Did HealthKick, a randomised controlled trial primary school nutrition intervention improve dietary quality of children in low-income settings in South Africa? *BMC Public Health* **2015**, *15*, 948. [CrossRef]
45. Jones, M.; Pitt, H.; Oxford, L.; Bray, I.; Kimberlee, R.; Orme, J. Association between Food for Life, a Whole Setting Healthy and Sustainable Food Programme, and Primary School Children's Consumption of Fruit and Vegetables: A Cross-Sectional Study in England. *Int. J. Environ. Res. Public Health* **2017**, *14*, 639. [CrossRef] [PubMed]
46. Larsen, A.L.; Robertson, T.; Dunton, G. RE-AIM analysis of a randomized school-based nutrition intervention among fourth-grade classrooms in California. *Transl. Behav. Med.* **2015**, *5*, 315–326. [CrossRef] [PubMed]
47. Shen, M.; Hu, M.; Sun, Z. Assessment of School-Based Quasi-Experimental Nutrition and Food Safety Health Education for Primary School Students in Two Poverty-Stricken Counties of West China. *PLoS ONE* **2015**, *10*, e0145090. [CrossRef]
48. Fairclough, S.J.; Hackett, A.F.; Davies, I.G.; Gobbi, R.; Mackintosh, K.A.; Warburton, G.L.; Stratton, G.; van Sluijs, E.M.; Boddy, L.M. Promoting healthy weight in primary school children through physical activity and nutrition education: A pragmatic evaluation of the CHANGE! randomised intervention study. *BMC Public Health* **2013**, *13*, 626. [CrossRef]
49. Cunha, D.B.; de Souza, B.d.S.N.; Pereira, R.A.; Sichieri, R. Effectiveness of a randomized school-based intervention involving families and teachers to prevent excessive weight gain among adolescents in Brazil. *PLoS ONE* **2013**, *8*, e57498. [CrossRef]
50. Ochoa-Avilés, A.; Verstraeten, R.; Huybregts, L.; Andrade, S.; Camp, J.V.; Donoso, S.; Ramirez, P.L.; Lachat, C.; Maes, L.; Kolsteren, P. A school-based intervention improved dietary intake outcomes and reduced waist circumference in adolescents: A cluster randomized controlled trial. *Nutr. J.* **2017**, *16*, 79. [CrossRef]
51. Muros, J.J.; Zabala, M.; Oliveras-López, M.J.; Ocaña-Lara, F.A.; de la Serra, H.L.G. Results of a 7-Week School-Based Physical Activity and Nutrition Pilot Program on Health-Related Parameters in Primary School Children in Southern Spain. *Pediatr. Exerc. Sci.* **2013**, *25*, 248–261. [CrossRef]
52. Moss, A.; Smith, S.; Null, D.; Long, R.S.; Tragoudas, U. Farm to School and Nutrition Education: Positively Affecting Elementary School-Aged Children's Nutrition Knowledge and Consumption Behavior. *Child Obes.* **2013**, *9*, 51–56. [CrossRef]
53. Zota, D.; Dalma, A.; Petralias, A.; Lykou, A.; Kastorini, C.M.; Yannakoulia, M.; Karnaki, P.; Belogianni, K.; Veloudaki, A.; Riza, E.; et al. Promotion of healthy nutrition among students participating in a school food aid program: A randomized trial. *Int. J. Public Health* **2016**, *61*, 583–592. [CrossRef] [PubMed]
54. Gold, A.; Larson, M.; Tucker, J.; Strang, M. Classroom Nutrition Education Combined With Fruit and Vegetable Taste Testing Improves Children's Dietary Intake. *J. Sch. Health* **2017**, *87*, 106–113. [CrossRef] [PubMed]
55. Mbhatsani, V.H.; Mbhenyane, X.G.; Mabapa, S.N. Development and Implementation of Nutrition Education on Dietary Diversification for Primary School Children. *Ecol. Food Nutr.* **2017**, *56*, 449–561. [CrossRef] [PubMed]
56. Hutchinson, J.; Christian, M.S.; Evans, C.E.L.; Nykjaer, C.; Hancock, N.; Cade, J.E. Evaluation of the impact of school gardening interventions on children's knowledge of and attitudes towards fruit and vegetables. A cluster randomised controlled trial. *Appetite* **2015**, *91*, 405–414. [CrossRef] [PubMed]
57. Viggiano, E.; Viggiano, A.; Costanzo, A.D.; Viggiano, A.; Viggiano, A.; Andreozzi, E.; Romano, V.; Vicidomini, C.; Tuoro, D.D.; Gargano, G.; et al. Healthy lifestyle promotion in primary schools through the board game Kaledo: A pilot cluster randomized trial. *Eur. J. Pediatr.* **2018**, *177*, 1371–1375. [CrossRef] [PubMed]
58. Waters, E.; Gibbs, L.; Tadic, M.; Ukoumunne, O.C.; Magarey, A.; Okely, A.D.; Silva, A.D.; Armit, C.; Green, J.; O'Connor, T.; et al. Cluster randomised trial of a school-community child health promotion and obesity prevention intervention: Findings from the evaluation of fun 'n healthy in Moreland! *BMC Public Health* **2017**, *18*, 92. [CrossRef] [PubMed]
59. Xu, F.; Ware, R.S.; Leslie, E.; Tse, L.A.; Wang, Z.; Li, J.; Wang, Y. Effectiveness of a Randomized Controlled Lifestyle Intervention to Prevent Obesity among Chinese Primary School Students: CLICK-Obesity Study. *PLoS ONE* **2015**, *10*, e0141421. [CrossRef]

60. Jung, T.; Huang, J.; Eagan, L.; Oldenburg, D. Influence of school-based nutrition education program on healthy eating literacy and healthy food choice among primary school children. *Int. J. Health Promot. Educ.* **2019**, *57*, 67–81. [CrossRef]
61. Zhou, W.-J.; Xu, X.; Li, G.; Sharma, M.; Qie, Y.-L.; Zhao, Y. Effectiveness of a school-based nutrition and food safety education program among primary and junior high school students in Chongqing, China. *Glob. Health Promot.* **2014**, *23*, 37–49. [CrossRef]
62. Anderson, E.L.; Howe, L.D.; Kipping, R.R.; Campbell, R.; Jago, R.; Noble, S.M.; Wells, S.; Chittleborough, C.; Peters, T.J.; Lawlor, D.A. Long-term effects of the Active for Life Year 5 (AFLY5) school-based cluster-randomised controlled trial. *BMJ Open* **2016**, *6*, e010957. [CrossRef]
63. Griffin, T.L.; Jackson, D.M.; McNeill, G.; Aucott, L.S.; Macdiarmid, J.I. A Brief Educational Intervention Increases Knowledge of the Sugar Content of Foods and Drinks but Does Not Decrease Intakes in Scottish Children Aged 10–12 Years. *J. Nutr. Educ. Behav.* **2015**, *47*, 367–373.e1. [CrossRef]
64. Kipping, R.R.; Howe, L.D.; Jago, R.; Campbell, R.; Wells, S.; Chittleborough, C.R.; Mytton, J.; Noble, S.M.; Peters, T.J.; Lawlor, D.A. Effect of intervention aimed at increasing physical activity, reducing sedentary behaviour, and increasing fruit and vegetable consumption in children: Active for Life Year 5 (AFLY5) school based cluster randomised controlled trial. *BMJ Br. Med J.* **2014**, *348*, g3256. [CrossRef]
65. Van de Gaar, V.M.; Jansen, W.; Grieken, A.V.; Borsboom, G.J.J.M.; Kremers, S.; Raat, H. Effects of an intervention aimed at reducing the intake of sugar-sweetened beverages in primary school children: A controlled trial. *Int. J. Behav. Nutr. Phys. Act.* **2014**, *11*, 98. [CrossRef]
66. Moore, G.F.; Murphy, S.; Chaplin, K.; Lyons, R.A.; Atkinson, M.; Moore, L. Impacts of the Primary School Free Breakfast Initiative on socio-economic inequalities in breakfast consumption among 9-11-year-old schoolchildren in Wales. *Public Health Nutr.* **2014**, *17*, 1280–1299. [CrossRef]
67. Nyberg, G.; Norman, Å.; Sundblom, E.; Zeebari, Z.; Elinder, L.S. Effectiveness of a universal parental support programme to promote health behaviours and prevent overweight and obesity in 6-year-old children in disadvantaged areas, the Healthy School Start Study II, a cluster-randomised controlled trial. *Int. J. Behav. Nutr. Phys. Act.* **2016**, *13*, 4. [CrossRef]
68. Mittmann, S.; Austel, A.; Ellrott, T. Behavioural effects of a short school-based fruit and vegetable promotion programme: 5-a-Day for kids. *Health Educ.* **2016**, *116*, 222–237. [CrossRef]
69. Huys, N.; Cardon, G.; Craemer, D.M.; Hermans, N.; Renard, S.; Roesbeke, M.; Stevens, W.; Lepeleere, S.D.; Deforche, B. Effect and process evaluation of a real-world school garden program on vegetable consumption and its determinants in primary schoolchildren. *PLoS ONE* **2019**, *14*, e0214320. [CrossRef]
70. Weber, K.S.; Spörkel, O.; Mertens, M.; Freese, A.; Strassburger, K.; Kemper, B.; Bachmann, C.; Diehlmann, K.; Stemper, T.; Buyken, A.E.; et al. Positive Effects of Promoting Physical Activity and Balanced Diets in a Primary School Setting with a High Proportion of Migrant School Children. *Exp. Clin. Endocrinol. Diabetes* **2017**, *125*, 554–562. [CrossRef]
71. Llargués, E.; Recasens, M.A.; Manresa, J.-M.; Jensen, B.B.; Franco, R.; Nadal, A.; Vila, M.; Recasens, I.; Perez, M.J.; Castel, C. Four-year outcomes of an educational intervention in healthy habits in schoolchildren: The Avall 3 Trial. *Eur. J. Public Health* **2016**, *27*, 42–47. [CrossRef]
72. Liz Martins, M.; Rodrigues, S.S.P.; Cunha, L.M.; Rocha, A. Strategies to reduce plate waste in primary schools–experimental evaluation. *Public Health Nutr.* **2016**, *19*, 1517–1525. [CrossRef]
73. Rosário, R.; Araújo, A.; Padrão, P.; Lopes, O.; Moreira, A.; Abreu, S.; Vale, S.; Pereira, B.; Moreira, P. Impact of a school-based intervention to promote fruit intake: A cluster randomized controlled trial. *Public Health* **2016**, *136*, 94–100. [CrossRef] [PubMed]
74. Zafiropulos, V.; Chatzi, V.; Petros, D.; Markaki, A.; Zacharias, F.; Nikolaos, T. Preliminary Results of A Dietary Intervention among Primary-School Children. In Proceedings of the European Congress on Obesity, Prague, Czech Republic, 6–9 May 2015.
75. Charlebois, J.; Gowrinathan, Y.; Waddell, P. A Review of the Evidence: School-based Interventions to Address Obesity Prevention in Children 6–12 Years of Age. *Tor. Public Health* **2012**, *48*, 102.
76. Delgado-Noguera, M.; Tort, S.; Martínez-Zapata, M.J.; Bonfill, X. Primary school interventions to promote fruit and vegetable consumption: A systematic review and meta-analysis. *Prev. Med.* **2011**, *53*, 3–9. [CrossRef] [PubMed]

77. Evans, C.E.; Christian, M.S.; Cleghorn, C.L.; Greenwood, D.C.; Cade, J.E. Systematic review and meta-analysis of school-based interventions to improve daily fruit and vegetable intake in children aged 5 to 12 y. *Am. J. Clin. Nutr.* **2012**, *96*, 889–901. [CrossRef]
78. Brown, E.C.; Buchan, D.S.; Baker, J.S.; Wyatt, F.B.; Bocalini, D.S.; Kilgore, L. A Systematised Review of Primary School Whole Class Child Obesity Interventions: Effectiveness, Characteristics, and Strategies. *BioMed Res. Int.* **2016**, *2016*, 4902714. [CrossRef]
79. Mikkelsen, B.E.; Kngesveen, K.; Afflerbach, T.; Barnekow, V. The human rights framework, the school and healthier eating among young people a European perspective. *Public Health Nutr.* **2016**, *19*, 15–25. [CrossRef]
80. Rashid, V.; Engberink, M.F.; Eijsden, M.V.; Nicolaou, M.; Dekker, L.H.; Verhoeff, A.P.; Weijs, P.J.M. Ethnicity and socioeconomic status are related to dietary patterns at age 5 in the Amsterdam born children and their development (ABCD) cohort. *BMC Public Health* **2018**, *18*, 115. [CrossRef]

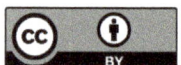

© 2020 by the authors. Licensee MDPI, Basel, Switzerland. This article is an open access article distributed under the terms and conditions of the Creative Commons Attribution (CC BY) license (http://creativecommons.org/licenses/by/4.0/).

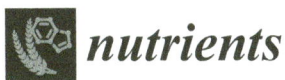

Article

Effects of the Preschool-Based Family-Involving DAGIS Intervention Program on Children's Energy Balance-Related Behaviors and Self-Regulation Skills: A Clustered Randomized Controlled Trial

Carola Ray [1,2,*], Rejane Figuereido [1,3], Henna Vepsäläinen [2], Reetta Lehto [1,2], Riikka Pajulahti [1,2], Essi Skaffari [1,2], Taina Sainio [1,4], Pauliina Hiltunen [1,2], Elviira Lehto [1,4], Liisa Korkalo [2], Katri Sääksjärvi [4], Nina Sajaniemi [4,5], Maijaliisa Erkkola [2] and Eva Roos [1,2,6]

1. Folkhälsan Research Center, Topeliuksenkatu 20, FI-00250 Helsinki, Finland; rejane.fig@gmail.com (R.F.); reetta.lehto@folkhalsan.fi (R.L.); riikka.pajulahti@helsinki.fi (R.P.); essi.skaffari@helsinki.fi (E.S.); taina.sainio@helsinki.fi (T.S.); pauliina.hiltunen@helsinki.fi (P.H.); elviira.lehto@helsinki.fi (E.L.); eva.roos@folkhalsan.fi (E.R.)
2. Department of Food and Nutrition, University of Helsinki, P.O. Box 66, FI-00014 Helsinki, Finland; henna.vepsalainen@helsinki.fi (H.V.); liisa.korkalo@helsinki.fi (L.K.); maijaliisa.erkkola@helsinki.fi (M.E.)
3. Clinicum, Faculty of Medicine, University of Helsinki, FI-00014 Helsinki, Finland
4. Department of Teacher Education, University of Helsinki, P.O. Box 9, FI-00100 Helsinki, Finland; katri.saaksjarvi@helsinki.fi (K.S.); nina.sajaniemi@helsinki.fi (N.S.)
5. School of Applied Educational Science and Teacher Education, Philosophical Faculty, University of Eastern Finland, P.O. Box 111, FI-80101 Joensuu, Finland
6. Department of Public Health, Clinicum, P.O. Box 63, University of Helsinki, FI-00014 Helsinki, Finland
* Correspondence: carola.ray@folkhalsan.fi; Tel.: +358-50-3705193

Received: 25 June 2020; Accepted: 24 August 2020; Published: 26 August 2020

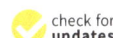

Abstract: The study examines the effects of a preschool-based family-involving multicomponent intervention on children's energy balance-related behaviors (EBRBs) such as food consumption, screen time and physical activity (PA), and self-regulation (SR) skills, and whether the intervention effects differed among children with low or high parental educational level (PEL) backgrounds. The Increased Health and Wellbeing in Preschools (DAGIS) intervention was conducted as a clustered randomized controlled trial, clustered at preschool level, over five months in 2017–2018. Altogether, 802 children aged 3–6 years in age participated. Parents reported children's consumption of sugary everyday foods and beverages, sugary treats, fruits, and vegetables by a food frequency questionnaire, and screen time by a 7-day diary. Physical activity was assessed by a hip-worn accelerometer. Cognitive and emotional SR was reported in a questionnaire by parents. General linear mixed models with and without repeated measures were used as statistical methods. At follow-up, no differences were detected in EBRBs or SR skills between the intervention and control group, nor did differences emerge in children's EBRBs between the intervention and the control groups when stratified by PEL. The improvement in cognitive SR skills among low PEL intervention children differed from low PEL control children, the significance being borderline. The DAGIS multicomponent intervention did not significantly affect children's EBRBs or SR. Further sub-analyses and a comprehensive process evaluation may shed light on the non-significant findings.

Keywords: energy balance-related behaviors; self-regulation skills; preschoolers; children; randomized controlled trial; intervention effects; parental educational level; intervention mapping; multicomponent intervention

1. Introduction

Young children's food intake, screen time, and physical activity (PA), commonly referred to as energy balance-related behaviors (EBRBs) [1], are of importance since they can predict the future weight status and health of children [2–4]. A socio-economic status (SES) gradient exists already in preschoolers' EBRBs; those with low SES family backgrounds tend to have less healthy EBRBs such as higher intake of sugary foods or beverages and excessive screen time [5–7].

Home and an early childhood education and care center, hereafter preschool, are the settings where three to six-year-olds spend most of their time, and it is therefore important that these environments promote healthy EBRBs including sufficient PA and fruit and vegetable (FV) consumption [8–10]. Reviews have concluded that EBRB interventions should be conducted at preschools and homes simultaneously in order to be successful [11,12]. Preschool-based family-involving interventions have been reported to be promising [12–15], although some studies show no effects on EBRBs [12,14,16]. This has raised discussion on intervention design and implementation in families [12]. When designing interventions for the general population, they should reach and show higher effects on those needing it most, namely those with low SES backgrounds [5,17]. To date, knowledge of the equity effectiveness of EBRB interventions among children is sparse [18,19]. Promoting several EBRBs simultaneously is challenging, as the aim can be to both promote healthy behaviors and discourage unhealthy behaviors. Strategies can differ, a review concluding that promoting PA among young children is successful when focusing on the preferred behavior, rather than focusing on decreasing sedentary time such as lying or sitting down [20].

Strengthening children's self-regulation (SR) skills in parallel to promoting children's healthy EBRBs could be an effective strategy in interventions [21,22]. Self-regulation is a multidimensional concept, briefly described as the capacity of a goal-directed behavior to regulate actions, emotions, and cognitions [23]. Cognitive SR skills refer to executive functioning such as self-monitoring to plan and proceed toward long-term goals [24–26], whereas emotional SR skills refers to capacities such as being able to recognize one's own feelings and staying calm in stressful situations [24,25]. Associations between children's SR skills and less favorable EBRBs and weight status have been found [21,22,24,25]. The Head Start study tested the strategy of strengthening young children's SR skills alongside promoting their healthy EBRBs [27]. The intervention included four arms: intervening on EBRBs and SR skills; intervening on EBRBs; intervening on SRs skills; and no intervention. Effects were seen in lower sugar-sweetened beverage consumption in the study arm promoting EBRBs and SR skills compared with the other arms [27].

The Increased Health and Wellbeing in Preschools (DAGIS) intervention aimed to promote preschoolers' (aged 3–6 years) healthy EBRBs and SR skills. The assumption was that there would be greater effects on children from families with low parental educational levels (PEL), also assuming a reduction in any health gaps between children with low and high PEL backgrounds [28]. The intervention development process was guided by the Intervention Mapping (IM) framework [29] and the process is described elsewhere [28]. A cross-sectional study served as the needs assessment [7,28], and based on these findings, there were three main aims: to reduce children's screen time; to reduce the consumption of sugary everyday foods and beverages; and to increase vegetable consumption. In these three behaviors, the needs assessment showed less favorable behaviors among children with low PEL background [28]. To promote alternatives to the reductions, additional aims were to increase fruit and berry consumption and total PA (light, moderate, and vigorous intensity) [28]. In addition, the intervention aimed to strengthen children's SR skills. Activities were planned to suit families with low PEL backgrounds.

In Finland, 78–86% of three to six year-olds attend municipality-driven preschools [30]. Therefore, preschools offer a good setting for interventions. As screen time and sugary food and beverage consumption occurs mostly at home [31], homes were considered as an equally important intervention setting. The developed program lasted 23 weeks, and was divided into five themes: SR skills; PA; fruit and vegetables; screen time; and sugary foods and beverages. Each theme was in focus for four to five weeks.

In this study, we aimed: (1) to evaluate the effects of a preschool-based family intervention on children's EBRBs and SR skills, and (2) to evaluate whether effects were stronger among children with low PEL background than among those with high PEL background.

2. Materials and Methods

The DAGIS intervention study is a preschool-level clustered randomized controlled trial (RCT) aimed to promote preschoolers' healthy EBRBs and SR skills so that those from low SES background would benefit most from the program. The study was conducted between September 2017 and May 2018 including baseline and follow-up measurements [28]. Early educators delivered the program and all included activities to all preschoolers independently of their participation in the study. Prospective trial registration number: ISRCTN57165350 (the 8th of January 2015).

2.1. Recruitment

We aimed to invite municipalities that had a high number of preschools and had a large variety in educational and income levels among inhabitants as well as being located within a convenient distance from the Helsinki region. Municipalities invited were selected by comparing municipality statistics from southern and western Finland [32], and excluded municipalities that were already part of the previous comprehensive DAGIS survey in 2015–2016 [7]. Power calculations prior to the recruitment for the intervention were based on the DAGIS survey results; specifically, we used the average (about 1.7 times/week for all and about 2 times/week for low PEL group) and standard deviations of children's sugary food and beverage consumption frequency [7]. Based on those values, we decided to aim at a decrease of 0.74 times/day in sugary foods and beverages consumption frequency. To detect a change of 0.74 times/day less sugary foods and beverages, the required sample size was calculated to be 432 children, considering an attrition rate of 70% (Fpower macro, SAS version 9.4.). The significance level was set at 5% and the power at 80%.

Altogether, seven municipalities were invited to participate in the study, and an oral presentation on the study was offered. Five municipalities had an oral presentation; two of these municipalities chose to participate. One municipality decided that all of its preschools ($n = 29$, preschool managers $n = 19$) would participate, whereas the other municipality allowed its preschool managers to make the decision individually, as such, the managers of three preschools chose to participate. We decided that these 32 preschools and 1702 eligible preschoolers were sufficient for our study (Figure 1).

Researchers visited each preschool to inform early educator professionals about the project and their role in the project. The recruitment phase lasted 1–2 weeks, and families returned informed consents (or refusals to participate) to preschools in sealed envelopes. Thereafter, the researchers returned to preschools to distribute the baseline research material for early educators, parents, and children.

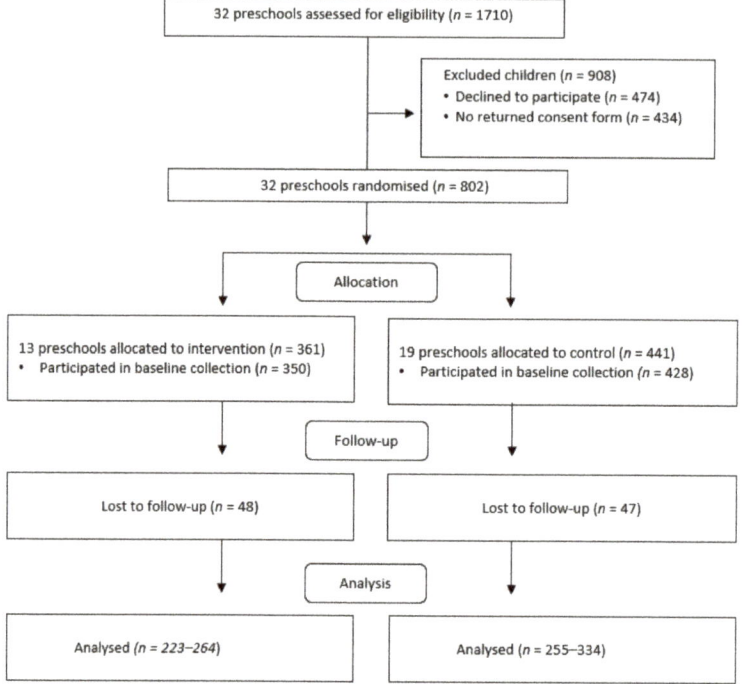

Figure 1. Flow chart in the Increased Health and Wellbeing in Preschools (DAGIS) intervention study, in accordance with the Consolidated Standards of Reporting Trials (CONSORT) 2010 statement [33].

2.2. Ethical Issues

The DAGIS intervention study received ethics approval from the Helsinki Ethics Review Board in humanities and social and behavioral sciences (22/2017; 16 May 2017). Early education professionals were informed about the study through site visits. The early educators' questionnaire stated that participation was voluntary and that the early educators had the option to withdraw at any stage of the study. Early educators gave their consent by filling in the questionnaire. Families returned written informed consent, and thereafter, the questionnaires were delivered.

2.3. Data Collection and Measurements

The baseline data collection occurred in four waves over five weeks and the follow-up data collection in three waves over five weeks. Data collection in waves was necessary due to the limited number of accelerometers available for measuring children's PA. Research staff visited each preschool to instruct early educators and left printed screen time diaries for families, study questionnaires for families who had requested paper copies, and accelerometers for children. These materials were picked up from preschools one week later. However, most parents requested that their questionnaires be sent electronically by sending the parent's main questionnaire as a personal link and the food frequency questionnaire link by email.

2.3.1. Measurements

Screen time was assessed by a printed screen time diary. In the diary, parents recorded their child's use of screens outside preschool time whenever the child used a screen for more than 10 min in a row. Screen use was recorded separately for different screens: TV, DVD, computer, tablet, or cell phone. The screen time diary was a slightly modified version from a previous validated diary [34], as the original did not include portable screens and questions about screen contexts. The screen time diary has shown good reproducibility [35]. Screen time was calculated for children who presented data for at least three weekdays, and one weekend day. Total screen time (min/day) was calculated as a weighted mean: (5 × weekday mean + 2 × weekend mean)/7.

Children's PA was assessed by a hip-worn accelerometer, the ActiGraph wGT3X-BT (ActiGraph, LLC, Pensacola, FL, USA), 24 h/day over seven consecutive days, and parents kept a screen time diary over the same days. A 15-s epoch length was used for data derived from accelerometers, and more than ten minutes of consecutive zeroes was set as non-wearing time [36]. In the analyses, the cut-off points of Evenson et al. [37] for children aged 5–15 years were used, which means that total PA including light, moderate, and vigorous intensity PA is defined as more than 100 counts/min. Inclusion criteria for the child's PA data to be in the analyses were that there were data for at least four days, of which one was a weekend day. In addition, each day needed to have 600 min or more of awake wearing time. The mean total PA (min/day) was used in the analyses.

The original 47-item food frequency questionnaire (FFQ) was designed for the DAGIS survey to particularly measure the consumption frequencies of vegetables and fruits as well as sugary foods and beverages [38]. It has shown acceptable validity for ranking food group consumption compared with 3-day food records [38], and testing the reproducibility of the items has yielded acceptable results [35]. In the DAGIS intervention, the FFQ was expanded into a 51-item FFQ that included six food groups (vegetables, fruit, and berries; dairy products; fish meat and eggs; cereal products; beverages; and other foods such as sweets and snacks). A link to the electronic 51-item FFQ was sent to all parents and hard copies were sent to those who did not fill in the electronic version. Parents reported how many times during the past week the child had consumed foods outside preschool hours. The FFQ included three answer options: not at all, times per week, and times per day. The instruction was to either tick the 'not at all' box or to write a number in one of the other columns. The FFQ was intentionally restricted to not cover municipality-provided foods and beverages consumed during preschool hours because parents would not have been able to reliably report these foods.

The three food consumption frequency variables ('sugary everyday foods and beverages', 'sugary treats', and 'fruit and vegetables (FV)') were formed by summing up the consumption frequencies (times/week). The sugary everyday foods and beverages variable included flavored yogurt and quark; puddings; sugar-sweetened cereals and muesli; berry, fruit, and chocolate porridge with added sugar; berry and fruit soups with added sugar; soft drinks; flavored and sweetened milk- and plant-based beverages; and sugar-sweetened juices. The sugary treats variable included ice cream, chocolate, sweets, cakes, cupcakes, sweet rolls, Danish pastries, pies and other sweet pastries, and sweet biscuits and cereal bars. The FV variable included fresh vegetables, cooked and canned vegetables, fresh fruit, and fresh and frozen berries.

Children's SR skills were assessed with 10 items derived from the Child Social Behavior Questionnaire, previously used in the Millennium Cohort Study on 3-year-olds [26]. Five items assessed cognitive skills and five items emotional SR skills. Each statement had three response options: disagree; agree to some extent; and fully agree. The mean points for each sub-dimension were calculated and used in the analyses. The internal consistency reliability as Cronbach's alphas was 0.68 for cognitive and 0.78 for emotional SR skills.

2.3.2. Parental Educational Level

The parent filling in the guardian's questionnaire reported his/her own highest educational achievement and the education of a partner living in the same household. The six answer options were categorized as follows: low educational level (comprising comprehensive school, vocational school, or high school); middle educational level (bachelor's degree or college); and high educational level (master's degree or licentiate/doctor). The highest educational level among parents was used as the parental educational level (PEL) variable in the analyses. In four cases, the highest education was not the education level of the mother or the father of the child, but that of a spouse living in the same household.

2.3.3. Confounding Factors

The parent reported the date of birth and gender of the participating child. In the statistical analysis, adjustments were made for the child's gender and age at baseline (continuous) for the categorical variable PEL and for the municipality.

2.4. Randomization, the Intervention, and the Program Content

Randomization was made at the preschool manager-level, separately for the two municipalities by an online randomization program (https://www.randomlists.com/team-generator). Preschools were divided into small and large preschools before randomization. After the baseline measurements, preschools were informed whether they had been randomized into the intervention ($n = 13$) or control ($n = 19$) group (Figure 1).

In intervention preschools, all early educators received program training. The training was split into a longer training session after the baseline measurements and a shorter training session around the middle of the 23-week program, in all, approximately 8 h [28]. Throughout the intervention, two researchers engaged with early educators conducting the program by email. Basically, the program at preschools was based on the international MindUp™ program [39]. Healthy EBRBs promoting strategies and methods were added to the existing ones in the program, and a program for families was developed [28]. The program was run in both preschools and homes and divided into five themes, all of which lasted 4–5 weeks: SR skills; physical activity; fruit and vegetables; screen time; and sugary foods and beverages. SR skills along with each EBRB were emphasized throughout the program in the preschool activities. SR skills were promoted by brain breaks, which were a few minutes' calming down and breathing sessions three times per day, led by early educators. In addition, early educators were trained to teach children to recognize and reflect on different feelings. In the family activities, focus was set on the children's EBRBs, and on how parents, by acting as role models and changing the availability and accessibility of the home environment, could influence their children's EBRBs. The methods used for families were, among others, information letters, emails containing videos or articles, bingos related to EBRBs, and two fairy tales written for the project. For each of the five themes, preschools arranged one activity afternoon. Early educators received the instructions and needed materials for the activities at the program training sessions. The activity afternoons were conducted as a workshop for children and parents to which all families were invited. An activity afternoon could consist of a working sheet about vegetable eating habits and favorite vegetables, or a vegetable tasting session that children and parents conducted together. Materials that were produced during the afternoons were expected to be displayed at the preschool, so that families could see each other's works. The early educators in the control preschools received training for the program after the intervention was finished.

2.5. Statistical Analyses

Differences between the participants' characteristics and the two groups (intervention/control) at baseline were analyzed by the Chi-square test (categorized variables) and t-test (continuous variables). Our main outcomes were total screen time (min/day), total PA (min/day), two variables related to sugar consumption (sugary everyday foods and beverages, and sugary treats, as times/week), total FV consumption frequency (times/week), and SR skills (cognitive and emotional dimensions, as scores). As a first step, a simple model was used to show the comparison between the intervention and control groups. To evaluate this, we used the general linear mixed models adjusted for baseline value of the outcome. This first model was used as a simple description of the results at follow-up. As a second step, a more complete and appropriate model was used with the major interest to evaluate the results between follow-up and baseline for the control and intervention groups. For this aim we used the linear mixed models with repeated measures for all outcomes, taking into account the interaction between the two groups and two time-points of baseline and follow-up. In the mixed models, normal distribution was visually checked. The preschool unit was used as a random effect in order to adjust for variability between the preschools. All aforementioned analyses were adjusted for child's gender, age at baseline, municipality, and PEL. Furthermore, accelerometer wearing time was included as an adjustment variable in the analyses where PA was the outcome. We also evaluated linear mixed models with three-level interactions: groups (intervention and control), time-points (baseline and post-intervention), and PEL. For these models, the results for the comparison between the two groups and time-points were presented as stratified by PEL group. In all analyses, multiple imputation was applied for independent variables with missing values. The number of children included in the analysis of each dependent variable and the missing values are presented in Supplementary Table S1 and the complete results for the linear mixed models with repeated measures and the respective effect size for interaction is presented in Supplementary Table S3.

All analyses were based on the intention-to-treat principle so that all randomized participants were included in the analysis in their randomized intervention group. General statistical analysis was performed and tables created using SPSS version 25. Mixed models, effect size for models' interaction, and multiple imputation analysis were conducted in R version 3.4.3 using the lme4, MuMIn, and MICE packages, respectively. For all analyses, a 5% statistical significance level was adopted.

3. Results

The average age of children in the study was 5.24 (±1.06) and 5.14 (±1.04) years for the control and intervention groups, respectively. Even though most characteristics were similar in the groups, a higher percentage of children with high educational level parents were found in the control group (26%) than in the intervention group (18%) (Table 1).

Table 1. Children's characteristics by the control and intervention group at baseline ($n = 802$).

		Control		Intervention		p-Value
		n	Mean ± SD *	n	Mean ± SD *	
Child's Age [c]		441	5.24 ± 1.06	360	5.14 ± 1.04	0.060 [a]
		n	%	n	%	
Child's gender	girl	203	46.0%	172	47.8%	0.496 [b]
	boy	238	54.0%	188	52.2%	
Parental educational level [d]	low	116	29.9%	109	35.4%	<0.001 [b]
	middle	169	43.6%	143	46.4%	
	high	103	26.5%	56	18.2%	
Municipality	Salo	357	81.0%	306	84.8%	0.040 [b]
	Riihimäki	84	19.0%	55	15.2%	

* SD, standard deviation; [a] comparison using t-test; [b] comparison using Chi-square test; [c] one missing value for age; [d] low educational level (comprehensive school, vocational school, or high school), middle (bachelor's degree or college), high (master's degree or licentiate/doctor).

Table 2 shows the descriptive results for children's EBRBs and SR skills according to the intervention and control group, at baseline and at follow-up, whereas the corresponding results according to PEL are presented in Supplementary Table S2. Children had about the same daily screen time in the intervention and control groups at baseline (Table 2), but low PEL children had higher screen time than the other groups (Supplementary Table S2). The FV consumption at baseline was higher in the high PEL groups than in the other groups (Supplementary Table S2).

Table 3 shows the comparison between the intervention and control groups at follow-up adjusted for respective baseline outcome values. Figures 2 and 3 present the mean of the main outcomes (descriptive values from Table 2) at the baseline and follow-up for the intervention and control groups, and for the PEL subgroups of the intervention group.

Table 2. Descriptors for children's EBRBs and self-regulation skills by control and intervention group.

EBRBs and SR Skills *	Baseline				Follow-Up			
	Control		Intervention		Control		Intervention	
	n	Mean ± SD **	n	Mean ± SD **	n	Mean ± SD **	n	Mean ± SD **
Total screen time (min/day)	370	84.87 ± 43.45	303	87.27 ± 44.06	325	88.84 ± 42.47	261	85.37 ± 41.34
Total physical activity [a] (min/day)	335	412.68 ± 48.40	282	405.66 ± 48.61	270	418.02 ± 45.34	210	414.42 ± 50.42
Sugary everyday food and beverages (times/week)	307	9.70 ± 6.89	293	10.53 ± 7.84	241	10.21 ± 8.96	200	9.76 ± 6.88
Sugary treats (times/week)	318	5.86 ± 3.99	299	5.77 ± 3.21	236	7.00 ± 5.34	192	6.99 ± 5.34
Fruit and vegetables (times/week)	323	21.79 ± 10.67	298	22.06 ± 13.12	258	22.26 ± 11.38	200	23.22 ± 13.39
Cognitive SR skills (scale 1–3)	383	2.31 ± 0.39	313	2.27 ± 0.43	324	2.32 ± 0.41	256	2.34 ± 0.43
Emotional SR skills (scale 1–3)	383	2.26 ± 0.51	313	2.25 ± 0.52	324	2.25 ± 0.51	256	2.29 ± 0.53

* EBRBs, energy balance-related behaviors; SR, self-regulation. ** SD, standard deviation.

Table 3. Comparison of EBRBs and SR skills between intervention and control, and changes within the groups *.

Children's EBRBs and SR Skills	General Linear Mixed Model [c]			Linear Mixed Models with Repeated Measures					
	Comparison between Intervention and Control Group at Follow-Up [c]			Change between Follow-Up and Baseline in Control Group			Change between Follow-Up and Baseline in Intervention Group		
		(95% C.I.)	p-Value	diff F-B	(95% C.I.)	p-Value	diff F-B	(95% C.I.)	p-Value
Total screen time (min/day) [a]	−4.20	(−9.86; 1.46)	0.146	4.46	(0.48; 8.44)	0.028	−1.42	(−5.86; 3.01)	0.529
Total physical activity (min/day) [b]	−0.56	(−6.65; 5.53)	0.858	23.77	(18.57; 28.97)	<0.001	27.30	(21.74; 32.86)	<0.001
Sugary food and beverage (times/week) [a]	−0.57	(−2.09; 0.96)	0.466	0.51	(−0.42; 1.43)	0.285	−0.79	(−1.77; 0.19)	0.112
Sugary treats (times/week) [a]	−0.13	(−1.03; 0.78)	0.781	1.20	(0.62; 1.77)	<0.001	1.28	(0.67; 1.90)	<0.001
Fruit and vegetables (times/week) [a]	1.43	(−0.64; 3.49)	0.176	−0.37	(−1.63; 0.89)	0.565	1.21	(−0.18; 2.61)	0.088
Cognitive SR skills (scale 1–3) [a]	0.02	(−0.04; 0.08)	0.505	0.01	(−0.03; 0.05)	0.574	0.06	(0.01; 0.11)	0.011
Emotional SR skills (1–3) [a]	−0.03	(−0.04; 0.10)	0.405	0.004	(−0.04; 0.05)	0.858	0.04	(−0.02; 0.09)	0.195

* (n = 645–737, estimates, and their 95% confidence intervals (C.I.); [a] models adjusted for gender, age, municipality, parental educational level; [b] models adjusted for gender, age, municipality, parental educational level, and accelerometer wear time; [c] models adjusted for gender, age, municipality, parental educational level, (accelerometer wear time in PA as behavior), and baseline value of the outcome.

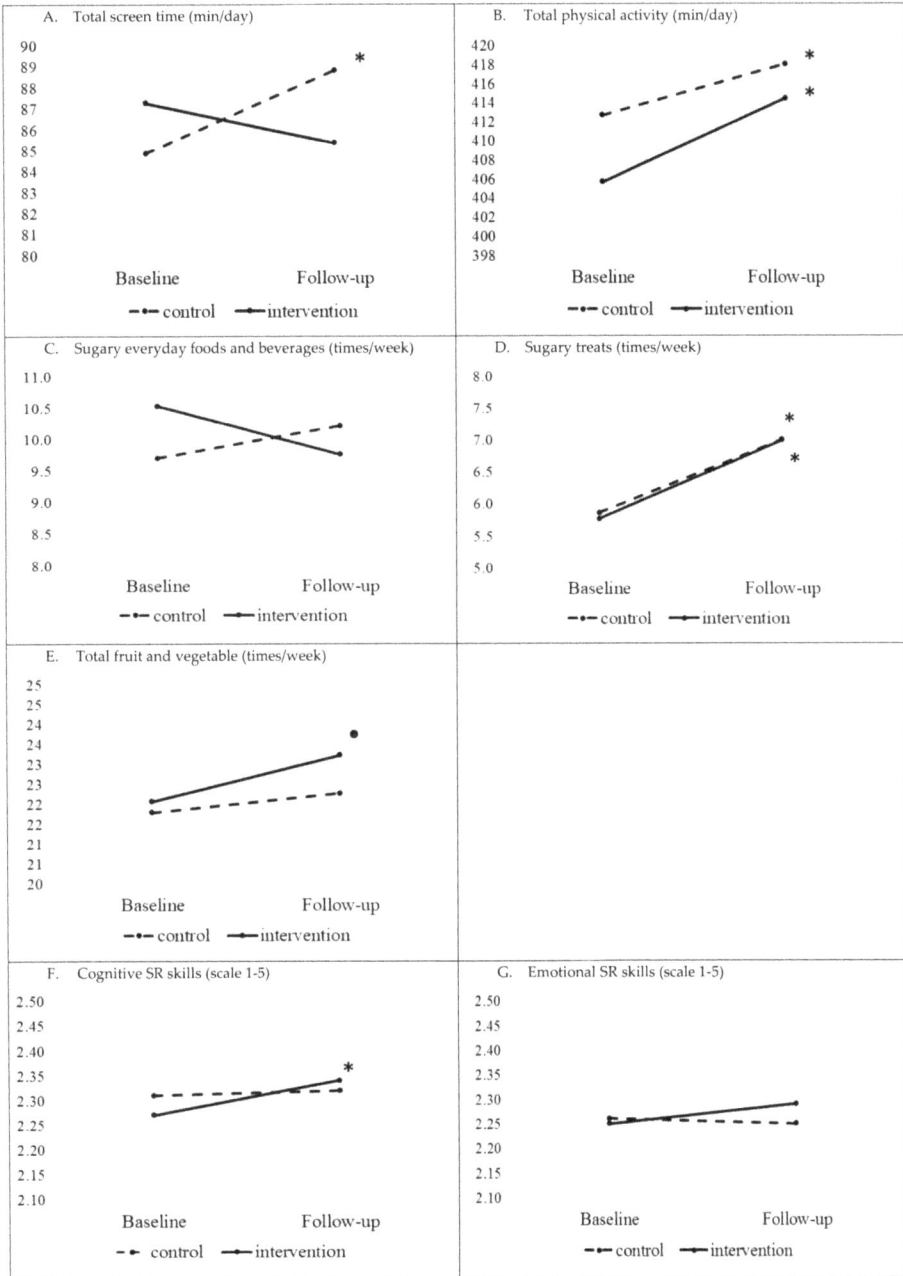

Figure 2. Children's EBRBs (heading (**A–E**)) and SR skills (headings (**F,G**)) at the baseline and follow-up in the intervention and control groups (means). For exact mean values, please see Table 2 (* p-value < 0.05, • p-value < 0.01 for the difference between the follow-up and baseline within the group).

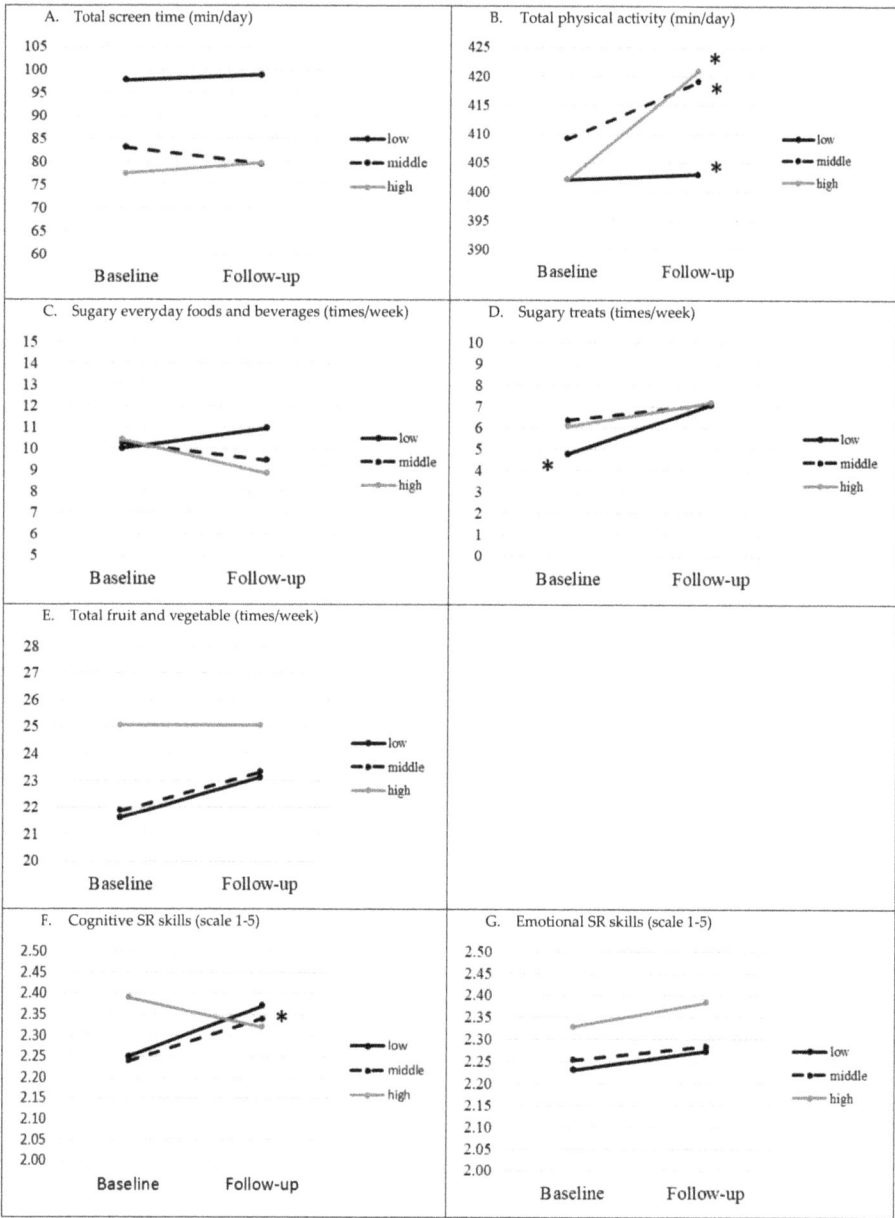

Figure 3. Children's EBRBs (headings (**A–E**)) and SR skills (headings (**F,G**)) within the intervention group separated by highest parental educational level (PEL) (means). For exact mean values, please see Supplementary Table S2 (* p-value < 0.05 for difference between follow-up and baseline within the group).

There were no significant differences detected in follow-up between the intervention and control groups for children's total screen time, total PA, consumption frequencies of sugary everyday foods and beverages, sugary treats, and FV, and cognitive and emotional SR skills (Table 3).

The results between the baseline and follow-up within the control and intervention groups differed for some EBRBs and SR skills (Table 3, see means in Figure 2). In the intervention group, the change between baseline and follow-up in total screen time was not significant, whereas there was a significant increase, approximately 4.5 min/day, in screen time in the control group ($p = 0.028$, Table 3, Figure 2A). The control group significantly increased in total PA on average by 24 min/day ($p < 0.001$), and the intervention group had a significant increase of 27 min/day ($p < 0.001$, Table 3 and Figure 2B). There was an increase in sugary treat consumption frequency in both groups ($p < 0.001$ in both groups, Table 3). In the intervention group, there was a trend, albeit not significant ($p = 0.088$), where FV consumption frequency increased (Table 3, Figure 2E). A positive significant change in points in cognitive SR skills was observed in the intervention group ($p = 0.011$, Table 3, Figure 2F).

Similar comparisons of children's EBRBs and SRs skills at follow-up stratified by PEL and the comparison between baseline and follow-up for intervention and control groups stratified by PEL are presented in Table 4. To illustrate the results within the separate PEL intervention groups, figures are presented with the mean of main outcomes at baseline and follow-up (Figure 3).

No significant differences were found when examining EBRBs and SR skills stratified by PEL (Table 4). In follow-up, there was a borderline significant result in cognitive SR skills when comparing low PEL intervention and control groups ($p = 0.051$).

Within the groups, the low PEL control group decreased their cognitive SR skills (borderline significance, $p = 0.052$). The total PA increased significantly within all intervention and control groups when stratified by PEL ($p < 0.001$ for all subgroups, Table 4, Figure 3B). The sugary treat consumption frequency increased within low PEL control and intervention groups ($p < 0.001$ in both groups), and in the middle PEL control group ($p = 0.027$, Table 4, Figure 3D). Cognitive SR skills strengthened in the middle PEL intervention group ($p = 0.038$, Table 4, Figure 3F).

Table 4. Comparison between the intervention and control group by parental educational level and changes within groups *.

Children's EBRBs and SR Skills	PEL	General Mixed Model		Linear Mixed Models with Repeated Measures					
		Comparison between Intervention and Control Group at Follow-Up [c]		Comparison between Follow-Up and Baseline in Control Group			Comparison between Follow-Up and Baseline in Intervention Group		
		(95% C.I.)	p-Value	diff F-B	(95% C.I.)	p-Value	diff F-B	(95% C.I.)	p-Value
Total screen time (min/day) [a]	low	−1.69 (−12.30; 8.92)	0.753	1.95	(−5.74; 9.64)	0.619	−3.42	(−11.23; 4.40)	0.391
	middle	−7.88 (−16.60; 0.84)	0.076	4.05	(−1.87; 9.98)	0.179	−2.00	(−8.57; 4.57)	0.551
	high	−3.73 (−16.13; 8.66)	0.553	7.65	(−0.10; 15.39)	0.053	2.95	(−6.86; 12.76)	0.555
Total physical activity (min/day) [b]	low	−7.17 (−24.15; 9.80)	0.404	21.41	(11.82; 31.00)	<0.001	22.10	(12.89; 31.32)	<0.001
	middle	1.86 (−11.90; 15.63)	0.787	26.61	(19.56; 33.66)	<0.001	30.89	(22.96; 38.83)	<0.001
	high	−0.77 (−19.96; 18.42)	0.937	21.10	(12.08; 30.13)	<0.001	27.66	(16.37; 38.95)	<0.001
Sugary foods and beverages (times/week) [a]	low	−0.15 (−2.70; 2.41)	0.909	0.83	(−1.07; 2.74)	0.392	0.10	(−1.71; 1.92)	0.911
	middle	−1.08 (−3.08; 0.93)	0.286	0.61	(−0.75; 1.96)	0.380	−0.88	(−2.26; 0.50)	0.210
	high	−1.34 (−4.14; 1.45)	0.344	0.09	(−1.64; 1.81)	0.920	−1.91	(−4.12; 0.31)	0.092
Sugary treats (times/week) [a]	low	−0.79 (−2.86; 1.29)	0.454	2.17	(0.97; 3.37)	<0.001	2.22	(1.15; 3.29)	<0.001
	middle	0.52 (−1.19; 2.22)	0.545	0.93	(0.10; 1.75)	0.027	0.74	(−0.17; 1.65)	0.109
	high	−0.07 (−2.32; 2.18)	0.954	0.89	(−0.18; 1.96)	0.103	1.02	(−0.34; 2.38)	0.140
Fruit and vegetables (times/week) [a]	low	2.99 (−1.00; 6.98)	0.141	−0.14	(−2.75; 2.47)	0.915	1.51	(−0.98; 3.99)	0.235
	middle	0.59 (−2.56; 3.74)	0.710	0.37	(−1.49; 2.23)	0.695	1.43	(−0.61; 3.48)	0.169
	high	1.03 (−3.30; 5.37)	0.638	−1.68	(−3.96; 0.60)	0.149	0.31	(−2.74; 3.36)	0.841
Cognitive SR skills (scale 1–3) [a]	low	0.11 (0.00; 0.21)	0.051	−0.11	(−0.22; 0.00)	0.052	0.04	(−0.08; 0.15)	0.513
	middle	0.001 (−0.09; 0.09)	0.987	−0.03	(−0.13; 0.06)	0.468	0.10	(0.01; 0.20)	0.038
	high	−0.06 (−0.18; 0.07)	0.380	0.04	(−0.09; 0.18)	0.536	−0.04	(−0.18; 0.09)	0.543
Emotional SR skills (scale 1–3) [a]	low	0.01 (−0.12; 0.13)	0.921	−0.02	(−0.11; 0.08)	0.750	0.03	(−0.07; 0.12)	0.563
	middle	0.05 (−0.05; 0.15)	0.313	−0.02	(−0.09; 0.05)	0.547	0.04	(−0.04; 0.12)	0.286
	high	0.01 (−0.13; 0.16)	0.861	0.07	(−0.02; 0.16)	0.141	0.03	(−0.09; 0.15)	0.611

* Estimates and their 95% confidence intervals (C.I.); [a] models adjusted for gender, age in years, municipality, and parental educational level; [b] models adjusted for gender, age in years, municipality, parental educational level, and accelerometer wear time; [c] models gender, age in years, municipality, parental educational level, (accelerometer wear time in PA as behavior), and for baseline value of outcome.

4. Discussion

We detected no differences in EBRBs or SR skills between the intervention and the control group in our preschool-based family-involving RCT. Furthermore, changes in children's EBRBs according to PEL did not differ between the intervention and control groups at follow-up, although a borderline significant result emerged in low PEL children in the intervention group, improving their cognitive SR skills compared with the corresponding control group ($p = 0.051$).

A possible reason for not detecting significant intervention effects might be that the goals set were unrealistic (0.74 times/day decrease in sugary foods and beverages), or it would have required a higher number of children. Our study was a complex multicomponent intervention of relatively short duration. Each of the five program themes were focused on for 4–5 weeks, which could have been too short a duration for changes to occur. Therefore, further evaluation of the effects is needed. Furthermore, the analysis did not show stronger intervention effects in low PEL children. Still, cognitive SR skills strengthened in the low PEL intervention group compared with the low PEL control group, and the results bordered on statistical significance. Within the low PEL control group, cognitive SR skills decreased; also here the results did border to reach statistical significance. However, a significant improvement in cognitive SR skills occurred among middle PEL intervention children. Since the above-mentioned increases in cognitive SR points when comparing control and intervention group were small, these results might lack practical implication. The Head Start intervention showed improvements in SR skills and a decrease in sugar-sweetened drink consumption in the group that received the intervention promoting both EBRBs and SR skills, compared with the other three groups [27]. Although the aims of that study and ours were similar, the results are not totally comparable. The age group in Head Start was slightly older (4–9 years), and SR skills were measured by another instrument. In both studies, activities to strengthen SR skills were mainly conducted in preschools, whereas parents were the main target when promoting healthy EBRBs. It was discussed that parents might not have been sufficiently engaged, which may have led to null results regarding the children's EBRBs, which may also be the case in the DAGIS.

Within the intervention and control group, several significant changes occurred in the EBRBs. The control group increased their screen time by approximately 4.5 min/day, whereas no changes were detected within the intervention group. For the control group, it had about a 30 min/week higher screen time, which might eventually harm energy balance, weight status, and development of SR skills. The results of the control children followed the trend that screen time increases with age among young children [40]. The ToyBox study also did not reveal an overall positive effect on screen time [16], nevertheless when including a process evaluation, a reduction in computer/video games time was shown [14]. Subgroup analyses in ToyBox showed less TV time during weekends in the intervention girls [16], and subgroup analyses should also be considered in the DAGIS study.

The total PA increased in the control and intervention group. A recently published European study reported that moderate-to-vigorous PA increased from the age group of 2–3 years to 4–5 years, and further to 6–7 years [41]. The trend might explain the results in the DAGIS. Moreover, the follow-up occurred in spring, when there are more daylight hours than at the baseline in autumn. Studies have revealed that the higher the temperature and the more daylight present, the higher the level of PA among children [42,43]. The municipality, in which all preschools participated, simultaneously runs a training program for all early educators aimed at increasing preschool PA, which has increased all children's preschool PA independently of intervention status. Previous interventions have reported no effects on children's PA [44–46], and discussion has ensued on whether short durations such as six weeks of promoting PA are sufficient to detect an increase in children's PA [16,47].

The follow-up results for sugary everyday food and beverage consumption outside preschool hours did not differ between the intervention and control groups. The reduction was mainly supposed to happen at home, as these foods are seldom served at Finnish preschools [31]. The program implementation in families might have been weak, leading to no changes. This needs to be further studied by analyzing the processes in the intervention. We found an increase in sugary treat consumption in both the control and intervention low PEL groups (Supplementary Table S2), but no changes in the middle or high intervention groups. It seems that as children grow older, the consumption increases, especially in low PEL groups, which might lead to a greater gap between the PEL groups. The change in FV consumption did not differ between the intervention and control groups. However, while the control group had a stable consumption of FV at both time-points, the consumption frequency in the intervention group increased by 1.3 times/week. Similarly, some intervention studies have shown improvements in FV consumption [48], although a systematic review concluded that multicomponent FV interventions have provided low evidence of increasing FV consumption [49].

When developing the DAGIS intervention, the focus was set on understanding the low educational level context and how to, by means of a universal intervention, reach those with low PEL backgrounds [28]. One strategy was to produce easy-to-read materials as the ToyBox intervention study discussed that the lack of significant results for children's food consumption might have been due to the intervention materials being insufficiently tailored to those with low education levels [13]. The DAGIS logic model of change included primary outcomes, which were seen as the most important determinants for explaining socio-economic differences in children's EBRBs. The main primary outcomes (i.e., adults role modeling and changes in the environment in availability and accessibility of, for example, foods and screens), should be examined next. It is more likely to see changes in these due to the relatively short duration of the intervention. Generally, it has been concluded that availability and accessibility (foods, screens) in the home environment would be of great importance for children's health behaviors in low PEL families [13].

As this study includes the intention-to-treat effect analysis, it was assumed that all intervention preschools and families conducted the program in the same manner and at the same intensity. Further analysis including fidelity and implementation degree of the program will yield a deeper understanding of the effects. The importance of the implementation degree has been discussed in conjunction with null results in multicomponent interventions [50].

The DAGIS intervention study had limitations that should be acknowledged. The short intervention time, in all, five months, was a limitation, but the project as a whole needed to be conducted during a preschool year. Previous discussion has questioned whether a short time period is adequate for children to change their EBRBs [13,44]. In addition, children's baseline consumption of FV, mean three times/day outside preschool time, was fairly high, which sets challenges for achieving an increase. Furthermore, reliably measuring food consumption is challenging. However, reproducibility and validity of our parental FFQ have been tested [36,38]. Still, the FFQ reflects the foods eaten during the last week outside preschool time and does not allow for analysis of whether food consumption changed at preschool. The 10-item questionnaire assessing two dimensions of children's SR skills had three answer categories, which might not have been sensitive enough to capture changes. Many instruments are available to assess children's SR skills, but no consensus exists on their validity in evaluating this multidimensional concept [51]. Finally, the sample size might not have been sufficiently large to detect significant results. The power calculations were conducted based on means and standard deviations from the DAGIS cross-sectional survey [7]. Some dissimilarities exist between these two studies such as the number of preschools and municipalities and the proportion of low PEL families participating, which might have led to an underpowered study.

A strength of the study is that the study development was guided by the IM framework [28], which enabled systematic planning. The logic model of change was formed on the best existing knowledge, and on a comprehensive evaluation of the Finnish preschool-family context [10,28]. This enables further systematic evaluations of the processes. The fairly high response rate of families, 47%, and having all preschools from one municipality participating including diverse preschools as well as diverse families can be seen as a strength. The high response rate indicates a lower selection bias among the participants. In addition, slightly more than 30% of the participating families had low education levels. It is often seen as a challenge that the less educated tend not to participate in intervention studies [52].

The study also included a combination of instruments such as the accelerometer for assessing PA, a validated screen time diary, and a validated FFQ for robust assessment [35,38].

The fairly new approach of simultaneously strengthening children's SR skills and promoting their EBRBs can be seen as a strength and also as a risk. To the best of our knowledge, this approach has been evaluated in one other study [27], where it was discussed that the next step should be integrating SR skill promotion into the EBRB context. In the DAGIS study, this can be seen as a strength as the program enhanced SR skills, while simultaneously promoting EBRBs by adding more materials to the existing program. The materials and methods for the program also underwent pretesting [28].

5. Conclusions

The DAGIS intervention study aimed to promote preschoolers' EBRBs and SR skills through a preschool-based family-involving intervention conducted as a clustered RCT. We detected no significant differences in the preschoolers' EBRBs between the intervention and control groups at follow up. No differences at follow-up between the PEL groups were found, except for the cognitive SR skills, where a borderline significant result emerged between low PEL control and intervention group. Within the middle PEL intervention group, there was an increase in cognitive SR skills. Even though the intervention did not achieve its goal and the aims were not attained, further analyses should examine whether changes can be seen in the determinants of children's EBRBs, especially those of importance for children with low PEL. In addition, a thorough process evaluation may provide insight into the non-significant findings.

Supplementary Materials: The following are available online at http://www.mdpi.com/2072-6643/12/9/2599/s1, Table S1: Number of children and missing values in each outcome, Table S2: Descriptors for study outcomes by the control and intervention groups and by parental educational level (PEL), Table S3: Adjusted differences and their 95% confidence interval (C.I.) between intervention and control group separated for baseline and follow-up; and adjusted differences between follow-up and baseline for each study group.

Author Contributions: Conceptualization, C.R., R.F., and E.R; Investigation, C.R., H.V., R.L., R.P., E.S., T.S., P.H., E.L., and L.K.; Formal analysis, R.F.; Data Curation, R.L.; Writing—Original Draft Preparation, C.R. and R.F.; Writing—Review & Editing C.R., R.F., H.V., R.L., R.P., E.S., T.S., P.H., E.L., L.K., K.S., N.S., M.E., and E.R.; Visualization, R.F.; Project Administration, C.R., Funding Acquisition, N.S., M.E., and E.R. All authors have read and agreed to the published version of the manuscript.

Funding: This study was financially supported by the Ministry of Education and Culture in Finland, The Ministry of Social Affairs and Health, The Academy of Finland (Grants: 285439, 287288, 288038, 315816), the Päivikki and Sakari Sohlberg Foundation, Signe and Ane Gyllenberg Foundation, and the Medicinska Föreningen Liv och Hälsa. Folkhälsan Research Center and University of Helsinki provided the infrastructure and the funding for PIs (N.S., M.E., E.R.) and key personnel (C.R., R.L.). Open access funding was provided by University of Helsinki. The funding bodies were not involved and did not interfere with the study at any stage.

Acknowledgments: The authors thank the preschools, the preschool personnel, and the families for their participation in the DAGIS study, and the research staff for the data collection. The authors thank the collaborating partners of the DAGIS study for providing assistance in designing the DAGIS study.

Conflicts of Interest: L.K. is a board member of the company TwoDads. The other authors declare that they have no competing interests.

References

1. Kremers, S.P.J.; de Bruijn, G.J.; Visscher, T.L.S.; van Mechelen, W.; de Vries, N.K.; Brug, J. Environmental Influences on Energy Balance-Related Behaviors: A Dual-Process View. *Int. J. Behav. Nutr. Phys. Act.* **2006**, *3*, 1–10. [CrossRef] [PubMed]
2. World Health Organization. *Report of the Comission on Ending Childhood Obesity*; WHO: Geneva, Switzerland, 2016.
3. Halfon, N.; Larson, K.; Slusser, W. Associations between Obesity and Comorbid Mental Health, Developmental, and Physical Health Conditions in a Nationally Representative Sample of US Children Aged 10 to 17. *Acad. Pediatr.* **2013**, *13*, 6–13. [CrossRef] [PubMed]
4. Reilly, J.J.; Methven, E.; Mcdowell, Z.C.; Hacking, B.; Alexander, D.; Stewart, L.; Kelnar, C.J.H. Health Consequences of Obesity. *Arch. Dis. Child.* **2003**, *88*, 748–752. [CrossRef] [PubMed]

5. Mantziki, K.; Vassilopoulos, A.; Radulian, G.; Borys, J.-M.; Du Plessis, H.; Gregorio, M.J.; Graca, P.; De Henauw, S.; Handjiev, S.; Visscher, T. Inequities in Energy-Balance Related Behaviours and Family Environmental Determinants in European Children: Baseline Results of the Prospective EPHE Evaluation Study. *BMC Public Health* **2015**, *15*, 1203. [CrossRef]
6. Fernandez-Alvira, J.; Mouratidou, T.; Bammann, K.; Hebestreit, A.; Barba, G.; Sieri, S.; Reisch, L.; Eiben, G.; Hadjigeorgiou, C.; Kovacs, E.; et al. Parental Education and Frequency of Food Consumption in European Children: The IDEFICS Study. *Public Health Nutr.* **2013**, *16*, 487–498. [CrossRef]
7. Lehto, E.; Ray, C.; Vepsäläinen, H.; Korkalo, L.; Lehto, R.; Kaukonen, R.; Suhonen, E.; Nislin, M.; Nissinen, K.; Skaffari, E.; et al. Increased Health and Wellbeing in Preschools (DAGIS) Study—Differences in Children's Energy Balance-Related Behaviors (EBRBs) and in Long-Term Stress by Parental Educational Level. *Int. J. Environ. Res. Public Health* **2018**, *15*, 2313. [CrossRef]
8. Gubbels, J.S.; Van Kann, D.H.H.; de Vries, N.K.; Thijs, C.; Kremers, S.P.J. The next Step in Health Behavior Research: The Need for Ecological Moderation Analyses—An Application to Diet and Physical Activity at Childcare. *Int. J. Behav. Nutr. Phys. Act.* **2014**, *11*, 52. [CrossRef]
9. Gubbels, J.S.; Stessen, K.; Van De Kolk, I.; De Vries, N.K.; Thijs, C.; Kremers, S.P.J. Energy Balance-Related Parenting and Childcare Practices: The Importance of Meso-System Consistency. *PLoS ONE* **2018**, *13*, e0203689. [CrossRef]
10. Määttä, S.; Lehto, R.; Nislin, M.; Ray, C.; Erkkola, M.; Sajaniemi, N.; Roos, E. Increased Health and Well-Being in Preschools (DAGIS): Rationale and Design for a Randomized Controlled Trial Health Behavior, Health Promotion and Society. *BMC Public Health* **2015**, *15*, 1–10. [CrossRef]
11. Biddle, S.J.H.; Petrolini, I.; Pearson, N. Interventions Designed to Reduce Sedentary Behaviours in Young People: A Review of Reviews. *Br. J. Sports Med.* **2014**, *48*, 182–186. [CrossRef]
12. Black, A.P.; D'Onise, K.; McDermott, R.; Vally, H.; O'Dea, K. How Effective Are Family-Based and Institutional Nutrition Interventions in Improving Children's Diet and Health? A Systematic Review. *BMC Public Health* **2017**, *17*, 1–19. [CrossRef] [PubMed]
13. Pinket, A.S.; De Craemer, M.; Huybrechts, I.; De Bourdeaudhuij, I.; Deforche, B.; Cardon, G.; Androutsos, O.; Koletzko, B.; Moreno, L.A.; Socha, P.; et al. Multibehavioural Interventions with a Focus on Specific Energy Balance-Related Behaviours Can Affect Diet Quality in Preschoolers from Six European Countries: The Toybox-Study. *Nutrients* **2017**, *9*, 479. [CrossRef] [PubMed]
14. Latomme, J.; Cardon, G.; De Bourdeaudhuij, I.; De Craemer, M.; Iotova, V.; Koletzko, B.; Socha, P.; Moreno, L.; Androutsos, O.; Manios, Y. Effect and Process Evaluation of a Kindergarten-Based, Family-Involved Intervention with a Randomized Cluster Design on Sedentary Behaviour in 4- to 6- Year Old European Preschool Children: The ToyBox-Study. *PLoS ONE* **2017**, *12*, e0172730. [CrossRef] [PubMed]
15. Duncan, S.; Stewart, T.; McPhee, J.; Borotkanics, R.; Prendergast, K.; Zinn, C.; Meredith-Jones, K.; Taylor, R.; McLachlan, C.; Schofield, G. Efficacy of a Compulsory Homework Programme for Increasing Physical Activity and Improving Nutrition in Children: A Cluster Randomised Controlled Trial. *Int. J. Behav. Nutr. Phys. Act.* **2019**, *16*, 80. [CrossRef] [PubMed]
16. De Craemer, M.; De Decker, E.; Verloigne, M.; De Bourdeaudhuij, I.; Manios, Y.; Cardon, G. The Effect of a Cluster Randomised Control Trial on Objectively Measured Sedentary Time and Parental Reports of Time Spent in Sedentary Activities in Belgian Preschoolers: The ToyBox-Study. *Int. J. Behav. Nutr. Phys. Act.* **2016**, *13*, 1–17. [CrossRef]
17. Marmot, M. Proportionate universalism. In *The Health Gap—The Challenge of an Unequal World*; Bloomsbury Publishing: London, UK, 2015; pp. 279–289.
18. Wijtzes, A.I.; Van De Gaar, V.M.; Van Grieken, A.; De Kroon, M.L.A.; Mackenbach, J.P.; Van Lenthe, F.J.; Jansen, W.; Raat, H. Effectiveness of Interventions to Improve Lifestyle Behaviors among Socially Disadvantaged Children in Europe. *Eur. J. Public Health* **2017**, *27*, 240–247. [CrossRef]
19. Love, R.E.; Adams, J.; van Sluijs, E.M.F. Equity Effects of Children's Physical Activity Interventions: A Systematic Scoping Review. *Int. J. Behav. Nutr. Phys. Act.* **2017**, *14*, 134. [CrossRef]
20. Downing, K.L.; Hnatiuk, J.A.; Hinkley, T.; Salmon, J.; Hesketh, K.D. Interventions to Reduce Sedentary Behaviour in 0–5-Year-Olds: A Systematic Review and Meta-Analysis of Randomised Controlled Trials. *Br. J. Sports Med.* **2018**, *52*, 314–321. [CrossRef]
21. Aparicio, E.; Canals, J.; Arija, V.; De Henauw, S.; Michels, N. The Role of Emotion Regulation in Childhood Obesity: Implications for Prevention and Treatment. *Nutr. Res. Rev.* **2016**, *29*, 17–29. [CrossRef]

22. Miller, A.L.; Lumeng, J.C. Pathways of Association from Stress to Obesity in Early Childhood. *Obesity* **2018**, *26*, 1117–1124. [CrossRef]
23. Nigg, J.T. Annual Research Review: On the Relations among Self-Regulation, Self-Control, Executive Functioning, Effortful Control, Cognitive Control, Impulsivity, Risk-Taking, and Inhibition for Developmental Psychopathology. *J. Child. Psychol. Psychiatry* **2017**, *58*, 361–383. [CrossRef] [PubMed]
24. Seeyave, D.M.; Coleman, S.; Appugliese, D.; Corwyn, R.F.; Bradley, R.H.; Davidson, N.S.; Kaciroti, N.; Lumeng, J.C. Ability to Delay Gratification at Age 4 Years and Risk of Overweight at Age 11 Years. *Arch. Pediatr. Adolesc. Med.* **2009**, *163*, 303–308. [CrossRef] [PubMed]
25. Liang, J.; Matheson, B.E.; Kaye, W.H.; Boutelle, K.N. Neurocognitive Correlates of Obesity and Obesity-Related Behaviors in Children and Adolescents. *Int. J. Obes.* **2014**, *38*, 494–506. [CrossRef] [PubMed]
26. Anderson, S.; Sacker, A.; Whitaker, R.; Kelly, Y. Self-Regulation and Household Routines at Age Three and Obesity at Age Eleven: Longitudinal Analysis of the UK Millennium Cohort Study. *Int. J. Obes.* **2017**, *41*, 1459–1466. [CrossRef]
27. Lumeng, J.C.; Miller, A.L.; Horodynski, M.A.; Brophy-Herb, H.E.; Contreras, D.; Lee, H.; Sturza, J.; Kaciroti, N.; Peterson, K.E. Improving Self-Regulation for Obesity Prevention in Head Start: A Randomized Controlled Trial. *Pediatrics* **2017**, *139*, e20162047. [CrossRef]
28. Ray, C.; Kaukonen, R.; Lehto, E.; Vepsäläinen, H.; Sajaniemi, N.; Erkkola, M.; Roos, E. Development of the DAGIS Intervention Study: A Preschool-Based Family-Involving Study Promoting Preschoolers' Energy Balance-Related Behaviours and Self-Regulation Skills. *BMC Public Health* **2019**, *19*, 1670. [CrossRef]
29. Eldredge, L.K.B.; Markham, C.M.; Ruiter, R.A.C.; Fernandez, M.E.; Parcel, G.S. *Planning Health Promotion Programs—An Intervention Mapping Approach*, 4th ed.; Jossey-Bass: San Fransisco, CA, USA, 2016.
30. Säkkinen, S.; Kuoppala, T. *Varhaiskasvatus 2017 (Children's Day Care 2018)*; National Institute of Health and Welfare: Helsinki, Finland, 2018. Available online: http://urn.fi/URN:NBN:fi-fe2018100937865 (accessed on 24 August 2020).
31. Korkalo, L.; Nissinen, K.; Skaffari, E.; Vepsäläinen, H.; Lehto, R.; Kaukonen, R.; Koivusilta, L.; Sajaniemi, N.; Roos, E.; Erkkola, M. The Contribution of Preschool Meals to the Diet of Finnish Preschoolers. *Nutrients* **2019**, *11*, 1531. [CrossRef]
32. National Institute for Health and Welfare. The Welfare Compass for Monitoring Regional Welfare. Available online: https://www.hyvinvointikompassi.fi/en/web/hyvinvointikompassi/etusivu (accessed on 21 March 2019).
33. Schulz, K.F.; Altman, D.G.; Moher, D. CONSORT 2010 Statement: Updated Guidelines for Reporting Parallel Group Randomised Trials. *BMJ* **2010**, *340*, c332. [CrossRef]
34. Wen, L.; van der Ploeg, H.; Kite, J.; Cashmore, A.; Rissel, C. A Validation Study of Assessing Physical Activity and Sedentary Behavior in Children Aged 3 to 5 Years. *Pediatr. Exerc. Sci.* **2010**, *22*, 408–420. [CrossRef]
35. Määttä, S.; Vepsäläinen, H.; Lehto, R.; Erkkola, M.; Roos, E.; Ray, C. Reproducibility of Preschool Personnel and Guardian Reports on Energy Balance-Related Behaviors and Their Correlates in Finnish Preschool Children. *Children* **2018**, *5*, 144. [CrossRef]
36. Cliff, D.; Okely, A.; Smith, L.; McKeen, K. Relationships between Fundamental Movement Skills and Objectively Measured Physical Activity in Preschool Children. *Pediatr. Exerc. Sci.* **2009**, *21*, 436–449. [CrossRef] [PubMed]
37. Evenson, K.; Catellier, D.; Gill, K.; McMurray, R. Calibration of Two Objective Measures of Physical Activity for Children. *J. Sports Sci.* **2008**, *26*, 1557–1565. [CrossRef] [PubMed]
38. Korkalo, L.; Vepsäläinen, H.; Ray, C.; Skaffari, E.; Lehto, R.; Hauta-alus, H.; Nissinen, K.; Meinilä, J.; Erkkola, M.; Roos, E. Parents' Reports of Preschoolers' Diets: Relative Validity of a Food Frequency Questionnaire and Dietary Patterns. *Nutrients* **2019**, *11*, 159. [CrossRef] [PubMed]
39. Maloney, J.E.; Lawlor, M.S.; Shonert-Reichl, K.A.; Whitehead, J. A universal, mindfulness-based social and emotional learning (SEL) Program designed to be implemented in schools by regular classroom teachers. In *Handbook of Mindfulness in Education—Integrating Theory into Practice*; Shonert-Reichl, K.A., Roeser, R.W., Eds.; Springer: New York, NY, USA, 2016; pp. 313–334.
40. Carson, V.; Lee, E.Y.; Hesketh, K.D.; Hunter, S.; Kuzik, N.; Predy, M.; Rhodes, R.E.; Rinaldi, C.M.; Spence, J.C.; Hinkley, T. Physical Activity and Sedentary Behavior across Three Time-Points and Associations with Social Skills in Early Childhood. *BMC Public Health* **2019**, *19*, 1–8. [CrossRef] [PubMed]

41. Steene-Johannessen, J.; Hansen, B.; Dalene, K.; Kolle, E.; Northstone, K.; Møller, N.; Grøntved, A.; Wedderkopp, N.; Kriemler, S.; Page, A.; et al. Variations in Accelerometry Measured Physical Activity and Sedentary Time across Europe—Harmonized Analyses of 47,497 Children and Adolescents. *Int. J. Behav. Nutr. Phys. Act.* **2020**, *17*, 38. [CrossRef] [PubMed]
42. Brusseau, T.A. The Intricacies of Children's Physical Activity. *J. Hum. Kinet.* **2015**, *47*, 269–275. [CrossRef] [PubMed]
43. Harrison, F.; Goodman, A.; van Sluijs, E.M.F.; Andersen, L.B.; Cardon, G.; Davey, R.; Janz, K.F.; Kriemler, S.; Molloy, L.; Page, A.S.; et al. Weather and Children's Physical Activity; How and Why Do Relationships Vary between Countries? *Int. J. Behav. Nutr. Phys. Act.* **2017**, *14*, 74. [CrossRef]
44. De Craemer, M.; Verloigne, M.; De Bourdeaudhuij, I.; Androutsos, O.; Iotova, V.; Moreno, L.; Koletzko, B.; Socha, P.; Manios, Y.; Cardon, G.; et al. Effect and Process Evaluation of a Kindergarten-Based, Family-Involved Cluster Randomised Controlled Trial in Six European Countries on Four- to Six-Year-Old Children's Steps per Day: The ToyBox-Study. *Int. J. Behav. Nutr. Phys. Act.* **2017**, *14*, 116. [CrossRef]
45. Bellows, L.; Davies, P.; Anderson, J.; Kennedy, C. Effectiveness of a Physical Activity Intervention for Head Start Preschoolers: A Randomized Intervention Study. *Am. J. Occup. Ther.* **2013**, *67*, 28–36. [CrossRef]
46. Reilly, J.; Kelly, L.; Montgomery, C.; Williamson, A.; Fisher, A.; McColl, J.; Lo Conte, R.; Paton, J.; Grant, S. Physical Activity to Prevent Obesity in Young Children: Cluster Randomised Controlled Trial. *BMJ Open* **2006**, *333*, 1041. [CrossRef]
47. Buscemi, J.; Odoms-Young, A.; Stolley, M.R.; Schiffer, L.; Blumstein, L.; Clark, M.H.; Berbaum, M.L.; McCaffrey, J.; Braunschweig, C.; Fitzgibbon, M.L. Comparative Effectiveness Trial of an Obesity Prevention Intervention in EFNEP and SNAP-ED: Primary Outcomes. *Nutrients* **2019**, *11*, 1012. [CrossRef] [PubMed]
48. Rios, L.M.; Serrano, M.M.; Aguilar, A.J.; Chacón, L.B.; Neria, C.R.; Monreal, L.A. Promoting Fruit, Vegetable and Simple Water Consumption among Mothers and Teachers of Preschool Children: An Intervention Mapping Initiative. *Eval. Program Plann.* **2019**, *76*, 101675. [CrossRef] [PubMed]
49. Wolfenden, L.; Barnes, C.; Jones, J.; Finch, M.; Wyse, R.; Kingsland, M.; Tzelepis, F.; Grady, A.; Hodder, R.; Booth, D.; et al. Strategies to Improve the Implementation of Healthy Eating, Physical Activity and Obesity Prevention Policies, Practices or Programmes within Childcare Services. *Cochrane Database Syst. Rev.* **2020**, *2*, CD011779. [CrossRef] [PubMed]
50. Steenbock, B.; Buck, C.; Zeeb, H.; Rach, S.; Pischke, C.R. Impact of the Intervention Program "JolinchenKids-Fit and Healthy in Daycare" on Energy Balance Related-Behaviors: Results of a Cluster Controlled Trial. *BMC Pediatr.* **2019**, *19*, 432. [CrossRef] [PubMed]
51. Halle, T.G.; Darling-Churchill, K.E. Review of Measures of Social and Emotional Development. *J. Appl. Dev. Psychol.* **2016**, *45*, 8–18. [CrossRef]
52. Prevo, L.; Kremers, S.; Jansen, M. Small Successes Make Big Wins: A Retrospective Case Study towards Community Engagement of Low-SES Families. *Int. J. Environ. Res. Public Health* **2020**, *17*, 612. [CrossRef]

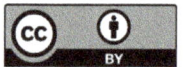

© 2020 by the authors. Licensee MDPI, Basel, Switzerland. This article is an open access article distributed under the terms and conditions of the Creative Commons Attribution (CC BY) license (http://creativecommons.org/licenses/by/4.0/).

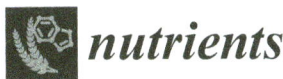

Review

Machine Learning Models to Predict Childhood and Adolescent Obesity: A Review

Gonzalo Colmenarejo

Biostatistics and Bioinformatics Unit, IMDEA Food, CEI UAM+CSIC, E28049 Madrid, Spain; gonzalo.colmenarejo@imdea.org

Received: 30 June 2020; Accepted: 13 August 2020; Published: 16 August 2020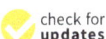

Abstract: The prevalence of childhood and adolescence overweight an obesity is raising at an alarming rate in many countries. This poses a serious threat to the current and near-future health systems, given the association of these conditions with different comorbidities (cardiovascular diseases, type II diabetes, and metabolic syndrome) and even death. In order to design appropriate strategies for its prevention, as well as understand its origins, the development of predictive models for childhood/adolescent overweight/obesity and related outcomes is of extreme value. Obesity has a complex etiology, and in the case of childhood and adolescence obesity, this etiology includes also specific factors like (pre)-gestational ones; weaning; and the huge anthropometric, metabolic, and hormonal changes that during this period the body suffers. In this way, Machine Learning models are becoming extremely useful tools in this area, given their excellent predictive power; ability to model complex, nonlinear relationships between variables; and capacity to deal with high-dimensional data typical in this area. This is especially important given the recent appearance of large repositories of Electronic Health Records (EHR) that allow the development of models using datasets with many instances and predictor variables, from which Deep Learning variants can generate extremely accurate predictions. In the current work, the area of Machine Learning models to predict childhood and adolescent obesity and related outcomes is comprehensively and critically reviewed, including the latest ones using Deep Learning with EHR. These models are compared with the traditional statistical ones that used mainly logistic regression. The main features and applications appearing from these models are described, and the future opportunities are discussed.

Keywords: childhood obesity; obesity; overweight; machine learning; deep learning; statistical models; data science; BMI

1. Introduction

Obesity and overweight prevalence among children and adolescents has increased to a large extent during the last four decades [1,2]. For instance, the prevalence of overweight and obese children and adolescents between 5 and 19 years has soared from about 4% in 1975 to 18% in 2016 [3]. This increase is especially dramatic in developing countries [4], while in developed countries it seems to be slowing down and affects mainly the low-income sub-populations [5]. In absolute numbers, it is currently estimated that about 38 million children under the age of 5 are overweight or obese, while about 340 million children and adolescents aged 5–19 years are overweight or obese [3].

This large prevalence poses a threat to the current and future health systems. Childhood and adolescent obesity is related to different comorbidities during this age [6–10], as well as to a lower quality of life [11], but, in addition, it is also associated to *adult* comorbidities, like metabolic syndrome and diabetes [12], cardiovascular risk [13,14], and death [15,16]. This is probably due to the difficulty in its eradication once it is established, justifying the adoption of childhood preventive measures, rather than therapeutic ones [9].

Obesity, that is, excess adipose tissue in the body [17], has a complex, multifactorial etiology. Among the factors involved in its development, the most important ones are genetics, physical activity, sedentary lifestyle, diet, etc. [18] In addition, obesity has additional complications for its analysis during childhood and adolescence. This is largely due to the huge changes in height and weight during this period. If we measure the Body Mass Index (BMI) through it, we see a pattern of an initial increase until reaching a first peak at about 1 year, followed by a decrease up to the age of about 6 years, where it starts to rise again (the so-called *adipose rebound*) [18]. So big are these changes that there is no universal consensus in the definitions of "overweight" and "obese" based on BMI at these ages [17], and in most cases, they are defined using sex-, age- and population-specific percentiles, normally ≥ 85th percentile for overweight, and ≥ 95th percentile for obese, as will be discussed in Section 4 in detail. (It must be noted that in this Review we use the concept "obesity" in two ways: one is as excess adipose tissue in the body in general, and the other is a BMI-based category to classify individuals, normally for adults BMI ≥ 30 kg/m^2 and for children with multiple definitions as described in the text.)

Therefore, during this period, there happen large metabolic and hormonal changes that largely influence the adiposity at different ages. On top of that, there is still a large influence of specific pre-gestational and gestational factors, especially during early childhood, that have a large impact at these ages. The additional risk factors for obesity in childhood-adolescence have been reviewed recently [18,19]. Some of the most outstanding ones are parent's BMI, gestational weight gain of the mother, gestational diabetes, maternal smoking, birth weight, rapid infant growth, and high protein and/or free sugars consumption. There are also psychological factors, especially during the adolescence period.

In order to prevent childhood and adolescent obesity, the development of predictive models to identify potential individuals of high risk is of great utility. This allows the focusing of preventive measures towards the high-risk subpopulation, allowing a more cost-effective and personalized approach to weight reduction interventions. In addition, the use of predictive models allows, by their analysis, to rank the different risk factors in order of importance, so that we can identify those that would be more effective in order to design these interventions. Moreover, the models can be used as simulation tools where "what-if" analyses can be conducted, by varying one or more predictor variables and seeing what would be the effect in obesity for particular sub-populations (defined by, e.g., sex, age, diet, etc.).

Given the large complexity of obesity, especially during the childhood and adolescence period, with a large number of multidomain influencing factors interacting in convoluted ways, traditional statistical methods like (generalized) linear models show limitations and have focused mainly in analyses with a reduced number of predictor variables and with limited predictive power. As we will see in Section 3, these models in most cases use more or less the same set of predictor variables transformed in one way or another and aggregated a linear functional form. Another limitation of these methods is their inability to deal with high-dimensional data, where the number of predictor variables (columns) is close or even much higher than that the number of dataset instances (rows), as they typically require many more instances than predictor variables in order to provide reliable inferences and avoid overfitting. Such situation makes them to need huge samples for they to be used with large sets of predictor variables, resulting in difficult practical implementations.

In this way, Machine Learning (ML) techniques are especially gifted modelling tools for these datasets, typically of high-dimensional nature and with complex relationships between many multidomain variables. This is due to their capacity to deal with high-dimensional data so that they can be applied to model relatively small datasets having large numbers of predictor variables and with reduced overfit. In addition, ML methods are able to find complex, nonlinear relationships between the predictor variables and these and the response variable or variables in an automated way, not requiring to manually predefine and test a large set of potential relationships between these variables. Therefore, the predictive capacity, ease of application, and robustness of these models for complex data far outclasses those of the traditional statistical models. This is even more in the case of the recent Deep Learning (DL) branch of ML, which can tap from huge datasets both in instances and predictor variables to obtain models with extremely good predictive capacities. DL methods, in addition, are able to directly use complex data like images, text, social media, time series, etc., avoiding the need of lengthy *feature engineering* processes, as we will see in Section 2. This is increasing dramatically the scope of data sources that can be used in this field, allowing to identify novel risk factors.

Given the above described advantages of ML over statistical methods for this problem, it is no surprise that ML have started to be used in the area. Thus, this paper attempts to conduct a critical and comprehensive review of the work done in ML models applied so far to the area of childhood and adolescent obesity. This will include a brief unbiased summary of each of the works available in the area to predict childhood or adolescent BMI and/or obesity/overweight with ML, followed by a thorough discussion of the collective patterns found, results obtained and novel risks factors identified, advantages and limitations of the approach, and future perspectives. The discussion will include also a comparison with the statistical models of the same outcomes, which will have been briefly reviewed previously. In addition, models to predict related outcomes (e.g., success of weight decreasing therapies, social obesogenic environments, pediatric attention to obesity, etc.) will also be reviewed, as they are of increasing interest especially in the area of preventive interventions. We will see that this is a new field that has experienced a recent explosion, especially during the last five years, mainly through the use of massive databases of Electronic Health Records (EHR) and the application for the first time of DL techniques, which is starting to allow a more systematic analysis of large cohorts with many multidomain predictor variables and the introduction of complex data sources as predictors. As the reader will see, this is also a very heterogeneous field, both in terms of type of model (cross-sectional, longitudinal), label predicted by the model (obesity, overweight, success of obesity therapies, pediatric attention to obesity, etc.), aim of the predictions (explanatory, predictive, and simulation), and application of the model (prediction of risk subpopulation, optimization of obesity therapy, suggestion of novel therapeutic approaches, etc.), further extending those typical of statistical models. It is expected to provide an updated view of the field to researchers within multiple disciplines and interests: statisticians, engineers, data scientists, epidemiologists, pediatricians, nurses, and nutritionists.

The article will be organized as follows: after this Introduction, first, a summary of the ML field will be conducted in order to provide some basic knowledge for readers not experts in the field, trying to make the work as much self-contained as possible; second, the procedure to search and select the reviewed works will be described; third, the statistical models in the childhood/adolescence obesity area will be reviewed, in order to set a comparison point with the ML models; fourth, ML models targeted to the prediction of BMI or categorized versions of BMI will be reviewed; fifth, ML models targeted to the prediction of related outcomes will be reviewed; sixth, a final wrap-up discussion of the main patterns in the models summarized will close the paper.

2. Basic Concepts in Machine Learning

Machine Learning (ML) exploded in the 90s of last century as a new field of data analysis at the interface between Statistics and Artificial Intelligence. Although the initial concepts like Rosenblatt's perceptron [20] (a basic, 1-layer artificial neural network to perform binary classification), Naïve Bayes [21], Decision Trees [21], and k-Nearest Neighbors date back to the 50s–60s of the 20th century, it was during the last decade of it when the field started to enter into full maturity and be massively applied. This happened with the appearance of multi-layer neural networks, thanks to the invention of the *backpropagation* training algorithm [22], as well as other ML paradigms like Support Vector Machines [23] and, in the first decade of the 21st century, Random Forests [24] and Gradient Boosting Machines [25]. This emergence has been fostered by the confluence of CPU miniaturization and cheapening, massive accessibility of computational capacity, and the development of completely new ideas for statistical modeling.

This explosion has been followed, in the second decade of the 21st century, by the one of *Deep Learning* (DL). DL is an outgrowth from ML that comprises mainly artificial neural networks of very large numbers of layers (the term "deep" comes from here), together with specialized layers, like *convolutional* and *recurrent* ones, and additional adaptations to allow the training of these huge neural networks: non-saturable activation functions; new weight initialization schemes; faster optimizers; and the training of the network in small, random batches of the data (the so-called *mini-batch* training). The DL models contain typically millions of training parameters. The specialized layers find directly from complex data like images, sounds, texts, music, etc., patterns ("feature maps") that are fed into multi-layer fully-connected perceptrons, allowing the direct modeling of this complex data, without the need of manually generating compressed representations of these data, the so-called "feature engineering".

Again, DL has benefited from an additional increase of computational power easily accessible, mainly though both the use of GPUs instead of CPUs, and of cloud computing, as well as the availability of huge public datasets (e.g., YouTube, San Bruno, CA, USA; Wikipedia, Facebook, Menlo Park, CA, USA; etc.) and open competitions (Kaggle, San Francisco, CA, USA, etc.).

Generally speaking, ML has put more emphasis in *prediction* rather than *testing of a predefined hypothesis* like traditional statistical models, where the emphasis is more in inference. In the same way, the focus is more in a practical, engineering-oriented approach rather than on a rigorous theoretical background. ML can be defined as a set of algorithms that *automatically learn simplified representations of the data*. For example, we can present the ML algorithm with a set of data instances, like pictures of animals, together with a label for the species present in each picture. The algorithm would then be *trained* by automatically learning some abstract internal rules to associate each image to each label, by minimizing some kind of measure of the prediction error or *loss*. When presented with new pictures, the algorithm would then be able to assign a label (species name) to each of them.

ML models are able to cope with very complex datasets, even those with many more predictor variables than instances (*high-dimensional datasets*). For this reason, they tend to be more difficult to interpret ("black-box" type of models), although as we will see later, new techniques have been developed to facilitate understanding the inner working of the model.

From our purposes in this Review, we can talk about two main groups of ML models: *supervised* and *unsupervised*. Supervised models are those that use datasets comprising both a set of *predictor variables* and one or more *target variables* or *labels*. The model would then be trained to be able to predict the label(s) from new instances of the predictor variables: for instance, to predict if a child will be obese or not from his age, sex, parent's BMI, and food consumption. The other type of ML models, *unsupervised ones*, attempt to find, without the use of labels, transformations of the input data with easier visualization, less noise, etc., or try to identify groups in the data. These techniques include *Dimensionality Reduction* and *Clustering* techniques.

Within the area of supervised models, which are the ones we will see in the Review, there are two main groups: *classification* models, those where the predicted label is a categorical one (e.g., obese child yes or not), and *regression* models, those where the label is a numeric one (e.g., BMI).

The most important type of classification models is *binary classification*, where the label has only two categories, for instance "+" and "−". In this case, the model frequently outputs a probability p of one of the two classes (e.g., "+"; the probability of the alternate class "−" would be $1 - p$). Once we define a threshold t for this probability, if $p \geq t$ for a new instance, we would assign the category "+" to that instance; if, on the contrary, $p < t$, we would assign the category "−". At this point, several concepts are used to characterize the performance of the model (Figure 1), depending on whether the real category is "+" or "−", and whether the predicted category is "+" or "−".

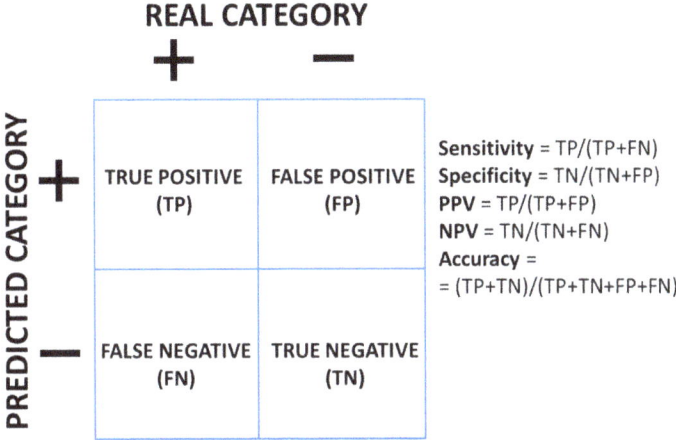

Figure 1. Measures of the performance of a binary classifier. Class labels are "+" and "−". Predicted category by the model is represented vs the real category, for all the possible situations.

Sensitivity (or *recall*) is the proportion of real positives that are predicted as positives. *Specificity* is the proportion of real negatives that are predicted as negatives. *Positive Predictive Value* (PPV), or *precision*, is the proportion of predicted positives that are real positives, and *Negative Predictive Value* (NPV) is the proportion of predicted negatives that are real negatives. *Accuracy* is the total proportion of correct predictions of all the predicted data.

A perfect model would have all these measures equal to 1. Obviously, this is almost never the case, and we have to cope with some proportion of errors. We can choose the threshold t so that it optimizes the purpose of our model. For example, if we are mainly interested in identifying as many real positives (e.g., future obese children) as possible, in order to apply to them some preventive weight-loss treatment, we would select a lower t and thus increase the sensitivity, even at the cost of increasing the false positives and, therefore, decreasing the specificity and the PPV. This approach would reach a point where we would identify so many false positives that would result in a prohibitive cost for treating many unnecessary cases or, if applying the treatment to a future normal-weight child has a negative effect, an unnecessary harm to too many members of our population. Alternatively, if we are more interested in finding a sample of children most of whom will be obese in the future, even if it is small (e.g., we can use it later for genotyping purposes), we would be more interested in optimizing the PPV; in this case, we would use a larger t, therefore increasing the false negatives. This would result in a decreased sensitivity and NPV. Again, we cannot increase t indefinitely, because there will be a point where the sample would be so small that would become useless. Therefore, there is always a balance between the cost and benefit, not just from the statistical point of view but also from the practical application of the model, which must be taken into consideration when optimizing the threshold of the model.

In order to characterize the discriminative capacity of the model, before selecting t, it is customary to use Receiver Operating Characteristic (ROC) curves. In this curve, the sensitivity is plotted against 1-specificity for all the values of the threshold (Figure 2).

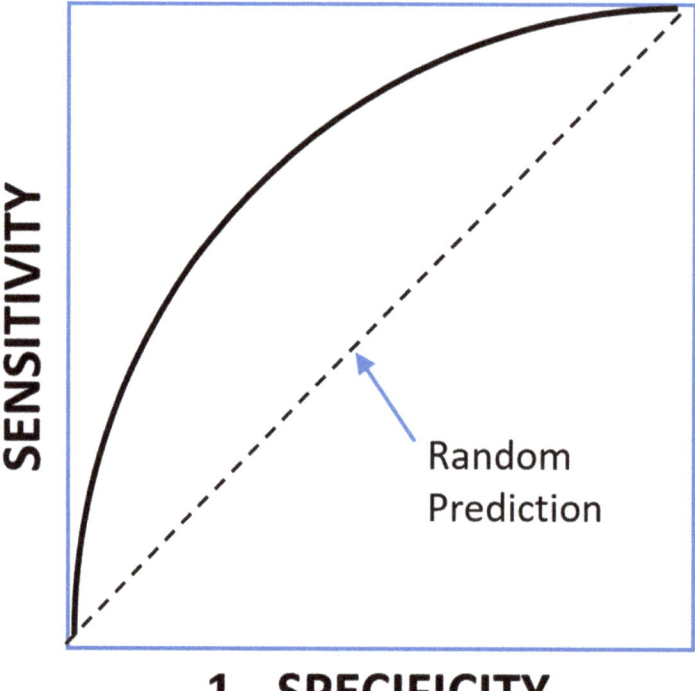

Figure 2. ROC curve of a binary classifier.

For a random classifier, the curve will be a diagonal going from (0, 0) to (1, 1). For a perfect classifier, the curve would go from (0, 0) to (0, 1) and then to (1, 1). Intermediate classifiers would have a curve in between these two extremes. A frequent measure of the discriminatory power of the classifier is the area under the curve of the ROC curve (AUCROC). A random classifier has an AUCROC of 0.5, and a perfect classifier has an AUCROC of 1. Real-life classifiers would have values in between, the better the closer to 1. The AUCROC equals the so-called *concordance index* or *c-index*.

When the classifier predicts a multi-class label, that is, with more than two classes, a measure of the prediction performance is the accuracy, defined above as the percentage of instances for which the label is predicted correctly. Another measure is the *categorical cross-entropy*. For a prediction instance i and an M-category label, it is defined as the Equation (1)

$$-\sum_{j=1}^{M} I_{ij} \log P_{ij} \qquad (1)$$

where I_{ij} is an indicator variable that is 0 if the predicted class j of instance i is not correct and 1 if it is. P_{ij} is the predicted probability for class j on the new instance i. For n predicted instances, the categorical cross-entropy would be the sum of each of the instances categorical cross-entropies. Therefore, it basically measures the match between the predicted probabilities for the different classes with the observed frequencies. The better the agreement between predicted and actual labels, the smaller the categorical cross-entropy, thus being an *error* or *loss* function that is minimized as the model is trained with the training data (in the case of accuracy, it would be maximized). For binary classifiers, the cross-entropy formula simplifies to $M = 2$, and we have the *binary cross-entropy*.

When we deal with regression, common measures of the error or loss are the *Mean Squared Error* (MSE, the Equation (2)):

$$MSE = \frac{1}{n}\sum_{i=1}^{n}(y_i - \hat{y}_i)^2 \qquad (2)$$

where n is the number of predicted instances, y_i is the actual continuous label for instance i, and $\hat{y}_i$ is the predicted value of the label for that instance. Another is the *Mean Absolute Error* (MAE, the Equation (3)):

$$MAE = \frac{1}{n}\sum_{i=1}^{n}|y_i - \hat{y}_i| \qquad (3)$$

where |.| means absolute value.

When training a model with training data, there is a risk that the model learns too many details of the latter, which makes it perform worse when presented with new data. In this case, we say that the model is *overfit*. Normally, all the models we fit will fit better the training data than new datasets. Therefore, in order to assess the *practical* prediction performance of a model, we need to *validate* it with new data. We will see that there are different approaches for validation of models, which can be divided in two groups: *internal validation* methods and *external validation* methods.

The main feature of internal validation methods is that we resample several times from the whole dataset, fit a new model with the resample, and evaluate the model with the instances left out from the resample. From this repeated resampling, model fit, and evaluation, we get an estimation of the predictive performance of the modeling *process* with new data, although we do not really test a final model with new data. Internal validations are used normally when the data is scarce, so it is very difficult to obtain a new data set to externally validate the model.

There are two main general approaches for internal validation: *cross-validation* and *bootstrap*. In the former case, in its *k-fold* version, what we do is divide the total sample into *k* random subsets ("folds"; as for *k*, normally 5 or 10 is used). Then what we do is, for each fold, validate with this fold a model fitted with the $k - 1$ remaining folds. The estimated validation measure of the performance of the model (accuracy, cross-entropy, MSE, etc.) will be the average of the performances of the *k* models fitted with each *k* subsamples, each having with $k-1$ folds and evaluated in the corresponding hold-out fold.

Cross-validation schemes can also be used to estimate *hyperparameters* of our model (e.g., number of nearest neighbors in the k-Nearest Neighbors method, see below). What we do then is perform the cross-validation with a double loop of folds; in one loop, we vary the hyperparameter among several options, and in the other, we estimate the validation performance within each hyperparameter selection. We will select the hyperparameter value that optimizes the cross-validation performance estimate, and at the same time that performance will serve as estimate of the external performance of the model (fitted with that optimal hyperparameter value).

It must be taken into account that the models fitted with cross-validation use a smaller dataset than the whole dataset, so this can be a source of error of estimation of the performance. The other approach for internal validation, bootstrap, avoids this issue by generating repeatedly samples of the same size of the original one by sampling with replacement (allowing randomly repeated instances). The model is refitted for each of these random samples and then evaluated in both that sample and in the original sample or the left-out instances. By averaging the difference between the training performance in each sample and the performance in the original sample, we get an estimation of the so-called *optimism* in the training performance. Then, we would derive the model with the whole dataset, evaluate its performance, and correct it by the estimated optimism.

We see that in both cross-validation and bootstrap, we do not make a real evaluation of the external performance of the model but rather make an estimation of it from data that is used at the end in the derivation of the final model. The alternative is to use an *external validation sample*. This is data that is not used in the derivation of the model and is only used for validating the model. A simple approach here is to randomly split the original sample into a training dataset (e.g., 60–80% of the data) to fit the model with it and then a validation/testing dataset (40–20% of the data) to evaluate external performance. This has two drawbacks when compared with internal validation methods: on one hand, we miss some of the data in the model derivation; on the other hand, we make the estimation of the external performance with a normally small dataset, which would result in an estimate with high variance (depending on how "lucky" we are in the random split, we can have very different estimates). This is not an issue if we have a very large dataset, and the validation set is quite large. However, in case we have a small dataset, it is preferable to use internal validation measures, despite being a bit more optimistic than external validations.

In addition, the random split approach has an additional problem in that both the training and the validation datasets come from the same sample, and thus, it is likely that they are very similar, a situation that quite possibly does not to occur when using the model in real life. There are ways to avoid this issue, like clustering the original sample and then generating training and validation datasets from different clusters. Another approach is to train the model with one dataset and then validate it with a different dataset, e.g., a posterior in time dataset, a dataset from another country, etc. This is a more demanding comparison but is probably the closest to the real performance of the model in production. Obviously, this approach is very expensive in terms of datasets, so it is only available in a reduced number of situations.

We will finish this section by briefly describing the ML models we will see in the Review.

2.1. Naïve Bayes (NB)

This method uses Bayes rule together with the approximation of conditional independence of predictor variables given the response class. Bayes rule establishes the posterior probability of the target variable y (label) taking the value j, conditioned to the predictor variables $x_1, \ldots, x_n$ (the Equation (4)):

$$P(y = j | x_1, \ldots, x_n) = \frac{P(x_1, \ldots, x_n | y = j) P(y = j)}{P(x_1, \ldots, x_n)} \quad (4)$$

where $P(y = j)$ is the prior probability of y taking the value j, $P(x_1, \ldots, x_n | y = j)$ is the posterior probability of the predictor variables conditioned to y taking the value j, and $P(x_1, \ldots, x_n)$ are the prior probabilities of the predictor variables. These prior and conditional probabilities can be estimated from the respective empirical frequencies when the predictor variables are categorical. When they are continuous, they can be approximated by different kernel functions. When the independence approximation is applied in NB, this simplifies largely (the Equation (5)):

$$P(y = j | x_1, \ldots, x_n) = \frac{P(y = j) \prod_1^n P(x_i | y = j)}{P(x_1, \ldots, x_n)} \quad (5)$$

The predicted class for a set of $x_1, \ldots, x_n$ predictor values will be the one that maximizes the productory above, since the other factors are constant.

2.2. k-Nearest Neighbors (kNN)

The idea of this method is quite simple: For a new instance with predictor variables $x_1, \ldots, x_n$, assign the label most frequent between the k instances in the training data with predictor variables less distant (more similar, the k-*nearest neighbors*) to the new instance predictor variables. This is called the *majority voting* class assignment. When the label is a continuous one (regression), the predicted value is the (weighted) average of the labels of the k-nearest neighbors. In order to measure the distance between sets of predictor variables, different metrics can be used. Probably the most frequent is the Euclidean one. The value of k can be quite variable and depends heavily on the dataset. It can be obtained through cross-validation techniques.

2.3. Decision Trees (DT)

This method can be used for both regression and classification. The idea here is to generate rectangular partitions of the space of predictor variables, by successive splitting the data by (usually binary) splits in one variable that optimize some loss function (e.g., minimization of MSE for regression). At the end, the label we assign to each partition is one function of the labels of the data instances belonging to each partition, e.g., its mean, or the majority voting class. Then, for new instances, we will find the partition it belongs to and assign the label that corresponds to that partition. A simple schema with only two predictor variables is depicted in Figure 3.

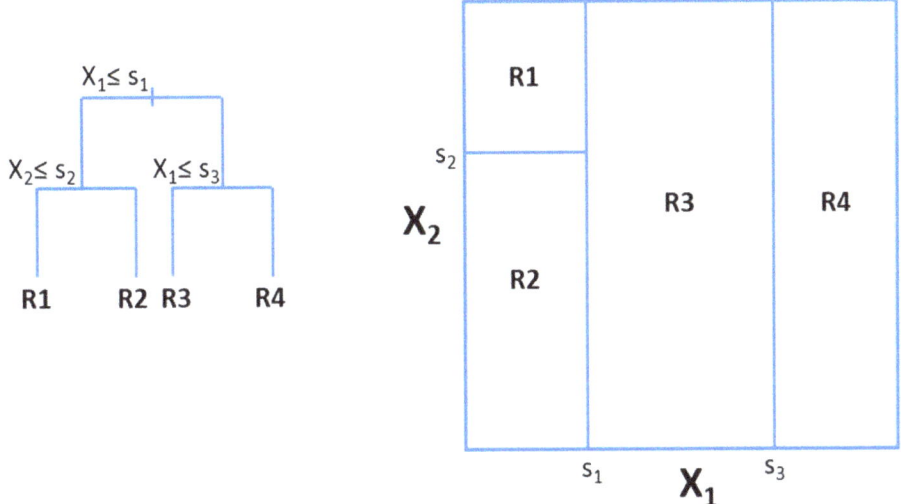

Figure 3. Depiction of Decision Tree for two variables, X_1 and X_2. R1, R2, R3, and R4 are partitions generated by the splits s_1, s_2, and s_3. The labels for the partitions would be a function of the labels of the instances in each partition in the training set.

Obviously, to grow a tree can become a very complicated task, given the combinatorial number of possible splits and variable sequences that can be created. Therefore, simplified algorithms for generating the tree have been devised. There are different ones, depending on the criteria for split, the selection of variables at each split, and the pruning of terminal nodes. These are CART [26], on one hand, and ID3 [27], which evolved to C4.5 (also called J48 in Weka's Java implementation) and later to C5.0. There is also the CHAID [28] algorithm, based on statistical tests and allowing non-binary splits.

The advantage of DT is the ease of interpretation, which can be aided by graphical displays; however, they are known for the high variance of their predictions, such that little variations of the dataset can result in very different trees and predictions.

2.4. Support Vector Machines (SVM)

This method was initially developed as a binary classifier. The approach is to build a hyperplane from the predictor variables with maximal margin, so that one half of the predictor space would result in a "+" label and the other in a "−" label. By maximal margin is meant a hyperplane that has the largest distance to the training instances of the infinite possible hyperplanes or, more correctly, the farthest minimum perpendicular distance to the training instances (since the "margin" is the minimum distance the training set points have to the hyperplane). Figure 4 displays a dataset of two predictor variables and the corresponding maximal margin hyperplane for the training instances.

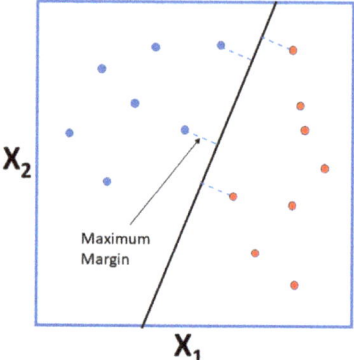

Figure 4. Maximum margin hyperplane for a predictor space of two variables. Two categories are perfectly classified by this hyperplane. The hashed lines indicate the maximum margin to the training set, obtained with this particular hyperplane. Training instances are presented as points in the plane, blue points corresponding to class "+" and red points to "−". The points located at a maximum margin to the hyperplane are the *support vectors*, since the plane only depends on these points of the training set.

For new testing instances, we just need to find which side of the hyperplane the new point lies in order to predict a label for it.

As a matter of fact, it is usually the case that the points are not perfectly separable. Therefore, instead of a maximum margin hyperplane, a "soft" margin one is obtained, by allowing some latitude for misclassified points with some specific criterion. This also makes the method more robust against small modifications of the dataset. In addition, in many situations, the boundary regions between the two classes are not linear. In this case, what we do is include as predictor variables additional specialized functions of these variables and instances, the so-called *kernels*, such that the dataset becomes linearly separable. There is a variety of kernels yielding different types of the SVM method: linear, polynomial, radial, etc. It turns out also that the computation of the hyperplane only requires the closest points to the boundary, which are called the *support vectors*, making the computation much faster. From this, the method takes its name.

Later developments of the method allowed it to deal with multiclass classification as well as regression.

2.5. Random Forest (RF)

RF are an example of ensemble methods, where a model of higher quality is built by aggregating multiple models of lower quality. The prediction for new instances will be obtained by averaging the prediction of all the simple models in the case of regression or, for classification problems, by the majority voting. In this way, we make predictions much more robust, with much less variance and with higher accuracy.

In the case of RF, we use an ensemble of hundreds or thousands of DTs. In addition, these DTs are built without pruning so that they will have little error, although large variance. However, since we are averaging many of them, the final variance will also be low. These DTs are built from bootstrap samples of the original training dataset (this is called *bagging* or bootstrap averaging). Moreover, to decorrelate the trees, at each split in the tree, only a random subset of predictor variables is used. In this way, the reduction of variance by averaging the trees is more efficient.

A very interesting property of the RFs is that they incorporate internally a direct estimation of the external validation error. Since the DT models are derived using bootstrap samples, for each instance in the training set, there will be a set of trees (approximately B/3, where B is the number of trees since they are fit using bootstrap samples) that will have been derived without that instance. By averaging the difference in label prediction for that instance in these trees and its actual label, we would have what is called an out-of-bag (OOB) estimate for that instance. Averaging over all the instances, results in an estimate of the external performance of the RF without the need to use cross-validation or bootstrap.

RFs are a very powerful predictive method, both for regression and classification, and very robust irrespective of the type of datasets. The issue with them is the difficulty of interpretation (this is general for all the ensemble methods), since they contain many different and decorrelated DTs using different predictor variables. An approach used to analyze them is the so-called *variable importance techniques*. The idea here is to analyze the effect that each predictor has (on average over all the DTs) on the error of the RF. One approach is to calculate, for each predictor, what error reduction it has had each time it has been used in the trees. This is summed for all the trees, and the largest sum will correspond to the most important predictor as on average it has produced the largest reduction of errors in all the trees. Another approach uses permutation of the variables. For each tree, we have its OOB prediction accuracy after applying it to its OOB samples. After that, the jth variable is permuted and the OOB prediction is recalculated and subtracted from the previous one. This is averaged over all the trees. This is also repeated for all the predictor variables. We would then obtain a ranking of the variables, with those with the largest reduction of OOB performance being the top ranked.

2.6. Gradient Boosting Machines (GBM)

This is another ensemble method, but one that uses *boosting* instead of bagging. By *boosting*, it is meant the iterative improvement of a weak model by adding sequentially new models that improve the previous fit. In the case of gradient boosting machines, normally the models are DTs, and the improvement is done by fitting the new model to the residuals of the model so far or, more generally, to the gradient of the loss function we are using. Newer versions, like XGboost, use the second derivatives instead of the first ones, in order to improve speed and performance.

GBM, especially XGBoost, are currently the most used ML algorithms for models using numeric tabular data or (when modeling more complex data) feature pre-engineered data. For problems using complex data directly (e.g., computer vision, speech recognition, natural language processing, etc.) Deep Learning methods are used instead (see below).

As it happens with RF, the interpretation of these ensemble models is complicated. However, in the same way, techniques like variable importance can be used to facilitate interpretation.

2.7. Regularized Linear Models (LASSO)

When fitting linear models, the residuals of the least squares fit decrease as we add more predictor variables. However, if the number of instances n is not so much larger than the number p of predictor variables, the estimates of the least squares increase their variance as p becomes closer to n so that the model becomes overfit, and the external or test performance of the model decreases. In the case of $n < p$, the variance become infinite, no unique fit exists, and the method becomes useless. However, this situation of high dimensionality is very typical in ML datasets. One way to fix this problem is to shrink or *regularize* the estimates, so they remain small and with low variance, and in some cases, they even become zero. One approach to regularization is *ridge regression*, where all predictor variables are maintained, but their betas are kept small by restraining the sum of squared betas to be less or equal than a small value. Although this approach improves external performance of the model, it keeps an interpretation issue as no irrelevant variables are removed. An alternative approach is the LASSO, where the sum of the absolute value of the betas is restrained to being less or equal than a small value. This has the advantage of making some betas equal to zero, thus performing an effective selection of important variables.

2.8. Bayesian Networks (BN)

A Bayesian Network is a directed acyclic graph of nodes that correspond predictor variables, plus one or more nodes that represent the label(s). The directed edges between the nodes represent causal relationships between the variables, through conditional dependence, and Bayes rule is used to determine the probability of the different possible values of the labels conditioned to particular values of the predictor variables. Nodes not connected would be conditionally independent. There is a large set of techniques to infer the structure and parameters of the network.

2.9. Artificial Neural Networks (ANN)

ANNs are ML methods that mimic the structure and mechanism of the nervous system. They are composed of layers of artificial neurons, with connections between neurons in consecutive layers. Each artificial neuron is an abstract unit that applies a weighted sum of its numeric inputs plus a bias parameter, and the resulting sum is passed to a so-called "activation function" to generate a numeric output. The first layer corresponds to the input variables; these variables are used as inputs of the next layer neurons, where each of its neurons generate an output, which is then used as input of the next layer neurons, and so on. The last layer contains typically one single neuron for one label or more for multilabel models. Figure 5 displays a typical fully connected, feedforward ANN (multilayer perceptron).

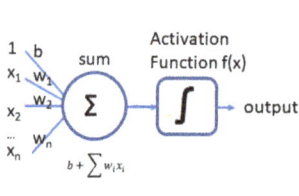
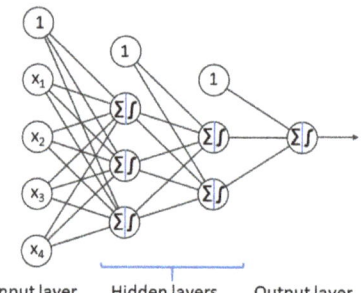

Figure 5. Typical structure of an artificial neuron and a fully connected feedforward neural network. The x_i are the predictor variables, the w_i are the weights and b is the biass.

The input layer contains the input variables (no transformation), while the last layer generates the output of the model and is called the output layer. In between, there are one or more layers, which are called "hidden" layers. Each neuron has a weight per input plus a bias parameter; all these weights and biases of all the neurons are the parameters of the network, which are optimized to minimize a loss function.

The first model or ANN was the perceptron by Rosenblat [20], which was designed as a one-neuron simple binary classifier after the mathematical neuron devised previously by McCulloh–Pitts [29]. The development of ANN to solve problems not linearly separable was allowed by the invention of the backpropagation algorithm [22], which allowed the training of multilayer perceptrons.

ANN became very popular in the 90s of last century, when they were amply used in many areas. At that time, they required feature engineering for many problems, and they were more or less abandoned in the first decade of the 21st century after the appearance of RF and GBM, since ANNs were slow to train, expensive computationally, and prone to overfitting. However, they have become very popular in the second decade of this century with the advent of the field of Deep Learning.

2.10. Deep Learning (DL)

The ML models we have seen so far have two main issues. On one hand, their performance in many cases shows *saturation*: This means that they reach a point when, irrespective of how big we grow the training set, the performance does not increase significantly. On the other hand, they work with numeric, tabular data, so they are unable to handle complex data like images, speech, text, etc. In order to model this type of data, it is required to convert it to numerical predictor variables in a very ad hoc and manual fashion. This is the so-called "feature engineering" problem. They are "shallow" methods, that is, unable to learn hierarchical representations of complex data.

These two problems are solved to a large extent with DL. DL consists mainly in ANNs with very large numbers of layers (that is the reason for the "Deep" in the name) and, therefore, huge numbers of training parameters. In this way, they are able to tap from huge datasets and increase steadily their performance without saturation.

On the other hand, some specialized layers have been developed that are able to automatically generate numerical representations (*feature maps*) of complex data. That is the case of *convolutional layers*, that are able to reformat tensor data of different dimensions. For example, in the case of 1D convolutional layers, they are able to find representations for serial data like text for language translation models; 2D convolutional layers are appropriate to model images like in computer vision models; while 3D layers can handle volumetric data like medical 3D images or video data.

Another specialized layers are the *recurrent layers*, where the output of the layer goes both to the next layer and to itself, allowing to find long-term and long-distance patterns by the use of ad hoc developed layers: Long Short-Term Memory (LSTM) [30] and Gated Recurrent Units (GRU) [31]. This type of layers is very appropriate also for serial data and is mostly used in natural language processing (NLP) applications.

Many of these specialized layers can be stacked sequentially and thus generate automatically hierarchies of representations with increasing levels of abstraction. This allows the model to learn very convoluted aspects of the data, which is not possible with the traditional ML methods. In addition, this hierarchical representation of the data can be applied to generate new specialized models with small datasets by reusing more general models fitted with much larger datasets. For example, we can develop one very efficient model to classify cats from a dataset of relatively few pictures of them by reusing some of the more abstract pre-fit layers of a more general model developed to classify animals from a huge dataset of pictures and adding to them some new layers that would be fit with the new small dataset of cat pictures. The previous layers would have learnt to identify the general shape of an animal, while the new layers would fit the specific features of cats. This is the process called *transfer learning*.

At the end of these layers, normally a multilayer perceptron is added to generate the output, whether numerical (regression) or categorical (classification).

DL is revolutionizing the ML area and is being applied in completely new fields, like drug discovery, music generation, self-driving cars, etc. They are also applied to biomedicine, [32,33] and as we will see, they have started to be used in the childhood obesity area.

After this summary of the main types of ML models, we proceed to describe the selection process of works reviewed in this paper.

3. Bibliographic Search and Selection of Works for Reviewing

An attempt was made for comprehensiveness in the bibliographic search, both in terms of time and publication media. Since the field of ML/DL applications is a very hot one, growing in an extremely fast way, it is not infrequent to find material published in congress proceedings, arXiv, etc. In addition, since this field shows a large interdisciplinarity, being at the interface between statistics, artificial intelligence, and biomedicine and including statisticians, engineers, pediatricians, nutritionists, and nurses in its research body, typical search engines used in biomedicine like Scopus, PubMed, etc., were not used in the search, as they missed many of the available references. Instead, Google Scholar was used for the bibliographic search. The search was performed by iteratively querying the engine with appropriate keywords in order to find papers that applied ML to predict childhood/adolescent obesity/overweight (e.g., childhood OR child OR adolescent AND machine learning OR data mining, etc.), extracting the matches and matching references in the corresponding bibliographies, and updating the queries after the titles of the matching references if necessary. This procedure was repeated until no new matches were obtained. Concept papers not applied to a particular dataset were not included.

On next section, the most outstanding statistical models in the literature to predict childhood and adolescent obesity will be briefly reviewed. These will be used as comparison point to the ML models, that will be reviewed afterwards.

4. Statistical Models to Predict Childhood/Adolescent Obesity

There has been a lot of work performed to derive statistical models to predict childhood/adolescent obesity [34–47]. Although in principle it is advisable not to categorize variables when deriving models, whether predictor or target ones, given that the process results in a loss of information, most of the work in this area has focused on classification models for overweight, obesity, or combinations of them. The reason is obviously that most of the clinical interest is in detecting the conditions that can lead to pathological complications, and these are overweight and obesity, not BMI or similar endpoints in general. Another pathological nutritional status is undernutrition, but it is outside the scope of this Review. In the case of children and adolescents, given the large variability of both height and weight during this period of life, there is no general consensus in the definitions of overweight and obese [17], and the single-cutoff definitions used with adults, namely BMI ≥ 25 kg/m^2 for overweight and BMI ≥ 30 kg/m^2 for obesity, following the WHO definition, [3] are not valid. Instead, the common practice in the case of children/adolescents is to refer the BMI to an age- and sex-based (in some cases ethnicity too) distribution of BMI of the population at hand. The most common criterion is to define as overweight a child whose BMI is equal or above the 85th percentile for that sex and age and as obese a child whose BMI is equal or above the 95th percentile. As we will see, in most of the cases, these percentiles are obtained from the Centers of Disease Control (CDC) data if the sample is from the US [48] or alternatively from WHO growth charts [3], charts from the International Obesity Task Force (IOTF) [49], or growth charts from samples in other countries (e.g., UK90 for UK [50]).

Previous recent reviews in the area are those of Butler et al. [51], Ziauddeen et al. [52], and Butler et al. [53], all of them from 2018. Here, we will briefly review all the works found there and additional ones, in order to provide some sort of baseline predictive models to compare with the ML ones. A total of 14 papers have been found. Table 1 summarizes the main features of these models.

The most used tool to develop the statistical models is logistic regression, which is applied to predict binary outcomes. Here, a linear equation is used to predict the log-odds of a binary variable displaying one of its two alternative categories vs. the other, like being obese or being overweight vs. normal weight. This is the case of all the works but two exceptions. One is the work by Cortés-Martín et al. [47], where proportional-odds ordinal logistic regression is used, which is an statistical model appropriate to predict ordinal variables. In this case, the predicted outcome was the three ordered categories of BMI, namely normal weight vs. overweight vs. obese for children and adolescents (5–17 years). The other case is the work by Mayr et al. [38] where the authors use quantile regression with boosting to derive prediction intervals (which are at the end quantiles of the BMI for future observations) for BMI at different ages in childhood.

In addition, in the paper by Pei et al. [40], the standardized BMI at 5 years was also predicted by means of linear regression, together with obesity at 10 years with logistic regression. Moreover, in the paper by Druet et al. [35], a metanalysis is performed from the odds-ratios obtained from several logistic regressions for 10 different cohorts of variable nationality to estimate an odds-ratio for childhood obesity as a function of the 0–1 year weight gain standard deviation score (SDS).

Table 1. Summary of statistical models.

Article (year)	Training Set Size	Number of Predictors	Country	Outcome Predicted *	Statistical Method	Validation	Type of Prediction **
Steur et al. [34] (2011)	1687	6	The Netherlands	OW 8 years	Stepwise Logistic Regression	Bootstrap	L
Druet et al. [35] (2012)	47,661; 8236	4	UK, France, Finland, Sweden, US, Seychelles	Childhood OB OR; Childhood OB	Metanalysis; Stepwise Logistic Regression	External	L
Levine et al. [36] (2012)	Not specified	5	UK	OB 5 years	Logistic regression	None	L
Morandi et al. [37] (2012)	4032	6	Finland	OB 7 years; OW 7 years; OB 16 years; OW 16 years; OB 7 and 16 years; OW 7 and 16 years	Stepwise Logistic Regression	External	L
Mayr et al. [38] (2012)	Not specified	10	Germany	Childhood OB prediction intervals	Quantile regression with boosting	Simulation and Internal	L
Manios et al. [39] (2013)	2294	5	Greece	OB 9–13 years	Logistic regression	None	L
Pei et al. [40] (2013)	1515	5	Germany	zBMI 10 years; OW 10 years	Linear regression; Logistic regression	Cross-validation	L
Weng et al. [41] (2013)	10,810	7	UK	OW 3 years	Stepwise Logistic Regression	External	L
Santorelli et al. [42] (2013)	1735	4	UK	OB 2 years	Stepwise Logistic Regression	External	L
Graversen et al. [43] (2015)	4111	3	Finland	OW adolescence	Logistic Regression	Bootstrap, External	L
Manios et al. [44] (2016)	5946	5	Greece	OB 6–15 years	Logistic Regression	None	L
Robson et al. [45] (2016)	166	5	US	OB 5 years	Stepwise Logistic Regression	Bootstrap	L
Redsell et al. [46] (2016)	980	7	UK	OW 5 years	Logistic regression	External validation of Weng et al. [41]	L
Cortés-Martin et al. [47] (2020)	415	7	Spain	NW/OW/OB 5–17 years	Ordinal Logistic Regression	Bootstrap	CS

* NW = normal weight; OW = overweight; OB = obese; ** L = longitudinal model; CS = cross-sectional model.

The rest of the papers aim at the prediction of overweight or obesity at one or several ages or a range of ages exclusively by means of logistic regression. Papers focused on the prediction of overweight are those of Steur et al. [34] (at 8 years), Weng et al. [41] (3 years), Graversen et al. [43] (at adolescence), and Redsell et al. [46] (5 years). Papers focused on the prediction of obesity are those of Druet et al. [35] (7–14 years), Levine et al. [36] (5 years, stratified by sex), Manios et al. [39,44] (9–13 years), Pei et al. [40] (10 years, as said before), Santorelli et al. [42] (2 years) and Robson et al. [45] (5 years). In the paper by Morandi et al. [37] both endpoints are predicted: overweight and obesity at both 7 and 16 years; in addition, predictions are made for *persistent* overweight and obesity, that is, overweight and obesity at *both* 7 and 16 years. By considering the definition of overweight and/or obesity in these works, some [34,35,37,39,41,46] used the IOTF criteria, others [40,44,47] used the WHO one, and other [45] used the CDC criteria.

When using logistic regression, in most of the cases, [34,35,37,41,42,45,46] a stepwise variable selection is performed from a pull of predictor variables to select the final ones to use in the definitive model or models. In one case [39,44], a score is derived "by hand" by combining odds-ratios obtained from simple logistic regressions of different variables and then used in a simple [39] or multiple [44] logistic regression to estimate its odds-ratio. In two other cases [36,43], the predictor variables are predefined, and in one case [40] several predefined predictor variables are used at the beginning, but then, the model is rederived with only the significant ones.

As regarding the predictor variables, the most popular ones, in decreasing order, are parental BMI (8 times), sex and birth weight (7 times), smoking mother during gestation (6 times), weight gain at some previous period (5 times), parental education (4 times), exclusive breastfeeding during some initial period (3 times), etc. Sometimes, versions of these variables are used, like categorized ones (e.g., obesity instead of BMI) or standardized ones. Some other times, mother's version (instead of parental ones) are used, e.g., mother's BMI, or mother's education. There are two cases where a set of genetic polymorphisms are used; in one case [37], incorporated as a score obtained as sum of risk alleles, they appeared to add no significant predictive capacity, but in the other, [47] in the form of components of a Multiple Component Analysis (MCA), they did.

The cohorts used in the derivation of the models are of variable origin: Netherlands [34], UK [36,41,42], Finland [37,43], Germany [38,40], Greece [39,44], USA (Latino community) [45], and Spain. [47] In the case of the metanalysis previously mentioned [35], the 10 different cohorts are also from multiple countries: UK, France, Finland, Sweden, USA, and Seychelles. We can see that most of the work has been performed in developed countries with mostly Caucasian samples, which limits their applicability. The sizes of the cohorts are also variable: They range from 166 [45] to around 13,000. [41] The metanalysis [35] includes more than 47,000 cases in the 10 cohorts.

In terms of model validation, some of the models [35,37,41,43,44,46] were externally validated (as a matter of fact, the works by Manios et al. [44] and Redsell et al. [46] are external validations of the previous models described in Manios et al. [39] and Weng et al. [41]), while other models were internally validated through bootstrap [34,45,47] or cross-validation [38,40]. In two cases, [42,43] both internal and external validation was used, while in one case [36] no validation was performed at all.

If we focus in the comparison of performances of the different logistic regression models, we can use the AUCROC (that equals the so-called c-index or concordance index) as a criterion for discrimination. Depending on where the linear predictor threshold of the model is set to assign one category or its alternative to the predictions, we can have very different sensitivities and specificities, as well as PPV (precision) and NPVs; to select the threshold we must take into account the purpose of the model, as well as the possible costs of false positives and/or false negatives. However, as a *global* measure of the discriminative capacity of the model, before its practical application by selecting a threshold, the AUCROC is a well-established criterion. Obviously, for two models with the same AUROC, one internally validated and the other externally validated, we will prefer the one externally validated, especially if it is with a large, unrelated cohort, because it will approximate more closely a real-life prediction than the internal validation that is based on data reutilization.

In this way, the models of the different works using external validation would be ranked in the following order of decreasing AUROC: Santorelli et al. [42] (0.89), Morandi et al. [37] (0.79), Druet et al. [35] (0.77), Weng et al. [41] (0.75), Redsell et al. [46] (0.67), and Manios et al. [44] (0.64). In the case of the paper by Graversen et al. [43], the AUROC is provided only for the internal validation. These values should be taken with caution, given that they do not compare the same "difficulty" in prediction, e.g., if the testing cohort is very similar to the training one, a very large AUROC could be obtained very easily; for example, an external validation with a different cohort to the training one is a more demanding task that an external validation with a random split of the same cohort, even if the latter is not used for training. Moreover, the difficulty depends on the relatedness between the predictor and target variables, e.g., the prediction of obesity at age 9 is more difficult if the predictor variable is weight gain between 0 and 1 years than if the predictor variable is weight gain between 7 and 8 years.

On the other hand, the ranking of models for internal validation by decreasing AUROC is Robson et al. [45] (0.78) and Steur et al. [34] (0.75). Mayr et al. [38] and Pei et al. [40] do not provide AUROC values. In principle, the evidence of predictive capacity of these models is weaker given that they have not been externally validated.

Finally, we should mention that, in terms of the type of prediction, all the models have a longitudinal setting, that is, they aim at predicting the endpoint *in the future* from *predictor variables taken in a previous point in time*, at least partially, e.g., predict overweight at 8 years using birth weight and mother smoking at gestation. These are designated in Table 1 as "L" type of prediction. The only exception is the work by Cortés-Marín et al., which has no predictive but explanatory purpose and therefore uses a cross-sectional setting, where the predictor variables are taken at the same time than the endpoint. This is designated in Table 1 as "CS" type of prediction. Here, the aim is to obtain the relative strengths of associations of variables of different domains with putative explanatory character (diet, age, sex, genetic polymorphisms, microbiota), although given the cross-sectional setting of the model, no demonstration of causality can be obtained from it but rather of putative variables to consider for a further test with a longitudinal setting.

5. Machine Learning Models to Predict Childhood/Adolescent Obesity Based on BMI

In this section, we will review the ML models derived to predict BMI (regression) and/or categorized versions of it (classification), e.g., normal-weight, overweight, obesity, etc.

To our knowledge, there are only two previous reviews of ML models to predict childhood/adolescent obesity. One early paper in 2010 by Adnan et al. [54] described the scarce work performed before it; another very recent paper [55] reviews the work up to 2020, together with the area of computerized decision support for the prevention and treatment of childhood obesity. However, the latter paper, being arranged as a systematic review, lacks many of the publications in the area of ML, and some of the ones described there could be more appropriately defined as statistical models (e.g., generalized linear mixed models and linear and logistic regression) or are targeted to the prediction of physical activity in children.

In what follows, we will use more or less a chronological order in the description of the works conducted in the area. As we will see, the field has experienced an explosion very recently, especially through the use of electronic health records (EHR) as sources of very large datasets. ML methods will be abbreviated as in Section 2. Table 2 summarizes the main features of the models that will be described.

The first attempts to use ML to predict childhood obesity are those of Novak and Bigec, back in 1995 [56] and 1996 [57]. In these papers, they describe the use of ANN to predict childhood obesity. However, the work is of preliminary nature and is more a description of the ANN theory and method, without providing a description of the results of a particular model derived from a particular sample.

This work was followed by that of Zhang et al. in 2009 [58]. Here, the aim is to compare the performance of ML models with the traditional logistic regression model. By using an UK cohort (the so-called Wirral database of >16,000 children), they developed several models to predict overweight at 3 years from previous data, using predictor variables available at 8 months or at 2 years. These variables were all child features like sex, BMI at 8 months, adjusted SDS of height at different visits, weight gain between pairs of visits, etc. Different ML methods were used: DT, Association Rules, ANN, Linear SVM, RFB (Radial Basis Function) SVM, BN, and NB. In the case of the prediction at 8 months, the ANN showed the largest accuracy, although the RBF (Radial Basis Function) SVM displayed the largest sensitivity (probably more useful for clinical purposes). For the prediction at 2 years, the largest accuracy was obtained with the Bayesian methods, although the largest sensitivity was observed in the case of RBF SVM again. Logistic regression had the largest specificity, but the sensitivity and accuracy were much worse than the ML models. They also derived models to predict obesity, but the quality of them was very low. No validation was performed in any of the models developed.

Table 2. Machine Learning (ML) models to predict BMI or its categories.

Article (year)	Training Set Size	Number of Predictors *	Country	Outcome Predicted **	ML Method	Validation	Type of Prediction ***
Novak and Bigec [56] (1995)	ND ****	ND	Slovenia	Childhood OB	ANN	Not described	ND
Novak and Bigec [57] (1996)	ND	ND	Slovenia	Childhood OB	ANN	Not described	ND
Zhang et al. [58] (2009)	16,523	10	UK	OW 3 years	DT; ANN; NB, BN, SVM, association rules, logistic regression	None	L
Rehkopf et al. [59] (2011)	2150	41	US	Girls Change in BMI percentile (9 to 19 years); onset of OW or OB	RF	None	L
Adnan et al. [60] (2012)	140	20	Malaysia	Children OB 9-11 years	NB	None	CS
Adnan et al. [61] (2012)	320	8	Malaysia	Children OW/OB	NB	None	CS
Adnan et al. [62] (2012)	180	19	Malaysia	Children OW/OB	NB	None	CS
Lazarou et al. [63] (2012)	600	5	Cyprus	OW 10-12 years	DT	Bootstrap	CS
Pochini et al. [64] (2014)	15,425	9	US	OW 14-18 years; OB 14-18 years	DT; Logistic Regression	External	CS
Dugan et al. [65] (2015)	7519	167	US	OB 2 years	DT; RF; NB; BN	Cross-validation	L
Lingren et al. [66] (2016)	5857	9	US	Severe OB 1-6 years	Rule based; SVM; NB	External	CS
Abdullah et al. [67] (2017)	4245	29	Malaysia	OB 12 years	BN; DT; NB; ANN; SVM	None	L
Rios-Julian et al. [68] (2017)	221	16	Mexico	OW 6-13 years	DT; Logistic Model Trees; ANN; RF; Logistic Regression	None	CS
Wiechmann et al. [69] (2017)	238	ND	US	OW 2-5 years	DT	None	CS
Zheng and Rugggiero [70] (2017)	5127	9	US	OB 14-18 years	Logistic Regression; DT; kNN; ANN	Cross-validation	CS
Gupta et al. [71] (2019)	40,817	1737	US	BMI and OB 3-20 years	DL(RNN)	External	L
Hammond et al. [72] (2019)	2759	19,290	US	OB 5 years	Logistic penalized Regression; RF; GBM; LASSO	Bootstrap cross-validation; External	L
Lee et al. [73] (2019)	~600,000	21	South Korea	OB 24-80 months	DT	External	L
Park et al. [74] (2019)	76	379	US	BMI progression in childhood	LASSO	Cross-validation; External	L
Singh and Tawfit et al. [75] (2019)	ND	ND	UK	BMI 14 years	Linear Regression; ANN	External	L
Kim et al. [76] (2019)	11,206	19	South Korea	BMI categories	BN	None	CS
Pang et al. [77] (2019)	10,881	102		OB 2-7 years	GBM	External	L

* When several models are derived, the largest number of predictors is reported; ** NW = normal weight; OW = overweight; OB = obese; *** L = longitudinal model; CS = cross-sectional model; **** ND = Not described. ML Method abbreviation as in Section 2.

A work in 2011 by Rehkopf et al. [59] used and American cohort (the NHLBI Growth and Health Study) of ca. 2000 white or black girls 8 or 9 years old that were followed for 10 years to predict the change from 9 to 19 years in the CDC BMI percentile and the transition from normal-weight to overweight or obese by means of RF models. They took 41 predictor variables from different domains: diet, physical activity, psychological, and social and parent health in order. They applied variable importance techniques by permutation to estimate the relative importance of these variables. For the first outcome, body dissatisfaction, drive for thinness, physical appearance (psychological), income and parental education (social), and other psychological variables were the most important variables. In the case of the transition to overweight or obesity, the most important predictor was income, followed by psychological variables. Again, no internal/external validation of the model was performed.

Following their review in 2010 [54], Adnan et al. published in 2012 three papers in this area [60–62] to predict the nutritional status (normal-weight, overweight and obese) by means of NB and a cohort of 140 Malaysian children 9–11 years old. They applied 19 predictor variables of different domains obtained from literature review: children features, lifestyle (including physical activity and diet), and family/environment. In the first work [60], they observed that the use of these variables improved the accuracy of obesity prediction by NB as compared to the work by Zhang et al. [58]. This approach was improved in the second paper [61] by using a genetic algorithm to select predictor variables in order to avoid the problem in NB with many variables where the predicted posterior probabilities turn to zero each time at least one of the predictor variables prior probability is zero. The third paper [62] adopted two additional methods for variable selection for NB models: variable importance with CART and Euclidean distances. The models were not validated in any of the papers.

Another work from 2012 is that of Lazarou et al., [63] where diet variables were used to predict overweight + obesity vs. normal-weight. A Cypriot cohort of ca. 600 children 10–12 years old was used with a cross-sectional setting. They used questionnaires of eating frequencies of food groups as predictor variables (fried food, fish and seafood, delicatessen meat, soft drinks, and sweets and junk food). By developing many DTs, for both boys and girls, they were able to derive rules of overweight + obesity risk as a function of diet patterns and sex. The approach was validated by bootstrap, but the results were not shown. Finally, they developed logistic regression models using as predictor variables PCA components of the diet variables; only one of the PC of the girls model was significant.

One paper in 2014 by Pochini et al. [64] predicted overweight and obesity in high-school students (14–18 years old) from 9 lifestyle predictor variables, using both logistic regression and DT, again, in a cross-sectional setting. The sample modeled was a cohort of ca. 15,000 high-school students in Columbia, USA (from the 2011 CDC Youth Behavior Risk Survey). For obesity, logistic regression significant factors were consumption of fruit/vegetables, smoking, being physically active, having regular breakfast, drinking fruit juice, and drinking soda; the remaining variables in the DT after pruning were physically active and tobacco. For the overweight prediction, the logistic significant variables were having regular breakfast and being physically active. For the DT, no variable remained after pruning; before pruning, the variables were breakfast, fruit juice, and sleep. In the case of the DT, the models were externally validated with a 30% of the original sample.

Dugan et al. [65], in 2015, used multiple ML methods to predict obesity at 2 years using predictor variables obtained before that age. The data came from a clinical decision support system, CHICA, that contained information from a multiethnic cohort in USA of >7000 children. Random Tree, RF, J48, ID3, NB, and BN were tried out. The best performing algorithm was ID3, with an accuracy of 85%, sensitivity of 89%, PPV of 84%, and NPV of 88%. Using some sort of variable importance by removing variable by variable, they found that the strongest predictors were overweight before 24 months, followed by being very tall before 6 months. All the models were internally validated through 10-fold cross-validation.

In 2016, a paper by Lingren et al. [66] was published aimed at the identification of putative cases of severe early childhood obesity from children 1–6 years old above the 99th BMI percentile, to separate them from those due to medications, pathologies, etc. The objective was to develop a cohort for further genotyping studies, in order to understand the genetic basis for severe early childhood obesity. Therefore, they attempted to optimize the PPV, in order to be most effective in the detection of these children. The dataset used corresponded to a cohort of >5000 of EHR from two children hospitals, one in Boston and another in Cincinnati. The predictor variables used were structured data (demographics, anthropometrics, ICD-9 diagnosis codes, and medications) as well as unstructured data (narrative) by NLP. They used both rule-based methods and ML methods (SVM and NB) that were tested in an external split of the original data. In general, the rule-based method worked better, but the ML one had more flexibility to leverage PPV and sensibility and to select variable sets.

Abdullah et al. published a paper [67] in 2017, where they used ML to predict obesity at 12 years from a Malaysian cohort of >4000 children 12 years old. The predictor variables were obtained from questionnaires and included three domains: socio-demographic, physical activity, and diet. Multiple methods for variable selection were tested, as well as multiple ML methods: BN, DT (J48), NB, ANN, and SVM. The best results were obtained with J48, together with consistency + linear forward variable selection. In this case, the models were not validated.

A later paper in the same year by Rios-Julián et al. [68] attempted to predict obesity + overweight (following the CDC criteria) vs. normal-weight by using BMI and other anthropometric variables in a community of Me'Phaa ethnicity in Mexico. They modeled a cohort of 221 children 6–13 years old by using different ML models: J48, logistic model trees, ANN, RF, and logistic regression. Three groups of variables were tried on: all; all but skinfold thickness; and sex, age, height, weight, BMI, and skinfold thickness. They obtained not very different results for the different variable groups and models, and in general, all the models yielded excellent predictions. All the models were internally validated by 10-fold cross-validation.

Moreover, in 2017 Wiechman et al. published a paper [69] that used DTs (C4.5 type) to gain insight on the factors influencing child obesity in Hispanic preschoolers in the USA. The sample analyzed was a cohort of children of 238 families, 2–5 years old, of Hispanic ethnicity. They develop shallow C4.5 decision trees to predict overweight by using variables from different domains: demographics, caregiver feeding style, feeding practices, home environment, dietary information, beverage consumption, social support, family life, integrated behavior model, and spousal support. They found some clues for obesity development: If the mother cares for the child or if she works but the father has high-level education, the child has less probability of being overweight. If the child is fed to avoid tantrums, the child tends to be more obese. The models were not validated.

The last paper in 2017 is that of Zheng and Ruggiero [70]. They used a dataset comprising a cohort of >5000 high-school (14–18 years) students in the USA. They predicted obesity between 14 and 18 years from 9 variables within three different domains: energy update, physical activity, and sedentary behavior. They used logistic regression, DT, kNN, and ANN. The best models were ANN and kNN, and all the ML models performed much better than logistic regression. All were internally validated by 10-fold cross-validation.

The year 2019 saw an explosion of ML and DL models to predict childhood obesity. We have identified up to 7 papers in this area, together with other aimed at related endpoints that will be described in the next section. Several of them make use of EHR as sources of data. We finish this section by describing these works.

An example of DL models is that of Gupta et al. [71] They used a cohort of EHR from ca. 68,000 children/adolescents with visits to medical centers for at least 5 years, in order to predict BMI and obesity from 3 to 20 years in groups of 3 consecutive years using data from the 3 previous years, resulting in multiple models. Recurrent NN of the LSTM type were used, with predictor variables from the EHR including medical conditions observed, drugs prescribed, procedures requested, and measurements taken, together with static demographic data. Data was split into three subsets: 60% for training, 20% for hyperparameter validation, and 20% for external validation. The whole training dataset was used to train a global model, and then, by transfer learning, specialized models for each sub-cohort were obtained by retraining the global model with the corresponding subset of data. In order to identify important variables, they used embedding, while to identify important time intervals, they used attention techniques. The RNN was compared with RF and linear regression, which do not take into account the longitudinal information, and the RNN gave a much better performance. The performance of the models decays with the temporal distance between the acquisition of the predictor variables and the time of BMI prediction in the future, as expected.

Another work that used EHR data is that of Hammond et al. [72], who used a multiethnic cohort obtained from multiple providers in a safety net in New York city that included >3000 children. The authors predict obesity at year 5 by using logistic penalized regression, RF, and GB. In addition, obesity was predicted by deriving regression models for z-BMI using LASSO, RF, and GB and applying an obesity cutoff for the z-BMI predicted. They used feature engineering to generate predictor variables from the EHR: demographic information, home address, vital signs, and medications from the children when they were < 2 years old and from the mother vital signs, diagnosis codes; procedures; and laboratory results before, during, and post-pregnancy. They developed different models for boys and girls. The most important predictors were weight-for-length z-score, BMI between 19 and 24 months, and the last BMI measure before age 2. The best models have an AUCROC of 81.7% for girls and 76.1% for boys. Internal validation was conducted by bootstrap CV and external validation with a previously selected test split.

One case of work aiming at understanding risk factors for childhood obesity is that of Lee et al. [73]. They used a South Korean longitudinal cohort of ca. 1 million children and used DT models to predict obesity vs. normal-weight between 24 and 80 months (overweight children are removed). They used a set of 21 predictor variables of different domains: socioeconomic status (SES (modelled after attending medical aid or not), maternal factors (e.g., pregestational obesity, abdominal obesity, hypertension, smoking, etc.), paternal factors (obesity, abdominal obesity, and hypertension), and child factors (preterm, exclusive breastfeeding, high consumption of sugar sweetened beverages, etc.)) The model was externally validated with a 40% test split, resulting in an accuracy of 93%. By using a CHAID-type of variable selection, the most important predictor variable was mother obesity, followed by parental obesity and SES; other important factors were old pregnancy and gestational diabetes and hypertension. Child factors were exclusive breastfeeding, consumption of sugar-sweetened beverages, and irregular breakfasting. Interestingly, they observed that child's z-score for weight at birth and z-score for weight-for-height were not selected.

A South-Korean dataset was also used in order to understand factors affecting obesity is that of Kim et al. [76], although in this case it deals with *adolescent* obesity. They used a cohort of >11,000 students from South Korea and 19 predictor variables from questionnaires of different domains: sociological, anthropometric, smartphone use, obesity, other. They predict the three categories of BMI: underweight, normal, and overweight, by means of a General Bayesian Network (GBN), and compare it with many different ML methods resulting in GBN displaying the best fit: the best accuracy is 53.7%, and the AUCROC is 0.758. No validation is performed. The variable most related to BMI class is pocket money. More interestingly, they use the GBN to perform a "what-if" analysis by modifying the values of different variables or combination of variables in order to get an understanding of putative mechanisms for risk of obesity. For instance, the combination of high pocket money and low wealth increases a lot the probability of obesity, etc.

An adolescent cohort was also used by Singh et al. [75] but in this case from the UK. The Millenium cohort of UK of children born between 2000 and 2001, particularly the subsets MC2 to MC5, was modeled in order to predict the BMI at 14 years (MC6). The data was externally validated with a test split of 25%. Linear SVM, linear regression, and ANN were tried, and the best performance was obtained by the ANN, followed by the SVM.

A work that uses XGBoost is that of Pang et al. [77]. The authors predict obesity in the period 2–7 years from data in windows in the 0–2 years period with a cohort of ca. 27,000 children from Philadelphia in the Pediatric Big Data repository. Variables included vital signs, laboratory values, and provider information, resulting in a total of 102 predictors. Data was divided into train 1 (40%), train 2 (40%), and hold-out (20%) to determine hyperparameters iteratively and train/test the model. Different ML models were tried, and the best was XGBoost, giving an AUCROC of 0.81, and for the threshold that gives a recall of 0.8, the precision, F1, accuracy, and specificity were 30.9%, 44.6%, 66.14%, and 63.27%, respectively. They analyzed the models with variable importance techniques, resulting in weight-for-height at month 24, weight at month 24, weight for height at month 18, and race being the most important ones. Different races, ethnicities, and caregivers had different importance distributions. Using sensitivity analysis, it was observed that the prediction of obesity at later times degrades, as expected.

An interesting alternative set of predictive variables to the ones described so far is the use of neuroimaging biomarkers. This is the case of the work by Park et al., [74] who used resting-state functional magnetic resonance imaging (rs-fMRI) to derive predictive models for BMI progression (and indirectly future BMI) of adolescents. A cohort of 76 individuals from the Enhanced Nathan Kline Institute Rockland Sample (NKI-RS) database of white and African American preadolescents (average age of 11.94 years) was used. Their BMI was measured in a first visit, followed by a second visit about 1.5 years later. From the fMRI of their brain in the first visit, both considering subcortical volume and cortical surface, 379 Degree-Centrality (DC) values of different parts of the brain were extracted. These were used with LASSO to predict the BMI progression (DeltaBMI/Deltat) and indirectly BMI in the second visit. Only six DC remained after the variable selection in the LASSO. These variables were entered in a linear regression model. The model was internally validated with leave-one CV, giving and Intra Class Correlation (ICC) for DeltaBMI of 0.70, and ICC for BMI of 0.98, and (when predicting the binary variable increase/decrease of BMI) an AUCROC of 0.82. Brain regions of the selected DCs were correlated with the eating disorder, anxiety, and depression. The approach was applied to a local South Korean dataset of 22 young adults (average age of 21.4), and the results were similar, suggesting robustness of the first model.

6. Machine Learning Models to Predict Related Outcomes

Some other works in the literature make use of ML to derive predictive models not of BMI or BMI categories, but of related endpoints. Table 3 summarizes these models.

Table 3. Summary of ML models to predict BMI-related outcomes.

Article (Year)	Training Set Size	Country	Outcome Predicted	ML Method	Validation
Nau et al. [78] (2015)	99 (communities)	US	Obesogenic environment	RF	None
Hasan et al. [79] (2018)	40191 (utterances)	US	Success of communication strategies to promote weight reduction behavior	DL	External
Öksüz et al. [80] (2018)	20	Switzerland	Success of weight decrease therapy	SVM, kNN, DT, GBM	Cross-validation
Turer et al. [81] (2018)	7192	US	Doctors attention to childhood obesity	Ad hoc algorithm	External
Duran et al. [82] (2019)	1333	US	Body fat% (excess)	ANN	External

ML Method abbreviation as in Section 2.

For instance, a work by Duran et al. [82] describes the use of ANN models to predict body fat percentage (BF%) and its excess (BF% above 85th percentile), which is an alternative measure of obesity to those based on BMI. A cohort ca. 2000 non-Hispanic white children less than 20 years old were used here. Different models were derived for boys and girls. The predictors used were age, height, weight, and waist circumference. The ANN were compared with the prediction using z-BMI and z-WC. In the case of boys, ANN has better accuracy, sensibility, and specificity than the simple models, especially the z-WC one; in the case of girls, the ANN performs similarly to the z-BMI one and better than the z-WC one. The models were internally validated and externally validated with a test split.

On the other hand, there are models aimed at the prediction of the success of therapies or treatments to decrease childhood obesity. One case is described in a work by Hasan et al. [79], where they used RNN (both LSTM and GRU types) and probabilistic models to try to predict the positive or negative reception by obese adolescents of communication sequences by a counselor in interviews to promote weight reduction behavior. The authors used a dataset of 129 motivational interviews between a counselor and an adolescent (accompanied by a caregiver) for promoting weight reduction behavior. These interviews included 50,239 encoded sequences of utterances ending or not in a positive change talk or positive commitment language by the adolescent or caregiver. Given the high imbalance of the sequences of utterances (most of them are successful ones), they evaluated the models through either synthetic oversampling of the negative sequences or under-sampling of the positive ones. The models were trained with 80% of the data and externally evaluated with 20% of the data. In the case of under sampling, the LSTM models with target replication (LSTM-TR) resulted in the best models in terms of F1, precision, and recall. The probabilistic models were much worse. When using oversampling, the LSTM-TR was again the best model. These models can therefore be used to design communication strategies that achieve the best success.

Another example of prediction of therapy success is the work by Öksüz et al. [80] They used a cohort of 20 overweight or obese children 11–16 years old in Switzerland to predict the success of a weight-decrease 6-months therapy (defined as BMI after therapy < 0.4 BMI units than before). As predictors, they measured the heart rate at several intervals during a run test and a cooldown period, plus weight, age, BMI, and height. They tried different ML methods: several SVM, kNN, DT, and GB. Nested cross validation was used to train and internally validate the models given the small sample size. The best model used linear SVM, giving an accuracy of 85%. They used permutation tests to estimate the relative importance of the predictors, and several heart rate ones are the most important. These ML models performed better than the prediction of two domain experts.

A related task is the detection from EHR of attention by pediatricians to childhood obesity and associated medical risks. This is the case of the paper by Turer et al. [81]. They used a dataset of doctor visits of >7000 overweight/obese children 6–12 years old in several centers in Texas. They developed a rule-based classification algorithm to detect from EHR doctor's behaviors that indicate therapeutic "attention towards excess BMI", "attention towards excess BMI + comorbidities (medical risk)", and "no attention". They used different types of evidence, in addition to pathology codes, from EHR indices: diagnosis codes, orders for laboratories, medications, and referrals. The algorithm was externally validated by manual review of EHR data of 309 additional visits. Sensitivity to BMI alone was 96%, while to BMI/Medical risk was 96.1%.

We end this section with an interesting paper by Nau et al. [78] describing a predictive model for obesogenic vs. obesoprotective community environments. Here, the aim is predicting not the obesity for a particular child or adolescent, but rather if the features of a community are those that foster childhood obesity within it, or on the contrary, they protect against it. These authors analyzed 99 communities in Pennsylvania, 50 of them in the high quartile of child obesity prevalence and 49 others other in the lowest quartile. Therefore, it uses community-aggregated data to try to predict obesogenic vs. obesoprotective communities. They used 44 variables as potential predictors in different domains: food services, social, physical activity establishments, and land use. They used variable importance measures with RF to identify the most important variables. A total of 13 were deemed important above noise; unemployment was the most important, followed by population density, social disorganization, proportion of people with less than high school education, population change, no car ownership, etc. These are physical activity and social variables. The most important food services variables are counts of snacks stores and counts of fast food chains score. Models were also obtained without social variables that are considered causal of the others; the results gave similar ranking of the other variables. It seems that well-off communities are more protected against obesity. It was also observed that classification accuracies were different for high and low obesity communities, indicating different structures/hierarchy of variables for these two groups. The models, however, were not internally or externally validated.

7. Discussion

In the present Review, we have seen a large amount of models to predict childhood/adolescent obesity. We have grouped them into two types: statistical ones and ML ones. The former models use traditional statistical techniques, mainly logistic regression, [34–37,39–46] although there are cases using linear regression [40], quantile regression [38], and ordinal logistic regression. [47] The ML models use a wide variety of ML methods: ANN [56–58,67,68,70,75], SVM [58,66,67], DT [58,64,65,67–70,73], NB [58,60–62,66,67], BN [58,65,67,76], LASSO [72,74], kNN [70], RF [59,65,68,72], GBM [72,77], and DL (RNN [71]).

In general, when in the same work logistic/linear regression is compared with ML models when fitting the same dataset [58,64,68,70,72,75], the latter give better results than the former in terms of prediction performance. This confirms that ML techniques are able to yield better predictions, not just by fitting better the training set but also through giving better results in internal and/or external validations.

On the other hand, if we analyze the models in terms of predictor variables, we see that the statistical models make use in most of the cases of a reduced set of well-established risk factors for childhood obesity: parental BMI, sex and birth weight, smoking mother during gestation, weight gain at some previous period, parental education, exclusive breastfeeding during some initial period, etc. Only the work by Cortés-Martín et al. [47] uses a wider set of predictor variables, including a Mediterranean diet score, multiple SNPs, and a marker of microbiota (urolithin metabotype), in addition to sex, age, and ethnicity. On the contrary, in multiple ML models, we observe other types of variables, alone or in combination with the "traditional" predictor variables. For example, the work of Rehkopf et al. [59] uses psychological predictor variables, that of Lazarou et al. [63] focuses mainly on diet, while that of Park et al. [74] utilizes rs-fMRI predictor variables. There are also several papers that use lifestyle variables (including both diet- and physical activity-related variables) [59–62,64,69,70]. Works that stand out for their use of specially wide sets of multidomain predictor variables are those of Rehkopf et al. [59] (diet; physical activity; and psychological, social, and parental health); Wiechman et al. [69] (demographics, caregiver feeding style, feeding practices, home environment, diet, social support, spousal support, family life, etc.); and Kim et al. [76] (wealth, smartphone use, pocket money, academic performance, sleeping quality, etc.) The latter work is interesting also because it makes a "what-if" analysis where some variables are modified, and their concerted effect on the predicted obesity is evaluated; this is an interesting approach to use ML models as simulation tools to suggest possible therapeutic or preventive interventions.

Therefore, we could say that the statistical models are probably more oriented towards earlier ages, where the number of factors affecting is less variable, or to predicting shorter times in the future. We would be mainly doing a short extrapolation of the BMI curve: Obese children would be those who were obese some short time before, and in the case of babies or early age children, gestational factors like smoking mother or gestational diabetes would also be of importance. These are simpler models with immediate implementation in the clinics, as they contain a small number of easily retrieved predictor variables. On the contrary, once the multidomain factors of obesity, like diet, physical activity, psychological variables, genetic, family environment, sociological, etc., enter the scene, which takes place in late childhood or adolescence, ML models are more appropriate. This is also for predictions spanning large periods of time, like the model by Gupta et al. that was developed to predict BMI and obesity from 3 to 20 years, or when we require higher accuracy in the prediction. In addition to prediction purposes, these ML models are useful in that they can be used to rank these wide sets of variables by importance, thus allowing to better identify the strongest risk factors and generate new ideas for future preventive interventions [59,71,73,74,77,83]. In the case of longitudinal models, the strongest influence times can also be derived through attention techniques [71].

A specially interesting situation from the point of view of predictor variables are the ML models that use EHR [65,66,71,72,77], since they appear as very powerful approaches to predict childhood/adolescent obesity by tapping from the large databases of medical records with many patients and extended sets of predictor variables, including measurements, drug prescriptions, conditions observed, and procedures requested. These are especially amenable of DL techniques of the RNN type, which are specialized in dealing with time serial data like this. As described above, one case in the models presented here is that of Gupta et al. [71], where they were able to deliver excellent predictions of BMI and obesity along the whole childhood and adolescence growth curve. Another interesting use of RNN in this framework would be the extraction of information from narrative data in the medical records by means of NLP; an example of predictor variables extracted through NLP is the work by Lingren et al. [66].

These ML/DL models using EHR could be implemented in hospitals and primary health care centers to provide predictions and alerts through *dynamic, online* training. By this, we mean a model that is fed continuously with new data and is retrained periodically to enhance its predictions with the new data. This is opposed to *static, offline* training where the model is fit with a definite dataset and only once and forever. All the models we have reviewed are in the last category.

EHR offer also very interesting opportunities as Big Data sources for remining through ML/DL models. For example, we have seen the case of the work by Lingren et al. [66] where the EHR was exploited to identify a cohort of severe early childhood obesity for further genotyping efforts. Many other applications are possible, like analyzing and predicting comorbidities through statistical network analysis [84–86], phenotyping, diagnosing, pharmacoepidemiology and pharmacovigilance, etc. [87].

In addition, we should mention the fruitful application of ML/DL models to the field of childhood obesity prevention, not just through the identification of risk subpopulations but through the analysis of different aspects of the preventive intervention. We have seen that these models can be useful to optimize obesity prevention strategies [79], predict its success [80], and identify doctor's behaviors attentive or not of childhood obesity and related risks in the clinics [81] and, from a community point of view, social environments with obesogenic properties that should be targeted with preventive governmental policies [78].

To summarize, ML/DL approaches offer extraordinary advantages and new insights for childhood and adolescent obesity prediction and prevention over statistical methods. The following points summarize them:

- They have increased the prediction accuracy over the statistical models, given their ability to model complex, nonlinear relationships between variables, as well as the very large number of parameters that they contain, especially in the case of DL, avoiding the saturation in prediction performance. This is always beneficial irrespective of the application, as the more accurate is a model the more practical it is in real life.
- They allow to model directly and automatically high-dimensional data, which is not possible in the case of traditional statistical models. For the latter, one has to make use of questionable variable selection techniques, and at the cost of making biased inferences.
- They have expanded the predictor variable set from the "traditional" one in statistical models (well-established risk factors) to a much wider, multidomain one: psychological, diet, social, lifestyle, smartphone use, academic performance, sleeping quality, drug prescriptions, spousal support, rs-fMRI, and other domains of variables. In this way, they have been able to find new insights about novel "risk" factors of a completely new nature.
- They are able to use new complex data sources other than numeric ones: text, images, RMN, social media, etc.; this is especially the case with DL, which can use that data directly, without previous "feature engineering". This is another way to expand the number and domain of predictor variables.

- They (especially DL) are appropriate tools for the modeling of EHR, as described in the examples reviewed. In particular, the EHR offer an incredible opportunity for remining efforts, in order to find new insights from these data sources that can suggest opportunities for further research and therapeutic approaches.
- They have provided new applications, besides the prediction of risk subpopulations, e.g., identification of samples for genotyping from EHR, optimization of utterances in counseling interventions to decrease adolescent obesity, analysis of pediatrician attention to obesity and related risks from EHR, etc.
- They have been used not just as prediction or explanatory tools but also as simulation tools, so that they can be used to get new insights about possible therapeutic approaches.

To be fully fair, we should as well mention the *disadvantages* of ML methods over statistical ones. The first one is that making statistical inferences (parameter estimation and hypothesis test) in these models is more complicated than in statistical models. However, it is not impossible, and resampling and simulation techniques could be used if required. Another drawback of ML models is that they are more difficult to interpret, and they are typically called "black-box" type of models. This is an area of intense research, and we have seen above several examples of techniques to solve this problem, namely, the techniques of variable importance, embedding, and attention.

Seeing the advantages and disadvantages of both types of methods, we can ask: when is ML more appropriate, and when are statistical models? The following patterns have emerged:

- If the interest is mainly in interpretability, inference, and simple models of reduced numbers of predictor variables, instead of predictive performance, statistical models should be more appropriate. Again, this is more the case with early childhood and for clinical applications not requiring high accuracy.
- The opposite is applicable: If we want to have very good predictive performance and are less worried about interpretability and inference, ML should be used.
- If we have a high-dimensional sample, ML should be used, for example, if we want to analyze a wide, multidomain set of predictor variables. This is more the case with exploratory studies from which we want to gain new insights about new risk factors: psychological, social, genetics or genomics, microbiome and metagenomics, neuroimaging, diet, lifestyle, etc. As said above, these models are more likely to be relevant as the child grows and especially during adolescence.
- If we want to use complex data as predictors (images, text, time series, social media, etc.) DL is the one to go for.
- If we want to use EHR, ML (DL) should be applied.
- It is likely that new applications will go mainly through the use of ML or DL, as these are more powerful to tap from Big Data sources: Internet, social media, mobile and wireless devices, sensors, etc. These applications would include computerized decision support systems, simulation applications, novel preventive interventions, analysis of social obesogenic environments, etc.

Hopefully this Review will help the wide set of researchers in the field, including pediatricians, nurses, nutritionists, statisticians, data scientists, engineers, and epidemiologists, to get an updated view of these novel approaches and the opportunities they open, in order to approach in a more effective and creative way the prevention of childhood and adolescent obesity. We are at the beginning of a qualitatively new phase that can revolutionize this field in the near future.

Author Contributions: Conceptualization and writing, G.C. The author has read and agreed to the published version of the manuscript.

Funding: This research received no external funding.

Acknowledgments: The author acknowledges the Community of Madrid Government for providing the funds for Open Access publication of this article.

Conflicts of Interest: The author declares no conflict of interests.

References

1. Abarca-Gómez, L.; Abdeen, Z.A.; Hamid, Z.A.; Abu-Rmeileh, N.M.; Acosta-Cazares, B.; Acuin, C.; Adams, R.J.; Aekplakorn, W.; Afsana, K.; Aguilar-Salinas, C.A.; et al. Worldwide trends in body-mass index, underweight, overweight, and obesity from 1975 to 2016: A pooled analysis of 2416 population-based measurement studies in 128·9 million children, adolescents, and Adults. *Lancet* **2017**, *390*, 2627–2642. [CrossRef]
2. Ng, M.; Fleming, T.; Robinson, M.; Thomson, B.; Graetz, N.; Margono, C.; Mullany, E.C.; Biryukov, S.; Abbafati, C.; Abera, S.F.; et al. Global, regional, and national prevalence of overweight and obesity in children and adults during 1980–2013: A systematic analysis for the global burden of disease study 2013. *Lancet* **2014**, *384*, 766–781. [CrossRef]
3. WHO. Obesity and Overweight. Available online: https://www.who.int/news-room/fact-sheets/detail/obesity-and-overweight (accessed on 15 June 2020).
4. De Onis, M.; Blössner, M.; Borghi, E. Global prevalence and trends of overweight and obesity among preschool children. *Am. J. Clin. Nutr.* **2010**, *92*, 1257–1264. [CrossRef]
5. Chung, A.; Backholer, K.; Wong, E.; Palermo, C.; Keating, C.; Peeters, A. Trends in child and adolescent obesity prevalence in economically advanced countries according to socioeconomic position: A systematic review. *Obes. Rev.* **2016**, *17*, 276–295. [CrossRef]
6. Kumar, S.; Kelly, A.S. Review of childhood obesity: From epidemiology, etiology, and comorbidities to clinical assessment and treatment. *Mayo Clin. Proc.* **2017**, *92*, 251–265. [CrossRef]
7. Gibson, L.Y.; Allen, K.L.; Davis, E.; Blair, E.; Zubrick, S.R.; Byrne, S.M. The psychosocial burden of childhood overweight and obesity: Evidence for persisting difficulties in boys and girls. *Eur. J. Pediatr.* **2017**, *176*, 925–933. [CrossRef] [PubMed]
8. Rankin, J.; Matthews, L.; Cobley, S.; Han, A.; Sanders, R.; Wiltshire, H.D.; Baker, J.S. Psychological Consequences of Childhood Obesity: Psychiatric Comorbidity and Prevention. Available online: https://www.dovepress.com/psychological--consequences-of-childhood-obesity-psychiatric-comorbidi-peer-reviewed-article-AHMT (accessed on 29 June 2020).
9. Pandita, A.; Sharma, D.; Pandita, D.; Pawar, S.; Tariq, M.; Kaul, A. Childhood Obesity: Prevention is Better Than Cure. Available online: https://www.dovepress.com/childhood-obesity-prevention-is-better-than-cure-peer-reviewed-article-DMSO (accessed on 29 June 2020).
10. Fox, C.K.; Ryder, J.R.; Gross, A.C.; Kelly, A.S. Obesity in children and adolescents. In *Obesity*; Sbraccia, P., Finer, N., Eds.; Endocrinology; Springer International Publishing: Cham, Switzerland, 2019; pp. 295–322. [CrossRef]
11. Anderson, Y.C.; Wynter, L.E.; Treves, K.F.; Grant, C.C.; Stewart, J.M.; Cave, T.L.; Wouldes, T.A.; Derraik, J.G.B.; Cutfield, W.S.; Hofman, P.L. Assessment of health-related quality of life and psychological well-being of children and adolescents with obesity enrolled in a New Zealand community-based intervention programme: An observational study. *BMJ Open* **2017**, *7*, e015776. [CrossRef] [PubMed]
12. Liang, Y.; Hou, D.; Zhao, X.; Wang, L.; Hu, Y.; Liu, J.; Cheng, H.; Yang, P.; Shan, X.; Yan, Y.; et al. Childhood obesity affects adult metabolic syndrome and diabetes. *Endocrine* **2015**, *50*, 87–92. [CrossRef] [PubMed]
13. Juonala, M.; Magnussen, C.G.; Berenson, G.S.; Venn, A.; Burns, T.L.; Sabin, M.A.; Srinivasan, S.R.; Daniels, S.R.; Davis, P.H.; Chen, W.; et al. Childhood adiposity, adult adiposity, and cardiovascular risk factors. *N. Engl. J. Med.* **2011**, *365*, 1876–1885. [CrossRef]
14. Twig, G.; Yaniv, G.; Levine, H.; Leiba, A.; Goldberger, N.; Derazne, E.; Ben-Ami Shor, D.; Tzur, D.; Afek, A.; Shamiss, A.; et al. Body-Mass index in 2.3 million adolescents and cardiovascular death in adulthood. *N. Engl. J. Med.* **2016**, *374*, 2430–2440. [CrossRef]
15. Abdullah, A.; Wolfe, R.; Stoelwinder, J.U.; de Courten, M.; Stevenson, C.; Walls, H.L.; Peeters, A. The number of years lived with obesity and the risk of all-cause and cause-specific mortality. *Int. J. Epidemiol.* **2011**, *40*, 985–996. [CrossRef] [PubMed]
16. Reilly, J.J.; Kelly, J. Long-term impact of overweight and obesity in childhood and adolescence on morbidity and premature mortality in adulthood: Systematic review. *Int. J. Obes.* **2011**, *35*, 891–898. [CrossRef]
17. Sweeting, H.N. Measurement and definitions of obesity in childhood and adolescence: A field guide for the uninitiated. *Nutr. J.* **2007**, *6*, 32. [CrossRef] [PubMed]

18. González-Muniesa, P.; Mártinez-González, M.-A.; Hu, F.B.; Després, J.-P.; Matsuzawa, Y.; Loos, R.J.F.; Moreno, L.A.; Bray, G.A.; Martinez, J.A. Obesity. *Nat. Rev. Dis. Primers* **2017**, *3*, 1–18. [CrossRef]
19. Larqué, E.; Labayen, I.; Flodmark, C.-E.; Lissau, I.; Czernin, S.; Moreno, L.A.; Pietrobelli, A.; Widhalm, K. From conception to infancy—Early risk factors for childhood obesity. *Nat. Rev. Endocrinol.* **2019**, *15*, 456–478. [CrossRef]
20. Rosenblatt, F. *The Perceptron—A Perceiving and Recognizing Automaton*; Cornell Aeronautical Laboratory: Buffalo, NY, USA, 1957.
21. Maron, M.E. Automatic indexing: An experimental inquiry. *J. ACM* **1961**, *8*, 404–417. [CrossRef]
22. Rumelhart, D.E.; Hinton, G.E.; Williams, R.J. Learning representations by back-propagating errors. *Nature* **1986**, *323*, 533–536. [CrossRef]
23. Cortes, C.; Vapnik, V. Support-vector networks. *Mach. Learn.* **1995**, *20*, 273–297. [CrossRef]
24. Breiman, L. Random forest. *Mach. Learn.* **2001**, *45*, 5–32. [CrossRef]
25. Friedman, J.H. Greedy Function Approximation: A Gradient Boosting Machine. *Ann. Stati.* **2001**, *29*, 1189–1232. [CrossRef]
26. Breiman, L.; Friedman, J.; Stone, C.J.; Olshen, R.A. *Classification and Regression Trees*; Taylor & Francis: New York, NY, USA, 1984.
27. Quinlan, J.R. Induction of decision trees. *Mach. Learn.* **1986**, *1*, 81–106. [CrossRef]
28. Kass, G.V. An exploratory technique for investigating large quantities of categorical data. *Appl. Stat.* **1980**, *29*, 119. [CrossRef]
29. McCulloh, W.S.; Pitts, W.H. A logical calculus of the ideas immanent in nervous activity. *Bull. Math. Biophys.* **1943**, *5*, 115–133. [CrossRef]
30. Hochreiter, S.; Schmidhuber, J. Long short-term memory. *Neural Comput.* **1997**, *9*, 1735–1780. [CrossRef] [PubMed]
31. Cho, K.; van Merrienboer, B.; Gulcehre, C.; Bahdanau, D.; Bougares, F.; Schwenk, H.; Bengio, Y. Learning Phrase Representations Using RNN Encoder-Decoder for Statistical Machine Translation. Available online: https://arxiv.org/abs/1406.1078 (accessed on 25 March 2019).
32. Wainberg, M.; Merico, D.; Delong, A.; Frey, B.J. Deep learning in biomedicine. *Nat. Biotechnol.* **2018**, *36*, 829–838. [CrossRef] [PubMed]
33. Mamoshina, P.; Vieira, A.; Putin, E.; Zhavoronkov, A. Applications of deep learning in biomedicine. *Mol. Pharm.* **2016**, *13*, 1445–1454. [CrossRef] [PubMed]
34. Steur, M.; Smit, H.A.; Schipper, C.M.A.; Scholtens, S.; Kerkhof, M.; de Jongste, J.C.; Haveman-Nies, A.; Brunekreef, B.; Wijga, A.H. Predicting the risk of newborn children to become overweight later in childhood: The PIAMA birth cohort study. *Int. J. Pediatr. Obes.* **2011**, *6*, e170–e178. [CrossRef]
35. Druet, C.; Stettler, N.; Sharp, S.; Simmons, R.K.; Cooper, C.; Davey Smith, G.; Ekelund, U.; Lévy-Marchal, C.; Jarvelin, M.-R.; Kuh, D.; et al. Prediction of childhood obesity by infancy weight gain: An individual-level meta-analysis: Infancy weight gain and childhood obesity. *Paediatr. Perinat. Epidemiol.* **2012**, *26*, 19–26. [CrossRef]
36. Levine, R.S.; Dahly, D.L.; Rudolf, M.C.J. Identifying infants at risk of becoming obese: Can we and should we? *Public Health* **2012**, *126*, 123–128. [CrossRef]
37. Morandi, A.; Meyre, D.; Lobbens, S.; Kleinman, K.; Kaakinen, M.; Rifas-Shiman, S.L.; Vatin, V.; Gaget, S.; Pouta, A.; Hartikainen, A.-L.; et al. Estimation of newborn risk for child or adolescent obesity: Lessons from longitudinal birth cohorts. *PLoS ONE* **2012**, *7*, e49919. [CrossRef]
38. Mayr, A.; Hothorn, T.; Fenske, N. Prediction intervals for future BMI values of individual children—a Non-parametric approach by quantile boosting. *BMC Med. Res. Methodol.* **2012**, *12*, 6. [CrossRef] [PubMed]
39. On behalf of the "Healthy Growth Study" Group; Manios, Y.; Birbilis, M.; Moschonis, G.; Birbilis, G.; Mougios, V.; Lionis, C.; Chrousos, G.P. Childhood obesity risk evaluation based on perinatal factors and family sociodemographic characteristics: Core index. *Eur. J. Pediatr.* **2013**, *172*, 551–555. [CrossRef] [PubMed]
40. For the GINIplus and LISAplus Study Group; Pei, Z.; Flexeder, C.; Fuertes, E.; Thiering, E.; Koletzko, B.; Cramer, C.; Berdel, D.; Lehmann, I.; Bauer, C.-P.; et al. Early life risk factors of being overweight at 10 years of age: Results of the German birth cohorts GINIplus and LISAplus. *Eur. J. Clin. Nutr.* **2013**, *67*, 855–862. [CrossRef] [PubMed]
41. Weng, S.F.; Redsell, S.A.; Nathan, D.; Swift, J.A.; Yang, M.; Glazebrook, C. Estimating overweight risk in childhood from predictors during infancy. *Pediatrics* **2013**, *132*, e414–e421. [CrossRef]

42. Santorelli, G.; Petherick, E.S.; Wright, J.; Wilson, B.; Samiei, H.; Cameron, N.; Johnson, W. Developing prediction equations and a mobile phone application to identify infants at risk of obesity. *PLoS ONE* **2013**, *8*, e71183. [CrossRef]
43. Graversen, L.; Sørensen, T.I.A.; Gerds, T.A.; Petersen, L.; Sovio, U.; Kaakinen, M.; Sandbaek, A.; Laitinen, J.; Taanila, A.; Pouta, A.; et al. Prediction of adolescent and adult adiposity outcomes from early life anthropometrics: Prediction of adolescent and adult adiposity. *Obesity* **2015**, *23*, 162–169. [CrossRef]
44. Manios, Y.; Vlachopapadopoulou, E.; Moschonis, G.; Karachaliou, F.; Psaltopoulou, T.; Koutsouki, D.; Bogdanis, G.; Carayanni, V.; Hatzakis, A.; Michalacos, S. Utility and applicability of the "Childhood Obesity Risk Evaluation" (CORE)-Index in predicting obesity in childhood and adolescence in Greece from early life: The "National Action Plan for Public Health". *Eur. J. Pediatr.* **2016**, *175*, 1989–1996. [CrossRef]
45. Robson, J.O.; Verstraete, S.G.; Shiboski, S.; Heyman, M.B.; Wojcicki, J.M. A risk score for childhood obesity in an urban Latino cohort. *J. Pediatr.* **2016**, *172*, 29–34.e1. [CrossRef]
46. Redsell, S.A.; Weng, S.; Swift, J.A.; Nathan, D.; Glazebrook, C. Validation, optimal threshold determination, and clinical utility of the infant risk of overweight checklist for early prevention of child overweight. *Child. Obes.* **2016**, *12*, 202–209. [CrossRef]
47. Cortés-Martín, A.; Colmenarejo, G.; Selma, M.V.; Espín, J.C. Genetic polymorphisms, mediterranean diet and microbiota-associated urolithin metabotypes can predict obesity in childhood-adolescence. *Sci. Rep.* **2020**, *10*, 7850. [CrossRef]
48. Ogden, C.L.; Flegal, K.M. Changes in Terminology for Childhood Overweight and Obesity. *Natl. Health Stat. Rep.* **2010**, *25*, 1–5.
49. Cole, T.J. Establishing a standard definition for child overweight and obesity worldwide: International survey. *BMJ* **2000**, *320*, 1240. [CrossRef]
50. Freeman, J.V.; Cole, T.J.; Chinn, S.; Jones, P.R.; White, E.M.; Preece, M.A. Cross sectional stature and weight reference curves for the UK, 1990. *Arch. Dis. Child.* **1995**, *73*, 17–24. [CrossRef] [PubMed]
51. Butler, É.M.; Derraik, J.G.B.; Taylor, R.W.; Cutfield, W.S. Prediction models for early childhood obesity: Applicability and existing issues. *Horm. Res. Paediatr.* **2018**, *90*, 358–367. [CrossRef]
52. Ziauddeen, N.; Roderick, P.J.; Macklon, N.S.; Alwan, N.A. Predicting childhood overweight and obesity using maternal and early life risk factors: A systematic review: Predicting childhood overweight. *Obes. Rev.* **2018**, *19*, 302–312. [CrossRef] [PubMed]
53. Butler, É.M.; Derraik, J.G.B.; Taylor, R.W.; Cutfield, W.S. Childhood obesity: How long should we wait to predict weight? *J. Pediatr. Endocrinol. Metab.* **2018**, *31*, 497–501. [CrossRef]
54. Adnan, M.H.B.M.; Husain, W.; Damanhoori, F. *A Survey on Utilization of Data Mining for Childhood Obesity Prediction*; IEEE: Kuching, Malaysia, 2010; pp. 1–6.
55. Triantafyllidis, A.; Polychronidou, E.; Alexiadis, A.; Rocha, C.L.; Oliveira, D.N.; da Silva, A.S.; Freire, A.L.; Macedo, C.; Sousa, I.F.; Werbet, E.; et al. Computerized decision support and machine learning applications for the prevention and treatment of childhood obesity: A systematic review of the literature. *Artif. Intell. Med.* **2020**, *104*, 101844. [CrossRef]
56. Novak, B.; Bigec, M. Application of artificial neural networks for childhood obesity prediction. In *Proceedings of the 1995 Second New Zealand International Two-Stream Conference on Artificial Neural Networks and Expert Systems*; IEEE Computer Society Press: Dunedin, New Zealand, 1995; pp. 377–380. [CrossRef]
57. Novak, B.; Bigec, M. Childhood obesity prediction with artificial neural networks. In Proceedings of the Ninth IEEE Symposium on Computer-Based Medical Systems; IEEE Computer Society Press: Ann Arbor, MI, USA, 1996; pp. 77–82. [CrossRef]
58. Zhang, S.; Tjortjis, C.; Zeng, X.; Qiao, H.; Buchan, I.; Keane, J. Comparing data mining methods with logistic regression in childhood obesity prediction. *Inf. Syst. Front.* **2009**, *11*, 449–460. [CrossRef]
59. Rehkopf, D.H.; Laraia, B.A.; Segal, M.; Braithwaite, D.; Epel, E. The relative importance of predictors of body mass index change, overweight and obesity in adolescent girls. *Int. J. Pediatr. Obes.* **2011**, *6*, e233–e242. [CrossRef]
60. Adnan, M.H.B.M.; Husain, W.; Rashid, N.A. *Parameter Identification and Selection for Childhood Obesity Prediction Using Data Mining*; IACSIT Press: Singapore, 2012; Volume 35, pp. 75–79.
61. Adnan, M.H.M.; Husain, W.; Rashid, N.A. Hybrid approaches using decision tree, naïve bayes, means and euclidean distances for childhood obesity prediction. *Int. J. Softw. Eng. Appl.* **2012**, *6*, 8.

62. Muhamad Adnan, M.H.B.; Husain, W.; Abdul Rashid, N. A hybrid approach using naïve bayes and genetic algorithm for childhood obesity prediction. In *2012 International Conference on Computer & Information Science (ICCIS)*; IEEE: Kuala Lumpur, Malaysia, 2012; pp. 281–285. [CrossRef]
63. Lazarou, C.; Karaolis, M.; Matalas, A.-L.; Panagiotakos, D.B. Dietary patterns analysis using data mining method. An application to data from the CYKIDS study. *Comput. Methods Programs Biomed.* **2012**, *108*, 706–714. [CrossRef]
64. Pochini, A.; Wu, Y.; Hu, G. Data mining for lifestyle risk factors associated with overweight and obesity among adolescents. In *2014 IIAI 3rd International Conference on Advanced Applied Informatics*; IEEE: Kokura Kita-ku, Japan, 2014; pp. 883–888. [CrossRef]
65. Dugan, T.M.; Mukhopadhyay, S.; Carroll, A.; Downs, S. Machine learning techniques for prediction of early childhood obesity. *Appl. Clin. Inform.* **2015**, *6*, 506–520. [CrossRef]
66. Lingren, T.; Thaker, V.; Brady, C.; Namjou, B.; Kennebeck, S.; Bickel, J.; Patibandla, N.; Ni, Y.; Van Driest, S.; Chen, L.; et al. Developing an algorithm to detect early childhood obesity in two tertiary pediatric medical centers. *Appl. Clin. Inform.* **2016**, *7*, 693–706. [CrossRef]
67. Abdullah, F.S.; Manan, N.S.A.; Ahmad, A.; Wafa, S.W.; Shahril, M.R.; Zulaily, N.; Amin, R.M.; Ahmed, A. Data mining techniques for classification of childhood obesity among year 6 school children. In *Recent Advances on Soft Computing and Data Mining*; Herawan, T., Ghazali, R., Nawi, N.M., Deris, M.M., Eds.; Springer International Publishing: Cham, Switzerland, 2017; Volume 549, pp. 465–474.
68. Rios-Julian, N.; Alarcon-Paredes, A.; Alonso, G.A.; Hernandez-Rosales, D.; Guzman-Guzman, I.P. Feasibility of a screening tool for obesity diagnosis in mexican children from a vulnerable community of me'phaa ethnicity in the state of Guerrero, Mexico. In *2017 Global Medical Engineering Physics Exchanges/Pan American Health Care Exchanges (GMEPE/PAHCE)*; IEEE: Tuxtla-Gutierrez, Mexico, 2017; pp. 1–6. [CrossRef]
69. Wiechmann, P.; Lora, K.; Branscum, P.; Fu, J. Identifying discriminative attributes to gain insights regarding child obesity in hispanic preschoolers using machine learning Techniques. In *2017 IEEE 29th International Conference on Tools with Artificial Intelligence (ICTAI)*; IEEE: Boston, MA, USA, 2017; pp. 11–15. [CrossRef]
70. Zheng, Z.; Ruggiero, K. Using machine learning to predict obesity in high school students. In *2017 IEEE International Conference on Bioinformatics and Biomedicine (BIBM)*; IEEE: Kansas City, MO, USA, 2017; pp. 2132–2138. [CrossRef]
71. Gupta, M.; Phan, T.-L.T.; Bunnell, H.T.; Beheshti, R. Obesity Prediction with EHR Data: A Deep Learning Approach with Interpretable Elements. Available online: https://arxiv.org/abs/1912.02655 (accessed on 25 March 2019).
72. Hammond, R.; Athanasiadou, R.; Curado, S.; Aphinyanaphongs, Y.; Abrams, C.; Messito, M.J.; Gross, R.; Katzow, M.; Jay, M.; Razavian, N.; et al. Predicting childhood obesity using electronic health records and publicly available data. *PLoS ONE* **2019**, *14*, e0215571. [CrossRef]
73. Lee, I.; Bang, K.-S.; Moon, H.; Kim, J. Risk factors for obesity among children aged 24 to 80 months in korea: A decision tree analysis. *J. Pediatr. Nurs.* **2019**, *46*, e15–e23. [CrossRef]
74. Park, B.; Chung, C.-S.; Lee, M.J.; Park, H. Accurate neuroimaging biomarkers to predict body mass index in adolescents: A longitudinal study. *Brain Imaging Behav.* **2019**. [CrossRef]
75. Singh, B.; Tawfik, H. A machine learning approach for predicting weight gain risks in young adults. In *2019 10th International Conference on Dependable Systems, Services and Technologies (DESSERT)*; IEEE: Leeds, UK, 2019; pp. 231–234. [CrossRef]
76. Kim, C.; Costello, F.J.; Lee, K.C.; Li, Y.; Li, C. Predicting factors affecting adolescent obesity using general bayesian network and what-if analysis. *Int. J. Environ. Res. Public Health* **2019**, *16*, 4684. [CrossRef]
77. Pang, X.; Forrest, C.B.; Le-Scherban, F.; Masino, A.J. Understanding early childhood obesity via interpretation of machine learning model predictions. In *2019 18th IEEE International Conference on Machine Learning and Applications (ICMLA)*; IEEE: Boca Raton, FL, USA, 2019; pp. 1438–1443. [CrossRef]
78. Nau, C.; Ellis, H.; Huang, H.; Schwartz, B.S.; Hirsch, A.; Bailey-Davis, L.; Kress, A.M.; Pollak, J.; Glass, T.A. Exploring the forest instead of the trees: An innovative method for defining obesogenic and obesoprotective environments. *Health Place* **2015**, *35*, 136–146. [CrossRef]
79. Hasan, M.; Kotov, A.; Carcone, A.I.; Dong, M.; Naar, S. Predicting the outcome of patient-provider communication sequences using recurrent neural networks and probabilistic models. *AMIA Jt. Summits Transl. Sci. Proc.* **2018**, *2018*, 64–73.

80. Öksüz, N.; Shcherbatyi, I.; Kowatsch, T.; Maass, W. A data-analytical system to predict therapy success for obese children. In Proceedings of the Thirty Ninth International Conference on Information Systems, San Francisco, CA, USA, 13–16 December 2018; pp. 1–16.
81. Turer, C.B.; Skinner, C.S.; Barlow, S.E. Algorithm to detect pediatric provider attention to high BMI and associated medical risk. *J. Am. Med. Inform. Assoc.* **2018**. [CrossRef]
82. Duran, I.; Martakis, K.; Rehberg, M.; Semler, O.; Schoenau, E. Diagnostic performance of an artificial neural network to predict excess body fat in children. *Pediatr. Obes.* **2019**, *14*, e12494. [CrossRef]
83. Marcos-Pasero, H.; Colmenarejo, G.; Aguilar-Aguilar, E.; Ramírez de Molina, A.; Reglero, G.; Loria-Kohen, V. Ranking of a wide multidomain set of predictors of children obesity by machine learning variable importance techniques. **2020**, submitted.
84. Capobianco, E.; Liò, P. Comorbidity networks: Beyond disease correlations. *J. Complex. Netw.* **2015**, *3*, 319–332. [CrossRef]
85. Brunson, J.C.; Agresta, T.P.; Laubenbacher, R.C. sensitivity of comorbidity network analysis. *JAMIA Open* **2020**, *3*, 94–103. [CrossRef]
86. Emmert-Streib, F.; Tripathi, S.; de Matos Simoes, R.; Hawwa, A.F.; Dehmer, M. The human disease network. *Syst. Biomed.* **2013**, *1*, 20–28. [CrossRef]
87. Bennett, T.D.; Callahan, T.J.; Feinstein, J.A.; Ghosh, D.; Lakhani, S.A.; Spaeder, M.C.; Szefler, S.J.; Kahn, M.G. Data science for child health. *J. Pediatr.* **2019**, *208*, 12–22. [CrossRef]

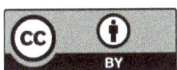

© 2020 by the author. Licensee MDPI, Basel, Switzerland. This article is an open access article distributed under the terms and conditions of the Creative Commons Attribution (CC BY) license (http://creativecommons.org/licenses/by/4.0/).

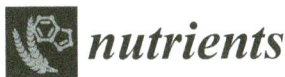

Article

The Effect of Supportive Implementation of Healthier Canteen Guidelines on Changes in Dutch School Canteens and Student Purchase Behaviour

Irma J. Evenhuis [1,*], Suzanne M. Jacobs [2], Ellis L. Vyth [1], Lydian Veldhuis [2], Michiel R. de Boer [1], Jacob C. Seidell [1] and Carry M. Renders [1]

[1] Department of Health Sciences, Faculty of Science, Vrije Universiteit Amsterdam, Amsterdam Public Health Research Institute, De Boelelaan 1085, 1081 HV Amsterdam, The Netherlands; info@ellisvyth.nl (E.L.V.); m.r.de.boer@umcg.nl (M.R.d.B.); j.c.seidell@vu.nl (J.C.S.); carry.renders@vu.nl (C.M.R.)
[2] Netherlands Nutrition Centre, PO Box 85700, 2508 CK The Hague, The Netherlands; jacobs@voedingscentrum.nl (S.M.J.); veldhuis@voedingscentrum.nl (L.V.)
* Correspondence: i.j.evenhuis@vu.nl

Received: 16 July 2020; Accepted: 10 August 2020; Published: 12 August 2020

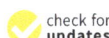

Abstract: We developed an implementation plan including several components to support implementation of the "Guidelines for Healthier Canteens" in Dutch secondary schools. This study evaluated the effect of this plan on changes in the school canteen and on food and drink purchases of students. In a 6 month quasi-experimental study, ten intervention schools (IS) received support implementing the guidelines, and ten control schools (CS) received only the guidelines. Changes in the health level of the cafeteria and vending machines were assessed and described. Effects on self-reported purchase behaviour of students were analysed using mixed logistic regression analyses. IS scored higher on healthier availability in the cafeteria (77.2%) and accessibility (59.0%) compared to CS (60.1%, resp. 50.0%) after the intervention. IS also showed more changes in healthier offers in the cafeteria (range −3 to 57%, mean change 31.4%) and accessibility (range 0 to 50%, mean change 15%) compared to CS (range −9 to 46%, mean change 9.7%; range −30 to 20% mean change 7% resp.). Multi-level logistic regression analyses on the intervention/control and health level of the canteen in relation to purchase behaviour showed no relevant relations. In conclusion, the offered support resulted in healthier canteens. However, there was no direct effect on students' purchase behaviour during the intervention.

Keywords: schools; nutrition; canteen; adolescents; implementation; purchase behaviour

1. Introduction

To support adolescents to make healthier food choices, many national governments have formulated food policies to encourage a healthy offering of foods and drinks in schools and their canteens [1]. To create healthier canteens, nudging strategies are used, by which the healthier option is made easier without restricting the freedom of choice [2]. Such strategies focus on availability and accessibility by offering mainly healthier products, discouraging the consumption of unhealthy foods by making them less readily available, making the healthier option the default, and promoting healthier products [3–6]. Evaluations of such strategies show improvements in food and drinks offered in schools, which is likely to influence students' consumption of healthier foods and drinks [4–7]. However, these results are only seen when the policy is implemented adequately [8,9], which can be increased with supportive implementation tools [10–12]. The provision and type of such tools differ within and across countries, though training, modelling, continuous support such as helpdesks and incentives are commonly provided [12].

In the Netherlands, most schools have no tradition of offering school meals, but do offer complementary foods and drinks in a cafeteria and/or vending machines. Most students bring their lunch from home, and buy additional food and drinks at school, or at shops around the school [13]. The national Healthy School Canteen Programme of the Netherlands Nutrition Centre, financed by the Dutch Ministry of Health, Welfare and Sports, provides schools with free support to create healthier canteens (cafeteria and/or vending machine) [14–16]. This includes, for example, a visit and advice from school canteen advisors (i.e., nutritionists), regular newsletters, and a website with information about and examples of healthier school canteens. The programme has been shown to lead to greater attention to nutrition in schools and a small increase in the offering of healthier food and drinks in the cafeterias, but not in vending machines [15,17,18]. However, until then, the programme only included availability criteria.

Based on literature and in collaboration with future users and experts in the field of nutrition, the Netherlands Nutrition Centre developed the "Guidelines for Healthier Canteens" in 2014, and updated them in 2017 [19]. These guidelines include criteria on both the availability and accessibility of healthier foods and drinks (including tap water) and an anchoring policy. The guidelines distinguish three incremental health levels: bronze, silver and gold [19]. Only silver (≥60%) and gold (≥80%) are qualified for the label "healthier school canteen". These guidelines define healthier products as food and drinks recommended in the Dutch Wheel of Five Guidelines, and products that are not included but contain a limited amount of calories, saturated fat and sodium [20]. To increase dissemination of the guidelines, an implementation plan was developed, based on experience within the Healthy School Canteen Programme and in collaboration with involved stakeholders from policy, practice and science [21]. This study investigated the effect of this implementation plan to support implementation of the Guidelines for Healthier Canteens in schools on both changes in the health level of the canteen and in purchase behaviour of students. Moreover, the relation between the health level of the canteen and purchase behaviour is determined.

2. Materials and Methods

2.1. Study Design

The effect of the implementation plan was evaluated in a 6 month quasi-experimental controlled trial with 10 intervention and 10 control schools, between October 2015 and June 2016. The control schools were matched to intervention schools on the pre-defined characteristics: school size (fewer or more than 1000 students); level of secondary education (vocational or senior general/pre-university); and how the catering was provided (by a catering company or the school itself). Additionally, we aimed to match the control schools to intervention schools on contextual factors: the availability of shops near the school and the presence of school policy to oblige students to stay in the schoolyard during breaks. Intervention schools received support to implement the Guidelines for Healthier Canteens according to the plan (the intervention), while control schools received only general information about the guidelines, although they also received the support after the intervention period. Further details about the study design are provided in the study protocol [22]. This study was registered in the Dutch Trial Register (NTR5922) and approved by the Medical Ethical Committee of the VU University Amsterdam (Nr. 2015.331).

2.2. Study Population

The schools, in western and central Netherlands, were recruited via the Netherlands Nutrition Centre and caterers. Inclusion criteria were (a) presence of a cafeteria, (b) willingness to create a healthier school canteen, and (c) willingness to provide time, space and consent for the researchers to collect data from students, employees and canteen workers. The exclusion criteria were (a) the school had already started to implement the Guidelines for Healthier Canteens, and (b) the school had already received personalized support on implementing a healthier canteen from a school canteen advisor from the Netherlands Nutrition Centre in 2015. In all participating schools, we recruited students per class. In each school, we recruited 100 second or third-year Dutch-speaking students (aged 13–15 years), equally distributed over the school's offered education levels. Parents and students received information about the study and the option to decline participation. Figure 1 shows the flow diagram of the inclusion of the schools and students.

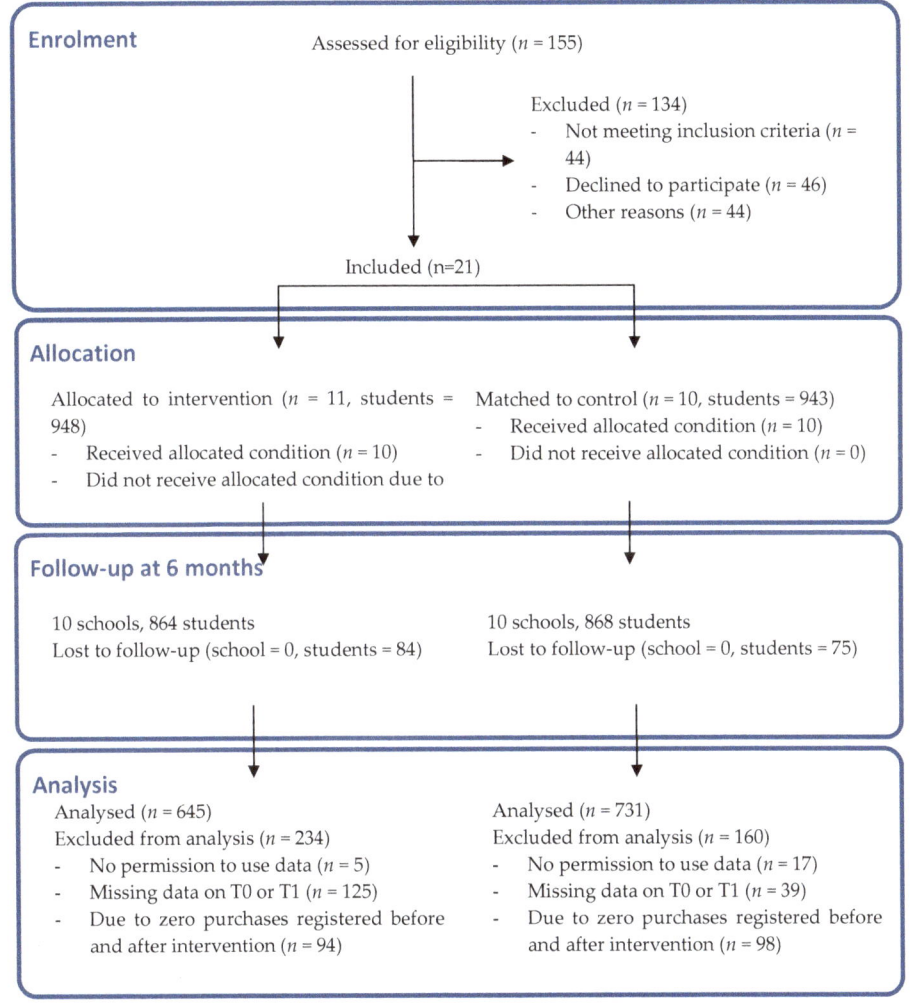

Figure 1. The CONSORT flow diagram of the present study [23].

2.3. Intervention

The intervention consisted of the implementation plan to support schools in creating a healthier school canteen, as defined by the Guidelines for Healthier Canteens. This plan was developed in a 3-step approach based on the "Grol and Wensing Implementation of Change model" [24] in collaboration with stakeholders, as described elsewhere [21], and delivered by school canteen advisors of the Netherlands Nutrition Centre, in collaboration with researchers of the Vrije Universiteit Amsterdam.

The intervention started with gaining insight into the context and current situation of the school and the canteen. For this purpose, involved stakeholders (e.g., teacher, school management, caterer, canteen employee) filled out a questionnaire on the schools' characteristics (educational level, number of students) and their individual (e.g., knowledge, motivation) and environmental (e.g., need for support, the innovation) determinants. School canteen advisors also measured the extent to which canteens met the Guidelines for Healthier Canteens, using the online tool "the Canteen Scan" [25]. Based on these findings, school canteen advisors provided tailored advice in an advisory meeting where all involved stakeholders discussed aims and actions to achieve a healthier canteen. Stakeholders also received communication materials about the Guidelines for Healthier Canteens, including a brochure with examples of, and advice on, how to promote healthier products. All stakeholders of all intervention schools were invited to a closed Facebook community to share experiences, ask questions and to support each other. In addition, to remind and motivate stakeholders, a newsletter with information and examples was sent by email once every 6 weeks. Finally, to gain insight into their students' opinion, students were asked to fill in a questionnaire (the same as used for the effect evaluation), and the results were fed back to schools in an attractive fact sheet.

2.4. Measurements

Measurements in the school canteens and among students were performed before and directly after the intervention period. The "health level" of the school canteen was measured in all participating schools using the online Canteen Scan [25], filled out by a school canteen advisor. The tool has been evaluated satisfactorily on inter-rater reliability and criterium validity if measured by a school canteen advisor, scoring > 0.60 on Weighted Cohen's Kappa [22]. Only intervention schools received the results of the Canteen Scan as part of the intervention.

Students reported their purchases via an online questionnaire filled out in a classroom under supervision of a teacher and/or researcher. Data on demographics and behavioural and environmental determinants were also collected [26]. The questions were derived from validated Dutch questionnaires [27–31], and the questionnaire was pretested for comprehensibility and length in a comparable population using the cognitive interview method think-aloud [32].

2.4.1. Health Level of the School Canteen

The Canteen Scan assessed the extent to which a canteen complies with the four subtopics of the Guidelines for Healthier Canteens: (1) a set of four basic conditions for all canteens, (2) the percentage of healthier foods and drinks available in the cafeteria (at the counter, display, racks) and (3) in vending machines and (4) the percentage of accessibility for healthier food and drink products [19,25]. According to these guidelines, a canteen is healthy if all basic conditions are fulfilled, if the percentage of healthier foods and drinks available is at least 60% in the cafeteria and in vending machines, if fruit or vegetables are offered, and if the percentage of fulfilled accessibility criteria is also at least 60%. As the basic conditions overlap with the availability and accessibility scores, this subtopic was not used in the analyses. For the other three subtopics, the change between pre- and post-measurement was calculated for each school.

In the Canteen Scan, all visible foods and drinks available in the cafeteria (counter, display, racks) and in vending machines were entered. The scan automatically identifies whether, according to the Dutch Wheel of Five Guidelines [30], an entered product is healthier or less healthy, and calculates the percentage of healthier products. In addition, to assess the accessibility for healthier foods and drinks, nine criteria (8 multiple choice, 1 multiple answer options) were answered, creating a score ranging from 0 to 90%. These questions relate to the attractive placement of healthier products in the cafeteria and vending machines; the offer at the cash desk; the offer at the route through the cafeteria; fruit and vegetables presented attractively; promotions for healthier products only; mostly healthier items at the menu/pricelist; and advertisements/visual materials only for healthier products. Questions include, for example, "Are only healthier foods and drinks offered at the cash desk?" and "Are fruit and vegetables presented in an attractive manner?"

2.4.2. Self-Reported Purchase Behaviour of Students

Purchase behaviour was measured by assessing the frequency of purchases per food group (sugary drinks, sugar free drinks, fruit, sweet snacks, etc.) over the previous week, for the cafeteria and the vending machines separately. If students stated that they had bought less than once per week, they answered the frequency of purchases in the last month. Students who did not buy anything at both time points were excluded ($n = 192$), as they do not provide information about the relation between the intervention and their purchases. Groups of foods and drinks were considered as healthier or less healthy, as defined by the Dutch Wheel of Five Guidelines [20]. All reported healthier purchases in the cafeteria and vending machines, respectively, were summed, as were the less healthy purchases. As the data were not normally distributed, we dichotomised the variable. Frequencies of the pre- and post-intervention survey were subtracted and categorized into the dichotomous variable indicating a healthy or unhealthy change in purchase behaviour. A healthy score was defined as (1) a higher increase in healthier products compared with less healthy products; (2) a higher decrease in less healthy products compared with healthier products; or (3) purchases remained stable over time and consisted mainly of healthier products. An unhealthy score was defined as (1) a higher increase in less healthy products compared with healthier products; (2) a higher decrease in healthier products compared with less healthy products; (3) purchases remained stable over time and consisted mainly of less healthy products or an equal number of healthier and less healthy products.

2.4.3. Other Student Variables

Demographic student variables included age (in years), gender and current school level (vocational (i.e., VMBO), senior general education (i.e., HAVO) or pre-university education (i.e., VWO)). Determinants of purchase behaviour included attitudes, subjective norms, perceived behavioural control and intention, all towards buying healthier products at school. For each variable, multiple questions (range 2–5) were asked on a 5-point Likert scale (answers ranging from, e.g., 1 = very unlikely to 5 = very likely) derived from existing validated Dutch questionnaires [27,28]. The mean score of each variable was calculated and the reliability of the measurements was assessed with Cronbach's alpha [33]. The measured environmental determinants were having breakfast (Yes, No); amount of money spent on food/drink purchases at school per week (<€1, €1–2, ≥€2); external food/drink purchase behaviour (<1 times p/w, 1–3 times p/w, ≥4 times p/w); and foods/drinks brought from home (<4 times p/w, ≥4 times p/w).

2.5. Sample Size

The sample size was calculated based on the outcome purchase behaviour, an expected 10% drop out, 80% power and 5% significance level [34]. The calculation showed that 20 schools and 100 students per school were necessary to be able to detect a 10% difference in purchase behaviour of students (continuous variable), with the expected multi-level structure (students within schools, intra-class correlation of 0.05).

2.6. Statistical Analyses

Student baseline characteristics and pre- and post-intervention canteen outcomes and student purchase behaviour were described by means and standard deviations. Canteen outcomes included three subtopics of the health level of the canteen: healthier food and drinks available in the cafeteria, in the vending machines and accessibility of healthier food and drinks. Mean (SD) pre- and post-intervention values and mean changes were described and changes in the subtopics per school were presented in a chart.

A mixed logistic regression analysis [35] was performed to investigate the effect of the intervention (independent variable) on purchase behaviour (dependent variable). Correlated errors of student scores (level 1) nested within schools (level 2) were taken into account by including a random intercept for schools in all analyses (model 1). The analyses were stratified by gender, as boys seems to react more to environmental changes than girls [36]. Models were first extended with demographic variables (model 2), secondly with students' behavioural determinants (model 3) and thirdly with students' environmental determinants (model 4).

The effect of a healthier canteen (independent variable) on student purchase behaviour (dependent variable) was also assessed using mixed logistic regression analyses with a random intercept for schools for boys and girls separately. We used the health level of the canteen at follow-up for each of the three subtopics of a healthier canteen. Due to non-linearity with student purchase behaviour, again a dichotomous variable was created, based on the guidelines, which state that 60% or higher is a healthier availability and accessibility, respectively. Again, the model was extended with demographic variables (model 2) and students' behavioural (model 3) and environmental determinants (model 4). Statistical analyses were performed using the IBM SPSS Statistics version 24.0 (IBM corporation (IBM Nederland), Amsterdam, The Netherlands. Odds ratios and 95% confidence intervals (CI's) are presented.

3. Results

3.1. Baseline Characteristics

We included data from 645 students of the intervention schools and 731 students of the control schools in the analyses (Table 1). Both groups consisted of more girls than boys (56% and 53%, respectively). The included schools offered education at the vocational ($n = 6$) level, the senior general/pre-university level ($n = 5$), or a combination of both levels ($n = 9$). The level of education was broadly similar for intervention and control schools. However, in intervention schools, slightly more girls followed the vocational education level (46.6%) compared to boys (41.4%), while the opposite was the case in control schools (girls, 39.5%; boys 46.2%). Most students indicated that they did bring food and drinks from home to school four or more times a week (for food, intervention schools (IS) 91.8 and control schools (CS) 89.2%; for drinks, IS 90.4% and CS 88.5%). The majority of students reported that they bought foods or drinks in the school cafeteria (IS 55.5%; CS 64.4%) or vending machine (IS 63.6%; CS 61.1%) less than once per week. During school time, 62.2% and 67.6% of the students in the IS reported buying food or drinks outside school less than once a week, compared to 65.6% and 73.6% in the CS.

Table 1. Baseline characteristics of students divided by intervention or control school and gender.

	Intervention Schools (N = 10)			Control Schools (N = 10)		
	Total	Boys	Girls	Total	Boys	Girls
Number of students—n (%)	645 (46.9)	302 (46.8)	343 (53.2)	731 (53.1)	318 (43.5)	413 (56.5)
Age (years)—mean (SD)	13.39 (0.62)	13.35 (0.55)	13.42 (0.68)	13.35 (0.62)	13.38 (0.66)	13.33 (0.59)
School level n (%)						
Vocational education	284 (44.0)	125 (41.4)	159 (46.4)	310 (42.4)	147 (46.2)	163 (39.5)
Senior general education	148 (22.9)	86 (28.5)	62 (18.1)	190 (26.0)	78 (24.5)	112 (27.1)
Pre-university education	213 (33.0)	91 (30.1)	122 (35.6)	231 (31.6)	93 (29.2)	138 (33.4)
Behavioural determinants—Mean (SD) [a]						
Attitude	2.81 (0.84)	2.73 (0.84)	2.88 (0.84)	2.91 (0.86)	2.67 (0.88)	3.09 (0.80)
Subjective norm	2.39 (0.64)	2.32 (0.64)	2.44 (0.63)	2.39 (0.68)	2.31 (0.71)	2.46 (0.66)
Perceived behavioural control	3.18 (0.92)	3.18 (0.95)	3.18 (0.89)	3.36 (0.89)	3.24 (0.93)	3.46 (0.84)
Intention	2.46 (0.94)	2.27 (0.97)	2.64 (0.88)	2.50 (0.89)	2.26 (0.87)	2.68 (0.87)
Environmental determinants—n (%)						

Table 1. Cont.

	Intervention Schools (N = 10)			Control Schools (N = 10)		
	Total	Boys	Girls	Total	Boys	Girls
Breakfast behaviour						
Yes, sometimes or always	610 (94.6)	294 (97.4)	316 (92.1)	705 (96.4)	311 (97.8)	394 (95.4)
No, never	35 (5.4)	8 (2.6)	27 (7.9)	26 (3.6)	7 (2.2)	19 (4.6)
Foods brought from home						
Less than four times per week	53 (8.2)	23 (7.6)	30 (8.7)	79 (10.8)	39 (12.3)	40 (9.7)
4 or more times per week	592 (91.8)	279 (92.4)	313 (91.3)	652 (89.2)	279 (87.7)	373 (90.3)
Drinks brought from home						
Less than four per week	62 (9.6)	30 (9.9)	32 (9.3)	84 (11.5)	45 (14.2)	39 (9.4)
4 or more times per week	583 (90.4)	272 (90.1)	311 (90.7)	647 (88.5)	273 (85.8)	374 (90.6)
Amount of money spent on food/drink purchases in school per week						
<€1	91 (14.1)	45 (14.9)	46 (13.4)	131 (17.9)	56 (17.6)	75 (18.2)
€1–2	354 (54.9)	154 (51.0)	200 (58.3)	442 (60.5)	180 (56.6)	262 (63.4)
≥€2	200 (31.0)	103 (34.1)	97 (28.3)	158 (21.6)	82 (25.8)	76 (18.4)
Food or drink purchases in school cafeteria						
Less than once per week	358 (55.5)	167 (55.3)	191 (55.7)	471 (64.4)	183 (57.5)	288 (69.7)
1 time per week	151 (23.4)	76 (25.2)	75 (21.9)	137 (18.7)	66 (20.8)	71 (17.2)
2 or more times per week	136 (21.1)	59 (19.5)	77 (22.4)	123 (16.8)	69 (21.7)	54 (13.1)
Food or drink purchases in school at vending machine [b,c]						
Less than once per week	410 (63.6)	196 (64.9)	214 (62.4)	447 (61.1)	183 (61.2)	264 (63.9)
1 time per week	123 (19.1)	48 (15.9)	75 (21.9)	147 (20.1)	62 (20.7)	85 (20.6)
2 or more times per week	112 (17.4)	58 (19.2)	54 (15.7)	101 (13.8)	54 (18.1)	47 (11.4)
Food purchases outside school						
Less than once per week	401 (62.2)	175 (57.9)	226 (65.9)	480 (65.6)	170 (53.5)	310 (75.1)
1 to 3 times per week	167 (25.9)	91 (30.1)	76 (22.2)	170 (23.3)	104 (32.7)	66 (16.0)
4 or more times per week	77 (11.9)	36 (11.9)	41 (12.0)	81 (11.1)	44 (13.8)	37 (9.0)
Drink purchases outside school						
Less than once per week	436 (67.6)	192 (63.6)	244 (71.1)	538 (73.6)	201 (63.2)	337 (81.6)
1 to 3 times per week	151 (23.4)	82 (27.2)	69 (20.1)	126 (17.2)	80 (25.2)	46 (11.1)
4 or more times per week	58 (9.0)	28 (9.3)	30 (8.7)	67 (9.2)	37 (11.6)	30 (7.3)

[a] Per variable, multiple questions (range 2–5) were asked on a 5-point Likert scale (answers ranging from 1 = very unlikely to 5 = very likely). [b] This variable was not used as confounder in the multi-level analyses due to the similarity with the outcome variable purchase behaviour per week. [c] On this variable, the control group has 40 students less (19 boys, 21 girls) as one school did not have a vending machine.

3.2. Intervention Effect on Health Level of the Canteen

Table 2 shows that intervention schools (IS) scored higher in terms of the healthier offering in the cafeteria (77.2%), compared to control schools (CS) (60.1%) after the intervention. Figure 2 confirms this and shows that nine of the ten IS increased the healthier offering (range of all IS: −3 to 57%, mean change 31.4%). In comparison, eight of the ten CS showed positive changes but the change (range of all CS: −9 to 46%, mean change 9.7%) was smaller compared to the IS. The healthier offering in vending machines increased in five of the ten IS (range of all IS: −15 to 33%, mean change 5.1%) and in three of the nine CS (range al all CS: −14 to 48%, mean change 5.3%) (Figure 3), although, on average, both groups made broadly similar changes in their offer (Table 2). With regard to the accessibility criteria, both groups showed overall increases, although two CS also showed decreases (Figure 4). The change in IS was higher compared to CS (range of all IS: 0 to 50%, mean change 15%; range of all CS −30 to 20%, mean change 7%), resulting in mean scores of 59% (IS) and 50% (CS) fulfilled accessibility criteria after the intervention.

Table 2. Subscores of a healthier canteen pre- and post-intervention, stratified by intervention and control schools.

	Intervention Schools (N = 10)			Control Schools (N = 10)		
	T0	T1	Mean Change	T0	T1	Mean Change
Healthier products available in the cafeteria [a,b]	45.80 (27.12)	77.20 (13.41)	31.4	50.40 (23.00)	60.10 (15.67)	9.7
Healthier products available at vending machine [a,b,c]	44.70 (19.40)	49.80 (20.33)	5.1	38.89 (24.30)	44.22 (22.99)	5.3
Fulfilled accessibility criteria [a,d]	44.00 (20.66)	59.00 (19.69)	15.0	43.00 (20.58)	50.00 (14.91)	20.0

[a] Mean score (SD). [b] Scores in percentage (0–100%). [c] One control school did not have a vending machine (N = 9, in control schools). [d] Nine criteria could be fulfilled, scoring 10% per criteria (0–90%).

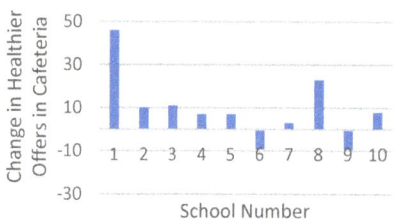

(a) Control Schools

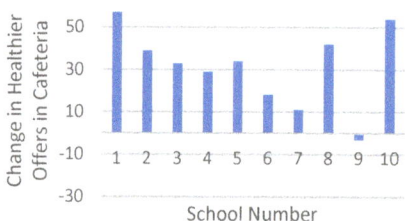

(b) Intervention Schools

Figure 2. Histogram of the changes in healthier products available in the cafeteria.

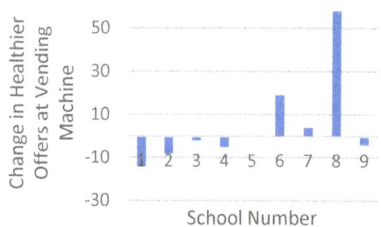

(a) Control Schools

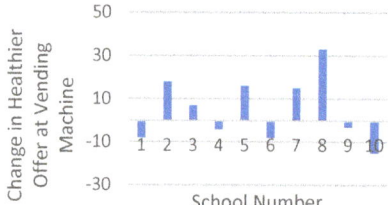

(b) Intervention Schools

Figure 3. Histogram of the changes in healthier products available at vending machines.

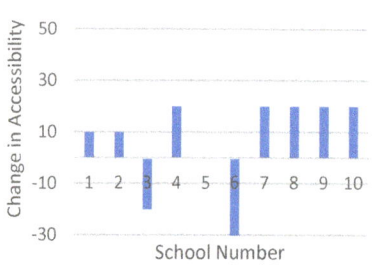

(a) Control Schools

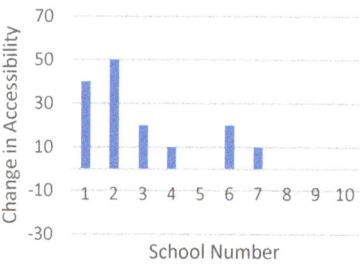

(b) Interventions Schools

Figure 4. Histogram of the changes in fulfilled accessibility criteria.

3.3. Purchases in the Cafeteria

Data on self-reported purchase behaviour at the cafeteria were included in the analysis from 1213 students (548 boys, 665 girls) (Table 3). Mean purchases of all foods and drinks per week varied between 0.46 and 1.72 per person. Both boys and girls bought more "less healthy" than healthier products. With regard to changes in weekly purchases in the cafeteria after 6 months, 50% of the boys of the IS maintained or changed to healthier purchase behaviour (Table 3). In boys of the CS, this percentage was 51.5%. Among girls, 53.6% maintained or changed to a healthier purchase behaviour in the IS, compared to 46.5% in the CS.

Table 3. Weekly food and drink purchases in the cafeteria.

	Intervention Schools				Control Schools			
	Boys (n = 276)		Girls (n = 308)		Boys (n = 272)		Girls (n = 357)	
	T0	T1	T0	T1	T0	T1	T0	T1
Purchase of less healthy products, mean (SD)	1.50 (3.84)	0.92 (1.39)	1.41 (2.11)	1.39 (4.20)	1.43 (2.63)	1.72 (4.97)	0.91 (1.34)	1.04 (3.71)
Purchase of healthier products, mean (SD)	0.85 (2.98)	0.51 (2.23)	0.80 (1.82)	1.17 (3.75)	0.82 (2.83)	1.17 (4.38)	0.46 (1.10)	0.59 (3.78)
Bought healthier products of total bought purchases, %	36.2%	35.7%	36.2%	45.7%	36.4%	40.5%	33.6%	36.2%
Changes in purchases per week over time [a]								
Healthy score [a], %	50.0%		53.6%		51.5%		46.5%	

[a] From each student, the difference between T0 and T1 has been calculated. Equal or bigger change in healthier products compared to less healthy products has been defined as a healthy score.

3.4. Purchases at the Vending Machines

Data on self-reported purchase behaviour at vending machines were available for 1217 students (542 boys, 675 girls) (Table 4). In the IS, the boys and girls, respectively, bought on average 0.79 and 1.48 healthier, and 0.88 and 1.40 less healthy products per week in vending machines after the intervention. Boys and girls in the CS bought on average 1.13 and 0.87 healthier, and 1.40 and 0.83 less healthy products per week in vending machines after the intervention, respectively. After 6 months, in both the IS and CS, half of the boys maintained or changed to a healthier purchase behaviour (both 49.3%). Among girls, approximately half of the girls in the IS (47.3%) and CS (52.0%) maintained or changed to a healthier purchase behaviour after 6 months.

Table 4. Weekly food and drink purchases at the vending machine.

	Intervention Schools				Control Schools			
	Boys (n = 270)		Girls (n = 311)		Boys (n = 272)		Girls (n = 364)	
	T0	T1	T0	T1	T0	T1	T0	T1
Weekly purchases of less healthy products, mean (SD)	1.41 (3.03)	0.88 (2.34)	1.60 (2.84)	1.40 (3.31)	1.51 (2.44)	1.40 (4.21)	0.94 (1.78)	0.83 (1.37)
Weekly purchases of healthier products, mean (SD)	1.11 (3.13)	0.79 (2.36)	1.43 (2.40)	1.48 (3.59)	1.26 (2.59)	1.13 (2.85)	0.97 (1.49)	0.87 (1.45)
Bought healthier products of total bought products, %	44.1%	47.3%	47.2%	51.4%	45.5%	44.7%	50.8%	51.2%
Changes in purchases per week over time [a]								
Healthy score [a], %	49.3%		47.3%		49.3%		51.6%	

[a] From each student, the difference between T0 and T1 has been calculated. Equal or bigger change in healthier products compared to less healthy products has been defined as a healthy score.

3.5. Purchase Behaviour Analysed by Mixed Logistic Regression Analyses

The results of the performed mixed logistic regression analyses showed that the odds for a healthier purchase behaviour compared to less healthy purchase behaviour is approximately equal for students in the intervention and control schools (Table 5). In boys, we found odds ratios of 0.92 (95%CI 0.62;

1.36) for cafeteria purchases and 1.02 (95%CI 0.62; 1.67) for vending machine purchases. Girls showed an odds ratio of 1.29 (95%CI 0.85; 1.96) for the cafeteria and 0.84 (95%CI 0.62; 1.14) in vending machines purchases. Adjustment for demographic (model 2), behavioural (model 3) and environmental variables (model 4) did not materially change the results.

Table 5. Mixed logistic regression analyses on the effect of the intervention (ref. group is control group) on changes in purchase behaviour.

		Model 1 [b]		Model 2 [c]		Model 3 [d]		Model 4 [e]	
		OR	95% CI	OR	95% CI	OR	95% CI	OR	95% CI
Purchases cafeteria [a]	Boys (n = 548)	0.92	0.62; 1.36	0.94	0.67; 1.32	0.96	0.68; 1.35	0.92	0.63; 1.34
	Girls (n = 665)	1.29	0.85; 1.96	1.29	0.83; 1.96	1.31	0.85; 2.02	1.30	0.85; 2.00
Purchases vending machine [a]	Boys (n = 542)	1.02	0.62; 1.67	1.00	0.60; 1.67	1.03	0.62; 1.69	1.03	0.62; 1.71
	Girls (n = 675)	0.84	0.62; 1.14	0.81	0.59; 1.11	0.85	0.61; 1.19	0.85	0.58; 1.23

[a] Dichotomous outcome: healthier vs. less healthy changes in purchases over time. [b] Model 1 = mixed logistic regression analysis, corrected for school. [c] Model 2 = Model 1, plus corrected for demographic variables (age, education). [d] Model 3 = Model 2, plus corrected for behavioural determinants (attitude, subjective norm, perceived behavioural control, intention); [e] Model 4 = Model 3, plus corrected for environmental determinants (amount of money spent in school p/w, breakfast, food purchases outside school, drink purchases outside school, food brought from home, drinks brought from home).

The analyses to the effect of a healthier canteen (healthier versus less healthy (ref. group) availability in the cafeteria, vending machine or accessibility) on purchase behaviour showed OR's ranging from 0.87 (95%CI 0.61–1.26) for combined purchases in girls, to 1.27 (95%CI 0.75–2.17) for purchases in vending machines in boys (Table 6). Adjustment for demographic (model 2), behavioural (model 3) and environmental variables (model 4) again did not materially change the results.

Table 6. Mixed logistic regression analyses on the effect of a healthier canteen (ref. group not healthy) on changes in purchase behaviour.

		Model 1 [e]		Model 2 [f]		Model 3 [g]		Model 4 [h]	
		OR	95% CI	OR	95% CI	OR	95% CI	OR	95% CI
Purchases cafeteria [ab]	Boys (n = 548)	0.93	0.60; 1.44	1.02	0.69; 1.52	1.03	0.69; 1.53	1.01	0.66; 1.55
	Girls (n = 665)	1.13	0.70; 1.83	1.14	0.70; 1.86	1.14	0.70; 1.88	1.13	0.69; 1.86
Purchases vending machine [ac]	Boys (n = 542)	1.27	0.75; 2.17	1.18	0.67; 2.05	1.18	0.68; 2.03	1.21	0.69; 2.12
	Girls (n = 675)	1.06	0.74; 1.50	1.14	0.77; 1.69	1.18	0.79; 1.75	1.15	0.75; 1.78
Purchases cafeteria and vending machine [ad]	Boys (n = 620)	1.17	0.84; 1.62	1.19	0.83; 1.73	1.19	0.83; 1.70	1.14	0.79; 1.65
	Girls (n = 756)	0.87	0.61; 1.26	0.89	0.61; 1.28	0.90	0.62; 1.30	0.90	0.61; 1.34

[a] Dichotomous outcome: healthier vs. less healthy changes in purchases over time. [b] Healthier canteen, measured with the subtopic healthier products available in cafeteria (≥60%, <60% (ref. group)). [c] Healthier canteen, measured with the subtopic healthier products available at vending machines (≥60%, <60% (ref. group)). [d] Healthier canteen, measured with the subtopic fulfilled healthier accessibility criteria (≥60%, <60% (ref. group)). [e] Model 1 = mixed logistic regression analysis, corrected for school. [f] Model 2 = Model 1, plus corrected for demographic variables (age, education). [g] Model 3 = Model 2, plus corrected for behavioural determinants (attitude, subjective norm, perceived behavioural control, intention); [h] Model 4 = Model 3, plus corrected for environmental determinants (amount of money spent in school p/w, breakfast, food purchases outside school, drink purchases outside school, food brought from home, drinks brought from home).

4. Discussion

We investigated the effect of support in implementing the "Guidelines for Healthier Canteens" on changes in the school canteen (cafeteria and vending machine) and on food and drink purchases of students. Our results show that the support has led to actual changes in the availability and accessibility of healthier products in the canteen. We did not observe changes in students' purchase behaviour. The large majority of the students (90%) reported that they usually bring food or drinks from home. Most (approximately 80%) students reported buying food or drinks in school only once a week or less.

Schools that received support showed a larger increase in the availability of healthier products in the cafeteria compared to control schools. The intervention schools also complied with more criteria for the accessibility of healthier products than the control schools. These results are in line with previous studies which also showed that implementation support is likely to increase the use of guidelines, especially if it consists of multiple components and is both practice and theory-based [24,37]. The support we offered was targeted at different stakeholder-identified impeding factors related to implementation of the guidelines, such as knowledge and motivation. The process evaluation already showed that our implementation plan favourably influenced these factors [38].

With regard to vending machines, changes were smaller and present in fewer schools compared to changes in the cafeteria. This result may be explained by the fact that schools do not always own nor regulate the content of the vending machines themselves, but outsource them to external parties such as caterers or vending machine companies. Some schools were therefore unable to change the offering and position of products in the machine within the study period. Previous research showed that vending machines were healthier if appointments about the healthy offer were included in agreements with caterers or vending machine companies [39]. Making agreements about the availability and accessibility of healthy products in the machines is therefore recommended.

In contrast to the changes in the canteen, we did not observe relevant differences in change of healthier purchases between students in intervention and control schools, nor between students from schools with a healthier canteen compared to students from schools with a less healthy canteen. An explanation for these results might be that the duration of the intervention was between four to six months, which proved to be short for the schools to make changes, as we noticed that in most canteens changes were made just before the post-measurements. As a result, students did not have enough time to get used to the new situation and to adapt their purchases. The effects of a healthier canteen on students' purchases remain therefore unknown. Our results are in contrast with many other studies that show that increasing the offering of healthier products and changes in placement and promotion in favour of healthier products are likely to lead to healthier food choices among customers [4,40–43]. However, reviews identified that investigations yielded contradictory results [44], and they emphasize the low quality of the studies [43], making more research needed.

Changing dietary behaviour is complex and affected by multiple individual, social and environmental factors [45–47]—for example, the palatability, price and convenience of foods offered in environments that youth visit regularly, including the school canteen and shops around schools [13,45,48]. During adolescence, many factors that influence youth's dietary choices are changing: they become more independent, parental influence decreases and influence of peers increases, living environments expand, and they have more money to spend [49,50]. These changes provide opportunities to develop healthy dietary habits which are likely to sustain over time [51]. Even though our study did not show a relation between a healthier canteen and healthier purchase behaviour, we would recommend that healthier food choices should be facilitated in school canteens, including vending machines, a place that students visit regularly and where students can autonomously choose what they buy. This might influence student purchase behaviour directly at the school canteen or in shops around schools, and foresees in educating adolescents on healthy norms [52]. This enables all youth to experience that healthy eating is important, tasty and very common, which they can use throughout their life.

A strength of our study is that the support consisted of multiple implementation tools which stakeholders could decide to use, as well as when and how. Moreover, our study included tailored advice. Previous research has shown that both a combination of components and tailored advice could increase the likelihood of an effective implementation plan [37,53]. Other strengths of our study are the measurement of outcomes both on the canteen and student level and the separate analyses for boys and girls. In general, boys are more likely to make impulsive, intuitive changes [41]. In contrast, girls are more likely to overthink their choices, limiting the effect of an attractive food offering. In our study, subtle differences across gender were observed, with boys indicating buying food and drinks outside the school more often. However, this finding should be further explored in future studies.

There are also some study limitations that should be mentioned. First, the use of self-reported questionnaires to investigate purchase behaviour. These measurements are potentially subject to reporting bias and socially desirable answers, likely leading to smaller number of reported purchases overall and larger number of reported healthier products. Possibilities to measure the dietary behaviour of student more objectively and regularly include, for example, the use of meal observations, sales data or Ecological Momentary Assessment (EMA) [54,55]. We could not use these options due to feasibility constraints, e.g., making use of sales data was not possible as due to different registration systems. Another limitation is the study duration, which was four to six months. A study duration of at least one school year will align to the schools' daily practice and will give schools the opportunity to create a team of involved people, to embed actions and to make changes.

The fact that the intervention was individualized to the contextual factors and needs of each school is both a strength and limitation. Alignment of the advices to a school's situation might lead to a more useful support but can also make it more difficult to compare results between different intervention schools. Therefore, it is important to (1) describe the core intervention functions of each tool of the implementation plan to be able to support schools with the same support and (2) to measure if the tools has been delivered and used as planned [12,56,57]. In our case, the core elements of the intervention have been described in the study design [34]. In addition to the effect evaluation, we also evaluated the quality of implementation to assess whether schools received each implementation tool [38].

A final limitation includes the fact that, due to the skewness of our purchase data and the non-linearity of some of the relations under study, we decided to dichotomize our data. This negatively influenced the power, and led to some loss of information.

Based on our results, we recommend that future studies investigate the sustainability of supportive implementation of food environment policy. In addition, we recommend longer-term studies that assess changes in students' purchases inside, and in shops around, school, that appear after an adaptation period.

Our results confirm that adolescents in the Netherlands bring most food and drinks from home and additionally buy their food inside as well as outside school. Attention to the home environment and the environment around school is therefore needed. The complexity of the food environment at schools within this broader food environment makes the use of whole system-based approaches important [13,46]. Different relevant stakeholders such as parents, shopkeepers, and local policy makers should be actively involved in this approach. Moreover, a healthy school environment not only consists of a healthy canteen, including vending machines, but also includes food education, integration with other health promotion school policies [58]. This is important, as schools contribute to the personal development of youth, wherein learning about making choices with regard to a healthy lifestyle in an obesogenic environment is an essential part.

5. Conclusions

This study investigated the changes in Dutch school canteens and self-reported student purchase behaviour after support to implement the Guidelines for Healthier Canteens compared to no support. We conclude that such support appears to contribute to healthier canteens. Our results did not show an effect of the implementation on healthier students' purchase behaviour, perhaps due to the short time between the changes made in the canteen and our follow-up measurements. Due to the fact that this study was performed in collaboration with the Netherlands Nutrition Centre and involved stakeholders, our research results are likely to lead to implementation in daily practice. More system-based approaches are warranted to be able to influence students' dietary behaviour. Additionally, long-term research to investigate the effects of healthier school canteens are needed.

Author Contributions: C.M.R., E.L.V. and J.C.S. designed the research. I.J.E. conducted the research, supported by S.M.J. and L.V. I.J.E. performed the data analysis, supported by M.R.d.B. I.J.E. drafted the manuscript, and all other authors helped refine the manuscript. All authors have read and agreed to the published version of the manuscript.

Funding: This research was funded by the Netherlands Organisation for Health Research and Development [ZonMw, Grant Number 50-53100-98-043].

Acknowledgments: We thank all schools, coordinators, school canteen advisors, students and other involved stakeholders who participated in this study. We also thank Renate van Zoonen and our Health Sciences students (Tamara Coppenhagen, Samantha Holt, Katelyn Sadee and Andrea Thoonsen) who supported us in the gathering of data.

Conflicts of Interest: The authors declare no conflict of interest. The funders had no role in the design of the study; in the collection, analyses, or interpretation of data; in the writing of the manuscript, or in the decision to publish the results.

References

1. Storcksdieck, S.; Kardakis, T.; Wollgast, J.; Nelson, M.; Caldeira, S. *Mapping of National School Food Policies across the EU28 Plus Norway and Switzerland*; European Commission, EUR 26621 EN, Joint Research Centre, Institute for Health and Consumer Protection: Luxembourg, 2014; ISSN 18319–42.
2. Thaler, R.H.; Sunstein, C.R. *Nudge: Improving Decisions about Health, Wealth, and Happiness*; Yale University Press: Connecticut, CT, USA, 2008.
3. Powell, L.M.; Chriqui, J.F.; Khan, T.; Wada, R.; Chaloupka, F.J. Assessing the potential effectiveness of food and beverage taxes and subsidies for improving public health: A systematic review of prices, demand and body weight outcomes. *Obes. Rev.* **2013**, *14*, 110–128. [CrossRef] [PubMed]
4. Grech, A.; Allman-Farinelli, M.A. Systematic literature review of nutrition interventions in vending machines that encourage consumers to make healthier choices. *Obes. Rev.* **2015**, *16*, 1030–1041. [CrossRef] [PubMed]
5. Driessen, C.E.; Cameron, A.J.; Thornton, L.E.; Lai, S.K.; Barnett, L.M. Effect of changes to the school food environment on eating behaviours and/or body weight in children: A systematic review. *Obes. Rev.* **2014**, *15*, 968–982. [CrossRef] [PubMed]
6. Kessler, H.S. Simple interventions to improve healthy eating behaviors in the school cafeteria. *Nutr. Rev.* **2016**, *74*, 198–209. [CrossRef]
7. Micha, R.; Karageorgou, D.; Bakogianni, I.; Trichia, E.; Whitsel, L.P.; Story, M.; Penalvo, J.L.; Mozaffarian, D. Effectiveness of school food environment policies on children's dietary behaviors: A systematic review and meta-analysis. *PLoS ONE* **2018**, *13*, e0194555. [CrossRef]
8. Masse, L.C.; Naiman, D.; Naylor, P.J. From policy to practice: Implementation of physical activity and food policies in schools. *Int. J. Behav. Nutr. Phys. Act.* **2013**, *10*, 71. [CrossRef]
9. de Silva-Sanigorski, A.; Breheny, T.; Jones, L.; Lacy, K.; Kremer, P.; Carpenter, L.; Bolton, K.; Prosser, L.; Gibbs, L.; Waters, E.; et al. Government food service policies and guidelines do not create healthy school canteens. *Aust. N. Z. J. Public Health* **2011**, *35*, 117–121. [CrossRef]
10. Leeman, J.; Wiecha, J.L.; Vu, M.; Blitstein, J.L.; Allgood, S.; Lee, S.; Merlo, C. School health implementation tools: A mixed methods evaluation of factors influencing their use. *Implement. Sci.* **2018**, *13*, 48. [CrossRef]
11. Wolfenden, L.; Nathan, N.K.; Sutherland, R.; Yoong, S.L.; Hodder, R.K.; Wyse, R.J.; Delaney, T.; Grady, A.; Fielding, A.; Tzelepis, F.; et al. Strategies for enhancing the implementation of school-based policies or practices targeting risk factors for chronic disease. *Cochrane Database Syst. Rev.* **2017**, *11*, Cd011677. [CrossRef]
12. McIsaac, J.-L.D.; Hernandez, K.J.; Kirk, S.F.L.; Curran, J.A. Interventions to Support System-level Implementation of Health Promoting Schools: A Scoping Review. *Int. J. Environ. Res. Public Health* **2016**, *13*, 200. [CrossRef]
13. Hermans, R.C.J.; Smit, K.; van den Broek, N.; Evenhuis, I.J.; Veldhuis, L. Adolescents' Food Purchasing Patterns in The School Food Environment: Examining the Role of Perceived Relationship Support and Maternal Monitoring. *Nutrients* **2020**, *12*, 733. [CrossRef]
14. Mensink, F.; Schwinghammer, S.A.; Smeets, A. The Healthy School Canteen programme: A promising intervention to make the school food environment healthier. *J. Environ. Public Health* **2012**, *2012*, 415746. [CrossRef] [PubMed]
15. Milder, I.E.; Mikolajczak, J.; van den Berg, S.W.; van de Veen-van Hofwegen, M.; Bemelmans, W.J. Food supply and actions to improve dietary behaviour of students—A comparison between secondary schools participating or not participating in the 'Healthy School Canteen Program'. *Public Health Nutr.* **2014**, *18*, 198–207. [CrossRef]
16. Van Rijn, M.J. Kamerbrief Over De Gezondheidseisen Van Schoolkantine [Letter to the Parlement about Health Regulations in School Canteens]. Available online: https://www.rijksoverheid.nl/documenten (accessed on 3 February 2017).

17. Geurts, M.; Brants, H.; Milder, I. De Voedingsomgeving op Scholen: De Stand Van Zaken in Het Voortgezet Onderwijs En Middelbaar Beroepsonderwijs Anno 2015. [the Food Environment at Schools: The State of Art in Secondary (Vocational) Education Anno 2015]. Available online: http://www.rivm.nl/Documenten_en_publicaties/Wetenschappelijk/Rapporten/2016/mei/De_voedingsomgeving_op_scholen_De_stand_van_zaken_in_het_voortgezet_onderwijs_en_middelbaar_beroepsonderwijs_anno_2015 (accessed on 7 December 2018).
18. iResearch, Inventarisatie Van Veranderingen in Schoolkantines Na Bezoek En Advies Van De Schoolkantine Brigade [Inventarisation of Changes in School Canteens after a Visit and Advise of the School Canteen Brigade, 2014]. Available online: https://static1.squarespace.com/static/5883d149e3df28fd7860bf14/t/590c4a96f7e0ab1d6d76a068/1493977754205/Inventarisatie+van+veranderingen+in+schoolkantine+%282014%29.pdf (accessed on 10 August 2020).
19. Veldhuis, L.; Mensink, F.; Wolvers, D. *Guidelines for Healthier Canteens, Fact Sheet*; Netherlands Nutrition Centre: The Hague, The Netherlands, 2017; Available online: https://www.voedingscentrum.nl/Assets/Uploads/voedingscentrum/Documents/Professionals/Pers/Factsheets/English/Fact%20sheet%20Guidelines%20for%20Healthier%20Canteens.pdf (accessed on 10 June 2020).
20. Brink, E.; van Rossum, C.; Postma-Smeets, A.; Stafleu, A.; Wolvers, D.; van Dooren, C.; Toxopeus, I.; Buurma-Rethans, E.; Geurts, M.; Ocké, M. Development of healthy and sustainable food-based dietary guidelines for the Netherlands. *Public Health Nutr.* **2019**, *22*, 2419–2435. [CrossRef] [PubMed]
21. Evenhuis, I.J.; Vyth, E.L.; van Nassau, F.; Veldhuis, L.; Westerman, M.J.; Seidell, J.C.; Renders, C.M. What do secondary schools need to create healthier canteens? The development of an implementation plan. Under review. 2020.
22. Evenhuis, I.J.; Veldhuis, L.; Jacobs, S.M.; Renders, C.M.; Seidell, J.C.; Schuit-Van Raamsdonk, H. Brengt de Kantinescan Aanbod En Uitstraling Goed in Kaart? [Is the Canteen Scan Able to Map the Availability and Accessibility Properly?]. Available online: https://gezondeschoolkantine.voedingscentrum.nl/Assets/Uploads/de-gezonde-kantine/Documents/Factsheet%20kantinescan.pdf (accessed on 23 November 2019).
23. Schulz, K.F.; Altman, D.G.; Moher, D. CONSORT 2010 Statement: Updated guidelines for reporting parallel group randomised trials. *BMC Med.* **2010**, *8*, 18. [CrossRef] [PubMed]
24. Grol, R.; Wensing, M.; Eccles, M.; Davis, D. *Improving Patient Care: The Implementation of Change in Health Care*; Wiley: Hoboken, NJ, USA, 2013.
25. Evenhuis, I.J.; Wezenbeek, N.L.W.J.; Vyth, E.L.; Veldhuis, L.; Poelman, M.P.; Wolvers, D.; Seidell, J.C.; Renders, C.M. Development of the 'Canteen Scan': An online tool to monitor implementation of healthy canteen guidelines. *BMC Public Health* **2018**, *18*, 1109. [CrossRef]
26. Kremers, S.P.; de Bruijn, G.J.; Visscher, T.L.; van Mechelen, W.; de Vries, N.K.; Brug, J. Environmental influences on energy balance-related behaviors: A dual-process view. *Int. J. Behav. Nutr. Phys. Act.* **2006**, *3*, 9. [CrossRef]
27. Janssen, E.H.; Singh, A.S.; van Nassau, F.; Brug, J.; van Mechelen, W.; Chinapaw, M.J. Test-retest reliability and construct validity of the DOiT (Dutch Obesity Intervention in Teenagers) questionnaire: Measuring energy balance-related behaviours in Dutch adolescents. *Public Health Nutr.* **2014**, *17*, 277–286. [CrossRef] [PubMed]
28. Singh, A.S.; Vik, F.N.; Chinapaw, M.J.; Uijtdewilligen, L.; Verloigne, M.; Fernandez-Alvira, J.M.; Stomfai, S.; Manios, Y.; Martens, M.; Brug, J. Test-retest reliability and construct validity of the ENERGY-child questionnaire on energy balance-related behaviours and their potential determinants: The ENERGY-project. *Int. J. Behav. Nutr. Phys. Act.* **2011**, *8*, 136. [CrossRef] [PubMed]
29. Van Assema, P.; Brug, J.; Ronda, G.; Steenhuis, I. The relative validity of a short Dutch questionnaire as a means to categorize adults and adolescents to total and saturated fat intake. *J. Hum. Nutr. Diet* **2001**, *14*, 377–390. [CrossRef] [PubMed]
30. Bogers, R.P.; Van Assema, P.; Kester, A.D.; Westerterp, K.R.; Dagnelie, P.C. Reproducibility, validity, and responsiveness to change of a short questionnaire for measuring fruit and vegetable intake. *Am. J. Epidemiol.* **2004**, *159*, 900–909. [CrossRef] [PubMed]
31. Martens, M.K.; van Assema, P.; Brug, J. Why do adolescents eat what they eat? Personal and social environmental predictors of fruit, snack and breakfast consumption among 12१-4-year-old Dutch students. *Public Health Nutr.* **2005**, *8*, 1258–1265. [CrossRef]
32. Drennan, J. Cognitive interviewing: Verbal data in the design and pretesting of questionnaires. *J. Adv. Nurs.* **2003**, *42*, 57–63. [CrossRef]

33. Tavakol, M.; Dennick, R. Making sense of Cronbach's alpha. *Int. J. Med. Educ.* **2011**, *2*, 53–55. [CrossRef] [PubMed]
34. Evenhuis, I.J.; Vyth, E.L.; Veldhuis, L.; Seidell, J.C.; Renders, C.M. Development and evaluation of the implementation of guidelines for healthier canteens in Dutch Secondary Schools: Study protocol of a Quasi-experimental trial. *Front. Public Health* **2019**, *7*, 254. [CrossRef] [PubMed]
35. Twisk, J.W.R. *Applied Multilevel Analysis: A Practical Guide for Medical Researchers*; Cambridge University Press: Cambridge, UK, 2006.
36. Khambalia, A.Z.; Dickinson, S.; Hardy, L.L.; Gill, T.; Baur, L.A. A synthesis of existing systematic reviews and meta-analyses of school-based behavioural interventions for controlling and preventing obesity. *Obes. Rev.* **2012**, *13*, 214–233. [CrossRef]
37. Powell, B.J.; Beidas, R.S.; Lewis, C.C.; Aarons, G.A.; McMillen, J.C.; Proctor, E.K.; Mandell, D.S. Methods to improve the selection and tailoring of implementation strategies. *J. Behav. Health Serv. Res.* **2015**, *44*, 117–194. [CrossRef]
38. Evenhuis, I.J.; Vyth, E.L.; Veldhuis, L.; Jacobs, S.M.; Seidell, J.C.; Renders, C.M. Implementation of guidelines for healthier canteens in Dutch Secondary Schools: A process evaluation. *Int. J. Environ. Res. Public Health* **2019**, *16*, 4509. [CrossRef]
39. Lane, C.; Naylor, P.-J.; Tomlin, D.; Kirk, S.; Hanning, R.; Masse, L.; Olstad, D.L.; Prowse, R.; Caswell, S.; Jarvis, S.; et al. Healthy vending contracts: Do localized policy approaches improve the nutrition environment in publicly funded recreation and sport facilities? *Prev. Med. Rep.* **2019**, *16*, 100967. [CrossRef]
40. Bucher, T.; Collins, C.; Rollo, M.E.; McCaffrey, T.A.; De Vlieger, N.; Van der Bend, D.; Truby, H.; Perez-Cueto, F.J. Nudging consumers towards healthier choices: A systematic review of positional influences on food choice. *Br. J. Nutr.* **2016**, *115*, 2252–2263. [CrossRef] [PubMed]
41. Arno, A.; Thomas, S. The efficacy of nudge theory strategies in influencing adult dietary behaviour: A systematic review and meta-analysis. *BMC Public Health* **2016**, *16*, 676. [CrossRef] [PubMed]
42. Grivois-Shah, R.; Gonzalez, J.R.; Khandekar, S.P.; Howerter, A.L.; O'Connor, P.A.; Edwards, B.A. Impact of healthy vending machine options in a large community health organization. *Am. J. Health Promot.* **2018**, *32*, 1425–1430. [CrossRef] [PubMed]
43. Hollands, G.J.; Carter, P.; Anwer, S.; King, S.E.; Jebb, S.A.; Ogilvie, D.; Shemilt, I.; Higgins, J.P.T.; Marteau, T.M. Altering the availability or proximity of food, alcohol, and tobacco products to change their selection and consumption. *Cochrane Database Syst. Rev.* **2019**, *9*, Cd012573.
44. von Philipsborn, P.; Stratil, J.M.; Burns, J.; Busert, L.K.; Pfadenhauer, L.M.; Polus, S.; Holzapfel, C.; Hauner, H.; Rehfuess, E. Environmental interventions to reduce the consumption of sugar-sweetened beverages and their effects on health. *Cochrane Database Syst. Rev.* **2019**, *6*, Cd012292. [CrossRef]
45. Story, M.; Kaphingst, K.M.; Robinson-O'Brien, R.; Glanz, K. Creating healthy food and eating environments: Policy and environmental approaches. *Annu. Rev. Public Health* **2008**, *29*, 253–272. [CrossRef]
46. Townsend, N.; Foster, C. Developing and applying a socio-ecological model to the promotion of healthy eating in the school. *Public Health Nutr.* **2013**, *16*, 1101–1108. [CrossRef]
47. Larson, N.; Story, M. A review of environmental influences on food choices. *Ann. Behav. Med.* **2009**, *38* (Suppl. S1), S56–S73. [CrossRef]
48. Hermans, R.C.J.; de Bruin, H.; Larsen, J.K.; Mensink, F.; Hoek, A.C. Adolescents' Responses to a school-based prevention program promoting healthy eating at school. *Front. Public Health* **2017**, *5*, 309. [CrossRef]
49. Draper, C.E.; Grobler, L.; Micklesfield, L.K.; Norris, S.A. Impact of social norms and social support on diet, physical activity and sedentary behaviour of adolescents: A scoping review. *Child Care Health Dev.* **2015**, *41*, 654–667. [CrossRef]
50. Meiklejohn, S.; Ryan, L.; Palermo, C. A systematic review of the impact of multi-strategy nutrition education programs on health and nutrition of adolescents. *J. Nutr. Educ. Behav.* **2016**, *48*, 631–646.e1. [CrossRef]
51. Craigie, A.M.; Lake, A.A.; Kelly, S.A.; Adamson, A.J.; Mathers, J.C. Tracking of obesity-related behaviours from childhood to adulthood: A systematic review. *Maturitas* **2011**, *70*, 266–284. [CrossRef] [PubMed]
52. Higgs, S. Social norms and their influence on eating behaviours. *Appetite* **2015**, *86*, 38–44. [CrossRef] [PubMed]

53. Yoong, S.L.; Nathan, N.; Wolfenden, L.; Wiggers, J.; Reilly, K.; Oldmeadow, C.; Wyse, R.; Sutherland, R.; Delaney, T.; Butler, P.; et al. CAFÉ: A multicomponent audit and feedback intervention to improve implementation of healthy food policy in primary school canteens: A randomised controlled trial. *Int. J. Behav. Nutr. Phys. Act.* **2016**, *13*, 126. [CrossRef] [PubMed]
54. Tugault-Lafleur, C.N.; Black, J.L.; Barr, S.I. A systematic review of methods to assess children's diets in the school context. *Adv. Nutr.* **2017**, *8*, 63–79. [CrossRef]
55. Mason, T.B.; Do, B.; Wang, S.; Dunton, G.F. Ecological momentary assessment of eating and dietary intake behaviors in children and adolescents: A systematic review of the literature. *Appetite* **2020**, *144*, 104465. [CrossRef]
56. van Nassau, F.; Singh, A.S.; van Mechelen, W.; Brug, J.; Chinapaw, M.J. Implementation evaluation of school-based obesity prevention programmes in youth; how, what and why? *Public Health Nutr.* **2015**, *18*, 1531–1534. [CrossRef]
57. Saunders, R.P.; Evans, M.H.; Joshi, P. Developing a process-evaluation plan for assessing health promotion program implementation: A how-to guide. *Health Promot. Pract.* **2005**, *6*, 134–147. [CrossRef]
58. Alaimo, K.; Oleksyk, S.C.; Drzal, N.B.; Golzynski, D.L.; Lucarelli, J.F.; Wen, Y.; Velie, E.M. Effects of changes in lunch-time competitive foods, nutrition practices, and nutrition policies on low-income middle-school children's diets. *Child. Obes.* **2013**, *9*, 509–523. [CrossRef]

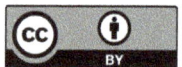

© 2020 by the authors. Licensee MDPI, Basel, Switzerland. This article is an open access article distributed under the terms and conditions of the Creative Commons Attribution (CC BY) license (http://creativecommons.org/licenses/by/4.0/).

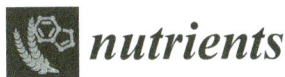

Article

Do Parent–Child Dyads with Excessive Body Mass Differ from Dyads with Normal Body Mass in Perceptions of Obesogenic Environment?

Karolina Zarychta [1,*], Anna Banik [1], Ewa Kulis [1], Monika Boberska [1], Theda Radtke [2], Carina K. Y. Chan [3], Karolina Lobczowska [1] and Aleksandra Luszczynska [1,4,*]

1. Wroclaw Faculty of Psychology, SWPS University of Social Sciences and Humanities, 53-238 Wroclaw, Poland; abanik@swps.edu.pl (A.B.); ekulis@swps.edu.pl (E.K.); mboberska@swps.edu.pl (M.B.); klobczowska@swps.edu.pl (K.L.)
2. School of Psychology and Psychotherapy, Witten/Herdecke University, 58456 Witten, Germany; Theda.Radtke@uni-wh.de
3. School of Psychology and Public Health, La Trobe University, Flora Hill, VIC 3550, Australia; Carina.Chan@latrobe.edu.au
4. Trauma, Health, & Hazards Center, University of Colorado at Colorado Springs, Colorado Springs, CO 80918, USA
* Correspondence: kzarychta1@swps.edu.pl (K.Z.); aluszczy@uccs.edu (A.L.)

Received: 15 June 2020; Accepted: 17 July 2020; Published: 19 July 2020

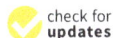

Abstract: Background: This study addressed differences between parent–child dyads with excessive body mass (overweight or obesity) and dyads with normal body mass in obesity determinants, derived from social-ecological models. It was hypothesized that parents and their 5–11 years-old children with excessive body mass would (1) report lower availability of healthy food at home, (2) perceive fewer school/local community healthy eating promotion programs, (3) report lower persuasive value of food advertising. Methods: Data were collected twice (T1, baseline; T2, 10-month follow-up), including $n = 129$ parent–child dyads with excessive body mass and $n = 377$ parent–child dyads with normal body mass. Self-reported data were collected from parents and children; with body weight and height assessed objectively. General linear models (including analysis of variance with repeated measures) were performed to test the hypotheses. Results: Compared to dyads with normal body mass, dyads of parents and children with excessive body mass perceived lower availability of healthy food at home and fewer healthy eating promotion programs at school/local community (T1 and T2). These effects remained significant after controlling for sociodemographic variables. No significant differences in persuasive value of food advertising were found. Conclusions: Perceptions of availability of healthy food at home and healthy nutrition promotion may be relatively low in parent–child dyads with excessive weight which, in turn, may constitute a risk factor for maintenance of obesity.

Keywords: childhood obesity; parent–child dyads; food availability; advertising; healthy diet; promotion programs

1. Introduction

The prevalence of overweight and obesity among children has doubled in recent decades, both in developed and developing countries [1,2]. Obesity is often considered as a result of an exposure of children to an unhealthy environment (also called obesogenic environment) and children's perceptions and responses to it [2,3]. The role of the obesogenic environment and the ways it is perceived are highlighted in several theoretical approaches explaining childhood obesity. For example, according to the ecological model of predictors of childhood obesity [4], characteristics of at-home-environment (e.g., types of food available at home), and out-of-home environment (e.g., community, demographic and societal characteristics, food policies at school or local community, policies regulating food advertising to children, etc.) represent the facets of a broader context, interacting with each other in the development and maintenance of childhood overweight/obesity.

Availability of various types of food at home is often considered a key determinant of children's nutrition behaviors [4,5]. In turn, unhealthy nutrition (diet low in fruit and vegetable intake, and high in energy-dense food intake) is significantly associated with excessive body mass [6]. Systematic reviews of environmental correlates of obesity-related behaviors in children showed that the availability of healthy food at home was associated with higher children's fruit and vegetable intake [7,8]. On the other hand, home availability of sugar-sweetened beverages was associated with a higher intake of these products by 8- to 13-year-olds [9], and intake of sweet and savory snacks among 12- to 13-year-old girls [10]. Lower perceived at-home availability of snacks and sweetened beverages was directly associated with lower intake of respective food among 10- to 11-year-olds [11]. Most of the studies, however, accounted only for children's perceptions of home food availability and did not consider parental perceptions. Parental perceptions may operate together with children's perceptions of availability, as parents are the key food gatekeepers at home. Furthermore, it is unclear whether children's and parental perceptions of availability of healthy food differ depending on body mass status of parent and child (normal body mass versus excessive body mass, i.e., overweight or obesity).

It is unclear if parents and their children with normal differ from those with excessive body mass in terms of their perceptions of availability of healthy food at home between. A cross-sectional study comparing 35 families with parents and children with excessive body mass with 47 families with normal body mass indicated that lower vegetable availability (rated by an independent observer) was associated with obesity issues [12]. This study, however, does not clarify how availability was perceived by parents and children. Determining the levels of parental and child perceptions of food availability at homes of families with overweight parents and children may be of practical relevance. Identifying if families differ in perceptions of at-home and out-of-home environment (depending on body mass status of family members) would allow designing more effective obesity prevention programs, targeting the general population, and family treatment programs for parents and children with excessive body mass [13].

Children's healthy nutrition and favorable changes in body mass are also shaped by perceptions of out-of-home environment, such as school and local community promotion of healthy eating which, in turn, may influence both parents' and children's behaviors and cognitions related to healthy food intake [4]. The World Health Organization [2] has recommended comprehensive programs promoting the intake of healthy food and a reduction of unhealthy food intake in schools as the key environmental strategies to address childhood obesity. An analysis of the effectiveness of 124 nutrition and physical activity programs indicated that the programs accounting for three settings (community, school, and home) were the most effective in terms of childhood obesity prevention [14]. The target population's awareness of out-of-home programs promoting healthy nutrition may be a condition for the successful implementation of such programs and their effectiveness [15]. Previous dyadic research has found out that parental perceptions of school and community-based physical-activity promotion programs are related to lower body mass in children [16]. It is unclear, however, whether perceptions of availability of nutrition programs may differ among parents and children with excessive body mass versus normal body mass.

Previous research investigating children's perception of healthy food environment indicated that those who are 5–9 years old perceive their parents and mass media as the primary source of nutrition information [17]. Thus, at-home availability of healthy food and perceptions of food advertising have been investigated in children as young as 5–9 years old [17,18]. Although teachers are reported by children as the source of information on healthy food, qualitative research did not elicit perceptions of programs at local community or at the school setting as relevant sources of information about health or healthy diet among young children [17]. Therefore, an adequate approach to investigate perceptions of

5–11 years old children may be to focus on at-home availability of food or perceptions of advertising, instead of testing young children's perceptions of a broader environment (e.g., local community).

In parallel to perceptions of food availability at home and availability of nutrition programs at the local community, perceptions of advertising have been shown to determine children's nutrition behaviors [19,20]. Food marketing practices are considered an environmental factor that can affect adults' and children's beliefs, attitudes, and knowledge about healthy eating, and their body mass [21]. Children's food decisions are made in an environment where food is extensively advertised to stimulate consumption at home, and where respective types of food are perceived as easily available [22,23]. Compared to children with normal body mass, 4–11-year-olds with excessive body mass had a higher recognition of energy-dense food advertisements [24] or food advertisements in general [25]. On the other hand, research suggested that children who are obese may know less about the persuasive value of food advertising [20]. Parents and their perceptions of advertising may play a role in modifying the impact of food advertising on children, e.g., through explaining the nature and selling intent of advertising [26,27]. To date, research has not clarified whether parental and child perceptions of advertising (e.g., its persuasiveness) of food may differ between families with parent and child with excessive body mass, compared to those with normal body mass.

This study investigated the differences between parent–child dyads with excessive body mass and parent–child dyads with normal body mass in terms of: perceptions of at-home environment (availability of healthy food at home) and out-of-home environment (perceptions of school and local community promotion of healthy eating, perceptions of advertising in terms of its persuasiveness). In particular, it was hypothesized that, compared to parents and children from dyads with normal body mass, parents and their 5–11-year-old children from dyads with excessive body mass would (1) report lower availability of healthy food at their homes, (2) perceive fewer healthy eating promotion programs at schools and local community, (3) report lower persuasive value of food advertising.

Moreover, we explored a 10-month stability of differences in perceptions of at-home and out-of-home environment, testing if any changes over time would occur in parent–child dyads with normal body mass and dyads with excessive body mass. During middle childhood (5–11 years old), children's perceptions of healthy food environment are influenced by their age and the developmental stage [28] and, in consequence, these perceptions may change over one year. Thus, it was investigated whether children's perceptions of at-home environment and perceptions of food advertising would change over a 10-month period. Finally, to account for the potential confounding effects of parental education, parental perceived economic status, and the location of the residence [29], the hypothesized effects were controlled for possible sociodemographic covariates.

2. Materials and Methods

2.1. Participants

Parents (98.6%) or legal guardians (1.4%; henceforth called "parents") that were the main caregivers in terms of preparing food and time spent with a child were included in the study as well as their 5–11-year-old children. The initially recruited sample included 924 dyads (1848 individuals) consisting of parents and their 5–11-year-old children participating in the measurement at Time 1 (T1, baseline), and 571 dyads (1142 individuals) at Time 2 (T2, 10-month follow-up). Data were collected as a part of a larger study testing parental and child psychosocial determinants of body mass [30,31].

At T1, the majority of parents ($n = 547$, 59.2%) from the initially recruited sample had normal body mass, $n = 355$ (38.4%) had excessive body mass, and $n = 22$ (2.4%) had underweight. Among children, $n = 617$ (66.8%) had normal body mass, $n = 222$ (24.0%) had excessive body mass, and $n = 85$ (9.2%) had underweight after adjusting for age and gender in relation to International Obesity Task Force cut-off points [32]. All participants were Caucasian (as 98% of Poland's population [33]).

Dyads in which either parent or child had underweight ($n = 126$ dyads) were excluded from further analyses, as the factors underlying underweight were not investigated in this study. The remaining sample was divided into the subgroups of parents and children recruited form dyads with a specific body mass composition (e.g., both parent and child with excessive body mass). The dyads with the mixed body mass composition (e.g., consisting of a parent with obesity and a child with normal body mass) were included in additional analyses only (see Appendix A). The mixed body mass composition dyads included n = 193 dyads with parents with excessive body mass and children with normal body mass as well as n = 88 dyads with parents with normal body mass and children with excessive body mass.

The main analyzed sample consisted of N = 506 parent–child dyads (1012 individuals), including n = 129 dyads with parent and child who both had excessive body mass and n = 377 dyads with parent and child who both had normal body mass. In this study, we use the term 'dyads', to highlight the specificity of the subgroup (dyads were not treated as the unit of analysis).

Demographic characteristics of the main analyzed sample (N = 506 dyads) and both subsamples (dyads with normal body mass, dyads with excessive body mass), as well as the differences between the subsamples are presented in Table A1.

2.2. Procedure

The convenience sample was recruited in 26 locations in six administrative regions of Poland representing three levels of the mean household income (the average, below the average, above the average [33]). Data from parents and children were collected at schools, in general practitioners' offices, or at participants' homes. In cases where a school was the location of data collection, dyads with children attending classes in the respective school (but also dyads with children attending other schools but living in the local community) were invited and recruited. In cases of dyads recruited via general practitioners' offices, children attended various schools in the respective city/town.

Study personnel informed participants about the research aims and procedure. Parents provided informed consent (with respect to their own and their child's participation) and the child gave assent to participate in the study. Afterward, de-identified codes were assigned to participants to secure their anonymity across the measurement points. Younger children (aged 5–8) were interviewed using a structured interview while older children (aged 9–11) completed a questionnaire. Parents completed the questionnaires separately from children (e.g., in a different room). Participants' body mass and height were measured with certified scales and rods at both T1 and T2.

At both T1 and T2 (10 months later), parents provided their data referring to their perceptions of at-home environment (perceptions of availability of healthy food at home) and out-of-home environment (perceptions of school and local community promotion of healthy eating, perceptions of advertising in terms of its persuasiveness). Children provided their data with reference to perceptions of availability of healthy food at home, and perceptions of food advertising at both T1 and T2. During the follow-up, study personnel revisited the study sites after contacting parents by phone. The attrition occurred due to parental decisions to change the school/general practitioner or parental or children's decisions to discontinue their participation at T2.

The study was approved by the Internal Review Board at SWPS University of Social Sciences and Humanities, Wroclaw, Poland. All procedures were in accordance with the ethical standards of the institutional research ethics committee and in line with the 1964 Helsinki declaration and its later amendments.

2.3. Materials

Variables measured in both members of the dyad were assessed with the same measures [34]. The feasibility of item-wording for children was tested in a pilot study with n = 18 children (aged 5–11 years old) and found to be satisfactory.

2.3.1. Parental and Child Perceptions of Availability of Healthy Food at Home (T1 and T2)

Parental and child perceptions of availability of healthy food at home were measured by four items, each based on Comprehensive Feeding Practices Questionnaire (CFPQ [35]), e.g., "Most of the food I keep in the house is healthy"). Participants were provided with a definition of healthy food, indicating that healthy meals include a lot of raw fruit and vegetable but limited amounts of products with added sugar or salt (e.g., limited amount of salty or sweet snacks) and a limited amount highly processed products (e.g., sausage, cheese). The responses ranged from 1 (*definitely not*) to 4 (*definitely yes*). Higher scores represent higher levels of parental or child perception of availability of healthy food at home. The mean item score for parents was $M = 3.05$, $SD = 0.40$, $\alpha = 0.54$ at T1 and $M = 3.07$, $SD = 0.32$, $\alpha = 0.56$ at T2; for children it was $M = 2.84$, $SD = 0.44$, $\alpha = 0.56$ at T1 and $M = 3.07$, $SD = 0.32$, $\alpha = 0.58$ at T2. Although the reliability coefficients are relatively low, they may be considered acceptable considering the scales had only 4 items [36].

2.3.2. Parental Perceptions of School and Local Community Promotion of Healthy Eating (T1 and T2)

Parental perceptions of school and local community promotion of healthy eating was measured with two items based on Stok et al. [37]: "At school my child draws attention to the issues of healthy revival" and "A lot of things are being done to help me and my child to eat more healthily". The responses ranged from 1 (*definitely not*) to 4 (*definitely yes*). Higher scores represent a higher level of parental perceptions of school and local community promotion of healthy eating. The mean item score was $M = 2.80$, $SD = 0.67$, $r_s = 0.58$ at T1 and $M = 2.81$, $SD = 0.53$, $r_s = 0.51$ at T2.

2.3.3. Parental and Child Perceptions of Food Advertising (T1 and T2)

Parental and child perceptions of food advertising (its persuasive value) were measured with one item each based on Food Advertising Questionnaire [38], e.g., "Advertising makes food products seem better than they really are". The responses ranged from 1 (*definitely not*) to 4 (*definitely yes*). The higher scores represent the higher levels of parental or child knowledge of persuasive value of food advertising. The item score for parents was $M = 2.42$, $SD = 0.98$ at T1 and $M = 2.51$, $SD = 1.06$ at T2; for children it was $M = 2.57$, $SD = 0.80$ at T1, and $M = 2.51$, $SD = 0.80$ at T2.

2.3.4. Body Weight and Height (T1)

Child and parental body weight and height were assessed with standard medically approved telescopic height measuring rods and floor scales (scale type: BF-100 or BF-25; Beurer, Germany, measurement error <5%). For children, age and gender specific BMI z-score values were calculated with WHO AnthroPlus macro [39]. For parents, BMI was calculated using body weight and height: $BMI = weight\ (kg)/height^2\ (m^2)$.

2.3.5. Sociodemographic Variables (T1)

Parental education was measured with a 5-point scale, ranging from 1 to 5 (primary, uncompleted secondary/vocational, secondary, ≤3 years of higher education, ≥4 years of higher education). Higher scores indicate higher education. Perceived economic status was assessed with one item, "Compared to the average economic situation of the family in the country, how would you rate the economic situation of your family", with responses ranging from 1 (*much below the average*) to 5 (*much above the average*). Higher scores indicate a higher economic status. The size of the place of residence was assessed with one question, "What is the number of inhabitants in the city/town/village where your family lives" with 4-item response scale (<10,000 inhabitants; between 10,000 and 100,000 inhabitants; between 100,000 and 500,000 inhabitants; >500,000 inhabitants). Higher scores indicate a larger population living in the place of residence.

2.4. Data Analysis

Assuming effect sizes of $f = 0.15$, power of 0.95, Type I error rate of 0.05, the sample size was estimated with G*Power calculator [40]. The estimation indicated that at least 120 dyads per a subsample should be recruited, if the analyses would be conducted accounting for potential covariates. Results yielding a *p*-value of 0.05 were considered to be statistically significant. Missing data were accounted for by using the full information maximum likelihood procedure performed in IBM AMOS 25 [41]. All analyses were conducted with SPSS version 25. Analyses of variance were performed to test the differences in parental and/or child perceptions of at-home (perceptions of availability of healthy food at home) and out-of-home environment (perceptions of school and local community promotion of healthy eating, perceptions of food advertising) between parent–child dyads with excessive body mass and dyads with normal body mass. General linear models with repeated measures were performed to test: (1) the time effects on perceptions of at-home and out-of-home environment measured at T1 and T2 in parent–child dyads with excessive body mass vs. dyads with normal body mass, as well as (2) the interaction effects of time and the type of subsample (excessive body mass vs. normal body mass dyads). Sensitivity analyses were conducted to test the robustness of findings [42] and to identify if the patterns of effects are similar when accounting for the effects of control variables (the parental education level, the parental perceived economic status, and the size of the place of residence).

3. Results

3.1. Preliminary Analysis

The differences between parents who participated at both T1 and T2 measurements and those who dropped out were not statistically significant in terms of perceptions of availability of healthy food at home, perceptions of school and local community promotion of healthy eating, perceptions of food advertising, age, BMI, all $Fs < 2.32$, $ps > 0.129$, or gender, $\chi^2(1) = 2.37$, $p = 0.306$. The differences between children who participated at both T1 and T2 measurements and those who dropped out were not statistically significant in terms of perceptions of availability of healthy food at home, perceptions of food advertising, age, or BMI, all $Fs < 2.36$, $ps > 0.137$. However, dyads with boys tended to drop out more often than dyads with girls, $\chi^2(1) = 3.26$, $p = 0.072$.

Parents from dyads with excessive body mass differed from parents from dyads with normal body mass in terms of gender, $\chi^2(1) = 12.83$, $p = 0.002$, education level, and economic status, all $Fs > 4.41$, $ps < 0.036$. Parents in dyads with excessive body mass were more often men, reported a lower level of education, and a lower perceived economic status than parents in dyads with normal body mass. The differences between two types of dyads were not statistically significant in terms of parental and child age, children's gender, or the size of the residence place. For details see Table A1.

Bivariate correlations between the study variables obtained for the main analyzed sample of $N = 506$ dyads ($N = 1{,}012$ individuals) are presented in Table A2. At both T1 and T2, healthy food availability and advertisement perceptions reported by parents were positively associated with children's perceptions of healthy food availability and perceptions of persuasiveness of advertisement. A higher level of parental education was related to higher availability of healthy food reported by children (T1 and T2). A higher level of parental perceived economic status (T1) was positively associated with healthy food availability, reported by parents and children (T1 and T2), and negatively with parental and children's BMI (T1 and T2).

3.1.1. Differences between Parent–Child Dyads with Excessive and Normal Body Mass: Perceptions of At-Home and Out-of-Home Environment

Compared to parents from dyads with normal body mass, parents from dyads with excessive body mass reported lower availability of healthy food at their homes (T1 and T2) and fewer school and local community promotion of healthy eating (T1 and T2). There were no statistically significant differences between parents from dyads with normal body mass and dyads with excessive body mass in terms of perceptions of persuasiveness of food advertisement (T1 and T2). The respective findings are reported in Table 1.

Table 1. Differences in at-home and out-of-home environment: Comparisons of dyads of parents and children with excessive body mass ($n = 129$) and dyads of parents and children with normal body mass ($n = 377$).

	M (SD) for Parent–child Dyads with Excessive Body Mass/M (SD) for Parent–child Dyads with Normal Body Mass	Between-Groups Differences		
		F (df) for the Model without Covariates/F (df) for the Model with Covariates	η^2 for the Model without Covariates/η^2 for the Model with Covariates	Cohen's d (95% CI)
Healthy food availability (P, T1)	2.94 (0.42)/3.08 (0.39)	13.01 (1, 504) ***/6.23 (4, 501) ***	0.025/0.047	0.35 (0.32, 0.39)
Healthy food availability (P, T2)	2.97 (0.33)/3.11 (0.30)	19.22 (1, 504) ***/7.74 (4, 501) ***	0.037/0.058	0.42 (0.39, 0.45)
School and local promotion (P, T1)	2.70 (0.66)/2.84 (0.67)	3.91 (1, 504) */2.44 (4, 501) *	0.008/0.019	0.21 (0.15, 0.27)
School and local promotion (P, T2)	2.73 (0.53)/2.83 (0.53)	3.69 (1, 504) †/2.96 (4, 501) †	0.007/0.008	0.19 (0.14, 0.24)
Advertisement perception (P, T1)	2.41 (0.98)/2.42 (0.98)	0.01 (1, 504)/0.42 (4, 501)	<0.001/0.003	0.01 (−0.08, 0.10)
Advertisement perception (P, T2)	2.48 (1.10)/2.52 (1.05)	0.11 (1, 504)/0.23 (4, 501)	<0.001/0.002	0.04 (−0.06, 0.13)
Healthy food availability (Ch, T1)	2.85 (0.46)/2.84 (0.44)	0.02 (1, 504)/3.18 (4, 501) *	<0.001/0.025	−0.02 (−0.06, 0.16)
Healthy food availability (Ch, T2)	2.75 (0.37)/2.82 (0.34)	3.24 (1, 504) †/5.36 (4, 501) ***	0.006/0.041	0.20 (0.17, 0.23)
Advertisement perception (Ch, T1)	2.54 (0.71)/2.59 (0.83)	0.34 (1, 504)/0.12 (4, 501)	0.001/0.002	0.06 (−0.01, 0.13)
Advertisement perception (Ch, T2)	2.49 (0.79)/2.52 (0.80)	0.23 (1, 504)/0.93 (4, 501)	<0.001/0.007	0.04 (−0.03, 0.11)

*** $p < 0.001$; * $p < 0.05$; † $p < 0.10$; P = parent; Ch = child; T1 = Time 1 (baseline); T2 = Time 2 (10-month follow-up); for all analyses $df = 1, 504$; Advertisement perception = perceptions of persuasiveness of food advertising; Local promotion = perceptions of school and local community promotion of healthy nutrition; Healthy food availability = perceptions of availability of heathy food at home. Covariates included: the parental education level, parental perceived economic status, and size of the place of residence. Significant differences (with both significant p-levels and significant 95% CI for Cohen's d) are marked in bold.

Compared to children from dyads with normal body mass, children from dyads with overweight/obesity reported lower availability of healthy food at their homes at T1 and T2 (see Table 1). However, there was no statistically significant difference between children from the two types of dyads in terms of perceptions of out-of-home environment (perceptions of persuasiveness of food advertisement at T1 and T2).

The same pattern of differences was found in sensitivity analysis, testing differences in parental and/or child perceptions of at-home (perceptions of availability of healthy food at home) and out-of-home environment (school and local community promotion of healthy eating, perceptions of persuasiveness of food advertising). In sensitivity analyses, parent–child dyads with normal body mass and dyads with excessive body mass were compared when controlling for parental education level, parental perceived economic status, and the size of the place of residence (see Table 1).

The results of additional analyses, comparing the four types of dyads (i.e., the dyads with normal body mass, dyads with excessive body mass, and the two types dyads with mixed body mass composition) are presented in Appendix A. The additional analyses showed only two significant differences, both referring to parental perceptions. Parents from dyads consisting of a parent with excessive body mass and a child with normal body mass reported lower healthy food availability (T1, T2), compared to parents from dyads with normal body mass.

3.1.2. Changes over Time in Perceptions of At-Home and Out-of-Home Environment among Parent–Child Dyads with Normal and Excessive Body Mass

Regarding the changes over the 10-month period, parental and children's perceptions remained stable over time. Furthermore, all Time x Group interactions were not significant, neither when tested without nor with control variables such as parental education, parental perceived economic status, or the place of residence (see Table A3). These findings suggest that the gap in perceptions of healthy nutrition options in at-home and out-of-home environment did not decrease over time, with families with excessive body mass perceiving a relatively low availability of healthy food and fewer school and local community promotion of healthy eating, controlling for confounding effects of socio-economic variables.

4. Discussion

This study examined the differences between parent–child dyads with excessive body mass versus normal body mass in terms of their perceptions of healthy food-promoting environment. The findings support the assumption that perceptions of factors related to at-home environment and out-of-home environment differ, depending on the body mass status [4]. In particular, parents and children from dyads with excessive body mass perceived lower availability of healthy food at home than parents and children from dyads with normal body mass status. Additionally, parents with excessive body mass status reported lower levels of school and local community promotion of healthy eating, compared to parents from dyads with normal body mass. These differences remained significant after controlling for the level of parental education and economic status, and the size of the place of residence. There were no statistically significant differences between parents and children from the two types of dyads (with excessive body mass versus with normal body mass) in terms of perceptions of persuasiveness of food advertisement.

The findings showing differences in perceived home availability of healthy food products are partially in line with the existing evidence [12]. Previous studies, however, used the ratings of external observers to assess availability of fresh vegetable in households [12]. Our study adds to these findings [12], clarifying that healthy food availability at home is observed differently in families with parents and children with overweight/obesity, compared to families with children and parents with normal body mass. Thus, dyads with excessive body mass are at risk of further body mass increase, due to perceptions of low availability of healthy food. As well documented in previous research, low perceived availability of healthy food may be a trigger for unhealthy nutrition habits [8], that in turn determine a further increase of body mass [13].

The present study also showed that parents from dyads with overweight/obesity perceived lower availability of community and school-based healthy nutrition programs. Previous longitudinal research showed that if parents perceive limited promotion of physical activity in local community or schools, then their overweight children gain even more weight [16]. Therefore, families with children and parents with excessive body mass, in which parents report low levels of community and school healthy nutrition programs, may be at risk of a further increase of body mass in children.

The results did not confirm statistically significant differences between the two types of parent–child dyads (with excessive body mass versus with normal body mass) in terms of perceptions of food advertisement. Previous research suggested that children who are obese know less about persuasive value of food advertising [20], yet the number of studies addressing this issue is limited. A lack of statistically significant differences in the present study was observed even when controlling for age, which is among key determinants of child food advertising knowledge and literacy [43]. Previous studies, however, did not account for parental perceptions of persuasiveness of food advertising. In turn, our study showed that the difference between parents from dyads with excessive body mass and parents with normal body mass was not statistically significant in terms of perceptions of persuasiveness of food advertising. It is possible that parents from both types of dyads interacted similarly with their children, for example when explaining the persuasive value of advertising.

Parents may use strategies such as mediation, including deliberate comments and judgments about TV commercials, or explaining the nature and purpose of advertising [26,44]. Similarities across dyads in terms of parental strategies may result in a lack of differences in children's perceptions of persuasiveness of advertising. Future research may also look more carefully into interactions between parental education [29] and parental practices [31] that may jointly predict children's perceptions of food advertising. Furthermore, perceptions or judgements other than persuasiveness of food advertising may better differentiate between dyads with excessive body mass and those with normal body mass. For example, recognition of logos (higher levels of fast food logos recognition compared to logos of other types of food among children with excessive body mass [24]), or the effect of exposure levels to food adverts on the energy intake in children with excessive body mass [45] were found to differentiate between the children with normal body mass and with overweight/obesity. Yet, the findings of the present study suggest that it may be relevant to account for the parental perceptions as well.

This study has several limitations. Only healthy food availability was assessed, whereas previous research suggested that assessing availability of both healthy and unhealthy food availability is relevant. Fruit and vegetable intake may be inversely associated with availability of unhealthy food; however, at the same time, higher low calorie and nutrient dense food availability was associated with higher child's intake of sweet and savory snack [18], which may suggest that certain products might be considered as less healthy than the others and that home environments might be healthy in some ways and at the same time unhealthy in another way (e.g., availability of healthy and unhealthy food products might be perceived as high). Future studies should account for perceptions of availability of healthy food and perceptions of availability of unhealthy food. Moreover, only self-reports of food availability were used. Perceived food availability is likely to be a different construct than the actual availability of food at home, and the two are only moderately related [46]. Therefore, the conclusions of the present study should not be generalized to the differences in actual availability of healthy food. A combination of subjective and objective indicators of at-home availability of food (e.g., photographs of food stored in the family's pantry or scanning food barcodes during grocery shopping) would be preferable [47]. Yet, the feasibility of using objective measures of food intake in large samples is limited. The study did not account for an actual school-based and local community promotion of healthy eating. Using such methods would allow for controlling whether parental and children's perceptions of at-home or out-of-home environment correspond with the actual presence of policies and programs at schools/communities. Moreover, the single-item measurement of perceptions of persuasiveness of food advertisement may have limited reliability. Future research could consider more complex measures of various aspects of perceptions of advertising to thoroughly examine if the differences between groups may depend on the content of investigated construct (e.g., perception of persuasiveness versus food advertising knowledge). The procedures for data collection did not allow for clustering children according to their schools; therefore, the analyses of the effects of the school-level variables could not be conducted. Next, this study accounted for excessive body mass status incorporating both overweight and obese individuals whereas previous research showed that the differentiation between overweight and obesity may be relevant. For example, studies showed that parents may misperceive their children's body mass, especially when it comes to differentiating between child being overweight or obese [46]. There is also evidence that obese children have more accurate perceptions of their body mass than overweight children [48,49]. Future studies should verify whether perceptions of availability of at-home and out-of-home environmental factors are different in parent–child dyads with overweight, compared to parent–child dyads with obesity. The sample was not representative for the general population of the country (e.g., in terms of parental education), which limits the generalizability of the findings. Any generalization to ethnically diverse populations should be made with caution as the analyzed sample was ethnically homogeneous (all participants were Caucasian).

To conclude, this is the first study to assess differences between parent–child dyads with normal body mass and dyads with excessive body mass in terms of perceptions of at-home (perceptions of the availability of healthy food at home) and out-of-home environment (perceptions of school and community promotion of healthy eating, perceptions of persuasiveness of food advertising). Future programs targeting obesity reduction may address specific perceptions of at-home and out-of-home environment, in particular when designing interventions targeting parents and children who already have excessive body weight. The perceptions of availability of healthy food at home, and perceptions of school and local community promotion of healthy eating may be relatively low in parent–child dyads with excessive weight, which in turn may constitute a risk factor for the maintenance of excessive body weight.

Author Contributions: Conceptualization, K.Z., A.B., E.K., M.B., T.R., C.K.Y.C., K.L. and A.L.; Data curation, K.Z. and A.L.; Investigation, K.Z., A.B., E.K., M.B., T.R., C.K.Y.C., K.L. and A.L.; Methodology, K.Z. and A.L.; Writing—original draft, K.Z., A.B., E.K., M.B., T.R., C.K.Y.C. and A.L.; Writing—review & editing, K.Z., A.B., E.K., M.B., T.R., C.K.Y.C., K.L. and A.L. All authors contributed to the manuscript revision, read and approved the submitted version. All authors have read and agreed to the published version of the manuscript.

Funding: This study was supported by grant no. 2017/27/B/HS6/00092 from National Science Centre, Poland, awarded to A.L. The contribution by A.B. was supported by grant no. 2017/27/N/HS6/0208 from National Science Centre, Poland. The contribution of M.B. was supported by a doctoral scholarship no. 2018/28/T/HS6/00021 from National Science Centre, Poland. Open access of this article was financed by the Ministry of Science and Higher Education in Poland under the 2019-2022 program "Regional Initiative of Excellence", project number 012/RID/2018/19.

Conflicts of Interest: The authors declare that the research was conducted in the absence of any commercial or financial relationships that could be construed as a potential conflict of interest.

Appendix A

Table A1. Demographic and clinical characteristics of $N = 798$ parent–child dyads and the main analyzed sample ($N = 506$ dyads) including, parent–child dyads with excessive body mass ($n = 129$) and parent–child dyads with normal body mass ($n = 377$).

	Parent–Child Dyads ($N = 798$)		Parent-Child Dyads with Excessive Body Mass ($n = 129$)		Parent–Child Dyads with Normal Body Mass ($n = 377$)		Parents from Dyads with Excessive Body Mass vs. Parents from Dyads with Normal Body Mass			Children from Dyads with Excessive Body Mass vs. Children from Dyads with Normal Body Mass		
	Parent	Child	Parent	Child	Parent	Child	χ^2 (df) or F (df)	η^2	Cohen's d (95% CI)	χ^2 (df) or F (df)	η^2	Cohen's d (95% CI)
	% or Range (M; SD)											
Gender							12.83 (1)**	0.025	0.04 (0.02, 0.06)	2.60 (1)⁺	0.005	0.04 (0.01, 0.07)
Female	$n = 707$ (88.6%)	$n = 433$ (54.3%)	$n = 108$ (83.7%)	$n = 80$ (62.0%)	$n = 354$ (93.9%)	$n = 203$ (53.8%)						
Male	$n = 91$ (11.4%)	$n = 365$ (45.7%)	$n = 21$ (16.3%)	$n = 49$ (38.0%)	$n = 23$ (6.1%)	$n = 174$ (46.2%)						
T1 Age	23–66 (36.40; 5.38)	5–12 (7.80; 1.46)	23–49 (36.03; 5.44)	5–11 (7.86; 1.38)	24–59 (36.22; 5.01)	5–10 (7.78; 1.51)	0.14 (1, 504)	<0.001	0.04 (−0.31, 0.39)	0.27 (1, 504)	0.001	−0.06 (−0.15, 0.04)
T2 Age	23–67 (36.82; 4.24)	6–12 (8.33; 1.12)	23–49 (36.49; 5.39)	6–12 (8.41; 1.38)	24–51 (36.79; 4.99)	6–11 (8.37; 1.46)	0.21 (1, 504)	0.001	0.06 (−0.29, 0.41)	0.05 (1, 504)	<0.001	−0.03 (−0.12, 0.07)
T1 BMI	18.50–46.87 (24.92; 4.43)	13.92–33.74 (17.60; 2.79)	25.08–46.87 (29.84; 4.11)	17.50–33.74 (21.49; 2.65)	18.50–24.92 (21.88; 1.70)	13.92–19.95 (16.18; 1.27)	945.89 (1, 504)***	0.652	2.74 (2.54, 2.93)	909.89 (1, 504)***	0.644	2.74 (2.61, 2.87)
T2 BMI	17.86–42.86 (24.91; 4.27)	11.96–30.56 (17.33; 3.04)	21.93–42.87 (29.50; 3.86)	17.01–30.56 (21.30; 3.02)	17.86–27.25 (22.00; 1.76)	13.06–20.93 (16.31; 1.46)	888.21 (1, 504)***	0.638	2.69 (2.50, 2.88)	371.57 (1, 504)**	0.552	2.69 (2.50, 2.88)
Education:												
Primary	$n = 20$ (2.5%)		$n = 4$ (3.1%)		$n = 11$ (2.9%)		4.41 (1, 504)*	0.009	0.21 (0.13, 0.30)			
Vocational	$n = 100$ (125%)		$n = 21$ (16.3%)		$n = 40$ (10.6%)							
Secondary	$n = 216$ (27.1%)		$n = 35$ (27.1%)		$n = 93$ (24.7%)							
Post-secondary	$n = 81$ (10.2%)		$n = 17$ (13.2%)		$n = 37$ (9.8%)							
Higher	$n = 381$ (47.7%)		$n = 52$ (40.3%)		$n = 195$ (51.7%)							
Economic status:												
Higher	$n = 68$ (8.5%)		$n = 37$ (28.7%)		$n = 127$ (33.7%)		4.98 (1, 504)*	0.010	0.22 (0.17, 0.27)			
Similar	$n = 483$ (60.5%)		$n = 74$ (57.4%)		$n = 224$ (59.5%)							
Lower	$n = 247$ (31.0%)		$n = 18$ (14.0%)		$n = 26$ (6.9%)							

Table A1. Cont.

	Parent–Child Dyads (N = 798)	Parent–Child Dyads with Excessive Body Mass (n = 129)	Parent–Child Dyads with Normal Body Mass (n = 377)	Parents from Dyads with Excessive Body Mass vs. Parents from Dyads with Normal Body Mass		Children from Dyads with Excessive Body Mass vs. Children from Dyads with Normal Body Mass
	% or Range (M; SD)					
Place of residence						
≤10,000 residents	n = 244 (30.6%)	n = 43 (33.3%)	n = 99 (26.3%)	1.18 (1, 504)	0.002	
10,000–100,000 residents	n = 172 (21.6%)	n = 26 (20.2%)	n = 88 (23.3%)			0.11 (0.03, 0.19)
100,000–500,000 residents	n = 114 (14.3%)	n = 21 (16.3%)	n = 67 (17.9%)			
≥500,000 residents	n = 268 (33.6%)	n = 39 (30.2%)	n = 123 (32.6%)			

*** $p < 0.001$; ** $p < 0.01$; * $p < 0.05$; † $p < 0.10$; T1 = Time 1 (baseline); T2 = Time 2 (10-month follow-up); BMI = body mass index; Education = the parental education level; Economic status = the parental perceived economic status (reports on comparison to the economic situations of the average family in the country). Significant differences (with significant $p = 0.05$ levels and significant 95% CI for Cohen's d) are marked in bold.

Table A2. Correlations and descriptive statistics for the study variables: Characteristics of the main analyzed sample (N = 506 parent–child dyads with normal body mass and parent–child dyads with excessive body mass) and for N = 798 (four types of dyads: parent with excessive body mass and child with normal body mass; parent with normal body mass and child with excessive body mass; parent–child dyads with excessive body mass; parent–child dyads with normal body mass).

		M (SD) for N = 506 Parent–child Dyads / M (SD) for N = 798 Parent–child Dyads	1	2	3	4	5	6	7	8	9	10	11	12	13	14	15	16	17	18	19	20
1	Healthy food availability (P, T1)	3.05 (0.40)/ 3.02 (0.40)																				
2	Healthy food availability (P, T2)	3.07 (0.32)/ 3.04 (0.31)	0.54/ 0.50																			
3	School and local promotion (P, T1)	2.80 (0.67)/ 2.76 (0.68)	0.01/ 0.02	0.02/ 0.05																		
4	School and local promotion (P, T2)	2.81 (1.53)/ 2.79 (0.52)	0.03/ 0.04	0.16/ 0.14	0.39/ 0.41																	
5	Advertisement perception (P, T1)	2.42 (0.98)/ 2.50 (0.98)	−0.05/ −0.06	0.01/ −0.01	0.01/ −0.02	−0.04/ −0.05																
6	Advertisement perception (P, T2)	2.51 (1.06)/ 2.56 (0.79)	−0.07/ −0.01	−0.09/ 0.01	−0.07/ 0.03	−0.06/ −0.05	0.39/ 0.33															
7	Healthy food availability (Ch, T1)	2.84 (0.44)/ 3.03 (0.47)	0.25/ 0.23	0.11/ 0.15	0.02/ 0.01	0.02/ −0.01	−0.02/ −0.03	−0.10/ −0.06														
8	Healthy food availability (Ch, T2)	3.07 (0.32)/ 3.17 (0.32)	0.29/ 0.20	0.39/ 0.31	0.06/ 0.03	0.11/ 0.12	−0.01/ 0.03	−0.09/ −0.05	0.32/ 0.34	0.10/ 0.10												
9	Advertisement perception (Ch, T1)	2.57 (0.80)/ 2.49 (1.04)	−0.01/ −0.07	0.01/ −0.02	0.05/ 0.04	0.09/ 0.04	0.30/ 0.27	0.11/ 0.06	0.08/ 0.09	−0.15/ −0.13	0.13/ 0.16											
10	Advertisement perception (Ch, T2)	2.51 (0.80)/ 2.53 (0.80)	−0.10/ −0.08	−0.15/ −0.10	−0.02/ −0.04	−0.01/ −0.03	0.04/ 0.03	0.30/ 0.24	−0.02/ −0.04	−0.06/ −0.03	−0.01/ −0.01											
11	BMI (P, T1)	23.91 (4.30)/ 24.92 (4.43)	−0.11/ −0.13	−0.17/ −0.14	−0.04/ −0.04	−0.06/ −0.06	−0.02/ −0.01	−0.06/ 0.01	−0.02/ −0.06	−0.04/ −0.04	−0.01/ −0.03	−0.02/ −0.02	0.98/ 0.98									
12	BMI (P, T2)	23.92 (4.10)/ 24.91 (4.27)	−0.12/ −0.14	−0.17/ −0.16	−0.06/ −0.04	−0.07/ −0.06	−0.03/ −0.03	−0.04/ 0.01	−0.02/ −0.06	−0.08/ −0.04	−0.01/ −0.02	−0.01/ −0.01	0.67/ 0.67	0.65								
13	BMI (Ch, T1)	17.53 (2.78)/ 17.60 (2.79)	−0.12/ −0.10	−0.15/ −0.11	−0.12/ −0.07	−0.07/ −0.06	−0.05/ −0.09	−0.06/ −0.01	0.03/ 0.04	−0.06/ −0.02	−0.02/ −0.02	−0.06/ −0.02	0.67/ 0.65	0.62/ 0.62	0.93/ 0.89							
14	BMI (Ch, T2)	17.43 (2.73)/ 17.33 (3.04)	−0.15/ −0.12	−0.21/ −0.22	−0.02/ 0.05	−0.01/ −0.02	0.04/ −0.11/	−0.08/ −0.02	−0.03/ −0.06	−0.09/ −0.05	−0.02/ −0.04	−0.09/ −0.07	0.62/ 0.62	0.62/ 0.01	0.89/ 0.07	0.01/ 0.03						
15	Age (P, T1)	36.17 (5.12)/ 36.40 (5.38)	0.14/ 0.11	0.16/ 0.12	−0.04/ −0.04	0.05/ 0.05	−0.11/ −0.07	−0.07/ −0.07	0.12/ 0.10	0.10/ 0.07	−0.01/ −0.01	−0.12/ −0.07	0.01/ 0.01	0.02/ 0.01	0.03/ 0.03	0.01/ 0.03						
16	Age (Ch, T1)	7.80 (1.48)/ 7.80 (1.46)	0.03/ 0.01	0.01/ −0.02	−0.07/ −0.06	0.05/ 0.01	−0.05/ −0.02	−0.09/ −0.04	0.01/ 0.04	0.01/ 0.02	−0.05/ −0.08	−0.16/ −0.14	0.04/ −0.02	0.05/ −0.01	0.25/ 0.27	0.22/ 0.13	0.23/ 0.20					
17	Gender (P, T1)	1.91 (0.28)/ 1.89 (0.32)	0.01/ 0.06	0.05/ 0.04	0.06/ 0.06	0.05/ 0.03	0.02/ −0.01	0.02/ 0.02	−0.06/ −0.06	−0.01/ 0.04	0.02/ 0.04	−0.04/ −0.03	−0.19/ −0.19	−0.18/ −0.18	−0.16/ −0.16	−0.08/ −0.03	−0.11/ −0.17	−0.04/ −0.07					
18	Gender (Ch, T1)	1.56 (0.50)/ 1.54 (0.50)	0.08/ 0.05	0.06/ 0.02	−0.01/ −0.03	−0.01/ 0.01	0.05/ 0.04	−0.01/ 0.02	0.14/ 0.07	0.08/ 0.08	0.02/ −0.02	−0.02/ −0.02	0.07/ 0.03	0.06/ 0.03	0.03/ −0.01	0.03/ 0.05	0.06/ 0.04	0.05/ 0.02	0.02/ 0.02				
19	Education	3.91 (1.22)/ 3.88 (1.21)	0.16/ 0.13	0.16/ 0.19	0.16/ 0.16	0.01/ 0.03	0.05/ 0.07	−0.02/ 0.06	0.10/ 0.07	0.15/ 0.09	0.04/ 0.07	−0.07/ −0.09	−0.14/ −0.13	−0.12/ −0.14	−0.12/ −0.09	−0.10/ −0.02	0.20/ 0.19	−0.06/ −0.02	−0.08/ −0.07	−0.01/ −0.01			
20	Economic status	2.70 (0.77)/ 2.72 (0.75)	0.08/ 0.08	0.04/ 0.04	0.03/ −0.04	−0.01/ −0.02	−0.01/ −0.01	0.03/ 0.03	0.13/ 0.14	0.16/ 0.15	−0.05/ −0.01	−0.05/ −0.09	−0.10/ −0.08	−0.10/ −0.08	−0.11/ −0.07	−0.11/ −0.07	0.04/ 0.04	−0.03/ −0.03	−0.05/ −0.04	0.02/ 0.03	0.25/ 0.24		
21	Place of residence	2.51 (1.23)/ 2.46 (1.24)	0.03/ 0.02	0.06/ 0.06	−0.05/ −0.04	0.01/ 0.02	−0.02/ 0.03	−0.01/ 0.01	−0.04/ −0.01	0.06/ 0.02	0.11/ 0.07	0.02/ 0.01	0.03/ 0.01	0.01/ −0.01	−0.07/ −0.08	−0.06/ −0.02	0.11/ 0.14	−0.07/ −0.08	−0.04/ −0.04	0.02/ 0.03	0.18/ 0.17	−0.04/ −0.03	

P = parent; Ch = child; T1 = Time 1 (baseline); T2 = Time 2 (10-month follow-up). BMI = body mass index; Advertisement perception = perception of persuasiveness of food advertising; School and local promotion = perception of school and local community promotion of healthy eating; Healthy food availability = perceptions of availability of healthy food at home; Education = the parental education level (1—primary, 2—uncompleted secondary/vocational, 3—secondary, 4—≤3 years of higher education, 5—≥4 years of higher education); Economic status = the parental perceived economic status (reports on comparison to the economic situations of the average family in the country; 1—much below the average, 2—below average, 3—similar to average, 4—above the average, 5—much above the average); Place of residence (1—<10,000 inhabitants, 2—between 10,000 and 100,000 inhabitants, 3—between 100,000 and 500,000 inhabitants, 4—>500,000 inhabitants); Gender (1—male; 2—female). Person's r for continuous variables and Spearman's rho for categorical variables are provided. Significant (at $p < 0.05$) coefficients are marked in bold.

Table A3. Differences in perceptions of at-home and out-of-home environment: Parent–child dyads with excessive body mass ($n = 129$) versus parent–child dyads with normal body mass ($n = 377$).

	M (SD) for Parent–child Dyads with Normal Body Mass at T1 → at T2/M (SD) for Parent–child Dyads with Excessive Body Mass at T1 → at T2	Time Effects (T1 Variable → T2 Variable)						Interaction Effects (Time*Group)	
		Parent–child Dyads with Excessive Body Mass			Parent–child Dyads with Normal Body Mass				
		F for the Model without Covariates/F for the Model with Covariates	η^2 for the Model without Covariates/η^2 for the Model with Covariates	Cohen's d (95% CI)	F for the Model without Covariates/F for the Model with Covariates	η^2 for the Model without Covariates/η^2 for the Model with Covariates	Cohen's d (95% CI)	F for the Model without Covariates/F for the Model with Covariates	η^2 for the Model without Covariates/η^2 for the Model with Covariates
1 Healthy food availability (P, T1) → Healthy food availability (P, T2)	3.08 (0.39) → 3.11 (0.30)/2.94 (0.42) → 2.97 (0.33)	0.96/<0.01	0.007/<0.001	0.08 (0.04, 0.11)	1.70/0.02	0.005/<0.001	0.08 (0.05, 0.11)	0.26/0.01	<0.001/<0.001
2 School and local promotion (P, T1) → School and local promotion (P, T2)	2.84 (0.67) → 2.83 (0.53)/2.70 (0.66) → 2.73 (0.53)	0.25/0.39	0.002/0.003	0.05 (−0.10, 0.01)	0.01/0.44	<0.001/0.001	0.02 (−0.04, 0.07)	0.20/0.52	<0.001/0.001
3 Advertisement perception (P, T1) → Advertisement perception (P, T2)	2.42 (0.98) → 2.52 (1.05)/2.41 (0.98) → 2.48 (1.10)	0.29/<0.01	0.002/<0.001	0.07 (−0.16, 0.02)	1.91/2.43	0.005/0.006	0.10 (0.01, 0.19)	0.03/0.05	<0.001/<0.001
4 Healthy food availability (Ch, T1) → Healthy food availability (Ch, T2)	2.84 (0.44) → 2.82 (0.34)/2.85 (0.46) → 2.75 (0.37)	2.28/2.59	0.019/0.023	0.23 (0.19, 0.27)	0.98/0.06	0.003/<0.001	0.05 (0.01, 0.08)	2.19/2.01	0.004/0.004
5 Advertisement perception (Ch, T1) → Advertisement perception (Ch, T2)	2.59 (0.83) → 2.52 (0.80)/2.54 (0.71) → 2.49 (0.79)	0.31/0.13	0.002/0.001	0.07 (0.01, 0.13)	1.25/1.33	0.003/0.007	0.09 (0.01, 0.16)	0.01/0.01	<0.001/<0.001

All F values reported in this table are not significant, $ps > 0.05$; P = parent; Ch = child; T1 = time 1 (baseline); T2 = time 2 (10-month follow-up); Advertisement perception = perceptions of persuasiveness of food advertising; Local promotion = perceptions of school and local community promotion of healthy eating; Healthy food availability = perceptions of availability of heathy food at home. Covariates included parental education level, parental perceived economic status and place of residence.

Table A4. Differences in the study variables and demographic variables between excessive body mass parent-normal body mass child dyads (n = 193), normal body mass child dyads (n = 88), parent-excessive body mass child dyads (n = 129), and parent–child dyads with normal body mass (n = 377).

M (SD) for (1) Excessive Body Mass Parent-Normal Body Mass Child Dyads/M (SD) for (2) Normal Body Mass Parent-Excessive Body Mass Child Dyads/M (SD) for (3) parent-Child Dyads with Excessive Body Mass/M (SD) for (4) Parent-Child Dyads with Normal Body Mass	Between Groups Differences F (df) or χ² (df)	η²	(1) vs. (2) Cohen's d (95% CI)	(1) vs. (2) Post-hoc THSD p (95% CI)	(1) vs. (3) Cohen's d (95% CI)	(1) vs. (3) Post-hoc THSD p (95% CI)	(1) vs. (4) Cohen's d (95% CI)	(1) vs. (4) Post-hoc THSD p (95% CI)	(2) vs. (3) Cohen's d (95% CI)	(2) vs. (3) Post-hoc THSD p (95% CI)	(2) vs. (4) Cohen's d (95% CI)	(2) vs. (4) Post-hoc THSD p (95% CI)	(3) vs. (4) Cohen's d (95% CI)	(3) vs. (4) Post-hoc THSD p (95% CI)
Healthy food availability (P, T1) 2.94 (0.41)/3.05 (0.34)/2.94 (0.42)/3.08 (0.39)	7.80 (3, 7787) ***	0.029	NS		−0.35 (−0.39, −0.32)	<0.001 (−0.23, −0.05)	NS		NS		NS		0.35 (0.32, 0.39)	0.002 (0.04, 0.25)
Healthy food availability (P, T2) 3.00 (0.31)/2.99 (0.30)/2.97 (0.33)/3.11 (0.30)	8.51 (3, 7787) ***	0.031	NS		−0.36 (−0.39, −0.34)	0.006 (−0.16, −0.02)	NS		NS		NS		0.42 (0.39, 0.45)	<0.001 (0.06, 0.22)
School and local promotion (P, T1) 2.70 (0.69)/2.67 (0.60)/2.70 (0.66)/2.84 (0.67)	2.97 (3, 7787) *	0.011	NS		NS		NS		NS		NS		0.21 (0.15, 0.27)	0.024 (0.02, 0.31)
School and local promotion (P, T2) 2.75 (0.53)/2.83 (0.43)/2.73 (0.53)/2.83 (0.53)	1.95 (3, 7787)	0.007	NS		NS		NS		NS		NS		0.19 (0.14, 0.24)	0.032 (0.04, 0.42)
Advertisement perception (P, T1) 2.62 (0.97)/2.66 (1.01)/2.41 (0.98)/2.42 (0.98)	3.03 (3, 7787)	0.001	NS		NS		NS		NS		NS		NS	
Advertisement perception (P, T2) 2.55 (0.78)/2.58 (0.70)/2.48 (1.10)/2.52 (1.05)	0.15 (3, 7787)	0.001	NS		NS		NS		NS		NS		NS	
Healthy food availability (Ch, T1) 2.84 (0.45)/2.95 (0.47)/2.85 (0.46)/2.84 (0.44)	1.70 (3, 7787)	0.005	NS		NS		NS		NS		NS		NS	
Healthy food availability (Ch, T2) 2.81 (0.44)/2.97 (0.40)/2.75 (0.37)/2.82 (0.34)	3.50 (3, 7787) †	0.009	NS		NS		NS		NS		NS		0.20 (0.17, 0.23)	0.039 (0.02, 0.24)
Advertisement perception (Ch, T1) 2.42 (0.99)/2.57 (1.05)/2.54 (0.71)/2.59 (0.83)	0.54 (3, 7787)	0.002	NS		NS		NS		NS		NS		NS	
Advertisement perception (Ch, T2) 2.53 (0.84)/2.60 (0.68)/2.49 (0.79)/2.52 (0.80)	0.34 (3, 7787)	0.001	NS		NS		NS		NS		NS		NS	
Gender (P, T1) 1.79 (0.41)/1.96 (0.21)/1.84 (0.37)/1.94 (0.24)	12.82 (3)	0.046	−0.47 (−0.52, −0.43)	<0.001 (−0.27, −0.07)	NS		−0.49 (−0.51, −0.46)	<0.001 (−0.22, −0.08)	0.38 (0.34, 0.42)	0.031 (0.01, 0.23)	NS		0.04 (0.02, 0.06)	0.008 (0.02, 0.18)
Age (P, T1) 38.01 (5.81)/35.41 (5.48)/36.03 (5.44)/36.22 (5.01)	1.56 (3, 7787)	0.002	NS		NS		NS		NS		NS		NS	
BMI (P, T1) 28.69 (3.14)/22.11 (1.71)/29.84 (4.11)/21.88 (1.70)	491.45 (3, 7787) ***	0.650	2.38 (2.06, 2.70)	<0.001 (5.72, 7.40)	NS		2.98 (2.79, 3.17)	<0.001 (6.22, 7.40)	−2.32 (−2.76, −1.87)	<0.001 (−8.67, −6.80)	NS		2.74 (2.54, 2.93)	<0.001 (7.28, 8.66)
BMI (P, T2) 28.55 (3.08)/22.26 (1.96)/29.50 (3.36)/22.00 (1.76)	458.07 (3, 7787) ***	0.634	2.27 (1.95, 2.60)	<0.001 (5.44, 7.16)	NS		2.86 (2.67, 3.05)	<0.001 (5.97, 7.13)	−2.25 (−2.68, −1.83)	<0.001 (−8.16, −6.32)	NS		2.69 (2.50, 2.88)	<0.001 (6.82, 8.18)
Education (P, T1) 3.83 (1.20)/3.85 (1.19)/3.71 (1.24)/3.97 (1.21)	1.72 (3, 7787)	0.006	NS		NS		NS		NS		NS		NS	
Economic status (P, T1) 2.77 (0.75)/2.73 (0.65)/2.83 (0.74)/2.66 (0.78)	2.10 (3, 7787)	0.008	NS		NS		NS		NS		NS		NS	
Place of residence (P, T1) 2.37 (1.27)/2.35 (1.24)/2.41 (1.26)/2.55 (1.22)	1.20 (3, 7787)	0.005	NS		NS		NS		NS		NS		NS	
Gender (Ch) 1.51 (0.50)/1.51 (0.50)/1.62 (0.49)/1.54 (0.50)	1.39 (3)	0.005	NS		NS		NS		NS		NS		NS	
Age (Ch, T1) 7.79 (1.42)/7.82 (1.29)/7.80 (1.48)/7.86 (1.38)	0.37 (3, 7787)	0.001	NS		NS		NS		NS		NS		NS	
BMI (Ch, T1) 16.42 (1.44)/20.71 (2.22)/21.49 (2.65)/16.18 (1.27)	432.61 (3, 7787) ***	0.621	−2.70 (−2.70, −2.30)	<0.001 (−4.86, −3.72)	−2.53 (−2.75, −2.31)	<0.001 (−5.67, −4.57)	NS		NS		3.04 (2.90, 3.17)	<0.001 (4.01, 5.06)	2.74 (2.61, 2.87)	<0.001 (4.86, 5.77)
BMI (Ch, T2) 16.88 (1.51)/20.62 (2.23)/21.30 (3.02)/16.31 (1.46)	418.16 (3, 7787) ***	0.549	−1.79 (−2.04, −1.55)	<0.001 (−3.25, −0.74)	−1.98 (−2.22, −1.74)	0.042 (−2.21, −0.03)	NS		NS		2.33 (2.16, 2.50)	<0.001 (0.73, 3.08)	2.69 (2.50, 2.88)	0.039 (0.03, 2.02)

*** $p < 0.001$; * $p < 0.05$; † $p < 0.10$; T1 = Time 1 (baseline); T2 = Time 2 (10-month follow-up); BMI = body mass index; Education = parental education level; Economic status = parental perceived economic status (reports on comparison to the economic situations of the average family in the country). Cohen's d is provided only for significant between groups differences. Significant differences ($p < 0.05$ and significant 95% CI for Cohen's d) are marked in bold.

References

1. Spinelli, A.; Buoncristiano, M.; Kovacs, V.A.; Yngve, A.; Spiroski, I.; Obreja, G.; Starc, G.; Pérez, N.; Rito, A.I.; Kunešová, M.; et al. Prevalence of Severe Obesity among Primary School Children in 21 European Countries. *OFA* **2019**, *12*, 244–258. [CrossRef] [PubMed]
2. World Health Organization. Commission on Ending Childhood Obesity. Available online: https://www.who.int/end-childhood-obesity/news/launch-final-report/en/ (accessed on 5 February 2020).
3. Lake, A.; Townshend, T. Obesogenic environments: Exploring the built and food environments. *J. R. Soc. Promot. Health* **2006**, *126*, 262–267. [CrossRef] [PubMed]
4. Davison, K.K.; Birch, L.L. Childhood overweight: A contextual model and recommendations for future research. *Obes. Rev.* **2001**, *2*, 159–171. [CrossRef] [PubMed]
5. Cullen, K.W.; Baranowski, T.; Owens, E.; Marsh, T.; Rittenberry, L.; de Moor, C. Availability, accessibility, and preferences for fruit, 100% fruit juice, and vegetables influence children's dietary behavior. *Health Educ. Behav.* **2003**, *30*, 615–626. [CrossRef]
6. Piernas, C.; Popkin, B.M. Trends in snacking among U.S. children. *Health Aff.* **2010**, *29*, 398–404. [CrossRef]
7. Pearson, N.; Biddle, S.J.H.; Gorely, T. Family correlates of fruit and vegetable consumption in children and adolescents: A systematic review. *Public Health Nutr.* **2009**, *12*, 267–283. [CrossRef]
8. van der Horst, K.; Oenema, A.; Ferreira, I.; Wendel-Vos, W.; Giskes, K.; van Lenthe, F.; Brug, J. A systematic review of environmental correlates of obesity-related dietary behaviors in youth. *Health Educ. Res.* **2007**, *22*, 203–226. [CrossRef] [PubMed]
9. Grimm, G.C.; Harnack, L.; Story, M. Factors associated with soft drink consumption in school-aged children. *J. Am. Diet. Assoc.* **2004**, *104*, 1244–1249. [CrossRef]
10. Campbell, K.J.; Crawford, D.A.; Salmon, J.; Carver, A.; Garnett, S.P.; Baur, L.A. Associations between the home food environment and obesity-promoting eating behaviors in adolescence. *Obesity* **2007**, *15*, 719–730. [CrossRef]
11. Luszczynska, A.; de Wit, J.B.F.; de Vet, E.; Januszewicz, A.; Liszewska, N.; Johnson, F.; Pratt, M.; Gaspar, T.; de Matos, M.G.; Stok, F.M. At-Home Environment, Out-of-Home Environment, Snacks and Sweetened Beverages Intake in Preadolescence, Early and Mid-Adolescence: The Interplay Between Environment and Self-Regulation. *J. Youth Adolesc.* **2013**, *42*, 1873–1883. [CrossRef]
12. Boles, R.E.; Scharf, C.; Filigno, S.S.; Saelens, B.E.; Stark, L.J. Differences in Home Food and Activity Environments between Obese and Healthy Weight Families of Preschool Children. *J. Nutr. Educ. Behav.* **2013**, *45*, 222–231. [CrossRef]
13. Cislak, A.; Safron, M.; Pratt, M.; Gaspar, T.; Luszczynska, A. Family-related predictors of body weight and weight-related behaviours among children and adolescents: A systematic umbrella review. *Child. Care Health Dev.* **2012**, *38*, 321–331. [CrossRef] [PubMed]
14. Wang, Y.; Wu, Y.; Wilson, R.F.; Bleich, S.; Cheskin, L.; Weston, C.; Showell, N.; Fawole, O.; Lau, B.; Segal, J. *Childhood Obesity Prevention Programs: Comparative Effectiveness Review and Meta-Analysis*; Agency for Healthcare Research and Quality (US): Rockville, MD, USA, 2013.
15. Horodyska, K.; Luszczynska, A.; Hayes, C.B.; O'Shea, M.P.; Langøien, L.J.; Roos, G.; van den Berg, M.; Hendriksen, M.; De Bourdeaudhuij, I.; Brug, J. Implementation conditions for diet and physical activity interventions and policies: An umbrella review. *BMC Public Health* **2015**, *15*. [CrossRef] [PubMed]
16. Horodyska, K.; Boberska, M.; Kruk, M.; Szczuka, Z.; Wiggers, J.; Wolfenden, L.; Scholz, U.; Radtke, T.; Luszczynska, A. Perceptions of Physical Activity Promotion, Transportation Support, Physical Activity, and Body Mass: An Insight into Parent-Child Dyadic Processes. *Int. J. Behav. Med.* **2019**, *26*, 255–265. [CrossRef] [PubMed]
17. Brindal, E.; Hendrie, G.; Thompson, K.R.; Blunden, S. How do Australian junior primary school children perceive the concepts of "healthy" and "unhealthy"? *Health Educ.* **2012**, *112*, 406–420. [CrossRef]
18. Bryant, M.; Stevens, J. Measurement of food availability in the home. *Nutr. Rev.* **2008**, *64*, 67–76. [CrossRef]
19. Buijzen, M.; Schuurman, J.; Bomhof, E. Associations between children's television advertising exposure and their food consumption patterns: A household diary–survey study. *Appetite* **2008**, *50*, 231–239. [CrossRef]
20. Tarabashkina, L.; Quester, P.; Crouch, R. Food advertising, children's food choices and obesity: Interplay of cognitive defences and product evaluation: An experimental study. *Int. J. Obes.* **2016**, *40*, 581–586. [CrossRef]

21. Contento, I.R. Nutrition education: Linking research, theory, and practice. *Asia Pac. J. Clin. Nutr.* **2008**, *17*, 176–179.
22. Boyland, E.J.; Halford, J.C.G. Television advertising and branding. Effects on eating behaviour and food preferences in children. *Appetite* **2013**, *62*, 236–241. [CrossRef]
23. Folkvord, F.; Anschütz, D.J.; Buijzen, M. The association between BMI development among young children and (un)healthy food choices in response to food advertisements: A longitudinal study. *Int. J. Behav. Nutr. Phys. Act.* **2016**, *13*, 16. [CrossRef] [PubMed]
24. Arredondo, E.; Castaneda, D.; Elder, J.P.; Slymen, D.; Dozier, D. Brand Name Logo Recognition of Fast Food and Healthy Food among Children. *J. Community Health* **2009**, *34*, 73–78. [CrossRef] [PubMed]
25. Halford, J.C.G.; Gillespie, J.; Brown, V.; Pontin, E.E.; Dovey, T.M. Effect of television advertisements for foods on food consumption in children. *Appetite* **2004**, *42*, 221–225. [CrossRef]
26. Buijzen, M. The effectiveness of parental communication in modifying the relation between food advertising and children's consumption behaviour. *Br. J. Dev. Psychol.* **2009**, *27*, 105–121. [CrossRef]
27. Buijzen, M.; van der Molen, J.H.W.; Sondij, P. Parental mediation of children's emotional responses to a violent news event. *Commun. Res.* **2007**, *34*, 212–230. [CrossRef]
28. Berk, L.E. *Child Development*; Allyn & Bacon: Boston, MA, USA, 2000; ISBN 0415276217.
29. Lissner, L.; Wijnhoven, T.M.A.; Mehlig, K.; Sjöberg, A.; Kunesova, M.; Yngve, A.; Petrauskienie, A.; Duleva, V.; Rito, A.I.; Breda, J. Socioeconomic inequalities in childhood overweight: Heterogeneity across five countries in the WHO European Childhood Obesity Surveillance Initiative (COSI–2008). *Int. J. Obes.* **2016**, *40*, 796–802. [CrossRef]
30. Liszewska, N.; Scholz, U.; Radtke, T.; Horodyska, K.; Luszczynska, A. Bi-directional associations between parental feeding practices and children's body mass in parent-child dyads. *Appetite* **2018**, *129*, 192–197. [CrossRef]
31. Zarychta, K.; Horodyska, K.; Gan, Y.; Chan, C.; Wiggers, J.; Wolfenden, L.; Boberska, M.; Luszczynska, A. Associations of Parental and Child Food and Exercise Aversion With Child Food Intake and Physical Activity. *Health Psychol.* **2019**, *38*, 1116–1127. [CrossRef]
32. Cole, T.J.; Lobstein, T. Extended international (IOTF) body mass index cut-offs for thinness, overweight and obesity. *Pediatric Obes.* **2012**, *7*, 284–294. [CrossRef]
33. Central Statistical Office. Demographic Yearbook of Poland. 2015. Available online: https://stat.gov.pl/en/topics/statistical-yearbooks/statistical-yearbooks/demographic-yearbook-of-poland-2015,3,9.html (accessed on 5 February 2020).
34. Kenny, D.A.; Kashy, D.A.; Cook, W.L. *Dyadic Data Analysis*; Guilford Press: New York, NY, USA, 2006; ISBN 9781572309869.
35. Musher-Eizenman, D.; Holub, S. Comprehensive Feeding Practices Questionnaire: Validation of a New Measure of Parental Feeding Practices. *J. Pediatric Psychol.* **2007**, *32*, 960–972. [CrossRef]
36. Cortina, J.M. What is coefficient alpha? An examination of theory and applications. *J. Appl. Psychol.* **1993**, *78*, 98–104. [CrossRef]
37. Stok, M.; Ridder, D.; De Vet, E.; Nureeva, L.; Luszczynska, A.; Wardle, J.; Gaspar, T.; Wit, J. Hungry for an intervention? Adolescents' ratings of acceptability of eating-related intervention strategies. *BMC Public Health* **2016**, 16. [CrossRef] [PubMed]
38. Zalma, A.R.; Safiah, M.Y.; Ajau, D.; Khairil Anuar, M.I. Reliability and validity of television food advertising questionnaire in Malaysia. *Health Promot. Int.* **2015**, *30*, 523–530. [CrossRef] [PubMed]
39. World Health Organization. Application Tools. Available online: http://www.who.int/growthref/tools/en (accessed on 10 February 2020).
40. Faul, F.; Erdfelder, E.; Lang, A.G.; Buchner, A. G_Power 3: A flexible statistical power analysis program for the social, behavioral, and biomedical sciences. *Behav. Res. Methods* **2007**, *39*, 175–191. [CrossRef] [PubMed]
41. Byrne, B.M. *Structural Equation Modeling with AMOS: Basic Concepts, Applications, and Programming*, 2nd ed.; Routledge/Taylor & Francis Group: New York, NY, USA, 2010; ISBN 9780203805534.
42. Thabane, L.; Mbuagbaw, L.; Zhang, S.; Samaan, Z.; Marcucci, M.; Ye, C.; Thabane, M.; Giangregorio, L.; Dennis, B.; Kosa, D.; et al. A tutorial on sensitivity analyses in clinical trials: The what, why, when and how. *BMC Med. Res. Methodol.* **2013**, *13*, 92. [CrossRef] [PubMed]

43. Livingstone, S.; Helsper, E. Does advertising literacy mediate the effects of advertising on children? A critical examination of two linked research literatures in relation to obesity and food choice. *J. Commun.* **2006**, *56*. [CrossRef]
44. Buijzen, M.; Valkenburg, P. Parental Mediation of Undesired Advertising Effects. *J. Broadcast. Electron. Media* **2005**, *49*, 153–165. [CrossRef]
45. Halford, J.C.; Boyland, E.J.; Hughes, G.M.; Stacey, L.; McKean, S.; Dovey, T.M. Beyond-brand effect of television food advertisements on food choice in children: The effects of weight status. *Public Health Nutr.* **2008**, *11*, 897–904. [CrossRef]
46. Campbell, M.W.C.; Williams, J.; Hampton, A.; Wake, M. Maternal concern and perceptions of overweight in Australian preschool-aged children. *Med. J. Aust.* **2006**, *184*, 274–277. [CrossRef]
47. Couch, S.C.; Glanz, K.; Zhou, C.; Sallis, J.F.; Saelens, B.E. Home Food Environment in Relation to Children's Diet Quality and Weight Status. *J. Acad. Nutr. Diet.* **2014**, *114*, 1569–1579. [CrossRef]
48. Hayward, J.; Millar, L.; Petersen, S.; Swinburn, B.; Lewis, A.J. When ignorance is bliss: Weight perception, body mass index and quality of life in adolescents. *Int. J. Obes.* **2014**, *38*, 1328–1334. [CrossRef] [PubMed]
49. Sarafrazi, N.; Hughes, J.P.; Borrud, L.; Burt, V.; Paulose-Ram, R. *Perception of Weight Status in U.S. Children and Adolescents Aged 8–15 Years, 2005–2012*; US Department of Health and Human Services, Centers for Disease Control and Prevention, National Center for Health Statistics: Hyattsville, MD, USA, 2014; pp. 1–7.

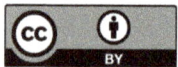

© 2020 by the authors. Licensee MDPI, Basel, Switzerland. This article is an open access article distributed under the terms and conditions of the Creative Commons Attribution (CC BY) license (http://creativecommons.org/licenses/by/4.0/).

Article

Importance of Self-Efficacy in Eating Behavior and Physical Activity Change of Overweight and Non-Overweight Adolescent Girls Participating in Healthy Me: A Lifestyle Intervention with Mobile Technology

Anna Dzielska [1,*], Joanna Mazur [1,2], Hanna Nałęcz [1], Anna Oblacińska [1] and Anna Fijałkowska [3]

1. Department of Child and Adolescent Health, Institute of Mother and Child, 17a Kasprzaka St., 01-211 Warsaw, Poland; j.mazur@cm.uz.zgora.pl (J.M.); hanna.nalecz@imid.med.pl (H.N.); anna.oblacinska@imid.med.pl (A.O.)
2. Department of Humanization in Medicine and Sexology, University of Zielona Gora, Collegium Medicum, Energetykow St. 2, 65-729 Zielona Gora, Poland
3. Department of Cardiology, Institute of Mother and Child, 17a Kasprzaka St., 01-211 Warsaw, Poland; anna.fijalkowska@imid.med.pl
* Correspondence: anna.dzielska@imid.med.pl; Tel.: +48-223277202

Received: 25 June 2020; Accepted: 15 July 2020; Published: 17 July 2020

Abstract: Very little is known about how multicomponent interventions directed to entire populations work in selected groups of adolescents. The aim was to evaluate the effectiveness of the Healthy Me one-year program on changes in healthy eating and physical activity among overweight and non-overweight female students. Randomization involved the allocation of full, partial or null intervention. The randomized field trial was implemented in 48 secondary schools (clusters) all over Poland among 1198 15-year-old girls. In this study, a sample of N = 1111 girls who participated in each evaluation study was analyzed. Using multimedia technologies, efforts were made to improve health behaviors and increase self-efficacy. The main outcome was a health behavior index (HBI), built on the basis of six nutritional indicators and one related to physical activity. HBI was analyzed before and immediately after intervention and at three months' follow-up, and the HBI change was modeled. Statistical analysis included nonparametric tests and generalized linear models with two-way interactions. Comparing the first and third surveys, in the overweight girls, the HBI index improved by 0.348 (SD = 3.17), while in the non-overweight girls it had worsened. After adjusting for other factors, a significant interaction between body weight status and level of self-efficacy as predictors of HBI changes was confirmed. The program turned out to be more beneficial for overweight girls.

Keywords: healthy lifestyle intervention; school-based intervention; eating behavior; MVPA; overweight and obesity; self-efficacy; adolescent girls

1. Introduction

According to the World Health Organization (WHO), adolescence starts in the second decade of life [1]. This period requires special attention because of its specific health and developmental needs and rights [2]. During adolescence, the transition period from childhood to adulthood, health behaviors are shaped and consolidated. Therefore, a healthy lifestyle is crucial for adolescents' proper growth and development. Moreover, targeting adolescents with health behavior-shaping intervention activities affects the burden of disease in adulthood, providing better health through the ripple effect [3,4].

Nearly 40 years of the cross-sectional Health Behavior in School-aged Children (HBSC) study has consistently identified burning problems and the most vulnerable groups of adolescents in the European region of WHO and Canada [5]. The comparison of health behaviors of adolescents of both sexes indicated a co-occurrence of positive trends in boys and negative in girls. That resulted in an elimination of gender-related differences in the frequency of many negative behaviors [6] and exposed the population of 15-year-old girls—the future mothers of the next generations—as extremely vulnerable, especially in the context of persistent disadvantages in girls' self-rated health, observed in many countries.

According to the international report from the HBSC study [5], obesity or overweight was found in 14% of 15-year-old girls and 36% consider themselves too fat. Moreover, girls aged 15 do not regularly eat breakfast on school days (52%) and do not eat fruit (62%) and vegetables (61%) every day, but every day they eat sweets (28%) and drink sweet carbonated drinks (15%). In addition, only 11% of them meet the recommendations for appropriate levels of moderate-to-vigorous physical activity.

Both systematic reviews of intervention programs [7] and guides for the prevention of obesity in children and adolescents [8] indicate the limited effectiveness of obesity prevention programs. Low effectiveness of these programs was found in children under 12 years of age and the introduction of interventions in young people aged 13–18 did not contribute to reducing BMI. Unfortunately, there is little research in this age group. Hence, it is difficult to give a reliable assessment of the effectiveness of the intervention [9].

Health-related behaviors are correlated, and many different consolidated patterns of behaviors can be observed in different environments [10]. Systematic reviews confirm that interventions aimed at improvement in moderate-to-vigorous physical activity have a simultaneous effect on empowering other health-related behaviors such as healthy eating or weight management [11]. Results of meta-analyses show that school-based interventions including a combination of healthy eating and physical activity may prevent overweight in the longer term [12] and also indicate moderate effectiveness of educational interventions in improving eating behaviors and ambiguous results concerning anthropometric changes [13].

Likewise, better intervention outcomes are associated with long-term interventions [14], as well as with the inclusion of a higher number of applied behavioral change techniques [15–17]. Incorporating behavioral change techniques focused on self-regulation into the intervention was found effective in changing physical activity and eating behaviors. Avery et al. (2012) confirmed this relationship in adult studies [18] and Martyn-Nemeth et al. (2009) in adolescents [19]. Furthermore, some studies demonstrate the effectiveness of interventions using interactive modern media to improve diet and physical activity of adolescents, although only a few indicate maintenance of the effect in the long term [20].

Effective behavior change requires the acquisition of appropriate skills that will allow activities to be initiated consistent with acquired knowledge. Moreover, it is extremely sensitive to environmental context [21]. One of the personal competences necessary to successfully implement changes in health behavior is self-efficacy, which has a proven link to motivation, behavior control and goal achievement [22]. By being convinced of one's own effectiveness, a person gains the ability to initiate and continue changes even when faced with emerging challenges [23].

To date, the assessment of the effectiveness of the Healthy Me program has been carried out in the whole study group, without distinguishing between girls with and without excess body weight [24]. The implemented program was a universal prevention aimed at the whole population of 15-year-old girls. In the reviews of systematic community obesity prevention programs, reducing the prevalence of obesity is often assumed to be the main outcome [25]. Less attention is paid to assessing the changes in health behavior of students with and without excess body weight. However, the question arises—to what extent do overweight teenagers use universal programs? Is it a group representing less advantageous health behaviors, and do any beneficial effects of the program remain in this group after its completion? The presented paper fills this knowledge gap, while at the same time providing a picture of the effectiveness of this innovative program, which tried to reach its addressees with the use of modern multimedia technologies.

The aim of the study was to evaluate the effectiveness of the Healthy Me intervention program on changes in the prevalence of healthy eating behaviors and the level of physical activity among 15-year-old girls in Poland. It has been hypothesized that the effectiveness of an intervention may differ in overweight and non-overweight girls, and the improvement of personal competence may be a factor strengthening the effectiveness of the intervention [26]. Therefore, the main issue was to determine in which groups of girls the Health Behavior Index (HBI), consisted of seven indicators of eating behaviors and physical activity, improved taking into consideration their body weight status, change in self-efficacy, the type of intervention provided and possible effect of school environment.

2. Materials and Methods

2.1. Study and Intervention Design

The data were obtained from the randomized field trial with cluster randomization by school and repeated measures. In total, 1198 15-year-old girls, from 48 randomly selected secondary schools all over Poland, participated in the one-year Healthy Me program in 2017–2018. Schools were randomly assigned to the subsequent groups: full intervention group (24 schools, 636 girls), partial intervention group (12 schools, 277 girls) and null intervention group (12 schools, 285 girls) (Figure 1).

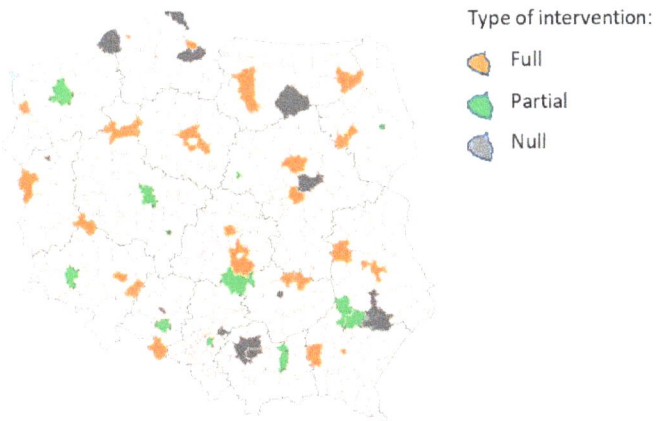

Figure 1. Location of schools participating in the Healthy Me program by the type of intervention.

The main area of interest was the improvement in physical activity, although the intervention activities were conducted in four thematic phases: physical activity, eating behavior, risk behavior and personal and social competencies. The multicomponent intervention used mobile technology (a dedicated mobile application and a fitness band) and involved a combination of techniques. The Healthy Me program used Social Cognitive Theory [27] as its theoretical foundation and was based on an interactive technology approach [26]. The intervention included behavioral and environmental components. Self-efficacy was shaped by setting goals, observing others and receiving feedback from the technologies (fitness band, app) that supported self-monitoring. However, the type of intervention depended on the type of intervention group, which made it possible to assess the effectiveness of particular sets of intervention methods and techniques (Table 1).

Table 1. Intervention components by type of intervention.

COMPONENTS	Full	Partial	Null
FITNESS BAND			
Objective measurement (steps, heart rate, sleep quality)	X	X	X
MOBILE APP			
Feedback from physical activity telemonitoring (steps, heart rate, distance, sleep quality)	X	X	X
Short messages (facts about a healthy lifestyle)	X	X	
Articles about a healthy lifestyle	X		
Gamification (challenges related to physical activity, nutrition, personal and social competences—individual and group, to be performed alone or in cooperation with family and friends)	X		
OTHER			
Workshops at school run by the project coordinator (health education)	X		
Promotion of the intervention theme (physical activity, eating behavior, risk behaviors, personal and social competences) at school and in the local environment—involvement of young people (e.g., preparation by girls of a poster promoting the program and the theme of intervention)	X	X	X
Promotional campaign via Facebook (closed group, competition)	X	X	X

The study and the intervention procedure were accepted by the Bioethics Committee of the Mother and Child Institute in Poland (number: 32/2017 from 22 June 2017) and the funding body (Ministry of Health in Poland, Grant no. 6/7/K/6/NPZ/2017/106/622).

2.2. Evaluation Surveys

The project has been fully evaluated, and as part of the evaluation of the intervention results, questionnaire surveys were conducted three times during the project implementation:

1. Study 1—at the beginning of the program implementation (November 2017).
2. Study 2—after the intervention completion (June 2018).
3. Study 3—three months after the intervention completion (September 2018).

Each questionnaire contained a similar set of questions to allow comparisons to be made about changes in subjective health, different health-related behaviors and related factors.

Anthropometric measurements (e.g., weight, height) were conducted three times by school nurses, once in each survey round.

2.3. Sample Characteristics

The present analyses cover girls (N = 1111) who have completed three rounds of the survey (Table 2). About half of the girls participated in the full intervention group, and half belonged to the partial and null intervention groups. Based on the WHO standards [28], almost a quarter of participants were assessed as overweight or obese (23.5%), and the frequency was higher than in the groups of similar age form cross-sectional HBSC, probably due to the different cut-off point used for the estimation of body weight status [6]. The percentage of BMI missing data in the studied sample was very low (0.8%). A similar percentage of girls with excess body weight occurred in each type of intervention group. At the baseline, the overweight and non-overweight groups did not differ in terms of the scores of the HBI or the general index of self-efficacy (GSE), both described below.

Table 2. Sample characteristics at the baseline.

	Total	Non-Overweight	Overweight
	N [1]	n (%)	n (%)
Total	1111	843(76.5)	259(23.5)
Type of intervention	n (%)	n (%)	n (%)
Full	597(53.7)	451(76.1)	142(23.9)
Partial	252(22.7)	190(76.3)	59(23.7)
Null	262(23.6)	202(77.7)	58(22.3)
	M ± SD	M ± SD	M ± SD
HBI [2]	13.69 ± 3.23	13.65 ± 3.19	13.81 ± 3.35
GSE [3]	34.69 ± 5.33	34.78 ± 5.40	34.37 ± 5.10

[1] Missing BMI data 0.8% (n = 9); [2] HBI—health behavior index; [3] GSE—general index of self-efficacy.

2.4. Measures

2.4.1. Health Behavior Indicators

Six indicators related to eating behaviors and one measure of physical activity were tested in these analyses.

1. Eating behaviors

    - Frequency of eating fruits, vegetables, sweets, drinking soft drinks with added sugar. Girls answered how often they eat or drink the products by choosing one answer from seven categories, from "never" to "daily, more than once".
    - Breakfast consumption. Girls were asked to answer the questions on the frequency of eating breakfast on schooldays, choosing from six answer categories, from "never" to "five days a week", and during the weekends, choosing from three options, from "never" to "both days".

2. Physical activity

    - Moderate-to-vigorous physical activity. Girls answered the question: "Over the past seven days, on how many days were you physically active for a total of at least 60 min per day? Please add up all the time you spent in physical activity each day". The questions had eight response categories: from "zero days" to "seven days".

The frequency distribution of girls undertaking the above-mentioned eating behaviors in subsequent study periods, by type of intervention and body weight status, is presented in the Supplementary Materials, Table S1. The above questions come from the HBSC study protocols and have been tested repeatedly in Poland in a population similar in age [6].

2.4.2. HBI

The summary HBI was estimated for all three study periods. The index consists of seven indicators of eating and physical activity behaviors mentioned above. The response categories in each behavior were recoded and scored from 0 to 3 points, as follows, with a higher value indicating a more favorable result:

- Fruit and vegetables: 0 points—never or less than once a week; 1 point—"once a week"; 2 points—"two to six days a week"; 3 points—"daily, at least once or daily more than once".
- Sweets and soft drinks consumption: 0 points—"daily, at least once or daily more than once"; 1 point—"two to six days a week"; 2 points—"once a week"; 3 points—"never or less than once a week".
- Breakfast consumption on schooldays: 0 points—"never"; 1 point—"one to two days"; 2 points—"three to four days"; 3 points—"daily".

- Breakfast consumption on weekends: 0 points—"never"; 1 point—"one day"; 3 points—"both days".
- Moderate-to-vigorous physical activity: 0 points—"zero days"; 1 point—"one to three days"; 2 points—"four to six days"; 3 points—"seven days".

The highest value (3 points) attributed to the recoded answers to the above questions was consistent with the national recommendations on the frequency of eating different groups of products and meals [29], as well as the global moderate-to-vigorous physical activity guidelines for children and adolescents [30].

The summary score of the HBI was from 0 to 21 points. HBI scores in each of the three evaluation surveys are presented in Tables 3 and 4.

Table 3. Health Behavior Index (HBI) change in 3 study periods by the body weight status.

	Total	Overweight	Non-Overweight	p^2
	M ± S	M ± SD	M ± SD	
Study 1	13.71 ± 3.30	13.81 ± 3.35	13.65 ± 3.19	0.405
Study 2	14.73 ± 4.11	15.12 ± 4.23	14.61 ± 4.07	0.052
Study 3	13.69 ± 3.23	14.16 ± 3.27	13.56 ± 3.29	0.008
p^1	<0.001	<0.001	<0.001	

[1] Differences in HBI between 3 study rounds—Kendall's W test for repeated measures. [2] Differences by the body weight status—U Mann–Whitney test for independent groups.

Table 4. Changes in the self-efficacy before and after the Healthy Me program by the body weight status.

Self-Efficacy	Total	Overweight	Non-Overweight	p^3
General self-efficacy (GSE) [1]				
Study 1	34.68 ± 5.33	34.36 ± 5.10	34.78 ± 5.40	0.206
Study 3	34.33 ± 5.13	33.99 ± 5.04	34.43 ± 5.16	0.228
p^2	0.027	0.677	0.030	
Domain of strength				
Study 1	17.38 ± 3.17	17.30 ± 3.07	17.42 ± 3.21	0.451
Study 3	17.16 ± 3.20	17.05 ± 3.30	17.19 ± 3.18	0.696
p^2	0.023	0.328	0.043	
Domain of perseverance				
Study 1	17.28 ± 3.33	17.06 ± 3.32	17.34 ± 3.33	0.227
Study 3	17.16 ± 3.13	17.02 ± 3.05	17.20 ± 3.15	0.608
p^2	0.191	0.831	0.165	

[1] Missing data in GSE 6.6% (Study 1) and 6.2% (Study 3). [2] Differences in self-efficacy between 1st and 3rd study rounds—Z Wilcoxon's test for repeated measures. [3] Differences by the body weight status—U Mann–Whitney test for independent groups.

In building the HBI, its six different variants were considered. Some factors were excluded, and attempts were made to additionally include intense physical activity and meals eaten together with parents. The psychometric properties of individual indices in three study periods and the significance of the level of their changes were evaluated. None of the analysed indices had a single factor structure, and the internal consistency was slightly below the recommended level of 0.70 which is accepted for larger sample analyses [31]. The advantage of the chosen index is the fact that it takes into account the level of physical activity, which was a key element of the intervention. Eating healthy food most strongly affects the variability of the selected index. Eating sweets appeared to be the weakest component. However, this element was not abandoned, due to a considerable decrease in the frequency of eating sweets during the project implementation period (Table S1). There was only one case of missing data in the HBI (n = 1).

2.4.3. Self-Efficacy—Personal Competence Scale

To measure the change in self-efficacy the KompOs scale was used. This is a two-dimension, 12-item, standardized questionnaire by Z. Juczynski, applied for younger and older adolescents to assess their self-efficacy [32]. In older adolescents (15–17 years) this tool has a two-dimensional structure and measures strength to initiate behavior and perseverance to sustain it. Psychometric analysis performed on our sample at the baseline revealed good reliability of the full scale, with Cronbach's α = 0.757, as well as the component scales: for strength Cronbach's α = 0.736 and for perseverance Cronbach's α = 0.677. In other studies, test–retest reliability of the scale, applied in older adolescents, was 0.51. The theoretical validity of the scale was tested and showed a positive correlation with General Self Efficacy [33] r = 0.43 and Coopersmith Self-Esteem Inventory (CSEI) [34,35] r = 0.30.

In the following description, instead of the national scale abbreviation (KompOs), the term self-efficacy is used. The general self-efficacy score (GSE), as well as two partial scores of strength and perseverance, were analyzed. The percentage of missing data in GSE was 6.6% and 6.2% in the first and third study, respectively.

2.4.4. Body Weight Status

Results from the anthropometric measurements (body weight, height) conducted by school nurses before the intervention (November 2017) were used. BMI classification was made using WHO standards [28]. For the analysis, the BMI variable was recoded into two categories of body weight status: (1) overweight (overweight and obese categories) and (2) non-overweight (other categories).

2.5. Statistical Analysis

A combined analysis of independent and dependent observations resulting from repeated measurements, which is an approach commonly used in the case of mixed data, was applied.

The HBI changes constituted the main outcome variable. They were analyzed by comparing successive measurements and examining the determinants of the changes themselves, which only required the technique of comparing independent samples. The most important variable was the HBI change between the first study and follow-up three months after intervention, because of simultaneous measurements of competence at these time points.

Due to the non-normal distribution of the HBI values and the HBI changes, non-parametric methods were used for two (BMI groups) and three (types of interventions) adolescent girls' groups, respectively. These were Wilcoxon and Kendall tests for dependent data and Mann–Whitney and Kruskal–Wallis tests for independent data.

The school effect was also examined by estimating the ICC (intraclass correlation coefficient). A mixed linear model with school as a random effect was used for this purpose. The ICC values for different types of interventions were compared separately for the absolute value of the HBI and the changes in this index.

In a multifactor analysis, a generalized linear model was estimated (GENLIN procedure in IBM SPSS software, v.23). It is a method that does not impose strict conditions as to the distribution of the analyzed variables, allowing various types of variables to be included as predictors (binary, categorical, continuous) and enabling a transparent analysis of the interaction effect.

Three GENLIN models were estimated, describing the determinants of the HBI change on the basis of the results of the Study 1 and Study 2, Study 2 and Study 3, and Study 1 and Study 3 evaluation surveys. After checking variants of the models, it was decided to include in the group of predictors the following: body weight status, the type of intervention and the interaction between the body weight status category and the change in self-efficacy. The analyses of the HBI change were also corrected with respect to the initial HBI level and the self-efficacy score. The overall quality of the models was measured by the omnibus test. It gives the answer to the question whether the explained variance in a set of data is significantly greater than the unexplained variance.

3. Results

3.1. HBI

The mean scores of the HBI in all three study periods in the overall sample, by body weight status are presented in Table 3, and by the type of intervention group in Table S2.

The HBI in Study 1 did not differ by body weight status. In Study 2, it was slightly higher in overweight than non-overweight girls, but the results were at the tendency to significance level ($p = 0.052$). Three months after the intervention (Study 3), the overweight girls presented significantly higher scores of HBI than non-overweight girls ($p < 0.01$). The highest HBI scores were indicated in the full and null intervention groups in all three study rounds, while the lowest occurred in the partial intervention group.

In the total sample, as well as in both groups distinguished by body weight status, significant differences were found in the HBI scores between the three rounds of the study. Comparing the initial level and results three months after the Healthy Me program completion, the crude level of change in HBI was equal to 0.026 (SD = 2.89). In the group of girls with overweight or obesity, an improvement was observed (0.348 ± 3.17), while in girls without excessive body mass health behaviors worsened.

3.2. Self-Efficacy—Personal Competence

Table 4 compares the distributions of self-efficacy indices, taking into account two available measurements, at the beginning of the Healthy Me program implementation (Study 1) and at follow-up after three months (Study 3). A decreasing trend in GSE was observed, which was caused by a considerably deteriorating assessment of the strength dimension, with slight changes in the level of perseverance. Unfavorable changes were observed only in non-overweight girls. In the overweight or obese group, changes in the general index and sub-indices were not statistically significant. These two groups of girls distinguished by body weight status did not differ considerably with regards to the general score, as well as regardless two dimensions of self-efficacy scale, both at the beginning of the program and three months after its completion.

Table S3 compares the results of non-parametric tests of the distribution of GSE, as well as the domains' scores in the three intervention groups. At the onset, the girls from the schools covered by full intervention achieved the best results, while in the control group (null intervention) those indices were the lowest. Observable differences concerned only Study 1, GSE and the dimension of strength. The third measurement point (three months' follow-up) did not reveal any significant differences between the intervention groups. Comparing the level of self-efficacy change in conjunction with the paired data test, a significant deterioration was shown in the full intervention group, which also concerned the overall score and the dimension of strength. A clear trend of a deterioration in competence level was also found with respect to the dimension of perseverance in the partial intervention group.

In reference to the initial hypothesis, HBI changes were checked depending on the level of GSE changes. It was contractually assumed that the deterioration and improvement would occur in case of a change by more than two points. In the three groups representing worsening, lack of change and improvement in GSE, there were 32.5%, 39.9% and 27.6% of girls, respectively. The percentage of girls with improved GSE was 28.4% in the overweight group and 27.0% in the non-overweight group ($p = 0.792$). According to the data presented in Figure 2, a significant change in GSE is associated with an improvement in dietary behavior and physical activity, measured by change in HBI. The impact of improved self-efficacy is more evident in overweight girls. In this group, even with a GSE change around zero, a slight improvement in HBI values has already been noted.

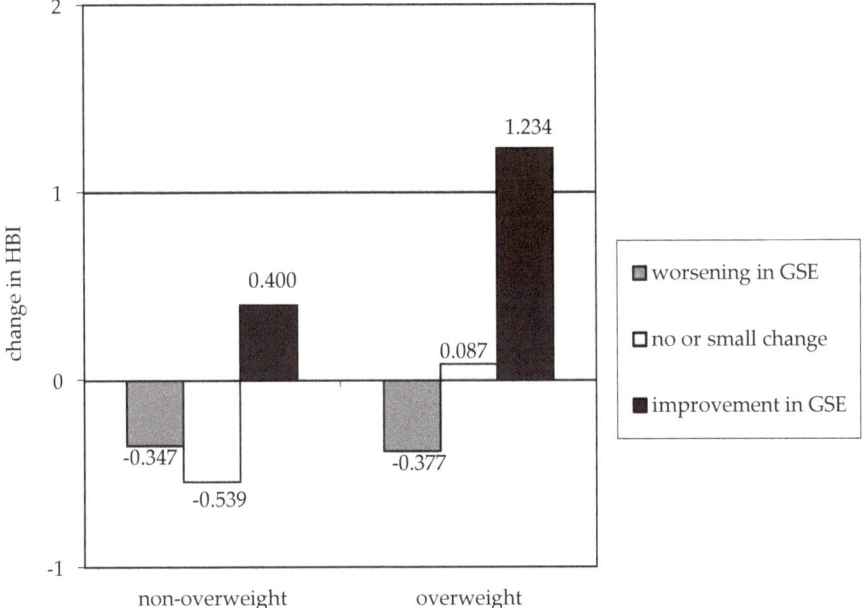

Figure 2. Change in HBI comparing baseline and 3 months' follow-up after intervention according to BMI group and change in self-efficacy (GSE).

3.3. School Effect

Taking the HBI change between the results of the first and the third evaluation study as the most important outcome, it was examined to what extent this change depends on local school conditions. The ICC index was calculated. In the whole sample of 48 schools, it equaled 0.012. For particular types of intervention, it was estimated at the level 0.006 (full), 0.020 (partial) and 0.015 (null). This means that the proportion of variance in the HBI change that lies between schools is very small and slightly varies depending on the type of intervention. At the same time, the low ICC value allows for the abandonment of multilevel analyses taking into account the hierarchical data structure.

For comparison, the school effect in the whole study group and in relation to the absolute HBI value at the onset (Study 1) equaled 0.031 and 0.044 in Study 1, and 0.039 in Study 3. An increase in the ICC may be a signal that schools were not implementing the intervention program to an equal extent over the entire duration of the program.

3.4. Independent Predictors of the Change in HBI

Table 5 shows the results of the estimation of generalized linear models in which the dependent variable was the HBI change, calculated on the basis of the results of different surveys (1 and 2; 2 and 3; 1 and 3).

The models were adjusted to the initial levels of the HBI and the self-efficacy score. The selected predictors accurately described the fluctuations of the HBI changes between first and second measurement points and between first and third points (deferred effect). The middle model (2 and 3) described to a small extent the determinants of the HBI changes immediately after the end of the program. The overweight girls achieved significantly higher HBI gains compared to peers without excess body weight in both extreme models (Table 5). The intervention effect was best demonstrated in the last model, describing the change between the first and third surveys. In the case of partial intervention, the changes were less beneficial. A significant interaction between the changes in self-efficacy and body weight was also shown. In the first and third models, among girls with excess body weight, the improvement in personal competence contributes more to the increase in the HBI value. For example, when comparing the first and third measurement points, an increase in the self-efficacy by one unit results in an increase in the HBI by 0.132 ($p = 0.006$) in the overweight and obese group. In the group of non-overweight girls, the HBI increase was only 0.037, and this parameter of regression function does not differ significantly from zero ($p = 0.198$).

Table 5. Determinants of change in the HBI around the period of Healthy Me intervention identified by generalized linear models.

Predictors	Dependent Variable								
	HBI Change Study 1–Study 2			HBI Change Study 2–Study 3			HBI Change Study 1–Study 3		
	Beta	SE	p	Beta	SE	p	Beta	SE	p
Constant	3.394	0.653	0.000	−1.332	0.908	0.142	4.738	0.899	0.000
Main effect:									
Body weight status									
Overweight	0.412	0.193	0.033	−0.113	0.269	0.674	0.539	0.266	0.043
Non-overweight				Reference category					
Type of intervention									
Full	−0.007	0.203	0.971	0.335	0.282	0.235	−0.357	0.280	0.201
Partial	−0.425	0.241	0.078	0.393	0.336	0.242	−0.833	0.332	0.012
Null (control)				Reference category					
Initial HBI [1]	−0.397	0.027	0.000	−0.018	0.037	0.618	−0.380	0.037	0.000
Initial GSE [2]	0.062	0.019	0.001	0.009	0.026	0.725	0.054	0.026	0.040
Interaction:									
Overweight with GSE	0.134	0.034	0.000	0.000	0.048	0.992	0.132	0.048	0.006
Non-overweight with GSE	0.096	0.021	0.000	0.060	0.029	0.038	0.037	0.029	0.198
Scale	6.393	0.291		12.352	0.562		12.106	0.551	
Omnibus test—p		0.000			0.455			0.000	

[1] HBI—health behavior index. [2] GSE—general index of self-efficacy.

On the basis of the above three models of the HBI change determinants, it is possible to estimate the theoretical values at the second and third measurement points in two groups of girls with different body weight statuses, starting from the actual initial value (Figure 3).

In both groups, an increase in the HBI was observed between the beginning and the end of the Healthy Me program, followed by a decrease, according to the measurement three months after the end of the program (Study 3). This initial improvement in health behaviors was clearly greater in the overweight group. Comparing the first and third measurement points, it is possible to draw a conclusion regarding the effectiveness of the program as a tool for improving health behaviors. In the group of girls without overweight or obesity, the effectiveness of the program is lower, and extreme measurements indicate a return to the baseline and even a slight deterioration in the HBI. Attempts to devise alternative models have not led to better results. Among other things, the independent influence of partial indices of self-efficacy (strength and perseverance) was studied, and attempts were made to include the main effect of self-efficacy in the model. The model that takes into account the interaction of body weight status with self-efficacy was considered optimal.

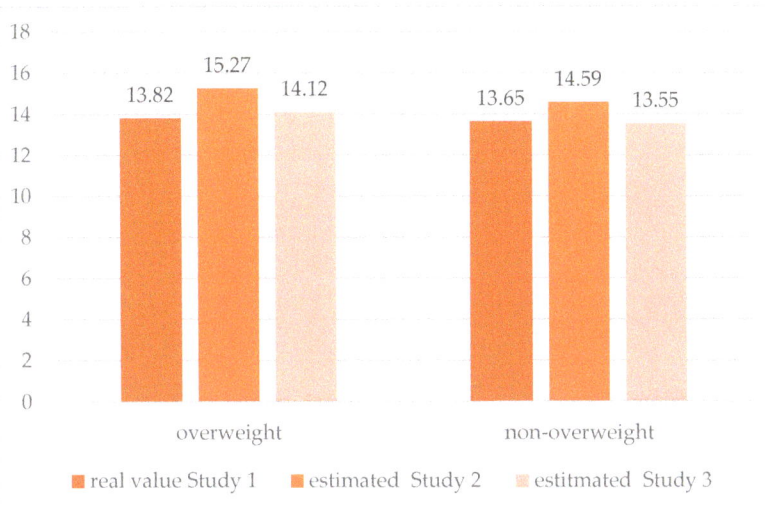

Figure 3. Changes in HBI in three waves of the survey under the Healthy Me program, according to body weight status groups adjusted for type of intervention, initial values of HBI, self-efficacy and interaction body weight status–self-efficacy.

4. Discussion

In our research, we assumed that a change in the level of HBI may be related to a change in the level of personal competence among girls participating in the Healthy Me intervention program, which used mobile technologies. Our analyses confirmed this assumption. The change in the HBI was explained by the interaction of the self-efficacy level with body weight status. Although there was no positive change in health behavior among girls without excess weight, girls with excess body weight (overweight or obesity) achieved a better score in the health behavior index in the follow-up study after three months of intervention.

Prior to the intervention, there were no observable differences in the values of health behavior indices between overweight and non-overweight adolescent girls. Taking into account the type of intervention, slightly lower values at the starting point occurred in the partial group than in the other two intervention groups. The other studies conducted among Polish schoolchildren also support our conclusion that maintaining a diet rich in beneficial products is not the domain of adolescents without overweight or obesity and even more often occurs in overweight or obese adolescents [36]. Conversely, some problems are more frequently observed in overweight teenagers compared to their peers without excess body weight, such as skipping meals [37], having fewer meals during the day [38] and lower physical activity [39,40].

The level of the HBI changed in the second evaluation study, but after three months from the end of the intervention, it returned to a level close to the initial level. It turns out that in girls without overweight or obesity, a slightly lower HBI score between extreme measurements was recorded, but in the group of girls with excess body weight, an improvement was observed. Moreover, the deferred effect revealed a significant difference in the average HBI indices in favor of overweight and obese teenagers. The result seems all the more interesting because our intervention was not aimed at changing behaviors of adolescents at risk—overweight, but at the general population of 15-year-old girls, which was selected because of the significant deterioration in health behavior for this age group. The aim of the program was to assess if the proposed intervention could help to slow down the unfavorable trend before they reached the age of 15. As effects were observed in the group of girls with excess body weight, it may be hypothesized that even if the study was not addressed to the adolescents from risk groups (selected prevention), the overweight participants may be more motivated to engage in prevention programs, which makes this group more vulnerable to benefits [41]. Based on our studies and thesis supported by other researchers, there is a need to cautiously draw conclusions about changes in health behavior induced by intervention, especially in the case of long-term programs carried out in the developmental period [42]. Among others, the negative changes resulting from developmental factors should be taken into account. Moreover, in a longer program, the rate of change could be altered by a number of interim measurements, promotion of the program before it starts, overlapping of other parallel trends or a negative effect of withdrawal from the program. Thus, the absence of a significant, positive change in the HBI in the general population of 15-year-old girls can be considered as a satisfactory result, taking into account developmental considerations, and a negative trend in health behaviors which increase with age, observed in other studies among girls [43].

The analysis of self-efficacy showed no differences among intervention types, nor the body weight status among the studied population at the starting point of the intervention. The main changes revealing the impact of the Healthy Me program concerned the general score and the self-efficacy dimension of strength (to initiate behavior) and showed the decrease in these scores among participants of the full intervention group. Within the partial intervention group, the dimension of perseverance also deteriorated, and this result supports the claim that the multicomponent, but moderate, intervention impacts have an exceptional effect on the participants' conviction about the possibility of sustaining behaviors. This result might be caused by an ongoing dynamic process of verification of self-efficacy during the program.

Based on Social Cognitive Theory, the self-efficacy building strategy is one of the most effective tools in the health behavior change programs targeting diet and/or physical activity among children [44]. Jacobson and Mazurek Melnyk (2011) concluded after their pilot study with overweight and obese school-age children that healthy lifestyle interventions that include cognitive behavior skill building may be the key to strengthening the child's healthy beliefs and facilitating healthy lifestyle choices and behaviors [45]. Morano et al. (2016) recommend that childhood obesity programs should target psychosocial correlates of physical activity [46], among which the crucial one, as Kołoło et al. (2010) indicate, is self-efficacy [47]. Higher self-efficacy is related to better decision-making and goal achievement [22]. Therefore, girls assessing their self-efficacy well are more likely to undertake (strength dimension of self-efficacy) and sustain (perseverance dimension) the health behaviors.

Our study shows significant interaction between self-efficacy and body weight. Among overweight girls, improvement in self-efficacy resulted in enhancement of health behaviors. The sense of interaction and the mediating role of self-efficacy and other social competences in the process of changing health behaviors is strongly established and widely proved in the literature. Especially regarding overweight and obesity, according to Goffman's spoiled identity theory [48], and further randomized control studies of the stigma effect on health behaviors [49], children with low social competence are at higher risk for obesogenic behaviors. That interaction was also confirmed in a national sample of Americans where nine-year-old children with lower social competence were at higher risk of becoming overweight or obese by age 11 [50]. In low social competence groups, avoiding stress caused by complex psychosocial factors with negative feedback related to excess body weight may manifest in unhealthy behaviors such as solitary, sedentary or unhealthy eating. According to Melnyk et al. (2009), psychosocial factors may inhibit or cause barriers to healthy behaviors in adolescents [51]. On the other hand, Vila et al. (2004), using a Child Behavior Checklist, found that obese adolescents demonstrated significantly poorer social skills [52]. These studies show the nature of the reciprocal relationship among competences, body weight and health behaviors.

Additionally, the school effect was measured in the analysis. Based on results obtained, the effect of the school has proved to be small, indicating quite a consistent approach by schools towards the implementation of intervention activities. Interventions to improve health behavior are largely implemented in the school environment, and many of them have a positive impact on nutrition and physical activity [53]. Due to the availability of target groups as well as methods, resources and qualified staff, the school seems to be an ideal environment for health promotion and education [54]. However, a lot depends on the quality of the proposed interventions, the way they are implemented, consistency of the activities [55], proper preparation of the contractors, financial possibilities and the duration of the intervention [54,56]. In this regard, the small school effect obtained in our study may be the result of how schools were prepared to implement the intervention activities. Preparations included providing clear instructions, training of direct executors, application of unified educational methods and contents and a strictly determined sequence of undertaken activities. Moreover, the high competences of physical education teachers responsible for coordination and carrying out activities at schools may have had an impact on the uniform implementation of the program at the school-setting.

Strengths and Limitations

We are aware of some limitations of our study, which were partly due to the schedule of the Healthy Me program, as well as the assumptions adopted in this article. First, the final deferred effect of the program should be assessed in the long term. Second, one of the most important variables, i.e., the level of self-efficacy, was not measured just after the end of the program but three months after the end of the intervention. Only a few factors were considered in the analyses, focusing on differences in the level of the HBI and its changes in the groups of overweight and non-overweight girls. The Healthy Me program was implemented in a variety of environments (48 schools all over Poland), over a long period of time (a year), covering a large group of girls ($n = 1111$). This environmental variability was undoubtedly an asset but also created additional limitations. In such a large and diverse group, it was difficult to control the involvement of individual schools in the implementation of the program, and the distinct differences are evidenced by the results of qualitative studies and different subjective evaluations of the program by its participants [24]. However, the low ICC values in this study may indicate quite consistent implementation of the intervention actions by the schools involved. It was not possible to analyze in detail the changes in the diet of the program participants. The main outcome variable, i.e., the HBI, contained a strong nutritional component but was corrected with respect to the level of physical activity. This version of HBI was chosen because improvement in physical activity was the main focus of the Healthy Me intervention.

Despite the above limitations, the analyses presented have a number of advantages and bring additional knowledge to research on the evaluation of multifaceted intervention programs. Attention was paid to the heterogeneity of the intervention group. Commonly, it is hypothesized that different intervention components will benefit equally different subgroups of participants in the hope of offering something for everyone. It has been proven that girls with excess body weight have benefited more from participation in the Healthy Me program, which is the main conclusion of these analyses. This was partly due to the change in their self-efficacy, which was at a relatively low level, but any improvement resulted in better health behaviors. Taking into account the aspect of personal competences is one of the strengths of this program. Self-efficacy was measured with a robust tool dedicated to the adolescents. Usually, the motivational and strengthening factors are only mentioned as a theoretical basis for intervention. In our program, this factor was one of the components to be evaluated. In addition, we have introduced an interaction effect into statistical analyses, which is now considered an important part of the search for an optimal intervention model [57].

5. Conclusions

In summary, our results demonstrate a significant effect of self-efficacy with the interaction of body weight status on improvement in eating behavior and physical activity among adolescent girls. The authors conclude that the positive impact of the intervention proved to be stronger for overweight girls. Girls with excess body weight, three months after intervention completion, presented a higher level of favorable health behaviors than girls without excess body weight. Further work is certainly required to disentangle these complexities in non-direct effects of interventions on health behavior change among adolescent girls. When analyzing the effects of such programs, it is necessary to take into account the multiplicity of interrelationships between different factors that may modify the effects obtained. Our paper opens new conceptual and practical fields in research on the evaluation of health interventions. Firstly, effective interventions targeting adolescent girls should include a strengthened element of developing personal competences, the growth of which appears to be most beneficial to girls at risk. Secondly, the level of change in personal competences should be monitored during the whole evaluation process. This seems to be far beyond including psychological factors as the only theoretical basis for the intervention.

Supplementary Materials: The following are available online at http://www.mdpi.com/2072-6643/12/7/2128/s1. Table S1: Prevalence of health behavior by the type of intervention and body weight status (%). Table S2: Health Behavior Index (HBI) change in 3 study periods by the type of intervention. Table S3: Changes in the self-efficacy before and after the Healthy Me program by the type of intervention.

Author Contributions: Conceptualization, A.D., J.M., H.N., A.O., A.F.; methodology, J.M., A.D.; analysis, J.M., A.D.; writing—original draft preparation, A.D., J.M., H.N., A.O., A.F.; writing—review and editing, A.D., J.M., H.N., A.O., A.F. All authors have read and agreed to the published version of the manuscript.

Funding: This research was funded by the National Health Program of the Ministry of Health in Poland (Grant no. 6/7/K/6/NPZ/2017/106/622).

Conflicts of Interest: The authors declare no conflict of interest. The funders had no role in the design of the study; in the collection, analyses or interpretation of data; in the writing of the manuscript or in the decision to publish the results.

References

1. Dick, B.; Ferguson, B.J. Health for the World's Adolescents: A Second Chance in the Second Decade. *J. Adolesc. Health* **2015**, *56*, 3–6. [CrossRef] [PubMed]
2. World Health Organization. *Sixty-Fourth World Health Assembly. Resolution WHA 64.28: Youth and Health Risks*; WHO: Geneva, Switzerland, 2011.
3. Sawyer, S.M.; A Afifi, R.; Bearinger, L.H.; Blakemore, S.-J.; Dick, B.; Ezeh, A.C.; Patton, G.C. Adolescence: A foundation for future health. *Lancet* **2012**, *379*, 1630–1640. [CrossRef]
4. Salam, R.A.; Das, J.K.; Ahmed, W.; Irfan, O.; Sheikh, S.S.; Bhutta, Z.A. Effects of Preventive Nutrition Interventions among Adolescents on Health and Nutritional Status in Low- and Middle-Income Countries: A Systematic Review and Meta-Analysis. *Nutrients* **2019**, *12*, 49. [CrossRef]
5. Inchley, J.; Currie, D.; Budisavljevic, S.; Torsheim, T.; Jåstad, A.; Cosma, A.; Kelly, C.; Már Arnarsson, Á. (Eds.) *Spotlight on Adolescent Health and Well-Being. - Findings from the 2017/2018 Health Behaviour in School-Aged Children (HBSC) Survey in Europe and Canada. International Report. Volume 1. Key Findings*; WHO Regional Office for Europe: Copenhagen, Denmark, 2020.
6. Mazur, J.; Małkowska-Szkutnik, A. (Eds.) *Zdrowie Uczniów w 2018 Roku na Tle Nowego Modelu Badań HBSC*; Instytut Matki i Dziecka: Warsaw, Poland, 2018.
7. Brown, T.; Moore, T.H.; Hooper, L.; Gao, Y.; Zayegh, A.; Ijaz, S.; Elwenspoek, M.; Foxen, S.C.; Magee, L.; O'Malley, C.; et al. Interventions for preventing obesity in children. *Cochrane Database Syst. Rev.* **2019**, *7*, CD001871. [CrossRef]
8. Blüher, S.; Kromeyer-Hauschild, K.; Graf, C.; Widhalm, K.; Korsten-Reck, U.; Jödicke, B.; Markert, J.; Müller, M.J.; Moss, A.; Wabitsch, M.; et al. Current Guidelines for Obesity Prevention in Childhood and Adolescence. *Obes. Facts* **2018**, *11*, 263–276. [CrossRef]
9. Waters, E.; De Silva-Sanigorski, A.; Burford, B.J.; Brown, T.; Campbell, K.J.; Gao, Y.; Armstrong, R.; Prosser, L.; Summerbell, C.D. Interventions for preventing obesity in children. *Cochrane Database Syst. Rev.* **2011**, CD001871. [CrossRef]
10. Mazur, J.; Kowalewska, A.; Baska, T.; Sigmund, E.; Nałęcz, H.; Nemeth, A.; Zawadzka, D. Patterns of physical activity and multiple risk behaviour in adolescents from Visegrad countries. *Zdr. Publiczne Zarządz.* **2014**, *12*, 56–67. [CrossRef]
11. Janssen, I.; Leblanc, A.G. Systematic review of the health benefits of physical activity and fitness in school-aged children and youth. *Int. J. Behav. Nutr. Phys. Act.* **2010**, *7*, 40. [CrossRef]

12. Brown, T.; Summerbell, C. Systematic review of school-based interventions that focus on changing dietary intake and physical activity levels to prevent childhood obesity: An update to the obesity guidance produced by the National Institute for Health and Clinical Excellence. *Obes. Rev.* **2009**, *10*, 110–141. [CrossRef] [PubMed]
13. Van Cauwenberghe, E.; Maes, L.; Spittaels, H.; Van Lenthe, F.J.; Brug, J.; Oppert, J.-M.; De Bourdeaudhuij, I. Effectiveness of school-based interventions in Europe to promote healthy nutrition in children and adolescents: Systematic review of published and 'grey' literature. *Br. J. Nutr.* **2010**, *103*, 781–797. [CrossRef] [PubMed]
14. Safron, M.; Cislak, A.; Sacchi, M.G.D.M.D.; Luszczynska, A. Effects of School-based Interventions Targeting Obesity-Related Behaviors and Body Weight Change: A Systematic Umbrella Review. *Behav. Med.* **2011**, *37*, 15–25. [CrossRef] [PubMed]
15. Hynynen, S.-T.; Van Stralen, M.M.; Sniehotta, F.F.; Araujo-Soares, V.; Hardeman, W.; Chinapaw, M.J.; Vasankari, T.; Hankonen, N. A systematic review of school-based interventions targeting physical activity and sedentary behaviour among older adolescents. *Int. Rev. Sport Exerc. Psychol.* **2015**, *9*, 22–44. [CrossRef] [PubMed]
16. Hendrie, G.A.; Brindal, E.; Corsini, N.; Gardner, C.; Baird, D.L.; Golley, R.K. Combined Home and School Obesity Prevention Interventions for Children. *Health Edu. Behav.* **2011**, *39*, 159–171. [CrossRef] [PubMed]
17. Owen, M.; Curry, W.; Kerner, C.; Newson, L.; Fairclough, S.J. The effectiveness of school-based physical activity interventions for adolescent girls: A systematic review and meta-analysis. *Prev. Med.* **2017**, *105*, 237–249. [CrossRef] [PubMed]
18. Avery, L.; Flynn, D.; Van Wersch, A.; Sniehotta, F.F.; Trenell, M.I. Changing Physical Activity Behavior in Type 2 Diabetes: A systematic review and meta-analysis of behavioral interventions. *Diabetes Care* **2012**, *35*, 2681–2689. [CrossRef]
19. Martyn-Nemeth, P.; Penckofer, S.; Gulanick, M.; Velsor-Friedrich, B.; Bryant, F.B. The relationships among self-esteem, stress, coping, eating behavior, and depressive mood in adolescents. *Res. Nurs. Health* **2009**, *32*, 96–109. [CrossRef]
20. Rose, T.; Barker, M.; Jacob, C.M.; Morrison, L.; Lawrence, W.; Strömmer, S.; Vogel, C.; Woods-Townsend, K.; Farrell, D.; Inskip, H.; et al. A Systematic Review of Digital Interventions for Improving the Diet and Physical Activity Behaviors of Adolescents. *J. Adolesc. Health* **2017**, *61*, 669–677. [CrossRef]
21. Teixeira, P.J.; Marques, M.M. Health Behavior Change for Obesity Management. *Obes. Facts* **2017**, *10*, 666–673. [CrossRef]
22. Bandura, A.; Freeman, W.H.; Lightsey, R. Self-Efficacy: The Exercise of Control. *J. Cogn. Psychother.* **1999**, *13*, 158–166. [CrossRef]
23. Mokhtari, S.; Grace, B.; Pak, Y.; Reina, A.; Durand, Q.; Yee, J.K. Motivation and perceived competence for healthy eating and exercise among overweight/obese adolescents in comparison to normal weight adolescents. *BMC Obes.* **2017**, *4*, 36. [CrossRef] [PubMed]
24. Mazur, J.; Dzielska, A.; Kleszczewska, D.; Oblacińska, A.; Fijałkowska, A. Changes in physical activity of adolescent girls in the context of their perception of the Healthy Me programme. *Eur. J. Public Health* **2020**, *30*, 461–466. [CrossRef] [PubMed]
25. Moores, C.; Bell, L.K.; Miller, J.; A Damarell, R.; Matwiejczyk, L.; Miller, M.D. A systematic review of community-based interventions for the treatment of adolescents with overweight and obesity. *Obes. Rev.* **2018**, *19*, 698–715. [CrossRef] [PubMed]
26. Whittemore, R.; Jeon, S.; Grey, M. An Internet Obesity Prevention Program for Adolescents. *J. Adolesc. Health* **2013**, *52*, 439–447. [CrossRef] [PubMed]
27. Bandura, A. *Social Foundations of Thought and Action: A Social Cognitive Theory*; Prentice-Hall: Englewood Cliffs, NJ, USA, 1986.
28. De Onis, M.; Lobstein, T. Defining obesity risk status in the general childhood population: Which cut-offs should we use? *Pediatr. Obes.* **2010**, *5*, 458–460. [CrossRef]
29. Jarosz, M.; Respondek, W.; Wolnicka, K.; Sajór, I.; Wierzejska, R. Zalecenia dotyczące żywienia i aktywności fizycznej. In *Normy Dla Populacji Polskiej—Nowelizacja*; Jarosz, M., Ed.; Instytut Żywności i Żywienia: Warsaw, Poland, 2012; pp. 158–163.
30. Global Recommendations on Physical Activity for Health. World Health Organization 2010. Available online: https://www.who.int/activities/developing-new-guidelines-on-physical-activity-and-sedentary-behaviour-for-youth-adults-and-sub-populations (accessed on 16 June 2020).

31. Peterson, R. A Meta-Analysis of Cronbach's Coefficient Alpha. *J. Consum. Res.* **1994**, *21*, 381–391. [CrossRef]
32. Juczynski, Z. *Narzędzia Pomiaru w Promocji i Psychologii Zdrowia*, 2nd ed.; Pracownia Testów Psychologicznych PTP: Warsaw, Poland, 2012.
33. Schwarzer, R.; Jerusalem, M. Generalized Self-Efficacy Scale. In *Measures in Health Psychology: A User's Portfolio. Causal and Control Beliefs*; Weinman, S., Wright, S., Johnston, M., Eds.; NFER-NELSON: Windsor, UK, 1995; pp. 35–37.
34. Goodman, N.; Coopersmith, S. The Antecedents of Self-Esteem. *Am. Sociol. Rev.* **1969**, *34*, 116. [CrossRef]
35. Coopersmith, S. *Revised Coopersmith Self-Esteem Inventory Manual*; Mind Garden: Redwood City, CA, USA, 2002.
36. Jodkowska, M.; Oblacińska, A.M.; Tabak, I.; Radiukiewicz, K. Differences in dietary patterns between overweight and normal-weight adolescents. *Med. Wieku Rozw.* **2011**, *15*, 266–273.
37. Monzani, A.; Ricotti, R.; Caputo, M.; Caputo, M.; Archero, F.; Bellone, S.; Prodam, F. A Systematic Review of the Association of Skipping Breakfast with Weight and Cardiometabolic Risk Factors in Children and Adolescents. What Should We Better Investigate in the Future? *Nutrients* **2019**, *11*, 387. [CrossRef]
38. Zalewska, M.; Maciorkowska, E. Selected nutritional habits of teenagers associated with overweight and obesity. *PeerJ* **2017**, *5*, 3681. [CrossRef]
39. Olds, T.S.; Ferrar, K.; Schranz, N.; Maher, C. Obese Adolescents Are Less Active Than Their Normal-Weight Peers, but Wherein Lies the Difference? *J. Adolesc. Health* **2011**, *48*, 189–195. [CrossRef]
40. Bullen, B.A.; Reed, R.B.; Mayer, J. Physical Activity of Obese and Nonobese Adolescent Girls Appraised by Motion Picture Sampling. *Am. J. Clin. Nutr.* **1964**, *14*, 211–223. [CrossRef] [PubMed]
41. Stice, E.; Shaw, H.; Marti, C.N. A meta-analytic review of obesity prevention programs for children and adolescents: The skinny on interventions that work. *Psychol. Bull.* **2006**, *132*, 667–691. [CrossRef]
42. Issel, L.M. *Health Program Planning and Evaluation. A Practical, Systematic Approach for Community Health*; Jones & Bartlett Learning: Burlington, MA, USA, 2018.
43. Inchley, J.; Currie, D.; Jewell, J.; Breda, J.; Barnekov, V. (Eds.) *Adolescent Obesity and Related Behaviours: Trends and Inequalities in the WHO European Region, 2002–2014; Observations from the Health Behaviour in School-Aged Children (HBSC) WHO Collaborative cross-National Study*; WHO: Copenhagen, Denmark, 2017.
44. Nixon, C.A.; Moore, H.J.; Douthwaite, W.; Gibson, E.L.; Vögele, C.; Kreichauf, S.; Wildgruber, A.; Manios, Y.; Summerbell, C. ToyBox-study group Identifying effective behavioural models and behaviour change strategies underpinning preschool- and school-based obesity prevention interventions aimed at 4-6-year-olds: A systematic review. *Obes. Rev.* **2012**, *13*, 106–117. [CrossRef] [PubMed]
45. Jacobson, D.; Mazurek Melnyk, B. Psychosocial Correlates of Healthy Beliefs, Choices, and Behaviors in Overweight and Obese School-Age Children: A Primary Care Healthy Choices Intervention Pilot Study. *J. Pediatr. Nurs.* **2011**, *26*, 456–464. [CrossRef]
46. Morano, M.; Rutigliano, I.; Rago, A.; Pettoello-Mantovani, M.; Campanozzi, A. A multicomponent, school-initiated obesity intervention to promote healthy lifestyles in children. *Nutrients* **2016**, *32*, 1075–1080. [CrossRef] [PubMed]
47. Kołoło, H.; Guszkowska, M.; Mazur, J.; Dzielska, A. Self-efficacy, self-esteem and body image as psychological determinants of 15-year-old adolescents' physical activity levels. *Hum. Mov.* **2012**, *13*, 264–270. [CrossRef]
48. Goffman, E. *Stigma. Notes on the Management of Spoiled Identity*; Penguin: London, UK, 1963.
49. Nolan, L.; Eshleman, A. Paved with good intentions: Paradoxical eating responses to weight stigma. *Appetite* **2016**, *102*, 15–24. [CrossRef] [PubMed]
50. Jackson, S.; Cunningham, S.A. Social Competence and Obesity in Elementary School. *Am. J. Public Health* **2015**, *105*, 153–158. [CrossRef] [PubMed]
51. Melnyk, B.M.; Jacobson, D.; Kelly, S.A.; O'Haver, J.; Small, L.; Mays, M.Z. Improving the Mental Health, Healthy Lifestyle Choices, and Physical Health of Hispanic Adolescents: A Randomized Controlled Pilot Study. *J. Sch. Health* **2009**, *79*, 575–584. [CrossRef]
52. Vila, G. Mental Disorders in Obese Children and Adolescents. *Psychosom. Med.* **2004**, *66*, 387–394. [CrossRef]
53. Racey, M.; O'Brien, C.; Douglas, S.; Marquez, O.; A Hendrie, G.; Newton, G. Systematic Review of School-Based Interventions to Modify Dietary Behavior: Does Intervention Intensity Impact Effectiveness? *J. Sch. Health* **2016**, *86*, 452–463. [CrossRef] [PubMed]

54. Wang, D.; Stewart, D.E. The implementation and effectiveness of school-based nutrition promotion programmes using a health-promoting schools approach: A systematic review. *Public Health Nutr.* **2012**, *16*, 1082–1100. [CrossRef] [PubMed]
55. Liu, Z.; Xu, H.-M.; Wen, L.-M.; Peng, Y.-Z.; Lin, L.-Z.; Zhou, S.; Li, W.-H.; Wang, H. A systematic review and meta-analysis of the overall effects of school-based obesity prevention interventions and effect differences by intervention components. *Int. J. Behav. Nutr. Phys. Act.* **2019**, *16*, 95. [CrossRef]
56. Cassar, S.; Salmon, J.; Timperio, A.; Naylor, P.-J.; Van Nassau, F.; Ayala, A.M.C.; Koorts, H. Adoption, implementation and sustainability of school-based physical activity and sedentary behaviour interventions in real-world settings: A systematic review. *Int. J. Behav. Nutr. Phys. Act.* **2019**, *16*, 1–13. [CrossRef] [PubMed]
57. Collins, L.M. Optimization of Behavioral, Biobehavioral, and Biomedical Interventions. In *Statistics for Social and Behavioral Sciences*; Springer Science and Business Media LLC: Berlin, Germany, 2018.

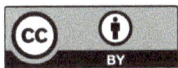

© 2020 by the authors. Licensee MDPI, Basel, Switzerland. This article is an open access article distributed under the terms and conditions of the Creative Commons Attribution (CC BY) license (http://creativecommons.org/licenses/by/4.0/).

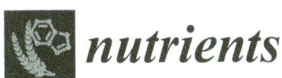

Article

Parent Stress as a Consideration in Childhood Obesity Prevention: Results from the Guelph Family Health Study, a Pilot Randomized Controlled Trial

Valerie Hruska [1], **Gerarda Darlington** [2], **Jess Haines** [3] **and David W. L. Ma** [1,*]
on behalf of the Guelph Family Health Study

[1] Department of Human Health and Nutritional Sciences, University of Guelph, Guelph, ON N1G2W1, Canada; vhruska@uoguelph.ca
[2] Department of Mathematics and Statistics, University of Guelph, Guelph, ON N1G2W1, Canada; gdarling@uoguelph.ca
[3] Department of Family Relations and Applied Nutrition, University of Guelph, Guelph, ON N1G2W1, Canada; jhaines@uoguelph.ca
* Correspondence: davidma@uoguelph.ca

Received: 7 May 2020; Accepted: 17 June 2020; Published: 19 June 2020

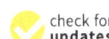

Abstract: Parents' stress is independently associated with increased child adiposity, but parents' stress may also interfere with childhood obesity prevention programs. The disruptions to the family dynamic caused by participating in a behaviour change intervention may exacerbate parent stress and undermine overall intervention efficacy. This study explored how family stress levels were impacted by participation in a home-based obesity prevention intervention. Data were collected from 77 families (56 fathers, 77 mothers) participating in the Guelph Family Health Study (GFHS), a pilot randomized control trial of a home-based obesity prevention intervention. Four measures of stress were investigated: general life stress, parenting distress, depressive symptoms, and household chaos. Multiple linear regression was used to compare the level of stress between the intervention and control groups at post-intervention and 1-year follow-up, adjusted for baseline stress. Analyses for mothers and fathers were stratified, except for household chaos which was measured at the family level. Results indicate no significant differences between intervention and control groups for any stress measure at any time point, indicating a neutral effect of the GFHS intervention on family stress. Future work should investigate the components of family-based intervention protocols that make participation minimally burdensome and consider embedding specific stress-reduction messaging to promote family health and wellbeing.

Keywords: stress; mental health; family; health behavior; childhood obesity; health intervention

1. Introduction

Childhood overweight and obesity are associated with several health concerns such as increased risk of chronic illnesses like cardiovascular disease, type 2 diabetes, cancer, and reduced overall lifespan, as well as increased risk of being bullied and developing disordered eating habits due to societal bias against those in larger bodies [1–4]. While there is a well-recognized genetic predisposition to body composition, the main focus of childhood obesity prevention has been on health behaviours such as dietary patterns, physical activity, sedentary or screen-based time, and sleep quality. There appears to be a critical window of development in early childhood where lifelong health behaviour patterns are largely established [5,6]. This presents an especially advantageous target for programs to focus on prevention in early life to maximize the preventative benefit of healthful behavioural patterns. Parental involvement has repeatedly been demonstrated to play a key role in the success of childhood obesity prevention programs [7–10]. These family-based behaviour change interventions typically focus on changing parenting practices and/or family behaviours such as eating meals as a family or group physical activities. However, parents engaged in a home-based childhood obesity prevention program manage several roles; they are participants making changes to their own behaviours plus being the taskmaster for their child's compliance, as well as the many other roles that they serve outside of the intervention context. The competing demands on parents' time and resources are numerous and dynamic, making it especially complex to effectively engage them in childhood obesity prevention programs.

Parents' stress may be an additional key consideration for family-based childhood obesity prevention programs for two key reasons. First, past research has established cross-sectional associations between parent stress or household dysfunction and several child health outcomes, including behaviours such as increased screen viewing [11], fast food consumption [12] as well as overall child weight status [12–15]. The second consideration is that parents who are overwhelmed may have difficulties adhering to an obesity prevention program, thus undermining the program's efficacy. It is well-understood that family routines are an important contributor to family well-being and positively influence children's development [16–19], but participation in a family-based childhood obesity prevention program is likely to impose substantial changes in the families' typical routines and activities. This perturbation of existing habits, even if intended for healthful changes, may inadvertently disrupt balances within the home. Alternatively, it is possible that promoting new behaviours as part of healthful routines could help families to establish more order and regularity within the home, thus decreasing overall family stress. The impact of health promotion programs on parents' wellbeing has not been widely explored.

In addition, dominant expectations of parenting place much more responsibility on mothers than fathers for active management of children's health and health behaviours [20,21]. Studies in Canada, the US, and Europe consistently demonstrate that, despite men's increasing involvement, women take on the bulk of responsibility for house and family work, including assuming responsibility for the health and well-being of family members, organizing their children's lives, and planning and preparing meals [20,21]. Thus, family-based health interventions may inadvertently reinforce the gendered division of labour and could result in an enhanced level of stress among mothers as compared to fathers. Additionally, perceptions and consequences of stress have repeatedly been demonstrated to differ between males and females [22–26], thus making gender an important consideration when exploring how participation in a family-based intervention may influence family stress.

The purpose of this study was to investigate the longitudinal changes in parents' perceived general life stress, parenting distress, depressive symptoms, and household chaos as a function of participation in a family-based health promotion intervention program among a cohort of Canadian mothers and fathers of young children. This study also examined whether these changes in family stress were moderated by parent gender.

2. Materials and Methods

2.1. Study Participants

This study used the Pilot phase 1 and 2 studies of the Guelph Family Health Study (GFHS), a pilot randomized control trial of a home-based obesity prevention intervention (clinical trials registration number NCT02223234, University of Guelph Research Ethics Board REB14AP008). The primary aim of the pilot studies was to test the feasibility of the intervention and assessment protocols. Detailed procedures of the pilot are published elsewhere [27] and briefly summarized below. Participants were recruited using posters and rack cards displayed at local family health team and early childhood education centres as well as posts to these agencies' social media accounts. To be eligible to participate, families had to have at least one child between the ages of 18 months to 5 years of age, live in Wellington

County, Ontario, Canada, with no plans to move in the following year, and have at least one parent able to respond to surveys in English.

Data for these analyses were collected at baseline, 6-months (post-intervention) and 18-months (1-year post-intervention). Participating families received grocery gift cards as compensation at each time point of assessment.

2.2. Exclusions and Losses to Follow-Up

As shown in Figure 1, 151 parent participants from 86 families met eligibility criteria and were enrolled in the study, though three families (three mothers, one father) later declined to participate before completing baseline assessment. The remaining 83 families (147 parents; 83 mothers, 64 fathers) were randomized to the three treatment groups: two home visits with a health educator (2HV), four home visits with a health educator (4HV), and a minimal-attention control, the protocols of which are explained further below. One family (one mother) randomized to the 4 HV group later declined to receive the intervention and was eventually lost to follow-up. The remaining 82 families (146 parents) completed all components of the intervention program, though five families (five mothers, six fathers) were later lost to follow-up, resulting in a 92.8% retention rate of the GFHS Pilot 1 and 2 cohorts at 1-year post-intervention. No harms of the intervention were detected.

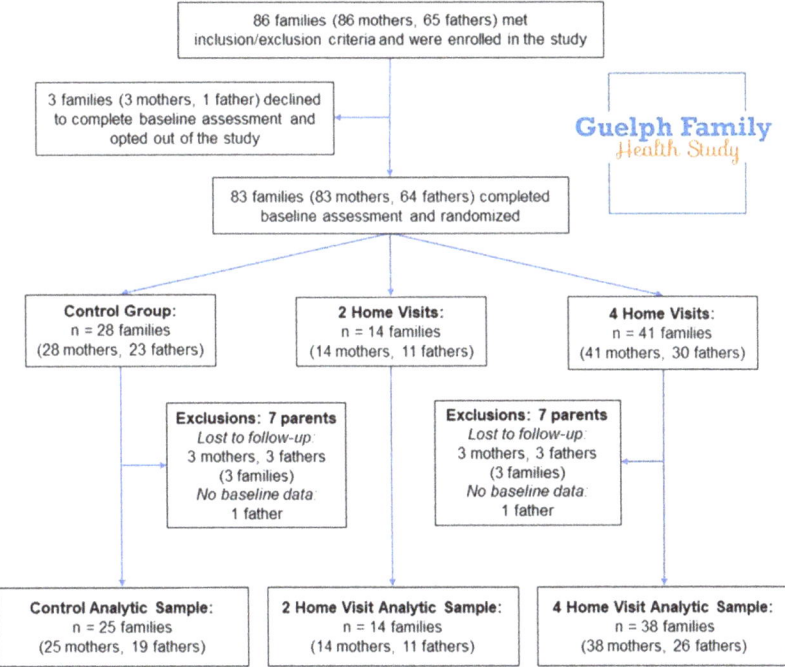

Figure 1. Study design and participant flow of the analytic sample from the Guelph Family Health Study Pilot Phase 1 and Phase 2 parent participants.

In addition to the 11 participants who were lost to follow-up, two fathers did not complete baseline stress measures and were therefore excluded from this analytic sample. Thus, a final analytic sample of 133 parent participants (77 mothers, 56 fathers) from 77 families was used for these analyses.

2.3. GFHS Intervention

The GFHS was designed as a home-based childhood obesity prevention program, informed by the Family Systems [28] and Self Determination [29] theories. The program used motivational interviewing, a collaborative and client-centred counselling technique that increases the likelihood of successful behaviour change by providing families with a sense of autonomy, confidence, and support with respect to health goals that the families set for themselves. Suggested goals in the GFHS included increasing fruit and vegetable intake, replacing sugar-sweetened beverages with water, reducing screen time, establishing a bedtime routine to promote adequate sleep, encouraging physical activity, or another goal of the family's own creation. The intervention program was delivered by a health educator, a registered dietitian trained in motivational interviewing, who worked with the families to develop personalized and self-directed health goals and provided support throughout the 6-month intervention period. These sessions were held in the family's home and typically were an hour in duration. Complementary to the home visits were a series of emails and mailed materials tailored to the family's goals, such as colourful plates to encourage more family meals or children's books to encourage regular sleep routines. Full details of the intervention protocol have been published previously [27].

All participants completed the baseline assessment, including a series of surveys and health visits at the University of Guelph, where measurements such as height, weight, blood pressure, and body composition were taken by trained research assistants. After baseline assessment families were randomized by the study coordinator into one of three parallel groups (in Pilot 1) or into one of two parallel groups (in Pilot 2) using a pseudo-random number generator. The three groups in Pilot 1 consisted of a minimal-attention control group (general health advice through monthly emails, such as current Canadian physical activity guidelines), a two home visit intervention group (home visits with a health educator, weekly emails, and monthly mailed incentives), and a four home visit intervention group (differing only in number of visits from the two home visit group). In Pilot 2, families were randomized to control or four home visits based on early feedback from Pilot 1 participants that two home visits were not preferred. Baseline data were collected between December 2014 and November 2016 at the University of Guelph, Ontario, Canada; follow-up data collection was completed by November 2018.

2.4. Stress Measures

Four different types of stress (general life stress, parenting distress, parental depression, and household chaos) were assessed via paper ($n = 152$) or online ($n = 238$) surveys. Data collection was conducted at baseline, then repeated post-intervention (6 months from baseline) and at 1-year post-intervention (18 months from baseline).

General life stress was examined with the question "Using a scale from 1 to 10, where 1 means 'no stress' and 10 means 'an extreme amount of stress', how much stress would you say you have experienced in the last year?" [12].

Levels of stress specific to the role of being a parent were examined using the 12-item Parent Distress subscale of the Parenting Stress Index (PSI) [30]. Participants were asked to respond on a 5-point Likert scale from 1 (strongly disagree) to 5 (strongly agree) to items such as "I often have the feeling that I cannot handle things very well", "I feel trapped by my responsibilities as a parent", and "Having a child has caused more problems than I expected in my relationship with my spouse (or male/female friend)". For parents who completed the paper version of the surveys, the response options were on a 4-point Likert scale (i.e., the neither disagree nor agree option was not included). This discrepancy in the response options between the paper and online surveys was managed by recoding the paper survey response options as 1 = strongly disagree, 2 = disagree, 4 = agree, and 5 = strongly agree. Analyses with the paper and online survey data together showed similar results to when only the online survey data were used; thus, results for the paper and online survey were combined for these analyses. A total score out of 60 was calculated by summing the responses; higher scores indicate greater parental distress. Standardized Cronbach's alpha for mothers in this sample at baseline, was 0.86; for fathers, 0.78. The PSI has been validated for use among both mothers [30] and fathers [31] of young children.

Parental depressive symptoms were assessed with the Andresen short form of the Centre for Epidemiological Studies Depression Scale (CES-D) [32]. Sample items include "My sleep was restless", "Everything I did was an effort", and "I felt fearful", and were scored as 0 (less than one day last week), 1 (1–2 days), 2 (3–4 days), or 3 (5–7 days). A total score out of 30 was calculated by summing the responses; higher scores indicate greater depressive symptoms. Standardized Cronbach's alpha for mothers in this sample at baseline was 0.87; for fathers, 0.80.

Household dynamic and chaos were examined using the 15-item Confusion, Hubbub, and Order Scale (CHAOS) [33]. This scale conceptualizes noisiness, disorganization, and confusion within the home environment. Participants responded to items such as "We almost always seemed to be rushed" or "It's a real zoo in our home" on a 4-point Likert scale from 1 (very much like your own home) to 4 (not at all like your own home). The CHAOS survey was asked only of Parent 1 in this sample (the first parent to sign up for the study, of whom 76% were female), and this was used as a family wide measure. Standardized Cronbach's alpha for this scale at baseline was 0.88.

2.5. Statistical Methods

In intent-to-treat complete case analyses, we used multiple linear regression models to examine differences between the study groups (control, 2HV, and 4HV) for post-intervention and for 1-year follow-up stress measures after controlling for baseline. Results for the 2HV and 4HV groups were not substantively different (see Table A1), thus, we present results with the two intervention groups combined. General stress, parenting distress, and depressive symptoms were analysed for each participant; household chaos was considered to be a shared variable among family measures and was analysed at the household-level. Data from males and females were analysed separately to account for potential gender-based differences in stress perception [22–26] and to better compare these results to the predominantly mother-focused parenting research in the field [34]. Household chaos was examined as one observation per family, regardless of the gender of the parent who reported it. No demographic covariates were included in the model. The use of a randomized design would mean that any difference in demographic characteristics across study groups would be due to chance. Statistical analyses were performed using SAS University Edition Version 3.6 [35]. A p-value of < 0.05 was considered statistically significant for all analyses.

3. Results

3.1. Descriptive Data

As shown in Table 1, this analytic sample contained 56 fathers (42%) and 77 mothers (58%). The average age of participants at baseline was 35 years. Over 80% of participants identified as white and over 40% had received postgraduate education. Of the 77 participating families, approximately 85% had parents who were married, nearly 80% contained two or more children, and 45% had an annual household income of $100,000 or more. Baseline characteristics (Table 1) and levels of stress (Table 2) were similar among the intervention and control groups.

Table 1. Baseline characteristics of parent participants in the Guelph Family Health Study.

Characteristic (Individual)	Overall n = 133 Parents	Control n = 44 Parents	Intervention n = 89 Parents
Baseline age (years), mean (SD)	35.5 (4.6)	34.8 (4.8)	35.9 (4.6)
Relation to child, n (%)			
Father	56 (42.1%)	19 (43.2%)	37 (41.6%)
Mother	77 (57.9%)	25 (56.8%)	52 (58.4%)
Ethnicity, n (%)			
White	109 (82.0%)	37 (84.1%)	72 (80.9%)
Other (e.g., Chinese, Latin American, South Asian, West Asian)	22 (16.5%)	5 (11.4%)	16 (18.9%)
Not reported	2 (1.5%)	2 (4.5%)	0 (0.0%)
Education, n (%)			
College diploma or less	30 (22.6%)	7 (15.9%)	23 (25.8%)
Some university or degree	35 (33.8%)	14 (38.1%)	31 (34.8%)
Postgraduate training	56 (42.1%)	21 (47.7%)	35 (39.3%)
Did not disclose	2 (1.5%)	2 (4.5%)	0 (0.0%)
Characteristic (Family Level)	**n = 77 families**	**n = 25 families**	**n = 52 families**
Marital status, n (%)			
Married	66 (85.7%)	22 (88.0%)	44 (84.6%)
Other (i.e., living with partner, divorced)	11 (14.3%)	3 (12.0%)	8 (15.4%)
Annual household income, n (%)			
< $60,000	16 (20.8%)	5 (20.0%)	11 (21.2%)
$60,000 to $99,999	24 (31.2%)	5 (20.0%)	19 (36.5%)
$100,000+	34 (44.2%)	14 (56.0%)	20 (38.5%)
Not reported	3 (3.9%)	1 (4.0%)	2 (3.8%)
Number of children, n (%)			
1	17 (22.1%)	7 (28.0%)	10 (19.2%)
2	45 (58.4%)	15 (60.0%)	30 (57.7%)
3 or more	15 (19.5%)	3 (12.0%)	12 (23.1%)

Table 2. Linear regression results comparing intervention and control groups with respect to stress levels at post-intervention and at 1-year follow-up after controlling for baseline, stratified by parent gender. Household chaos model analysed at the family level (one observation per household).

Measure	Intervention Group	Baseline Mean (SD)	Post-Intervention Mean (SD)	Difference from Control [1] β (95% CI) p value	1-Year Follow-Up Mean (SD)	Difference from Control [1] β (95% CI) p Value
		Analysis of mothers in the home visit groups (n = 52) compared to the control group (n = 25)				
General Stress	Intervention	6.60 (2.02)	6.02 (2.10)	−0.60 (−1.47, 0.27) 0.18	6.55 (1.89)	−0.15 (−1.13, 0.83) 0.76
	Control	6.32 (2.12)	6.63 (1.69)		6.63 (1.92)	
Parenting Distress	Intervention	28.04 (9.70)	26.80 (8.91)	−0.62 (−4.90, 3.65) 0.77	28.49 (8.91)	−1.92 (−5.37, 1.53) 0.27
	Control	29.68 (6.64)	28.13 (9.28)		30.91 (8.26)	
Depressive Symptoms	Intervention	6.78 (5.39)	5.98 (5.23)	−0.57 (−2.98, 1.84) 0.64	6.00 (4.48)	−0.92 (−2.87, 1.04) 0.35
	Control	6.80 (4.34)	6.67 (5.01)		6.73 (4.73)	
		Analysis of fathers in the home visit groups (n = 37) compared to the control group (n = 19)				
General Stress	Intervention	6.78 (1.86)	6.72 (1.63)	0.56 (−0.43, 1.56) 0.26	6.03 (2.14)	−0.90 (−2.08, 0.27) 0.13
	Control	6.26 (2.10)	5.88 (2.20)		6.57 (2.06)	
Parenting Distress	Intervention	29.03 (8.03)	27.81 (7.16)	−1.28 (−4.60, 2.04) 0.44	28.03 (8.12)	−0.41 (−4.56, 3.74) 0.84
	Control	27.53 (5.50)	28.65 (5.72)		27.57 (4.38)	
Depressive Symptoms	Intervention	7.19 (5.25)	6.13 (4.63)	−0.91 (−3.48, 1.67) 0.48	6.57 (4.31)	−0.70 (−2.98, 1.58) 0.54
	Control	7.63 (3.39)	7.06 (4.38)		7.86 (3.23)	
		Analysis of families in the home visit groups (n = 52) compared to control group (n = 25)				
Household Chaos	Intervention	31.02 (8.39)	30.92 (8.07)	0.65 (−3.06, 1.77) 0.60	30.29 (7.89)	−2.57 (−5.34, 0.21) 0.07
	Control	31.04 (6.31)	31.74 (6.45)		33.00 (6.20)	

[1] Linear regression coefficient after controlling for baseline.

3.2. Mean Stress Levels

As shown in Table 2, mothers and fathers reported moderate levels of stress on all measures at all time points and across all treatment groups. Across the three timepoints, mothers' general stress means ranged from 6.0 to 6.6 out of a maximum score of 10. Fathers' general stress scores ranged from 5.9 to 6.8. Mothers' parenting distress mean scores ranged from 26.8 to 30.9 out of a maximum score of 60, which ranks between the 59th and 68th percentiles of the PSI scoring reference [30]. Fathers' parenting distress scores ranged from 27.5 to 29.0, which falls within the 62nd and 64th percentiles. Mothers' depressive symptoms scores ranged from 6.0 to 6.8; fathers' scores ranged from 6.1 to 7.9. While these CES-D means may seem low in relation to the maximum score of 30 points, they should be interpreted as moderate given that a CES-D score of 10 or greater indicates significant depressive symptomology consistent with clinical diagnosis [32]. Household chaos means ranged from 30.3 to 33.0 out of a maximum score of 60 points.

3.3. Post-Intervention

No intervention effect was observed for any of the stress measures among mothers or fathers at post-intervention after controlling for baseline measures. Among mothers randomized to the intervention, there was a non-significant difference of −0.60 (95% CI: −1.47, 0.27) compared to control, after adjustment for baseline. Among fathers, there was a non-significant difference of 0.56 (95% CI: −0.43, 1.56) in the intervention compared to control, after adjustment for baseline. For parenting distress, mothers randomized to the intervention had a non-significant difference of −0.62 (95% CI: −4.90, 3.65) to control, after adjustment for baseline. Among fathers in the intervention, there was a non-significant difference of −1.28 (95% CI: −4.60, 2.04) compared to the control after adjustment for baseline. Differences in depressive symptoms followed a similar trend; no significant differences were found for either mothers or fathers. Among mothers randomized to the intervention, there was a non-significant difference of −0.57 (95% CI: −2.98, 1.84) compared to the control, after adjustment for baseline. As was found for mothers' depressive symptoms scores, there was no significant difference between fathers in the intervention compared to those in the control after controlling for baseline (−0.91, 95% CI: −3.48, 1.67).

At the family level, household chaos scores were similar at baseline and post-intervention. The difference of 0.65 (95% CI: −3.06, 1.77) was not statistically significant.

3.4. 1-Year Follow-Up

Similar to the results at post-intervention, no intervention effect was observed for any of the stress measures among mothers or fathers at 1-year follow-up after controlling for baseline (Table 2). Specifically for general stress, the difference between the intervention and control was not significant (−0.15, 95% CI: −1.13, 0.83) after controlling for baseline. Among fathers, there was a non-significant difference in general stress at 1-year post-intervention after controlling for baseline (−0.90, 95% CI: −2.08, 0.27). The mean parental distress score at 1-year follow-up among mothers randomized to the intervention compared to the control yielded a non-significant difference of −1.92 (95% CI: −5.37, 1.53). Likewise, for fathers, the mean parental distress among those randomized to the intervention was not significantly different from the control at 1-year after controlling for baseline (−0.41, 95% CI: −4.56, 3.74). Among mothers randomized to the intervention, the mean depressive symptoms score was not significantly different from mothers randomized to the control (−0.92, 95% CI: −2.87, 1.04) after controlling for baseline. Among fathers, comparison of mean depressive symptoms scores at 1-year follow-up for the intervention and control resulted in a non-significant difference of −0.70 (95% CI: −2.98, 1.58) after controlling for baseline.

At 1-year follow-up, mean household chaos among families randomized to the intervention compared to the control resulted in a non-significant difference of −2.57 (95% CI: −5.34, 0.21) after controlling for baseline.

4. Discussion

The purpose of this study was to investigate differences in family-based stress between intervention and control groups at post-intervention and 1-year follow-up in a sample of Canadian mothers and fathers participating in the GFHS, a home-based obesity prevention randomized control trial. Our results suggest no harmful impact of the intervention program on the family environment across the four dimensions examined.

The GFHS pilot studies demonstrated success in increasing children's fruit and vegetable consumption [36] and at post-intervention, children and parents had lower indices of body fat [27,37]. This suggests that the GFHS intervention program did meaningfully change some family behaviours, but until the present study, it was unknown how these changes could impact families' stress levels.

The program may have encouraged families to implement more structured, organized behavioural patterns focused around these health goals, thus calming the home environment and increasing parenting confidence; however it is also possible that the program may have caused conflict or confusion from the disruptions to the families' typical behaviours. Our results suggest that family stress levels were not different when comparing intervention to control families, despite evidence that behavioural changes did indeed occur among both parents and children [27,36,37].

There are several potential explanations for these results. Careful planning and consideration went into designing the GFHS intervention to have a minimal burden on participants, such as the health educator visits occurring within the family's home instead of at a research centre, the use of online surveys to allow for more convenient completion, and financial compensation for the family's time. Thus, participation in the study may not have been particularly burdensome to families. In addition, the use of motivational interviewing, a client-centred counselling technique that empowers participants to choose their own goals and strategies to achieve them [38], may have helped to relieve the burden from the participants compared to other more expert-led intervention techniques. The exact characteristics of the intervention protocol that contributed to these effects would require further research to disentangle but likely all factors had an influence.

The current body of evidence on household stress is based mostly on clinical populations such as children with behavioural problems, developmental delays, or chronic illness [39–42], or special interest family situations such as parents who are military servicemembers or incarcerated [43–45], including the few studies that have examined family stress over the course of an intervention program [46–49]. This study extends evidence in the literature by providing insight into the impact of a home-based health intervention on the family environment in a community-based non-clinical sample of families. Additionally, our inclusion of both mothers' and fathers' perceptions addresses a substantial gap in the literature [34]. The present study also includes follow-up beyond the post-intervention period to better understand the nature of these associations.

Despite this study's many strengths, there are some limitations that merit consideration. First, these analyses are based on a small cohort of families because the GFHS pilot was not designed as a fully powered study; thus, there is a risk that important effects were not identified. Second, with respect to the general stress measure, a single item may not be sufficient to capture the many dimensions of everyday stress. Third, our protocol is to ask only Parent 1 (defined as the first parent to enrol in the study) items relating to the household; as such, it is possible that perceptions of the home environment chaos may differ between cohabitants. Fourth, the majority of families in our sample identified as Caucasian and nearly half had an annual household income of over $100,000, which limits the generalizability of our results. Additional research with a diverse sample of families is needed because the socio-cultural environment, including ethnic and economic factors, is an important consideration for parenting practices and family stress [50–52]. Finally, while it is most likely that any differences in stress due to the intervention would be evident in the post-intervention period, it is possible that the true nature of these associations requires a longer follow-up period to be discovered. Continued longer-term monitoring of the participants' stress may be an important consideration for our participants' retention in the study. Indeed, any family-focused or home-based intervention program should consider how disruptions to the family dynamic may influence participants' willingness to adhere to the program.

5. Conclusions

The GFHS has several behaviour change goals aimed at preventing childhood obesity; however, reducing family stress levels was not among the primary intentions of the program. While these results show no differences in family stress between the intervention and control groups, the overall mean stress levels seen here indicate that families may benefit from intervention strategies specifically aimed at reducing family stress. Program designs that integrate family physical and mental health promotion should be further investigated. In conclusion, these results demonstrate a need for continued research into how home-based health interventions influence the family environment. In particular, there is a need for intervention programs that incorporate specific stress-reduction messaging into family health programs.

Author Contributions: Conceptualization, V.H. and J.H.; Formal Analysis, V.H.; Writing—Original Draft Preparation, V.H.; Writing—Review & Editing, V.H., G.D., J.H., and D.W.L.M.; Visualization, V.H.; Supervision, J.H. and D.W.L.M.; Project Administration, J.H. and D.W.L.M.; Funding Acquisition, J.H. and D.W.L.M. All authors have read and agreed to the published version of the manuscript.

Funding: This research was partially supported by the University of Guelph's Health for Life Initiative.

Conflicts of Interest: The authors declare no conflict of interest. The funders had no role in the design of the study; in the collection, analyses, or interpretation of data; in the writing of the manuscript, or in the decision to publish the results.

Appendix A

Table A1. Linear regression results comparing intervention (two home visit and four home visit groups) and control groups with respect to stress levels at post-intervention and at 1-year follow-up after controlling for baseline, stratified by parent gender. Household chaos model analysed at the family level (one observation per household).

Measure	Intervention Group	Baseline Mean (SD)	Post-Intervention Mean (SD)	Difference from Control [1] B (95% CI) p Value	1-Year Follow-Up Mean (SD)	Difference from Control [1] β (95% CI) p Value
	Analysis of mothers in the 2 home visit (n = 14) and 4 home visit (n = 37) groups compared to the control (n = 25)					
General Stress	Control	6.32 (2.12)	6.63 (1.69)		6.64 (1.92)	
	2HV	5.92 (2.33)	5.21 (2.01)	−1.07 (−2.27, 0.13) 0.08	6.29 (2.33)	−0.34 (−1.68, 1.01) 0.62
	4HV	6.84 (1.88)	6.33 (2.08)	−0.42 (−1.35, 0.51) 0.37	6.66 (1.71)	−0.08 (−1.13, 0.97) 0.88
Parenting Distress	Control	29.68 (6.64)	28.13 (9.28)		30.91 (8.26)	
	2HV	23.07 (5.86)	26.14 (8.20)	0.71 (−5.31, 6.72) 0.81	25.36 (6.06)	−3.01 (−7.74, 1.73) 0.21
	4HV	29.92 (10.25)	27.06 (9.27)	−1.10 (−5.65, 3.45) 0.63	29.74 (7.57)	−1.52 (−5.18, 2.14) 0.41
Depressive Symptoms	Control	6.80 (4.34)	6.67 (5.01)		6.73 (4.73)	
	2HV	4.71 (4.38)	5.43 (4.57)	−0.50 (−3.80, 2.79) 0.76	4.57 (2.53)	−0.35 (−1.67, 0.97) 0.60
	4HV	7.58 (5.58)	6.19 (5.51)	−0.60 (−3.19, 2.00) 0.65	6.57 (4.97)	0.06 (−1.00, 1.12) 0.91
	Analysis of fathers in the 2 home visit (n = 11) and 4 home visit (n = 26) groups compared to the control (n = 19)					
General Stress	Control	6.26 (2.10)	5.88 (2.20)		6.57 (2.06)	
	2HV	6.82 (1.78)	6.60 (1.58)	0.32 (−1.01, 1.66) 0.63	6.33 (2.29)	−0.57 (−2.13, 0.99) 0.46
	4HV	6.77 (1.69)	6.77 (1.69)	0.66 (−0.41, 1.74) 0.22	5.90 (2.11)	−1.05 (−2.31, 0.22) 0.10

Table A1. Cont.

Measure	Intervention Group	Baseline Mean (SD)	Post-Intervention Mean (SD)	Difference from Control [1] B (95% CI) p Value	1-Year Follow-Up Mean (SD)	Difference from Control [1] β (95% CI) p Value
	Analysis of fathers in the 2 home visit (n = 11) and 4 home visit (n = 26) groups compared to the control (n = 19)					
Parenting Distress	Control	27.53 (5.50)	28.65 (5.72)	−1.62 (−6.07, 2.83) 0.47	27.57 (4.38)	−1.24 (−6.77, 4.29) 0.65
	2HV	28.27 (9.33)	27.10 (4.89)		27.33 (6.36)	
	4HV	29.35 (7.59)	28.14 (8.07)	−1.12 (−4.74, 2.49) 0.54	28.33 (8.89)	−0.06 (−4.52, 4.41) 0.98
Depressive Symptoms	Control	7.63 (3.39)	7.06 (4.38)	−0.78 (−4.26, 2.71) 0.66	7.86 (3.23)	−0.10 (−1.97, 1.78) 0.92
	2HV	5.82 (3.52)	5.70 (3.89)		4.00 (2.35)	
	4HV	7.77 (5.80)	6.32 (5.01)	−0.97 (−3.78, 1.84) 0.49	7.67 (4.53)	−0.61 (−2.11, 0.89) 0.42
	Analysis of families in the 2 home visit (n = 14) and 4 home visit (n = 36) groups compared to control (n = 24)					
Household Chaos	Control	31.04 (6.31)	31.74 (6.45)	−0.43 (−3.66, 2.81) 0.79	33.00 (6.20)	−3.42 (−7.16, 0.32) 0.07
	2HV	30.50 (8.48)	31.00 (8.17)		29.54 (8.08)	
	4HV	31.22 (8.47)	30.89 (8.14)	−0.74 (−3.33, 1.86) 0.57	30.57 (7.92)	−2.22 (−5.19, 0.73) 0.14

[1] Linear regression coefficient after controlling for baseline.

References

1. Pont, S.J.; Puhl, R.; Cook, S.R.; Slusser, W. Stigma Experienced by Children and Adolescents with Obesity. *Pediatrics* **2017**, *140*, e20173034. [CrossRef] [PubMed]
2. Tsiros, M.D.; Olds, T.; Buckley, J.D.; Grimshaw, P.; Brennan, L.; Walkley, J.; Hills, A.P.; Howe, P.R.C.; Coates, A.M. Health-related quality of life in obese children and adolescents. *Int. J. Obes.* **2009**, *33*, 387–400. [CrossRef] [PubMed]
3. Lobstein, T.; Baur, L.; Uauy, R. Obesity in children and young people: A crisis in public health. *Obes. Rev.* **2004**, *5*, 4–85. [CrossRef] [PubMed]
4. *World Health Organisation Prioritizing Areas for Action in the Field of Population-Based Prevention of Childhood Obesity: Report of a WHO Forum and Technical Meeting*; WHO: Geneva, Switzerland, 2009.
5. Singer, M.R.; Moore, L.L.; Garrahie, E.J.; Ellison, R.C. The tracking of nutrient intake in young children: The Framingham Children's Study. *Am. J. Public Health* **1995**, *85*, 1673–1677. [CrossRef]
6. Moore, L.L.; Nguyen, U.S.D.T.; Rothman, K.J.; Cupples, L.A.; Ellison, R.C. Preschool physical activity level and change in body fatness in young children: The Framingham Children's Study. *Am. J. Epidemiol.* **1995**, *142*, 982–988. [CrossRef]
7. Wang, Y.; Cai, L.; Wu, Y.; Wilson, R.F.; Weston, C.; Fawole, O.; Bleich, S.N.; Cheskin, L.J.; Showell, N.N.; Lau, B.D.; et al. What childhood obesity prevention programmes work? A systematic review and meta-analysis. *Obes. Rev.* **2015**, *16*, 547–565. [CrossRef]
8. Hendrie, G.A.; Brindal, E.; Corsini, N.; Gardner, C.; Baird, D.; Golley, R.K. Combined Home and School Obesity Prevention Interventions for Children. *Health Educ. Behav.* **2012**, *39*, 159–171. [CrossRef]
9. Lindsay, A.C.; Sussner, K.M.; Kim, J.; Gortmaker, S.L. The role of parents in preventing childhood obesity. *Future Child.* **2006**, *16*, 169–186. [CrossRef] [PubMed]
10. Favaro, A.; Santonastaso, P. Effects of parents' psychological characteristics and eating behaviour on childhood obesity and dietary compliance. *J. Psychosom. Res.* **1995**, *39*, 145–151. [CrossRef]
11. Walton, K.; Simpson, J.R.; Darlington, G.; Haines, J. Parenting stress: A cross-sectional analysis of associations with childhood obesity, physical activity, and TV viewing. *BMC Pediatrics* **2014**, *14*, 244. [CrossRef] [PubMed]
12. Parks, E.P.; Kumanyika, S.; Moore, R.H.; Stettler, N.; Wrotniak, B.H.; Kazak, A. Influence of stress in parents on child obesity and related behaviors. *Pediatrics* **2012**, *130*, e1096–e1104. [CrossRef] [PubMed]
13. Halliday, J.A.; Palma, C.L.; Mellor, D.; Green, J.; Renzaho, A.M.N. The relationship between family functioning and child and adolescent overweight and obesity: A systematic review. *Int. J. Obes.* **2014**, *38*, 480–493. [CrossRef]

14. Bates, C.R.; Buscemi, J.; Nicholson, L.M.; Cory, M.; Jagpal, A.; Bohnert, A.M. Links between the organization of the family home environment and child obesity: A systematic review. *Obes. Rev.* **2018**, *19*, 716–727. [CrossRef] [PubMed]
15. Tate, E.B.; Wood, W.; Liao, Y.; Dunton, G.F. Do stressed mothers have heavier children? A meta-analysis on the relationship between maternal stress and child body mass index. *Obes. Rev.* **2015**, *16*, 351–361. [CrossRef]
16. Fiese, B.H.; Hooker, K.A.; Kotary, L.; Schwagler, J.; Rimmer, M. Family Stories in the Early Stages of Parenthood. *J. Marriage Fam.* **1995**, *57*, 763–770. [CrossRef]
17. Fiese, B.H.; Tomcho, T.J.; Douglas, M.; Josephs, K.; Poltrock, S.; Baker, T. A review of 50 years of research on naturally occurring family routines and rituals: Cause for celebration? *J. Fam. Psychol.* **2002**, *16*, 381–390. [CrossRef] [PubMed]
18. Markson, S.; Fiese, B.H. Family Rituals as a Protective Factor for Children with Asthma. *J. Pediatrics Psychol.* **2000**, *25*, 471–480. [CrossRef]
19. Everhart, R.S.; Fiese, B.H.; Reis, H.; Sprecher, S.; Everhart, R.S.; Fiese, B.H. Family Routines and Rituals. *Encycl. Hum. Relatsh.* **2013**, *20*, 284–299.
20. Beagan, B.; Chapman, G.E.; D'Sylva, A.; Bassett, B.R. "It's just easier for me to do it": Rationalizing the family division of foodwork. *Sociology* **2008**, *42*, 653–671. [CrossRef]
21. Ristovski-Slijepcevic, S.; Chapman, G.E.; Beagan, B.L. Being a 'Good Mother': Dietary governmentality in the family food practices of three ethnocultural groups in Canada. *J. Soc. Study Health Illn. Med.* **2010**, *14*, 467–483. [CrossRef]
22. Ayanian, J.Z.; Block, J.P.; He, Y.; Zaslavsky, A.M.; Ding, L. Psychosocial stress and change in weight among US adults. *Am. J. Epidemiol.* **2009**, *170*, 181–192.
23. Lee, M.R.; Cacic, K.; Demers, C.H.; Haroon, M.; Heishman, S.; Hommer, D.W.; Epstein, D.H.; Ross, T.J.; Stein, E.A.; Heilig, M.; et al. Gender differences in neural–behavioral response to self-observation during a novel fMRI social stress task. *Neuropsychologia* **2014**, *53*, 257–263. [CrossRef]
24. Meshefedjian, G.A.; Fournier, M.; Blanchard, D.; Frigault, L.-R.R. Gender-specific correlates of perceived life stress: A population-based study, Montreal, Canada, 2012. *Can. J. Public Health* **2019**, *110*, 563–574. [CrossRef] [PubMed]
25. Shivpuri, S.; Gallo, L.C.; Crouse, J.R.; Allison, M.A. The association between chronic stress type and C-reactive protein in the multi-ethnic study of atherosclerosis: Does gender make a difference? *J. Behav. Med.* **2012**, *35*, 74–85. [CrossRef] [PubMed]
26. Steptoe, A.; Hamer, M.; Chida, Y. The effects of acute psychological stress on circulating inflammatory factors in humans: A review and meta-analysis. *Brain Behav. Immun.* **2007**, *21*, 901–912. [CrossRef]
27. Haines, J.; Douglas, S.; Mirotta, J.A.; O'Kane, C.; Breau, R.; Walton, K.; Krystia, O.; Chamoun, E.; Annis, A.; Darlington, G.A.; et al. Guelph Family Health Study: Pilot study of a home-based obesity prevention intervention. *Can. J. Public Health* **2018**, *109*, 549–560. [CrossRef]
28. Ackerman, N.W. *The Psychodynamics of Family Life*; Basic Books: New York, NY, USA, 1958.
29. Ryan, R.M.; Deci, E.L. Self-determination theory and the facilitation of intrinsic motivation, social development, and well-being. *Am. Psychol.* **2000**, *55*, 68–78. [CrossRef]
30. Abidin, R.R. *Parenting Stress Index Professional Manual*; Par Inc.: Lutz, FL, USA, 2012.
31. McKelvey, L.M.; Whiteside-Mansell, L.; Faldowski, R.A.; Shears, J.; Ayoub, C.; Hart, A.D. Validity of the Short Form of the Parenting Stress Index for Fathers of Toddlers. *J. Child Fam. Stud.* **2009**, *18*, 102–111. [CrossRef]
32. Andresen, E.M.; Byers, K.; Friary, J.; Kosloski, K.; Montgomery, R. Performance of the 10-item Center for Epidemiologic Studies Depression scale for caregiving research. *SAGE Open Med.* **2013**, *1*, 205031211351457. [CrossRef] [PubMed]
33. Matheny, A.P.; Wachs, T.D.; Ludwig, J.L.; Phillips, K. Bringing order out of chaos: Psychometric characteristics of the confusion, hubbub, and order scale. *J. Appl. Dev. Psychol.* **1995**, *16*, 429–444. [CrossRef]
34. Davison, K.K.; Kitos, N.; Aftosmes-Tobio, A.; Ash, T.; Agaronov, A.; Sepulveda, M.; Haines, J. The forgotten parent: Fathers' representation in family interventions to prevent childhood obesity. *Prev. Med. (Baltimore)* **2018**, *111*, 170–176. [CrossRef]
35. SAS Institute Inc. *SAS/IML®14.1 User's Guide*; SAS Institute Inc.: Cary, NC, USA, 2015.
36. Mirotta, J.A.; Darlington, G.A.; Buchholz, A.C.; Haines, J.; Ma, D.W.L.; Duncan, A.M. Guelph Family Health Study's Home-Based Obesity Prevention Intervention Increases Fibre and Fruit Intake in Preschool-Aged Children. *Can. J. Diet. Pract. Res.* **2018**, *79*, 86–90. [CrossRef] [PubMed]

37. Krystia, O.; Ambrose, T.; Darlington, G.; Ma, D.W.L.; Buchholz, A.C.; Haines, J. A randomized home-based childhood obesity prevention pilot intervention has favourable effects on parental body composition: Preliminary evidence from the Guelph Family Health Study. *BMC Obes.* **2019**, *6*, 10. [CrossRef] [PubMed]
38. O'Kane, C.; Irwin, J.D.; Morrow, D.; Tang, L.; Wong, S.; Buchholz, A.C.; Ma, D.W.L.; Haines, J. Motivational interviewing with families in the home environment. *Patient Educ. Couns.* **2019**, *102*, 2073–2080. [CrossRef] [PubMed]
39. Rao, P.A.; Beidel, D.C. The Impact of Children with High-Functioning Autism on Parental Stress, Sibling Adjustment, and Family Functioning. *Behav. Modif.* **2009**, *33*, 437–451. [CrossRef]
40. Hayes, S.A.; Watson, S.L. The Impact of Parenting Stress: A Meta-analysis of Studies Comparing the Experience of Parenting Stress in Parents of Children With and Without Autism Spectrum Disorder. *J. Autism Dev. Disord.* **2013**, *43*, 629–642. [CrossRef]
41. Barroso, N.E.; Mendez, L.; Graziano, P.A.; Bagner, D.M. Parenting Stress through the Lens of Different Clinical Groups: A Systematic Review & Meta-Analysis. *J. Abnorm. Child Psychol.* **2018**, *46*, 449–461.
42. Levine, A.; Zagoory-Sharon, O.; Feldman, R.; Lewis, J.G.; Weller, A. Measuring cortisol in human psychobiological studies. *Physiol. Behav.* **2007**, *90*, 43–53. [CrossRef]
43. Besemer, K.L.; Dennison, S.M. Family Imprisonment, Maternal Parenting Stress and Its Impact on Mother-Child Relationship Satisfaction. *J. Child Fam. Stud.* **2018**, *27*, 3897–3908. [CrossRef]
44. Malia, J.A. A reader's guide to family stress literature. *J. Loss Trauma* **2007**, *12*, 223–243. [CrossRef]
45. Dekel, R.; Goldblatt, H.; Keidar, M.; Solomon, Z.; Polliack, M. Being a Wife of a Veteran with Posttraumatic Stress Disorder. *Fam. Relat.* **2005**, *54*, 24–36. [CrossRef]
46. Schwichtenberg, A.; Poehlmann, J. Applied behaviour analysis: Does intervention intensity relate to family stressors and maternal well-being? *J. Intellect. Disabil. Res.* **2007**, *51*, 598–605. [CrossRef]
47. Rickards, A.L.; Walstab, J.E.; Wright-Rossi, R.A.; Simpson, J.; Reddihough, D.S. One-year follow-up of the outcome of a randomized controlled trial of a home-based intervention programme for children with autism and developmental delay and their families. *Child Care Health Dev.* **2009**, *35*, 593–602. [CrossRef]
48. Toth, S.L.; Sturge-Apple, M.L.; Rogosch, F.A.; Cicchetti, D. Mechanisms of change: Testing how preventative interventions impact psychological and physiological stress functioning in mothers in neglectful families. *Dev. Psychopathol.* **2015**, *27*, 1661–1674. [CrossRef] [PubMed]
49. Lester, P.; Liang, L.-J.; Milburn, N.; Mogil, C.; Woodward, K.; Nash, W.; Aralis, H.; Sinclair, M.; Semaan, A.; Klosinski, L.; et al. Evaluation of a Family-Centered Preventive Intervention for Military Families: Parent and Child Longitudinal Outcomes. *J. Am. Acad. Child Adolesc. Psychiatry* **2016**, *55*, 14–24. [CrossRef] [PubMed]
50. Harkness, S.; Super, C. Culture and Parenting. In *Handbook of Parenting*; Lawrence Erlbaum Associates Publishers: Mahwah, NJ, USA, 1995; Volume 2, pp. 253–280.
51. Hoff, E.; Laursen, B.; Tardiff, T. Socioeconomic Status and Parenting. In *Handbook of Parenting*; Lawrence Erlbaum Associates Publishers: Mahwah, NJ, USA, 1995; pp. 231–252.
52. Nomaguchi, K.; House, A.N. Racial-Ethnic Disparities in Maternal Parenting Stress. *J. Health Soc. Behav.* **2013**, *54*, 386–404. [CrossRef] [PubMed]

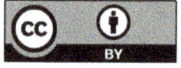

© 2020 by the authors. Licensee MDPI, Basel, Switzerland. This article is an open access article distributed under the terms and conditions of the Creative Commons Attribution (CC BY) license (http://creativecommons.org/licenses/by/4.0/).

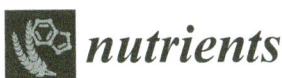

Article

Eating Vegetables First at Start of Meal and Food Intake among Preschool Children in Japan

Jiaxi Yang [1], Yukako Tani [2], Deirdre K. Tobias [3,4], Manami Ochi [5] and Takeo Fujiwara [2,*]

1. Department of Epidemiology, Harvard T. H. Chan School of Public Health, 677 Huntington Ave, Boston, MA 02215, USA; jiaxiyang@g.harvard.edu
2. Department of Global Health Promotion, Tokyo Medical and Dental University, 1-5-45 Yushima, Bunkyo-ku, Tokyo 113-8510, Japan; tani.hlth@tmd.ac.jp
3. Department of Nutrition, Harvard T. H. Chan School of Public Health, 677 Huntington Ave, Boston, MA 02215, USA; dtobias@bwh.harvard.edu
4. Division of Preventive Medicine, Department of Medicine, Brigham and Women's Hospital, 900 Commonwealth Avenue, Boston, MA 02215, USA
5. Department of Health and Welfare Services, National Institute of Public Health, 2-3-6 Minami, Wako-shi, Saitama 351-0197, Japan; ochi.m.aa@niph.go.jp
* Correspondence: fujiwara.hlth@tmd.ac.jp; Tel.: +81-3-5803-5187

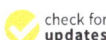

Received: 13 May 2020; Accepted: 11 June 2020; Published: 12 June 2020

Abstract: Eating behavior is an important aspect for dietary quality and long-term health. This study examined associations between eating vegetables first at a meal and food intakes among preschool children in Tokyo, Japan. We used cross-sectional data of 135 preschool children from seven nursery schools in Adachi City, Tokyo, Japan. Caregivers completed a survey on child's eating behaviors and a diet questionnaire. Linear regression was used to examine frequency of eating vegetables first at a meal and food intakes; percent difference and the corresponding 95% confidence interval (95% CI) were presented. Overall, 25.2% of children reported eating vegetables first at a meal every time, 52.6% sometimes, and 22.2% not often or never. In the multivariate analysis, higher vegetable intake remained significant after adjusting for other covariates (compared with the group of eating vegetables first not often or never, the group reported sometimes: 27%, 95% CI: 0–63%; the group reported every time: 93%, 95% CI: 43–159%). No significant difference in intake by frequency categories of eating vegetables first was observed for other food groups, including fruits, meat, fish, cereals, and sweets. Children eating vegetables first at a meal more was associated with higher total intake of vegetables compared with children who did not eat vegetables first, among Japanese preschool children.

Keywords: dietary habit; vegetable consumption; food intake; preschool children; Japan; nutrition

---

1. Introduction

A healthy diet is an essential component for meeting proper nutrition requirement for optimal body growth and body weight during childhood [1–3]. A poor diet can be a result of an imbalanced diet by overeating low-nutrient-dense foods such as refined carbohydrates and sweets and failing to consume other foods with high nutrient density, such as fruits, vegetables, and healthy meats [4]. Having a poor diet by consuming an excessive amount of unhealthy food and an insufficient amount of healthy food can lead to both short-term and long-term negative consequences on children development, such as obesity, nutrition deficiency, and insufficient body growth [5–7]. In addition to its beneficial role on body growth in childhood, a healthy diet pattern formed in childhood will also benefit long-term health if the pattern is maintained in later life [8,9].

Eating behaviors can reflect and even potentially influence overall dietary quality [10,11]. Particularly, choice of foods consumed during the early phase of a meal with respect to energy intake and intakes of different food groups has been examined in several studies conducted in the United States (U.S.) among people of different age groups. For instance, a randomized cross-over study conducted among adults in the U.S. found that consuming a first course with low-energy-dense salad enhanced satiety and led to reduced energy intake in the subsequent courses [12]. The beneficial role of consuming low-energy-dense foods at the beginning of a meal, particularly vegetables, has also been examined among children. More importantly, studies have revealed that consuming vegetables during the early phase of a meal led to not only reduced meal energy intake but also increased vegetable intake. A study conducted at a daycare center in Pennsylvania by the same research group found that serving low-energy-dense vegetable soup during the early phase of a meal led to reduced intake of energy-dense entrée and increased vegetable consumption at the meal [13]. Another cross-over study examined portion size of vegetables served at the start of meal among preschool children and reported that increasing portion size of vegetables at the start of a meal led to greater vegetable consumption without increasing meal energy intake [14]. Therefore, serving vegetables at the start of a meal and avoiding presence of competing foods that are less healthy may be advocated as an effective strategy to promote higher vegetable intake in preschool children [14].

Lately, there has been a trend of decreasing in vegetable intake and increasing in meat intake among the general Japanese population. The annual survey on citizens' health and nutrition published by the Ministry of Health, Labor and Welfare in Japan suggested that, compared with 10 years ago, the daily intakes of vegetables and fruits among Japanese had been decreasing (277.4 g/day for vegetables with a drop of 18.4 g/day, 110.3 g/day for fruits with a drop of 22.0 g/day), whereas the daily intake of meat had been increasing (80.7 g/day with an increase of 6.7 g/day) [15]. Since one's dietary habit is often formed as early as in childhood, identifying children with insufficient vegetable intake and subsequently developing dietary guidelines and interventions that will likely lead to increased vegetable intake and other healthy food intakes should be considered as a useful strategy to address the current diet problem in Japan [9,16].

A typical Japanese meal set usually consists of a staple food (mostly rice), three side dishes, and a soup served all at once [17]. Therefore, the sequence of food consumed can vary from person to person. As suggested by the earlier studies conducted in the U.S. on consuming vegetables during early phase of a meal, evaluating frequency of eating vegetables first at a meal with respect to various food intakes will be useful to determine if early consumption of vegetables at a meal is informative of assessing vegetable consumption and possibly overall dietary quality among Japanese children.

We used data from a cross-sectional study of preschool children in Japan and evaluated the association between frequency of eating vegetables first at a meal and intakes of different food groups, including vegetables, fruits, meat, fish, cereal, and sweets. We hypothesized that frequently consuming vegetables first at a meal would be associated with higher intake of vegetables and other healthier foods.

2. Materials and Methods

2.1. Study Population

We used data from a cross-sectional study of 135 preschool children from Adachi City, Tokyo, Japan in 2017. The study was initiated as a component of a health promotion campaign known as "Eat Vegetable First at Meals", which was launched in Adachi City in 2013. Children in 5-year-old class from seven licensed public nursery schools in Adachi City were invited to participate in the study. Teachers at the nursery schools explained to the children's caregivers about the study and distributed the study questionnaires. The questionnaires included a survey on regular eating behaviors of the participated child and a brief-type diet history questionnaire developed for Japanese preschool children aged 3–6 years (BDHQ3y) [18]. Participants were informed that participation in the study was voluntary and returning the completed questionnaires indicated their consent to participating in the study. The questionnaires were distributed to 165 caregivers, out of which 135 caregivers returned the questionnaires in sealed envelopes via each nursery school (response rate: 81.8%). Use of the data for this study was approved by the Ethics Committee of Tokyo Medical and Dental University (No. M2016-284).

2.2. Survey on Dietary Behavior

The dietary behavior survey was filled out by the caregiver of the participated child. It aimed to assess the regular eating and cooking behaviors of both the caregiver and the child. For our study, we were particularly interested in the frequency of eating vegetables first at a meal. In the dietary behavior survey, frequency of eating vegetables first at a meal was assessed in the following question: "how often does your child eat the first bite from vegetables at a given meal?" The caregiver was asked to circle the answer that best applied to his or her child from the following options: "every time", "sometimes", "not often", or "never". Since there were only 4 children who reported "never" for consuming the first bite from vegetables at a meal, we collapsed the groups of children who reported "not often" or "never" into one group in the analysis.

2.3. Survery on Food Intake

Food intakes were assessed using a brief-type diet history questionnaire for Japanese preschool children aged 3–6 years (BDHQ3y), which was developed based on the adult version of a self-administered diet history questionnaire that has been widely used in a range of epidemiologic studies for assessing food intakes in Japanese adults [19]. The caregiver reported the regular food intakes of his or her child during the preceding month by filling out BDHQ3y. The validity of BDHQ3y has been previously tested [18]. Details of BDHQ3y have been described elsewhere [18,20]. Briefly, BDHQ3y is a four-page questionnaire which reflects the typical Japanese dietary pattern, and it includes four sections to assess the food intake frequency: (1) 57 food and nonalcoholic beverage items; (2) daily intakes of rice (the most widely consumed staple food in Japan) and miso soup (widely consumed soup type in Japan); (3) usual cooking methods; and (4) general dietary behaviors. The daily intakes of 66 food items, total energy intake, and nutrient values are then estimated using an ad hoc computer algorithm, which takes into account the age-specific portion size using a specific weighting factor to adjust for the effect of age on the portion size consumed.

We considered the following food groups in our analysis: vegetable, fruit, meat (excluding fish), fish, cereal (including rice, noodles, and bread), and sweets. In the BDHQ3y, vegetable intake was collected based on the consumptions of dark green-leaf vegetables, cabbage, carrots, pumpkins, rooted vegetables, tomatoes, and mushrooms. Fruit intake was collected based on the commonly consumed fruits, except juice and jam made from fruits. Meat intake was collected based on the consumptions of chicken, pork, beef, processed meat, and animal liver. Fish intake was collected based on the intakes from fresh fish, canned fish, dried and salted fish, and food made from fish. Cereal intake was categorized into three sub-groups, and the intake of each group was calculated respectively: rice (including plain white rice, barley, whole grain rice, brown rice, and multigrain rice); noodles (including buckwheat noodles, Japanese wheat noodles, Chinese noodles, fried noodles, instant noodles, and western-style noodles); and bread. Intake on sweets was assessed from the following food sources: western sweets, Japanese sweets, ice cream, chocolate, and other sweet snacks. For each of the food groups, daily intakes of the food items were then summed and a value of total daily intake (g/day) was obtained, respectively. The summed value of the daily intakes from rice, noodles, and bread was reported as the daily intake of cereal. In addition, total energy intake (kcal/day) was also assessed in our study.

For each of the food groups, from the value of daily intake (g/day) estimated based on the nutrient database, we divided the food intake by the total energy intake and then multiplied the value by 1000 to derive the nutrient density (g/1000 kcal per day), so the food intake was represented as a dietary composition (a percentage from daily energy intake) rather than the absolute intake value for each child [4,21]. Nutrient density values were then log-transformed to account for potential non-normality.

2.4. Covariates

Information on the child's date of birth, sex, height, and weight were filled out by the caregiver in the BDHQ3y questionnaire. Information on the following covariates was additionally collected from the dietary behavior survey: number of people in the household, household economic status (in good standing, normal, indigent), parents' job (self-owned business, full-time, part-time, other), caregiver-rated child's physical health (good, normal, poor), and child's physical activity status, which was assessed by the frequency of conducting physical exercise that was longer than 30 min (almost every day, 5–6 times a week, 3–4 times a week, 1–2 times a week, rarely or never). In addition, the caregiver was asked to recall the average frequency of the child's vegetable consumption (almost at every meal, twice in a day, less than once in a day). We considered the covariates mentioned above as potential confounders for the association between frequency of eating vegetables first at a meal and food intakes and subsequently examined them in the analysis. For any question that was not answered by the caregiver, the missing value was set to the most commonly reported response.

2.5. Statistical Analysis

The main exposure of interest was frequency of eating vegetables first at a meal. The exposure was evaluated as a categorical variable with the following category: every time, sometimes, and not often or never. The group of children reported as not often or never eating vegetables first at a meal was set as the reference category. We first examined the association between frequency of eating vegetables first at a meal and other demographic or lifestyle-related covariates by conducting a chi-square test for a categorical covariate and analysis of variance for a continuous covariate. For the univariate analysis, the frequency of eating vegetables first at a meal was included as the only predictor in the univariate model. For the multivariate analysis, covariates with a p-value less than 0.05 from the chi-square test or the analysis of variance test were considered as significant and were subsequently adjusted in the multivariate model: age (months), physical health status (good, normal, poor), frequency of consuming vegetables (almost at every meal, twice in a day, less than once in a day). For both univariate and multivariate analyses, we used a linear regression model and examined the association between frequency of eating vegetables first at a meal and intake of the food groups. Since the outcome of food intake was on a logarithmic scale, coefficients and standard errors were back-transformed to the original scale with an interpretation of percent difference in the daily nutrient density for a given group compared to the reference group. All analyses were conducted using STATA version 13 (STATA Statistical Software: Release 13. College Station, TX, USA: StataCorp LP).

3. Results

Characteristics of the overall study sample by the reported frequency of eating vegetables first at a meal are summarized in Table 1. Our study included 135 Japanese preschool children with average age of 6.4 years (SD = 0.3 years) and average body mass index (BMI) of 15.5 kg/m^2 (SD = 1.8 kg/m^2). With respect to the frequency of eating vegetables first at a meal reported by the caregiver, 34 (25.2%) participants reported "every time", 71 (52.6%) participants reported "sometimes", and 30 (22.2%) participants reported "not often or never". Compared with the other two groups, the group of children reported as eating vegetables first at a meal every time had slightly higher BMI, a greater proportion of parents who owned self-business or had full-time job, better caregiver-rated physical health, more frequent physical activity, as suggested by a lower proportion of children who rarely or never conducted exercise that was longer than 30 min, and more frequent vegetable consumption (Table 1).

Table 1. Population characteristics and characteristics by frequency of eating vegetables first at a meal.

| | Total (n = 135) | Every Time (n = 34, 25.2%) | Frequency of Eating Vegetables First at a Meal | | p-Value [1] |
			Sometimes (n = 71, 52.6%)	Not Often or Never (n = 30, 22.2%)	
			Mean (SD) [2]		
Age (years) [3]	6.4 (0.3)	6.3 (0.3)	6.4 (0.3)	6.5 (0.3)	0.03
BMI (kg/m^2) [4]	15.5 (1.8)	15.9 (1.7)	15.4 (1.6)	15.3 (2.2)	0.42
Family size [5]	3	3	3	3	0.08
			Count (percent)		
Male	67 (49.6%)	15 (44.1%)	34 (47.9%)	18 (60.0%)	0.41
Economic status					0.89
In good standing	13 (9.6%)	3 (8.8%)	6 (8.5%)	4 (13.3%)	
Normal	93 (68.9%)	24 (70.6%)	48 (67.6%)	21 (70.0%)	
Indigent	29 (21.5%)	7 (20.6%)	17 (23.9%)	5 (16.6%)	
Job of mother					0.38
Self-owned business	10 (7.4%)	3 (8.8%)	4 (5.6%)	3 (10.0%)	
Full-time	63 (46.7%)	20 (58.8%)	32 (45.1%)	11 (36.7%)	
Part-time	53 (39.3%)	10 (29.4%)	28 (39.4%)	15 (50.0%)	
Other	9 (6.7%)	1 (2.9%)	7 (9.9%)	1 (3.3%)	
Job of father					0.64
Self-business	15 (11.1%)	3 (8.8%)	6 (8.5%)	6 (20.0%)	
Full-time	94 (69.6%)	25 (73.5%)	52 (73.2%)	17 (56.7%)	
Part-time	6 (4.4%)	1 (2.9%)	3 (4.2%)	2 (6.7%)	
Other	20 (14.8%)	5 (14.7%)	10 (14.1%)	5 (16.7%)	
Physical health status					0.01
Good	106 (78.5%)	33 (97.1%)	50 (70.4%)	23 (76.7%)	
Normal	21 (15.6%)	1 (2.9%)	17 (23.9%)	3 (10.0%)	
Poor	8 (5.9%)	0	4 (5.6%)	4 (13.3%)	
Frequency of conducting physical activity (longer than 30 min)					0.69
Almost every day	17 (12.6%)	5 (14.7%)	6 (8.5%)	6 (20.0%)	
5–6 times a week	9 (6.7%)	3 (8.8%)	5 (7.0%)	1 (3.3%)	
3–4 times a week	24 (17.8%)	8 (23.5%)	13 (18.3%)	3 (10.0%)	
1–2 times a week	66 (48.9%)	14 (41.2%)	36 (50.7%)	16 (53.3%)	
Rarely or never	19 (14.1%)	4 (11.8%)	11 (15.5%)	4 (13.3%)	
Frequency of consuming vegetables					<0.01
Almost at every meal	57 (42.2%)	20 (58.8%)	29 (40.9%)	8 (26.7%)	
Twice in a day	60 (44.4%)	13 (28.2%)	35 (49.3%)	12 (40.0%)	
Less than once in a day	18 (13.3%)	1 (2.9%)	7 (9.8%)	10 (33.3%)	

[1] p-value from chi-square test for categorical covariate and analysis of variance for continuous covariate is presented. [2] SD: standard deviation. [3] Age is presented in years by dividing age in months by 12. [4] BMI: body mass index. [5] Median is presented for the number of people in the household.

Daily intakes of the major food groups (g/1000 kcal, except for total energy intake) with respect to the frequency of eating vegetables first at a meal are summarized in Table 2. As Table 2 suggests, we observed higher total vegetable intake independent of total energy intake in the groups of children reported as more frequently eating vegetables first at a meal (every time: 147.8 g/1000 kcal, sometimes: 88.7 g/1000 kcal, not often or never: 68.0 g/1000 kcal). Higher intakes of fruits and fish and lower intakes of cereal and sweets were also observed in the group of eating vegetables first every time compared with the other two groups with the lower frequency. We did not observe a difference in total energy intake across the three groups (Table 2).

Table 2. Summary of major food group intakes by frequency of eating vegetables first at a meal.

Daily Food Intake	Total (n = 135)	Frequency of Eating Vegetables First at a Meal		
		Every Time (n = 34, 25.2%)	Sometimes (n = 71, 52.6%)	Not Often or Never (n = 30, 22.2%)
		Mean (SD)		
Total energy intake (kcal)	1427.1 (471.7)	1442.6 (408.1)	1405.51 (445.9)	1460.5 (596.9)
Vegetables (g/1000 kcal)	99.0 (68.5)	147.8 (88.5)	88.7 (50.1)	68.0 (51.7)
Fruits (g/1000 kcal)	40.9 (29.4)	56.6 (31.1)	33.8 (24.5)	39.9 (32.0)
Meat excluding fish (g/1000 kcal)	32.3 (14.3)	33.7 (12.8)	33.3 (13.9)	31.2 (16.9)
Fish (g/1000 kcal)	31.4 (16.0)	34.6 (15.1)	30.9 (15.8)	28.6 (17.4)
Cereal (g/1000 kcal) [1]	240.7 (63.4)	230.7 (59.1)	241.9 (56.7)	549.5 (81.4)
Rice	189.3 (66.1)	188.4 (59.6)	188.3 (59.9)	192.7 (86.5)
Noodles	32.5 (20.1)	27.5 (14.6)	33.56 (18.7)	35.4 (27.2)
Bread	19.0 (13.1)	14.7 (11.3)	20.0 (13.8)	21.4 (12.5)
Sweets (g/1000kcal)	34.8 (21.5)	29.1 (17.5)	36.8 (21.4)	36.4 (25.1)

[1] Cereal intake was calculated as the summed value of intakes from rice, noodles, and bread.

We present our main analysis results in Table 3. In the univariate analysis, we observed a significant association between frequently eating vegetables first at a meal and higher total vegetable intake (Table 3). Compared with the group of eating vegetables first at a meal not often or never, we observed 46% (95% CI: 14–88%) higher vegetable intake in the "sometimes" group and 139% (95% CI: 79–219%) higher vegetable intake in the "every time" group. In addition, significantly higher intakes of fruits and fish and lower intake of bread were also observed in the group of eating vegetables first at a meal every time compared with the reference group (Table 3).

After adjusting for the relevant covariates (age, physical health status, frequency of consuming vegetables) in the multivariate model, the association between frequently eating vegetables first at a meal and higher intake of vegetables was slightly attenuated, but it still remained statistically significant (Table 3). Compared with the group of children reported as eating vegetables first at a meal not often or never, the "sometimes" group had 27% (95% CI: 0–63%) higher vegetable intake, and the "every time" group had 93% (95% CI: 43–159%) higher vegetable intake. We did not observe significant associations between frequency of eating vegetables first at a meal and food intake for the remaining food groups that we examined, including fruits, meat, fish, cereal, and sweets (Table 3).

Table 3. Results on association between frequency of eating vegetables first at a meal and types of food intake [1].

Daily Food Intake [1]	Frequency of Eating Vegetables First at a Meal	Univariate Model [2] Percent Difference (95% CI)	Multivariate Model [3] Percent Difference (95% CI)
Vegetables	Not often or never	Reference	
	Sometimes	46% (14%, 88%)	27% (0%, 63%)
	Every time	139% (79%, 219%)	93% (43%, 159%)
Fruits	Not often or never	Reference	
	Sometimes	−9% (−34%, 26%)	−21% (−43%, 11%)
	Every time	51% (4%, 118%)	23% (−17%, 82%)
Meat excluding fish	Not often or never	Reference	
	Sometimes	12% (−8%, 35%)	8% (−12%, 32%)
	Every time	15% (−8%, 43%)	9% (−15%, 39%)
Fish	Not often or never	Reference	
	Sometimes	14% (−12%, 49%)	15% (−13%, 52%)
	Every time	36% (1%, 86%)	30% (−7%, 82%)
Cereal [4]	Not often or never	Reference	
	Sometimes	0% (−12%, 14%)	3% (−10%, 19%)
	Every time	−5% (−18%, 10%)	0% (−16%, 17%)
Rice	Not often or never	Reference	
	Sometimes	4% (−13%, 25%)	3% (−16%, 25%)
	Every time	4% (−15%, 28%)	5% (−17%, 33%)
Noodles	Not often or never	Reference	
	Sometimes	−5% (−26%, 23%)	3% (−22%, 35%)
	Every time	−20% (−40%, 8%)	−15% (−39%, 19%)
Bread	Not often or never	Reference	
	Sometimes	−13% (−38%, 21%)	3% (−28%, 48%)
	Every time	−40% (−59%, −11%)	−31% (−55%, 5%)
Sweets	Not often or never	Reference	
	Sometimes	8% (−18%, 43%)	3% (−24%, 39%)
	Every time	−13% (−37%, 20%)	−15% (−41%, 22%)

[1] Food intake was calculated as nutrient density (g/1000 kcal per day) for each food type on the natural log scale (nutrient density was calculated by dividing reported daily food intake (g/day) by total energy intake and then multiplying by 1000). [2] Frequency of eating vegetables first at a meal was included in the univariate model. [3] Multivariate model was adjusted for age (months), physical health status (good, normal, poor), and frequency of consuming vegetables (almost every meal, twice in a day, less than once in a day). [4] Cereal intakes were calculated as the summed value of intakes from rice, noodles, and bread.

4. Discussion

In our analysis of 135 Japanese preschool children, we found that frequently eating vegetables first at a meal was associated with higher intake of vegetables, and suggestively higher intakes of fruits and fish and lower intake of bread, independent of energy intake. To our knowledge, this is the first study examining frequency of eating vegetables first at a meal and its association with intake of various food groups among Japanese preschool children. The multi-dish style in the Japanese meal culture allowed us to closely examine the role of eating vegetables first at a meal on the intakes of commonly consumed foods among Japanese preschool children.

Our results were consistent with the previous study findings on consuming vegetables during early phase of a meal and greater vegetable consumption. A cross-over study conducted among preschool children in the U.S. found that doubling the portion size of vegetables as the first course led to a subsequent 47% increase in vegetable consumption at a given meal [14]. The same research group conducted other studies examining the role of serving vegetable dishes in the early phase of a meal. They reported similar findings that consuming a vegetable dish early led to increased meal vegetable intake and decreased meal energy intake [12,13]. Based on these study findings, placing vegetable dishes earlier during the course of a meal can be advocated as a strategy to encourage vegetable intake among children who have insufficient vegetable consumptions. Indeed, serving-vegetable-first has been demonstrated as an effective way to increase vegetable consumption among school children in other settings [22].

In addition to the significant association with higher vegetable intake, we also observed that frequently eating vegetables first at a meal was associated with suggestively higher intakes of fruits and fish, and it was not associated with higher intakes of the food groups that were considered less healthy, such as bread and sweets. In fact, compared with the group of children reported as not often or never eating vegetables first at a meal, the group of children eating vegetables first every time had suggestive lower intakes in bread and sweets (Tables 2 and 3). Further, eating vegetables first more frequently at a given meal did not seem to be associated with increased meal energy intake, which was also consistent with the previous study findings (Table 2) [14]. Therefore, it may be implied that frequently eating vegetables first at a meal was not associated with higher intake of unhealthy food or higher intake of energy. Considering the healthy benefits of eating vegetables, fruits, and fish and current dietary guidelines on limiting intake of refined carbohydrates, our results suggested the possibility of using frequency of eating vegetables first at a meal as a useful tool to assess the overall dietary quality among Japanese preschool children [16,23–31].

Our study provided preliminary evidence that assessing frequency of eating vegetables first at a meal might serve as a convenient and useful method for the policymakers to identify the population of children with generally low vegetable consumption and possibly suboptimal diet quality, and to subsequently develop community interventions or guidelines to improve their diet. Findings from our study also provide useful insights for future interventional studies to further pursue this area of research in order to draw causal conclusions on frequency of eating vegetables first at a meal and increasing total vegetable intake among preschool children in Japan.

There are some limitations in our study. First, with a small sample size ($n = 135$), the statistical power of our study was limited. Therefore, the null associations observed in some food groups may be interpreted as either no association or a possible association but underpowered. In addition, since we collapsed the groups of "not often" and "never" into one group due to the limited sample size, we were unable to separately examine the food intakes for those two groups. Furthermore, a small sample size may limit the generalizability of our results. Therefore, future studies with greater sample size and sufficient statistical power should be conducted to address such limitations. Second, given the cross-sectional nature of the study, our results can only be interpreted as findings of associations. Therefore, we cannot make the causal interpretation that eating vegetables first at a meal will lead to higher vegetable intake. However, our results still suggest that frequently eating vegetables first at the start of a meal is informative of higher total vegetable consumption among Japanese preschool children. Lastly, similar to other nutritional studies, diet was likely to be measured with errors, as the validity and reliability of BDHQ3y filled out by the caregiver may not be high enough to accurately capture the regular dietary pattern of the Japanese preschool children. With respect to the dietary behaviors survey, since it was structured as questions with a reasonable number of choices, misclassification was likely to be low.

5. Conclusions

In conclusion, our study on 135 Japanese preschool children suggested that compared with children who did not eat vegetables first, eating vegetables first at a meal more was associated with a higher total vegetable intake. Larger-scale studies with a geographically diverse population of preschool children should be conducted to further confirm our findings. Future intervention studies or randomized trials are warranted to further examine the causal role of eating vegetables first at a meal on increasing healthy foods consumptions among Japanese preschool children.

Author Contributions: All authors contributed to the study design. T.F., Y.T., and M.O. collected the data. J.Y. conducted data analysis and led the writing of the manuscript. T.F., Y.T., and D.K.T. provided input into data analysis approach. All authors provided input into interpretation of the study results and have read and approved the final manuscript. All authors have read and agreed to the published version of the manuscript.

Funding: This study was funded by a Grant-in-Aid for Scientific Research from the Japan Society for the Promotion of Science (JSPS KAKENHI Grant Number 16H03276, 19K14029, and 16K21669).

Acknowledgments: The authors thank all the individuals who participated in the study.

Conflicts of Interest: The authors declare no conflict of interest.

References

1. Emmett, P.M.; Jones, L.R. Diet, growth, and obesity development throughout childhood in the Avon Longitudinal Study of Parents and Children. *Nutr. Rev.* **2015**, *73* (Suppl. 3), 175–206. [CrossRef]
2. Wu, X.Y.; Zhuang, L.H.; Li, W.; Guo, H.W.; Zhang, J.H.; Zhao, Y.K.; Hu, J.W.; Gao, Q.Q.; Luo, S.; Ohinmaa, A.; et al. The influence of diet quality and dietary behavior on health-related quality of life in the general population of children and adolescents: A systematic review and meta-analysis. *Qual. Life Res.* **2019**, *28*, 1989–2015. [CrossRef] [PubMed]
3. Alimujiang, A.; Colditz, G.A.; Gardner, J.D.; Park, Y.; Berkey, C.S.; Sutcliffe, S. Childhood diet and growth in boys in relation to timing of puberty and adult height: The Longitudinal Studies of Child Health and Development. *Cancer Causes Control.* **2018**, *29*, 915–926. [CrossRef]
4. Willett, W.C.; Howe, G.R.; Kushi, L.H. Adjustment for total energy intake in epidemiologic studies. *Am. J. Clin. Nutr.* **1997**, *65*, S1220–S1228. [CrossRef] [PubMed]
5. Dehghan-Kooshkghazi, M.; Akhtar-Danesh, N.; Merchant, A.T. Childhood obesity, prevalence and prevention. *Nutr. J.* **2005**, *4*, 24. [CrossRef] [PubMed]
6. Rogol, A.D.; A Clark, P.; Roemmich, J.N. Growth and pubertal development in children and adolescents: Effects of diet and physical activity. *Am. J. Clin. Nutr.* **2000**, *72*, S521–S528. [CrossRef]
7. Scaglioni, S.; Agostoni, C.; De Notaris, R.; Radaelli, G.; Radice, N.; Valenti, M.; Giovannini, M.; Riva, E. Early macronutrient intake and overweight at five years of age. *Int. J. Obes.* **2000**, *24*, 777–781. [CrossRef]
8. Kelder, S.H.; Perry, C.L.; I Klepp, K.; Lytle, L.L. Longitudinal tracking of adolescent smoking, physical activity, and food choice behaviors. *Am. J. Public Health* **1994**, *84*, 1121–1126. [CrossRef]
9. Reilly, J.J. Physical activity, sedentary behaviour and energy balance in the preschool child: Opportunities for early obesity prevention. *Proc. Nutr. Soc.* **2008**, *67*, 317–325. [CrossRef]
10. Patrick, H.; Nicklas, T.A. A review of family and social determinants of children's eating patterns and diet quality. *J. Am. Coll. Nutr.* **2005**, *24*, 83–92. [CrossRef]
11. Bellisle, F. Meals and snacking, diet quality and energy balance. *Physiol. Behav.* **2014**, *134*, 38–43. [CrossRef] [PubMed]
12. Rolls, B.J.; Roe, L.S.; Meengs, J.S. Salad and satiety: Energy density and portion size of a first-course salad affect energy intake at lunch. *J. Am. Diet. Assoc.* **2004**, *104*, 1570–1576. [CrossRef] [PubMed]
13. Spill, M.K.; Birch, L.L.; Roe, L.S.; Rolls, B.J. Serving large portions of vegetable soup at the start of a meal affected children's energy and vegetable intake. *Appetite* **2011**, *57*, 213–219. [CrossRef] [PubMed]
14. Spill, M.K.; Birch, L.L.; Roe, L.S.; Rolls, B.J. Eating vegetables first: The use of portion size to increase vegetable intake in preschool children. *Am. J. Clin. Nutr.* **2010**, *91*, 1237–1243. [CrossRef]
15. Ministry of Health, Labour and Welfare (Japan). Japan National Health and Nutrition Survey. 2011. Available online: https://www.mhlw.go.jp/bunya/kenkou/eiyou/h23-houkoku.html (accessed on 19 September 2019).
16. Mikkila, V.; Räsänen, L.; Raitakari, O.; Pietinen, P.; Viikari, J. Consistent dietary patterns identified from childhood to adulthood: The Cardiovascular Risk in Young Finns Study. *Br. J. Nutr.* **2005**, *93*, 923–931. [CrossRef] [PubMed]
17. Ministry of Agriculture, Forestry and Fisheries (Japan). WASHOKU. Available online: http://www.maff.go.jp/j/keikaku/syokubunka/culture/pdf/guide_all.pdf (accessed on 19 September 2019).
18. Asakura, K.; Haga, M.; Sasaki, S. Relative Validity and Reproducibility of a Brief-Type Self-Administered Diet History Questionnaire for Japanese Children Aged 3–6 Years: Application of a Questionnaire Established for Adults in Preschool Children. *J. Epidemiol.* **2015**, *25*, 341–350. [CrossRef]

19. Kobayashi, S.; Murakami, K.; Sasaki, S.; Okubo, H.; Hirota, N.; Notsu, A.; Fukui, M.; Date, C. Comparison of relative validity of food group intakes estimated by comprehensive and brief-type self-administered diet history questionnaires against 16 d dietary records in Japanese adults. *Public Health Nutr.* **2011**, *14*, 1200–1211. [CrossRef]
20. Kano, M.; Tani, Y.; Ochi, M.; Sudo, N.; Fujiwara, T. Association Between Caregiver's Perception of "Good" Dietary Habits and Food Group Intake Among Preschool Children in Tokyo, Japan. *Front. Pediatr.* **2019**, *7*, 554. [CrossRef]
21. Willett, W. *Nutritional Epidemiology*; Oxford University Press: Oxford, UK, 2012; Volume 40.
22. Elsbernd, S.; Reicks, M.; Mann, T.; Redden, J.P.; Mykerezi, E.; Vickers, Z. Serving vegetables first: A strategy to increase vegetable consumption in elementary school cafeterias. *Appetite* **2016**, *96*, 111–115. [CrossRef]
23. Slavin, J.L.; Lloyd, B. Health Benefits of Fruits and Vegetables1. *Adv. Nutr.* **2012**, *3*, 506–516. [CrossRef]
24. Aune, D.; Giovannucci, E.; Boffetta, P.; Fadnes, L.T.; Keum, N.; Norat, T.; Greenwood, D.C.; Riboli, E.; Vatten, L.J.; Tonstad, S. Fruit and vegetable intake and the risk of cardiovascular disease, total cancer and all-cause mortality-a systematic review and dose-response meta-analysis of prospective studies. *Int. J. Epidemiology* **2017**, *46*, 1029–1056. [CrossRef] [PubMed]
25. Yip, C.S.C.; Chan, W.; Fielding, R. The Associations of Fruit and Vegetable Intakes with Burden of Diseases: A Systematic Review of Meta-Analyses. *J. Acad. Nutr. Diet.* **2019**, *119*, 464–481. [CrossRef] [PubMed]
26. DeSalvo, K.B.; Olson, R.; Casavale, K.O. Dietary Guidelines for Americans. *JAMA* **2016**, *315*, 1. [CrossRef] [PubMed]
27. Frost, L.; Vestergaard, P. n-3 Fatty acids consumed from fish and risk of atrial fibrillation or flutter: The Danish Diet, Cancer, and Health Study. *Am. J. Clin. Nutr.* **2005**, *81*, 50–54. [CrossRef] [PubMed]
28. Jacobs, D.R.; Marquart, L.; Slavin, J.; Kushi, L.H. Whole-grain intake and cancer: An expanded review and meta-analysis. *Nutr. Cancer* **1998**, *30*, 85–96. [CrossRef] [PubMed]
29. Gaesser, G.A. Carbohydrate Quantity and Quality in Relation to Body Mass Index. *J. Am. Diet. Assoc.* **2007**, *107*, 1768–1780. [CrossRef]
30. Steyn, N.P.; Mann, J.; Bennett, P.H.; Temple, N.; Zimmet, P.; Tuomilehto, J.; Lindstrom, J.; Louheranta, A. Diet, nutrition and the prevention of type 2 diabetes. *Public Heal. Nutr.* **2004**, *7*, 147–165. [CrossRef]
31. Burke, J.D. Dietary Guidelines for Americans. *Nutr. Today* **2015**, *50*, 174–176. [CrossRef]

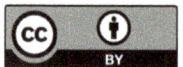

© 2020 by the authors. Licensee MDPI, Basel, Switzerland. This article is an open access article distributed under the terms and conditions of the Creative Commons Attribution (CC BY) license (http://creativecommons.org/licenses/by/4.0/).

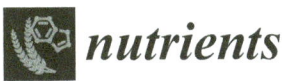 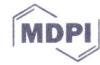

Article

Dietary Habits in Children with Respiratory Allergies: A Single-Center Polish Pilot Study

Eliza Wasilewska [1,*], **Sylwia Małgorzewicz** [2], **Marta Gruchała-Niedoszytko** [2], **Magdalena Skotnicka** [3] **and Ewa Jassem** [1]

1 Department of Pulmonology and Allergology, Medical University of Gdansk, Debinki str 7, 90-211 Gdańsk, Poland; ejassem@gumed.edu.pl
2 Department of Clinical Nutrition, Medical University of Gdansk, Debinki str 7, 90-211 Gdańsk, Poland; sylwia.malgorzewicz@gumed.edu.pl (S.M.); marta.gruchala@gumed.edu.pl (M.G.-N.)
3 Department of Food Commodity Science, Medical University of Gdansk, Debinki str 7, 90-211 Gdańsk, Poland; skotnicka@gumed.edu.pl
* Correspondence: ewasilewska@gumed.edu.pl

Received: 13 May 2020; Accepted: 21 May 2020; Published: 23 May 2020

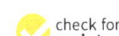

Abstract: Background: The rising trend in allergic diseases has developed in parallel with the increasing prevalence of obesity, suggesting a possible association. The links between eating habits and allergies have not been sufficiently clarified. Aim: To evaluate the nutritional status, eating habits, and risk factors of obesity and pulmonary function in children with allergic rhinitis. Materials and methods: We evaluated 106 children with allergic rhinitis (mean age 12.1 ± 3.4 years; M/F 60/46) from the Department of Allergology. Clinical data were collected regarding allergies, physical activity, nutritional status (Bodystat), dietary habits (Food Frequency Questionnaire validated for the Polish population), skin prick test with aeroallergens (Allergopharma), and spirometry (Jaeger). Results: All children suffered from allergic rhinitis; among them, 43 (40.6%) presented symptoms of asthma. There were differences between children with only allergic rhinitis (AR group) and children with both rhinitis and asthma (AA group) in pulmonary function (forced expiratory volume in one second (FEV_1) 100 ± 11 vs. 92.1 ± 15.0; $p < 0.05$). A total of 84 children (79%) presented a normal body mass index (BMI) (10–97 percentile), 8 (7.5%) were underweight, and 14 (13.5%) were overweight or obese. There were no differences in body composition between the AR and AA groups. Incorrect eating habits were demonstrated by most of the children, e.g., consumption of three or fewer meals in a day (38%), sweets every day (44%), snacking between meals every day (80%), and eating meals less than 1 h before bedtime (47%). Compared to the AR group, the AA group was more likely to eat more meals a day ($p = 0.04$), snack more often ($p = 0.04$), and eat before sleeping ($p = 0.005$). Multiple regression analysis showed a significant association between high BMI and snacking between meals and low physical activity (adjusted $R^2 = 0.97$; $p < 0.05$). Conclusions: The risk factors for obesity in children with allergies include snacking and low physical activity. Most children with respiratory allergies, especially those with asthma, reported incorrect eating habits such as snacking and eating before bedtime. A correlation between pulmonary function and body composition or dietary habits was not found.

Keywords: nutritional status; obesity; dietary habits; allergy; pulmonary function; allergic rhinitis; asthma

1. Introduction

The incidence of allergic diseases in Poland is increasing concomitantly with improvements in living standards and the adoption of a Western lifestyle. The most common clinical manifestation of hypersensitivity to inhalant allergens is allergic rhinitis (AR), which is one of the strongest factors affecting the quality of life and contributing to missed or unproductive time at work and school. In Europe and the United States, a significant increase in allergic diseases has been observed in recent decades [1,2]. In addition, the multicenter, standardized, randomized Epidemiology of Allergic Disorders in Poland (ECAP) study showed a prevalence of AR among the Polish population of 36% based on self-reported nasal symptoms, and 29% as diagnosed by physicians [3].

Among children with allergies, decreased involvement in outdoor activities and increased problems with concentration, sleep problems, and headaches are seen; moreover, children with AR often also suffer from asthma [4]. It is estimated that up to 40% of people with AR also have asthma, and almost 70% of asthmatics present coexisting AR [5,6]. In the Polish population, the asthma rate was 8% in children and adolescents according to the ECAP study, of which 70% of asthmatics presented with AR, while asthma occurred in 40% of patients with AR [7].

It is known that not only hygiene habits and exposure to allergens, tobacco smoke, and environmental pollution, but also a poor-quality diet, high caloric intake, overweight, and obesity in children and adolescents are important environmental factors that are conducive to the development of allergies [8,9]. Epidemiological and clinical studies suggest a relationship between obesity and allergic rhinitis as well as bronchial asthma [10,11].

In recent years, a significant increase has been noted in the incidence of obesity in children and adolescents in many European countries [12]. Excess body mass was diagnosed in 2% of Polish children in the 1990s, and in 15% of children 20 years later [13–15]. The authors of these studies indicated increased changes in lifestyle and nutritional habits as the causes of increased childhood obesity, i.e., consumption of sweets and unhealthy food; limited consumption of fruits, vegetables, and whole grains; and limited physical activity. In recent decades, fast foods have become a significant component of the diet in Westernized high-income countries, and now also for young people in Poland.

Children with allergic diseases present numerous risk factors for poor nutrition status. There are few studies describing dietary habits and their impact on the nutritional status of people with respiratory allergies. Although allergies are chronic and common diseases, these issues have not yet been clarified. Moreover, early diagnosis of excess body weight in children with allergic diseases, including asthma, seems to be important due to the course and treatment of the disease [16]. Therefore, the aim of this work was to evaluate the pulmonary function, nutritional status, eating habits, and risk factors of obesity in children and adolescents with AR.

2. Methods

2.1. Study Design

In this single-center, cross-sectional study, we evaluated, for the first time pediatric patients with symptoms of persistent rhinitis who visited the Department of Allergology of the Medical University in Gdańsk, Poland, between 2015 and 2017. The study was performed in compliance with the Code of Ethics of the World Medical Association (Declaration of Helsinki). The study protocol was approved by the Gdańsk Medical University Ethics Committee, and written informed consent was obtained from the parents of each patient. The study was supported by local research grant no. ST-554.

2.2. Patients

Inclusion criteria for the study were as follows: (1) age 7–18 years old, (2) persistent allergic rhinitis (duration at least 6 months in the last 12 months) never diagnosed and never treated with antihistamine drugs, (3) ability to perform spirometry, and (4) signed consent from parents to participate in the study.

Patients were evaluated according to the study protocol by a multidisciplinary team (allergologist, pediatrician, dietician). Children with persistent rhinitis symptoms in the last 12 months who had never been diagnosed and treated with anti-allergic or anti-asthmatic drugs were enrolled in the study (Visit 1, screening). During the next visit (Visit 2), allergy was confirmed by skin prick test,

AR was diagnosed according to Allergic Rhinitis and Its Impact on Asthma (ARIA) [6], and asthma according to Global Initiative for Asthma (GINA) guidelines [17]. The medical history and spirometry results indicated newly diagnosed asthma in 43 patients; therefore, patients were divided into two groups: allergic rhinitis (AR group), and allergic rhinitis and asthma (AA group). Anthropometry, bioimpedance assessment, and dietary habits based on Food Frequency Questionnaire (FFQ-6) were collected and compared between the two groups. The scheme of the study is presented in Figure 1.

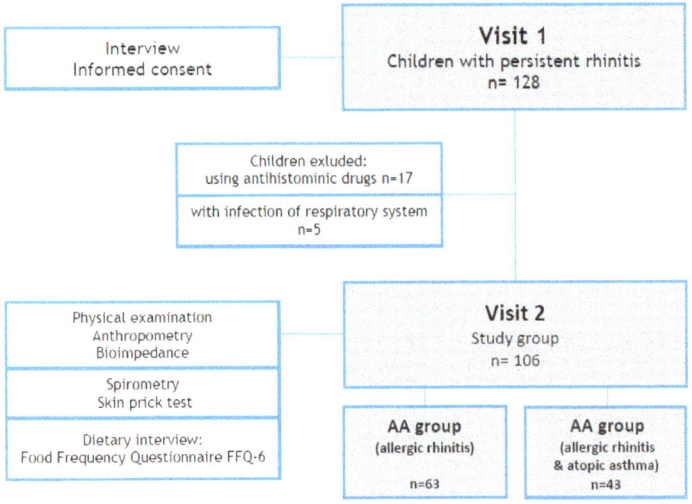

Figure 1. Study design.

Allergy background was confirmed with skin prick test to aeroallergens (*Dermatophagoides pteronyssinus, Dermatophagoides farinae*; cat, dog; *Alternaria alternata, Cladosporium herbarum*; pollens: grass mix, rye, birch pollen, alder, hazel; Allergopharma, Germany). Children with food allergies and atopic dermatitis were excluded from the study because of the frequent use of elimination diets.

Spirometry with a reversibility test (400 µg salbutamolum) was performed using a MasterScreen Pneumo spirometer, Jaeger Company, Germany. Forced expiratory volume in one second (FEV_1), forced vital capacity (FVC) and forced expiratory flow (FEF_{25-75}) were measured in accordance with the procedures recommended by the European Respiratory Society [18] and presented as percentage of predicted value (pv).

2.3. Nutritional Habits

Data were collected by face-to-face interviews using a researcher-designed standardized questionnaire based on the Food Frequency Questionnaire (FFQ-6) and validated for the Polish population [19]. The FFQ-6 is the most common dietary assessment tool used in large epidemiological studies of diet and health and is validated for the population. The self-administered FFQ-6 asks participants to report the frequency of consumption of approximately 62 line items over a defined period of time (last year). Each line item is defined by a series of foods or beverages. The FFQ-6 includes an assessment of eight food groups (sweets and snacks, dairy products and eggs, grain products, fats, fruits, vegetables and grains, meat products and fish, drinks). Respondents have a choice of six categories of food consumption frequency: (1) never or almost never, (2) once a month or less often, (3) several times a month, (4) several times a week, (5) daily, and (6) several times a day. The FFQ-6 also includes questions on eating habits, i.e., meal intake frequency and snacking between meals.

The following information was obtained: the number of meals in a day, amount of sweets consumed in a week, amount of fast-food eaten in a month, time of last meal before bedtime, and snacking between meals. Fast food was defined as mass-produced food prepared and served very quickly, with poor nutritional quality (hamburgers, takeaways, and carbonated soft drinks).

2.4. Physical Activity

The subjects were assigned to four categories depending on their level of physical activity: sedentary lifestyle (up to 2 h per week), low (3–5 h per week), moderate (6–7 h per week), and high (more than 8 h per week). One hour of physical activity corresponded to one hour of classroom attendance (45 min). Subjects were classified as having a sedentary lifestyle if only sometimes present during gym classes or not exercising at all. The low physical activity group attended gym class in school and an additional hour, e.g., swimming. Children identified as high activity trained in some kind of sport.

2.5. Nutritional Status

Body height was measured by stadiometer and body mass by electronic scale (Tanita Inc., Amsterdam, The Netherlands) by a nurse during the first visit. Body mass index (BMI) was calculated by dividing body mass in kilograms by the square of height in meters. Based on centile charts for sex and age for the Polish population—OLAF/OLA project—percentiles of BMI were specified [20]. According to the OLAF/OLA charts, above the 90th percentile is overweight, above the 97th percentile is obese, and below the 10th percentile is underweight. Body composition values of fat mass (FAT), fat-free mass (LEAN), and water content were measured via the bioimpedance method using a BodyStat 1500 (Bodystat Ltd., Ballafletcher, UK).

2.6. Statistical Analysis

Differences for somatic traits and between AR and AA groups were evaluated using Student's t-test or using the Mann-Whitney test for asymmetrical distributions. Distributions of values for somatic traits were evaluated using the Kołmogorov-Smirnov test. Differences between qualitative data were compared using the χ^2 test. The association between obesity risk factors and BMI percentile was determined using linear multivariate regression analysis. Differences were considered significant at $p < 0.05$. All analyses were carried out using the Statistica 10.0 software package.

3. Results

3.1. Patients

Allergic rhinitis was diagnosed in all 106 patients included in the study; among them, asthma was newly diagnosed in 43 (40.6%). Subjects with only allergic rhinitis were classified into the AR group and those with both allergic rhinitis and atopic asthma into the AA group (see Figure 1). All 106 children (100%) had a positive skin prick test to house dust mite (HDM; *D. farinae* and/or *D. pteronyssimus*), among which 40 (37.7%) were also positive to grass pollen ($n = 29$) and animals ($n = 11$).

Children in the AA group had a positive reversibility test and lower FEV_1 % predicted volume than children in the AR group. The basic characteristics of the study groups and the spirometry parameters are presented in Table 1.

3.2. Eating Habits and Physical Activity

The results of the eating habits and physical activity assessment are presented in Table 2.

Table 1. Clinical and lung function characteristics of patients.

Parameters	All Children * n = 106	AR Group n = 63	AA Group n = 43	p-Value AR vs. AA
M/F	60/46	38/25	22/21	0.34
Age (years) mean ± SD (range)	12.2 ± 3.5 (7–18)	13.3 ± 3.5 (7–18)	11.5 ± 3.2 (7–18)	0.01
Tobacco smoking exposure n (%)	21 (19.8%)	15 (24%)	6 (28%)	0.21
Animal at home n (%)	49 (50.7%)	32 (50.7%)	17 (39.5%)	0.25
Family allergies n (%)	65 (61%)	34 (53%)	31 (72%)	0.09
	Spirometry mean % pv ± SD			
FEV_1	95.4 ± 16.3	100.0 ± 11.1	92.1 ± 15.0	0.05
FVC	95.1 ± 10.0	97.1 ± 10.1	94.0 ± 10.9	0.13
FEV_1%FVC	108.8 ± 9.9	102.0 ± 4.4	99.0 ± 9.2	0.16
PEF	86.7 ± 16.0	90.2 ± 15.4	84.2 ± 15.9	0.06

AR: allergic rhinitis; AA: atopic asthma; FEV_1: forced expiratory volume in one second; FVC: forced vital capacity; PEF: peak expiratory flow; pv: predicted value; n: number of subjects. * All children (n = 106) had a positive skin prick test.

Table 2. Eating habits and physical activity assessment.

Parameters	All Patients n = 106	AR Group n = 63	AA Group n = 43
	Meals (number per day)		
2	4 (3.7%)	3 (4.7%)	1 (2.3%)
3	35 (33.0%)	19 (30.1%)	16 (37.2%)
4	31 (29.2%)	16 (25.6%)	15 (34.8%)
5 or more	36 (34.1%)	25 (39.6%)	11 (25.7%)
	Sweets (days per week)		
1	12 (11.5%)	7 (11.1%)	5 (11.6%)
2–3	29 (27.3%)	19 (30.1%)	10 (23.2%)
4–6	18 (16.9%)	10 (15.8%)	8 (18.6%)
every day	47 (44.3%)	27 (43.0%)	20 (46.6%)
	Fast food (days per month)		
never	17 (16.0%)	12 (19.0%)	5 (11.6%)
1	52 (49.0%)	32 (50.7%)	20 (46.6%)
2–3	27 (25.4%)	13 (20.6%)	14 (32.5%)
4–6	9 (8.7%)	6 (9.7%)	3 (7.0%)
every day	1 (0.9%)	0 (0.0%)	1 (2.3%)
	Last meal before sleep (hours to bedtime)		
<1	52 (49.0%)	30 (47.6%)	22 (51.1%)
1	20 (18.8%)	7 (11.1%)	13 (30.2%)
2	13 (12.4%)	11 (17.4%)	2 (4.6%)
>2	21 (19.8%)	15 (23.9%)	6 (14.1%)
	Snacking between meals		
yes	85 (80%)	50 (79.3%)	35 (81.4%)
no	21 (20%)	13 (20.7%)	8 (18.6%)
	Physical activity		
sedentary lifestyle	9 (8.4%)	4 (6.3%)	5 (11.6%)
low	58 (54.7%)	40 (63.4%)	18 (42.0%)
moderate	27 (25.4%)	12 (19.2%)	15 (34.8%)
high	12 (11.5%)	7 (11.1%)	5 (11.6%)

AR: allergic rhinitis; AA: atopic asthma; n: number of subjects.

3.2.1. Number of Meals

The majority of children reported eating three (33.4%), four (29.2%), or five (34.1%) meals per day. Children with AA ate more frequently than children with AR ($\chi^2 = 12.9; p = 0.04$).

Thirty-five children (34%) did not eat regularly; their meals were at different hours each day. There was no difference in meal regularity between AR and AA groups ($\chi^2 = 0.26; p = 0.60$).

3.2.2. Sweets

Almost half of the patients (47; 44.3%) ate sweets every day, in comparison to 12 (11.5%) who consumed sweets only one day per week. There was no difference in the consumption of sweets between AR and AA groups ($\chi^2 = 2.5; p = 0.88$).

3.2.3. Snacks

Eight-seven children (80%) snacked (sweet and salty snacks) between meals, 81.4% in the AA group and 79.3% in the AR group. There was no difference in snack consumption, but deeper analysis showed the AA group consumed more salty snacks than AR group ($\chi^2 = 0.59; p = 0.04$).

All overweight and obese children (AR and AA) snacked significantly more often between meals ($\chi^2 = 9.46, p = 0.01$) than children with normal BMI.

3.2.4. Fast Food

Seventeen patients (16.0%) had never eaten fast food. Most of the children (84%) ate fast food; half of them ($n = 52$) ate it very rarely (once a month) and 8.7% ate it 4–6 times per month. There was no difference in fast food consumption between AR and AA groups ($\chi^2 = 6.3; p = 0.50$).

3.2.5. Meals before Bedtime

It was found that children most often consumed their last meal of the day 0.5–2 h before bedtime; a total 12.4% ($n = 13$) did so 2 h before falling asleep, 19.8% ($n = 21$) did so much earlier (from 2.5 to 3 h before bedtime), and 49% ($n = 52$) ate the last meal <1 h before sleeping. Children with AA ate the last meal 1 h before sleep more frequently than those in the AR group ($\chi^2 = 19.4; p = 0.005$).

3.3. Physical Activity

The mean physical activity was 5 h per week. Most children (55%) reported 3–5 h/week physical activity. These children had only physical education (PE) at school and 1 h of additional activities after school (swimming or games). Children with AR reported low (63.4%; $n = 40$) and moderate (19.2%; $n = 12$) physical activity; similarly, children with AA reported low (42.0%; $n = 8$) and moderate (34.8%; $n = 15$) activity. There was no difference in physical activity between the AR and AA groups ($\chi^2 = 13.1; p = 0.15$). There was a negative correlation between physical activity level and BMI centile in the whole study population (Spearman's R = –0.19; $p < 0.05$).

3.4. Nutritional Status and Body Composition

Obesity was diagnosed in six children (6.0%) and eight were overweight (7.5%). In the AA group, obesity was present in 4.7% compared to 6.9% in the AR group ($\chi^2 = 3.58; p = 0.30$). The results of body composition measurement are presented in Table 3. There was no difference between the AR and AA groups.

3.5. The Multifactorial Linear Regression Analysis

Multifactorial linear regression analysis showed an association (independent of age) between BMI percentile and both snacking and physical activity level (see Figure 2 and Table 4).

Table 3. Nutritional status and body composition in studied groups.

Parameters	All Patients	AR Group n = 63	AA Group n = 43	p-Value AR vs. AA
Anthropometric data, mean ± SD (range)				
Weight (kg)	47.1 ± 17.9 (18–98.2)	51.3 ± 17.9 (21–95)	44.5 ± 17 (18–92)	0.06
Height (cm)	154.6 ± 19.1 (110–185)	160.3 ± 17.1 (116–182)	151.4 ± 19.2 (110–185)	0.03
BMI (percentile)	45.5 ± 32.1 (1–99)	41.6 ± 31.1 (5–99)	47.9 ± 33.1 (1–99)	0.63
BMI, n (%)				
Underweight BMI <10th percentile	8 (7.5%)	5 (7.9%)	3 (6.9%)	0.81
Normal BMI, 10th–90th percentile	84 (79.0%)	52 (82.5%)	32 (74.4%)	0.43
Overweight BMI, 90th–97th percentile	8 (7.5%)	3 (6.9%)	5 (11.0%)	0.57
Obesity BMI, >97th percentile	6 (6.0%)	3 (4.7%)	3 (6.9%)	0.89
Body composition; mean ± SD (range)				
Body fat (%)	29.6 ± 20.6 (1–90)	20 ± 15.4 (3–70)	21.5 ± 17 (1–90)	0.14
Body fat (kg)	9.2 ± 4.8 (1–30)	8.2 ± 4.7 (2–31)	7.9 ± 3.9 (1–17)	0.94
LEAN (%)	70.3 ± 20.6 (8.9–89)	79 ± 16.5 (21–89)	78.1 ± 17.1 (8.9–56)	0.42
LEAN (kg)	27.9 ± 17.3 (2–24)	39.5 ± 17.6 (6–24)	36.8 ± 17.4 (2–24)	0.23

AR: allergic rhinitis; AA: atopic asthma; BMI: body mass index; LEAN: lean body mass.

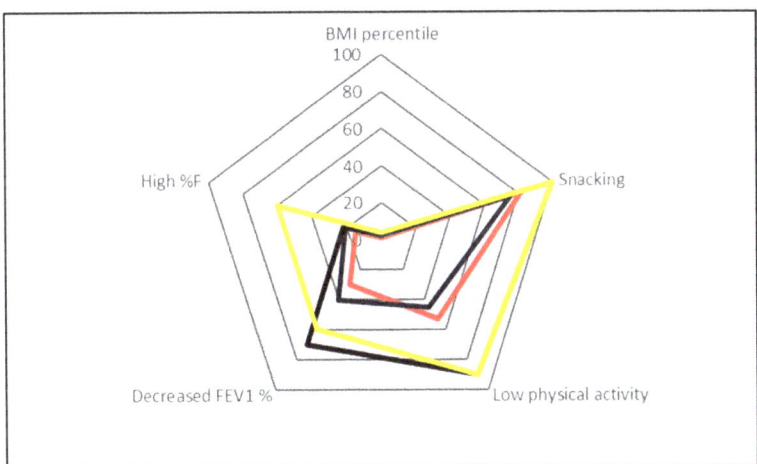

Figure 2. Association between body mass index (BMI) percentile and risk factors for obesity in all studied groups (adjusted R^2 = 0.97; $p < 0.05$). %F: percentage of body fat; FEV_1: forced expiratory volume in one second. Legend: red line means < 25th percentile, black line 25th–89th percentile, grey line 90th–97th percentile and yellow line >97th percentile.

Table 4. Multivariate regression model predicting BMI value (adjusted R^2 of the model was 0.97, $p < 0.05$).

Regression Model	B	Standard Error	Beta	p-Value
Constant	16.7	2.84		<0.001
Snacking	2.07	0.94	0.21	0.03
Fat%pv	−0.05	0.02	−0.21	0.058
FEV_1%pv	0.03	0.02	0.11	0.23
Physical activity	−1.02	0.46	−0.21	0.028

FEV_1: forced expiratory volume in one second; B: Regression coefficient B; Beta: beta standardized regression coefficient.

4. Discussion

In the present study, we evaluated the nutritional status and dietary habits of Caucasian children with allergic rhinitis alone or with co-existing asthma. Although all of the children presented respiratory allergy symptoms at least 12 months before the study, they were never diagnosed with allergies and had not previously been treated with an antihistamine or anti-asthmatic drugs before.

The most important finding of the study is that the majority of children with respiratory allergies reported incorrect eating habits and low physical activity, with 7.5% being overweight and 6.0% being obese. In the study population, excess body weight was significantly associated with snacking between meals and low physical activity.

4.1. Nutritional Status

Unexpectedly, the prevalence of overweight and obesity among allergic children was similar to the population of healthy children in Poland [13,14,21,22]. This aligned with data from the International Obesity Task Force (IOTF) showing that approximately 10% of children worldwide are overweight [12].

Although AR is a common disease, most authors focus on children with food allergies or asthma. These studies have suggested that adiposity indicators are associated with asthma, asthma severity, and atopy [23,24]. It is obvious that a positive energy balance is associated with changes in immune system functioning, including chronic inflammation, which is clearly an unfavorable phenomenon [22]. Overweight and obese children with allergic diseases have metabolic derangements, and obesity may have an impact on inflammation and clinical symptoms in asthma. The cause of impact of the obesity on asthma risk is still unknown. Potential etiologies include airway smooth muscle dysfunction from thoracic restriction, obesity-related circulating inflammation priming the lung, and obesity-related comorbidities mediating asthma symptom development. Studies suggest that obesity in children with asthma appears to be associated with greater airflow obstruction and a mildly diminished response to inhaled corticosteroids [25]. Additionally, anti-allergic and anti-asthmatic medications may be risk factors for obesity and physiological factors associated with puberty, also intensifying the tendency to gain weight in adolescents [23]. In our study, we did not take into account the effects of medicines because all of the children were newly diagnosed with respiratory allergies and had not been treated with an antihistamine or anti-asthmatic drugs. This may be one of the reasons for the relatively small number of children with obesity observed in our study.

Recent prospective evidence supports the notion that increased body weight precedes asthma development, but there is an ongoing debate as to whether obesity directly increases this risk or whether patients first experience asthma and then become overweight or obese, possibly because of respiratory constraints and reduced physical activity [26].

There are only a few studies on nutritional status and allergic rhinitis. A cross-sectional study of obesity indicators and AR in 8165 participants from the 2005–2006 National Health and Nutrition Examination Survey (NHANES) showed that overweight and obesity were associated with increased risk of AR in adults, but no such evidence was found among children [27].

Interestingly, in our study, although children with co-existing asthma were younger than and not as tall as the children with only AR, they had similar weight. However, there were no statistical differences between the number of overweight and obese children and body composition (FAT, LEAN) in the two groups. This is interesting because other authors have reported more than 50% of children with excessive body weight among children with asthma [28]. Spirometry parameters also did not correlate to BMI, body fat, and lean body mass content in the whole study group, although pulmonary function tests were lower in asthmatics. There were no differences in terms of family burden between allergy, asthma, obesity, exposure to tobacco smoke, and pet allergens.

4.2. Dietary Habits

Our study showed that incorrect eating habits were reported by most of the children with allergies, such as frequent consumption of fast foods and sweets, snacking between meals, and eating meals less than 1 h before bedtime.

Many studies have confirmed that fast-food consumption is linked to childhood obesity [29,30]. The multicenter International Study of Asthma and Allergies in Children (ISAAC) showed that fast food consumption is high in childhood (6–7 years), increases in adolescence (13–14 years), and is associated with higher BMI [31]. In our study, 35% of the children reported fast food consumption at least several times a month. This result is similar to the ISAAC results, showing that 27% of children and 52% of adolescents reported more than weekly fast food consumption [31]. We did not find an association between dietary habits and pulmonary function. There were also no differences in fast food consumption between children with asthma and those with only rhinitis. These results are different from those reported by other authors, suggesting that fast food consumption may contribute to the increasing prevalence of asthma, rhinoconjunctivitis, and eczema in adolescents and children [31]. Other results from case-control [32–34] and cross-sectional [35–40] studies indicate that consumption of fast foods is significantly related to current asthma and allergic rhinitis (pollen fever). Wang et al. suggested that the amount of processed foods eaten correlates with the frequency and severity of asthma [29].

Another important finding from this study was that approximately 80% of children with respiratory allergies snacked between meals every day. Moreover, although all children with excess body mass consumed more snacks compared to normal-weight patients and reported low physical activity, asthmatics consumed snacks more frequently ($\chi^2 = 0.59$; $p = 0.04$) and were more likely to eat their last meal of the day 1 h before sleeping ($\chi^2 = 19.4$; $p = 0.001$). Similar results were seen in the PANACEA study, which showed that among a population of 700 Greek children 10–12 years old with a 23.7% prevalence of asthma symptoms, almost half the children reported salty snack consumption ≥1 times/week [41]. In the cited study, consumption of salty snacks >3 times/week (vs. never/rarely) was associated with a 4.8 times higher likelihood of having asthma symptoms, irrespective of potential confounders. The authors noted that the association of salty snack eating and asthma symptoms was more prominent in children who watched television or played video games >2 h/day [41].

Unlike other researchers, we studied the times of meals consumed and found, interestingly, that almost half of the children ate in the last hour before bedtime. This incorrect habit was more common in children with asthma symptoms. There are well-known factors that affect and exacerbate inflammation in the lower respiratory tract in asthmatics, such as infection or gastroesophageal reflux. Eating immediately before bed might have contributed to the formation of gastroesophageal reflux and bronchial hyperreactivity in the studied group of children with AR. This is also interesting because children with AR differed compared to asthmatics in lung function ($FEV_1\%pv$), but not in nutritional status or other eating habits except for snacking and meals consumed less than 1 h before bedtime. Unfortunately, we did not study the symptoms of gastroesophageal reflux, and we, therefore, cannot form any specific conclusions.

Braithwaite et al. [31] postulated some possible mechanisms to explain the relationship between asthma and allergic disease and the consumption of fast food, which may involve higher concentrations of saturated fatty acids, trans fatty acids, sodium, carbohydrates, and sugar, as well as preservatives that may modulate immune reactions. Consumption of processed foods reduces the consumption of foods that are rich in protective nutrients, such as fruits and vegetables. A reduced intake of fruits and vegetables, which have antioxidative and anti-inflammatory properties, is likely to have an unfavorable impact on asthma prevalence/management [42]. Additionally, indications are that a diet poor in antioxidants is a key factor influencing the development of allergic diseases; a Western lifestyle and processed food consumption can also cause reduced exposure to microbial products and a changed microbiome, which are thus possible causes of the increase in allergic disease [43].

4.3. Physical Activity

In our study, children from both groups (AR and AA) in over 50% reported low physical activity. It is well known that a lack of exercise increases the risk of obesity. This was confirmed by research in the Phase 3 ISAAC trial, in which television viewing (5+ h/day vs. <1 h/day, $p < 0.001$) (the group with low physical activity) was statistically significantly associated with higher BMI in comparison to vigorous physical activity (3+ h/week vs. never, $p < 0.001$) (the group with high physical activity) in adolescents. The authors also suggested that current behaviors are more important than other factors such as birth weight, breastfeeding, current maternal or paternal smoking in early childhood in the development of obesity [24].

A few studies have shown a relationship between physical activity and allergy. In the ISAAC study, associations were found between vigorous physical activity and a sedentary lifestyle for 13-year-olds with allergic rhinoconjunctivitis. Mitchell et al. showed that several hours of TV viewing was associated with symptoms of current asthma in adolescents [24]. Similarly, studies indicate that physical activity could be protective against the development of asthma [44]. On the other hand, Byberg et al. found no association between physical activity and allergic rhinoconjunctivitis [45].

Our results do not contradict the association between pulmonary function and physical activity but show a correlation between physical activity level and BMI percentile in the whole study population (Spearman's $R = -0.19$; $p < 0.05$).

Our study provides two very important issues in the study of respiratory affections such as allergy and asthma. These are the fact that this is the first study on nutrition carried out in newly diagnosed AR teenagers, before any medication that could mislead any result and the fact that this is another study from a few existent about nutrition in respiratory allergy. The limitation of our study is the relatively small group of patients; therefore, a more accurate analysis was not possible, for example based on age or sex. This study is not generalizable to the Polish population because it was performed in a clinical sample of children. Although the relationship between incorrect dietary habits, low physical activity, and obesity in children with respiratory allergies is supported by our findings, no conclusions about causality can be made due to the cross-sectional design.

Further studies with large groups are necessary to determine the relationship between respiratory allergy, body weight, and diet.

5. Conclusions

The risk factors of obesity in allergic children were found to be snacking and low physical activity. Most children with respiratory allergies, especially asthmatics, reported incorrect eating habits such as snacking and eating before bedtime. A correlation between pulmonary function and body composition or dietary habits was not found.

Our study also indicated that in groups of children with respiratory allergies, there is a need for correction of diet and lifestyle. We suggest that early dietary correction may be helpful for children with allergic rhinitis and a high risk of asthma.

Author Contributions: E.W.: S.M., M.S. designed the study. E.W., S.M. collected and analysed the data. M.S., M.G.-N. and E.J. carried out independent internal peer review of the data. All authors agreed the final version of the manuscript submitted for publication.

Funding: The study was supported by local research grant no ST-554.

Conflicts of Interest: The authors declare no conflict of interest.

References

1. McNeill, G.; Tagiyeva, N.; Aucott, L.; Russell, G.; Helms, P.J. Changes in the prevalence of asthma, eczema and hay fever in pre-pubertal children: A 40-year perspective. *Paediatr. Perinatal. Epidemiol.* **2009**, *23*, 506–512. [CrossRef] [PubMed]

2. Masoli, M.; Fabian, D.; Holt, S.; Beasley, R. Global Initiative for Asthma (GINA) Program. Global burden of asthma developed for the Global Initiative for Asthma. *Allergy* **2004**, *59*, 469–478. [CrossRef] [PubMed]
3. Samoliński, B.; Sybilski, A.J.; Raciborski, F.; Tomaszewska, A.; Samelkowalik, P.; Walkiewicz, A.; Lusawa, A.; Borowicz, J.; Gutowskaślesik, J.; Trzpil, L.; et al. Prevalence of rhinitis in Polish population according to the ECAP (Epidemiology of Allergic Disorders in Poland) study. *Otolaryngol. Pol.* **2009**, *63*, 324–330. [CrossRef]
4. Bousquet, P.J.; Demoly, P.; Devillier, P.; Mesbah, K.; Bousquet, J. Impact of allergic rhinitis symptoms on quality of life in primary care. *Int. Arch. Allergy. Immunol.* **2013**, *160*, 393–400. [CrossRef]
5. Guerra, S.; Sherrill, D.L.; Martinez, F.D.; Barbee, R.A. Rhinitis is an independent risk factor for adult-onset asthma. *J. Allergy Clin. Immunol.* **2002**, *109*, 419–425. [CrossRef]
6. Bosquet, J.; Van Cauwenberge, P.; Khaltaev, N. ARIA Workshop Group. Allergic rhinitis and its impact on asthma. *J. Allergy Clin. Immunol.* **2001**, *108*, 147–334. [CrossRef]
7. Samoliński, B.; Raciborski, F.; Lipiec, A.; Tomaszewska, A.; Krzych-Fałta, E.; Nowicka, A. Epidemiology of allergic diseases in Poland. *Pol. J. Allergol.* **2014**, *1*, 10–18.
8. Nagel, G.; Weinmayr, G.; Kleiner, A.; Garcia-Marcos, L.; Strachan, D.P. Effect of diet on asthma and allergic sensitisation in the International Study on Allergies and Asthma in Childhood (ISAAC) phase two. *Thorax.* **2010**, *65*, 516–522. [CrossRef]
9. Rosenheck, R. Fast food consumption and increased caloric intake: A systematic review of a trajectory towards weight gain and obesity risk. *Obes. Rev.* **2008**, *9*, 535–547. [CrossRef]
10. Leynaert, B.; Neukirch, C.; Liard, R.; Bousquet, J.; Neukirch, F. Quality of life in allergic rhinitis and asthma: A population-based study of young adults. *Am. J. Respir. Crit. Care. Med.* **2000**, *162*, 1391–1396. [CrossRef]
11. Bernstein, J.A. Allergic and mixed rhinitis: Epidemiology and natural history. *Allergy Asthma Proc.* **2010**, *31*, 365–369. [CrossRef] [PubMed]
12. International Obesity Task Force. Prevalence of overweight and obesity in a number of countries (global prevalence database) [in:] European Union Public Health Information System 2007. Available online: http://www.euro.who.int/__data/assets/pdf_file/0005/96980/2.3.-Prevalence-of-overweight-and-obesity-EDITED_layouted_V3.pdf (accessed on 12 June 2018).
13. Oblacinska, A.; Wroclawska, M.; Woynarowska, B. Frequency of overweight and obesity in the school-age population in Poland and health care for pupils with these disorders. *Ped. Pol.* **1997**, *72*, 241–245.
14. Mazur, A.; Malecka-Tendera, E.; Lewin-Kowalik, J. Overweight and obesity in primary school children from the Podkarpatian Region. *Ped. Pol.* **2001**, *76*, 743–748.
15. Lipowicz, A.; Opuszalska, M.; Kolodziej, H.; Szklarska, A.; Bielicki, T. Secular trends in BMI and the prevalence of obesity in young Polish males from 1965 to 2010. *Eur. J. Public Health* **2015**, *25*, 279–282. [CrossRef]
16. De, A.; Rastogi, D. Association of pediatric obesity and asthma, pulmonary physiology, metabolic dysregulation, and atopy; and the role of weight management. *Expert Rev. Endocrinol. Metab.* **2019**, *14*, 335–349. [CrossRef]
17. Global Initiative for Asthma. Global Strategy for Asthma Management and Prevention. 2020. Available online: www.ginasthma.org (accessed on 3 April 2018).
18. Miller, M.R.; Crapo, R.; Hankinson, J.; Brusasco, V.; Burgos, F.; Casaburi, R.; Coates, A.; Enright, P.; van der Grinten, C.P.M.; Gustafsson, P.; et al. General consideration for lung function testing. *Eur. Respir. J.* **2005**, *26*, 153–161. [CrossRef]
19. Niedzwiedzka, E.; Wadolowska, L.; Kowalkowska, J. Reproducibility of a Non-Quantitative Food Frequency Questionnaire (62-Item FFQ-6) and PCA-Driven Dietary Pattern Identification in 13–21-Year-Old Females. *Nutrients* **2019**, *11*, 2183. [CrossRef]
20. Kułaga, Z.; Litwin, M.; Tkaczyk, M.; Palczewska, I.; Zajączkowska, M.; Zwolińska, D.; Krynicki, T.; Wasilewska, A.; Moczulska, A.; Morawiec-Knysak, A.; et al. Pan HPolish 2010 growth references for school-a-ged children and adolescents. *Eur. J. Pediatr.* **2011**, *170*, 599–609.
21. Stankiewicz, M.; Pieszko, M.; Sliwińska, A.; Małgorzewicz, S.; Wierucki, Ł.; Zdrojewski, T.; Wyrzykowski, B.; Łysiak-Szydlowska, W. Obesity and diet awareness among Polish children and adolescents in small towns and villages. *Cent. Eur. J. Public Health.* **2014**, *22*, 12–16. [CrossRef]
22. Chrzanowska, M.; Suder, A. Changes in central fatness and abdominal obesity in children and adolescents from Cracow, Poland 1983–2000. *Ann. Hum. Biol.* **2010**, *37*, 242–252. [CrossRef]

23. Forno, E.; Acosta-Pérez, E.; Brehm, J.; Han, YY.; Alvarez, M.; Colón-Semidey, A.; Canino, G.; Celedón, J. Obesity and adiposity indicators, asthma, and atopy in Puerto Rican children. *J. Aller. Clin. Immunol.* **2014**, *133*, 1308–1314. [CrossRef]
24. Mitchell, E.A.; Stewart, A.W.; Braithwaite, I.; Murphy, R.; Hancox, R.J.; Wall, C.; Beasley, R. ISAAC Phase Three Study Group. Factors associated with body mass index in children and adolescents: An international cross-sectional study. *PLoS ONE* **2018**, *2*, e0196221. [CrossRef]
25. Lang, J.E. Obesity, Nutrition, and Asthma in Children. *Ped. Allerg. Immunol. Pulmonol.* **2012**, *25*, 64–75. [CrossRef]
26. Papoutsakis, C.; Priftis, K.N.; Drakouli, M.; Prifti, S.; Konstantaki, E.; Chondronikola, M.; Antonogeorgos, G.; Matziou, V. Childhood overweight/obesity and asthma: Is there a link? A systematic review of recent epidemiologic evidence. *J. Acad. Nutr. Diet.* **2013**, *113*, 77–105. [CrossRef]
27. Han, Y.Y.; Forno, E.; Gogna, M.; Celedón, J. FAAAAI Obesity and rhinitis in a nationwide study of children and adults in the United States. *J. Allerg. Clin. Immunol.* **2016**, *137*, 1460–1465. [CrossRef]
28. Evans, E.W.; Koinis-Mitchell, D.; Kopel, S.J.; Jelalian, E. Lung Function, Dietary Intake, and Weight Status in Children with Persistent Asthma from Low-Income, Urban Communities. *Nutrients* **2019**, *3*, 2943. [CrossRef]
29. Wang, C.S.; Wang, J.; Zhang, X.; Zhang, L.; Zhang, H.P.; Wang, L.; Wood, L.G.; Wang, G. Systematic Review Free Access Is the consumption of fast foods associated with asthma or other allergic diseases? *Respirology* **2018**, *23*, 901–913. [CrossRef]
30. Wickens, K.; Barry, D.; Friezema, A.; Rhodius, R.; Bone, N.; Purdie, G.; Crane, J. Fast foods—Are they a risk factor for asthma? *Allergy* **2005**, *60*, 1537–1541. [CrossRef]
31. Braithwaite, I.; Stewart, A.; Hancox, R.J.; Beasley, R.; Murphy, R.; Mitchell, E.A. ISAAC Phase Three Study Group. Fast-food consumption and body mass index in children and adolescents: An international cross-sectional study. *BMJ Open* **2014**, *8*, 4.
32. Lawson, J.A.; Rennie, D.C.; Dosman, J.A.; Cammer, A.L.; Senthilselvan, A. Obesity, diet, and activity in relation to asthma and wheeze among rural dwelling children and adolescents. *J. Obes.* **2013**, *2013*, 315096. [CrossRef]
33. Mai, X.M.; Becker, A.B.; Liem, J.J.; Kozyrskyj, A.L. Fast foods consumption counters the protective effect of breastfeeding on asthma in children? *Clin. Exp. Allergy* **2009**, *39*, 556–561. [CrossRef] [PubMed]
34. Hijazi, N.; Abalkhail, B.; Seaton, A. Diet and childhood asthma in a society in transition a study in urban and rural Saudi Arabia. *Thorax* **2000**, *55*, 775–779. [CrossRef] [PubMed]
35. Kim, J.L.; Elfman, L.; Mi, Y.; Johansson, M.; Smedje, G.; Norbäck, D. Current asthma and respiratory symptoms among pupils in relation to dietary factors and allergens in the school environment. *Indoor Air.* **2005**, *15*, 170–182. [CrossRef] [PubMed]
36. Garcia-Marcos, L.; Canflanca, I.M.; Garrido, J.B.; Varela, A.L.; Garcia-Hernandez, G.; Grima, F.G.; Gonzalez-Diaz, C.; Carvajal-Urueña, I.; Arnedo-Pena, A.; Busquets-Monge, R.M.; et al. Relationship of asthma and rhinoconjunctivitis with obesity, exercise and Mediterranean diet in Spanish school children. *Thorax* **2007**, *62*, 503–508. [CrossRef] [PubMed]
37. Huang, S.L.; Lin, K.C.; Pan, W.H. Dietary factors associated with physician-diagnosed asthma and allergic rhinitis in teenagers: Analyses of the first nutrition and health survey in Taiwan. *Clin. Exp. Allergy* **2001**, *31*, 259–264. [CrossRef] [PubMed]
38. Takaoka, M.; Norback, D. Diet among Japanese female university students and asthmatic symptoms, infections, pollen and furry pet allergy. *Respir. Med.* **2008**, *102*, 1045–1054. [CrossRef]
39. Norbäck, D.; Zhao, Z.H.; Wang, Z.H.; Wieslander, G.; Mi, Y.H.; Zhang, Z. Asthma, eczema, and reports on pollen and cat allergy among pupils in Shanxi province, China. *Int. Arch. Occup. Environ. Health* **2007**, *80*, 207–216. [CrossRef]
40. Awasthi, S.; Kalra, E.; Roy, S. Prevalence and risk factors of asthma and wheeze in school-going children in Lucknow, North India. *Indian Pediatr.* **2004**, *41*, 1205–1210.
41. Arvaniti, F.; Priftis, K.N.; Papadimitriou, A.; Yiallouros, P.; Kapsokefalou, M.; Anthracopoulos, M.B.; Panagiotakos, D.B. Salty-Snack Eating, Television or Video-Game Viewing, and Asthma Symptoms among 10-to 12-Year-Old Children: The PANACEA Study. *J. Am. Diet. Assoc.* **2011**, *111*, 251–257. [CrossRef]
42. Wood, L.G.; Garg, M.L.; Gibson, P.G. A high-fat challenge increases airway inflammation and impairs bronchodilator recovery in asthma. *J. Allergy Clin. Immunol.* **2011**, *127*, 1133–1140. [CrossRef]

43. Weiland, S.K.; von Mutius, E.; Hüsing, A.; Asher, M.I. Intake of trans fatty acids and prevalence of childhood asthma and allergies in Europe. ISAAC Steering Committee. *Lancet* **1999**, *353*, 2040–2041. [CrossRef]
44. Eijkemans, M.; Mommers, M.M.; Draisma, J.; Thijs, C.; Martin, H. Physical Activity and Asthma: A Systematic Review and Meta-Analysis. *PLoS ONE* **2012**, *7*, e50775. [CrossRef] [PubMed]
45. Byberg, K.K.; Eide, G.E.; Forman, M.R.; Júlíusson, P.B.; Øymar, K. Body mass index and physical activity in early childhood are associated with atopic sensitization, atopic dermatitis and asthma in later childhood. *Clin. Trans. Allergy* **2016**, *6*, 33. [CrossRef] [PubMed]

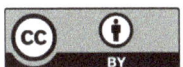

© 2020 by the authors. Licensee MDPI, Basel, Switzerland. This article is an open access article distributed under the terms and conditions of the Creative Commons Attribution (CC BY) license (http://creativecommons.org/licenses/by/4.0/).

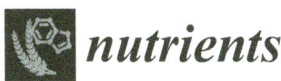

Article
A Serious Game Approach to Improve Food Behavior in Families—A Pilot Study

Sigrid Skouw, Anja Suldrup and Annemarie Olsen *

Food Design and Consumer Behavior Section, Department of Food Science, University of Copenhagen, Rolighedsvej 26, 1958 Frederiksberg C, Denmark; ssn@food.ku.dk (S.S.); clg487@alumni.ku.dk (A.S.)
* Correspondence: ano@food.ku.dk; Tel.: +45-3533-1018

Received: 15 April 2020; Accepted: 9 May 2020; Published: 14 May 2020

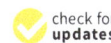

Abstract: The objective of this pilot study was to investigate the effect of a specially developed serious game to improve food behavior in families with children aged 5–13 years using mixed methods. Fourteen families were randomized into a game-group and a non-game-group and divided into age groups (game-children (GC), game-parents (GP), non-game-children (nGC), and non-game-parents (nGP)). The families completed a baseline test, a three-week intervention period with or without a game element, and a follow-up test. Qualitative results showed a positive change in food behavior in all families. Quantitative results mainly showed an effect in food neophobia as a decrease was seen in all groups; however, it was only significant ($p < 0.05$) in three groups (GP, nGC, nGP). No changes were seen in willingness to taste, and only limited changes in liking and number of words used to describe the stimuli. In conclusion, qualitative results showed positive change in the children's food behavior in most families, indicating a positive effect of performing tastings and tasks together as a family—regardless of the presence of a game element. However, this was not as clear in the quantitative data, indicating that current quantitative tools are less suited to measure complex concepts like willingness to taste.

Keywords: serious game; gamification; eating behavior; food neophobia; willingness to taste

1. Background

Low intake of fruit and vegetables (F&V) was according to WHO among the top 10 leading risk factor causes of death in middle- and high-income countries and among 6 diet-related risks of disability-adjusted life years in 2004 [1]. Surveys from 2005 [2] and 2014 [3] showed F&V intake among European 11-year-old children to be below the recommended levels of 400 g/day [4].

Issanchou and Nicklaus [5] put together a conceptual framework showing a number of different concepts determining children's food choice, one of these being experience and social influence from parents and peers. Genetics will affect children's sensory perceptions, and parenting style will further be determining preferences, choices, and intake [5]. This has also been shown in experimental research, like a recent review of different strategies to change children's eating behavior [6]. Parental control and using rewards/instrumental feeding was shown to largely impact eating behavior both positively and negatively. Examples of such strategies are availability of food in the household, restriction of the amount of food a child is allowed to eat, and use of rewards to get children to eat particular foods [6].

A report on vegetable consumption in Denmark showed intake to be limited to only a few types of vegetables such as carrot, onion, and tomato [7]. The most limiting factors of vegetable purchase in Danish families were found to be the lack of ideas on how to use and to get children to eat different and new vegetables [7]. Children's limited food choices are also a challenge in other countries. For instance, a survey from Uruguay found similar results of low variety of vegetable intake and low liking, and some vegetables were never offered to the children due to either parents not eating them themselves or not knowing how to prepare them [8]. To meet the national recommendations for fruit and vegetable intake and to prevent picky eating and food neophobia (reluctance to eat new foods [9]), these limiting factors should be addressed. Encouraging families to approach novel or disliked F&V in a more explorative manner may reduce these limitations, e.g., through sensory exploration and involvement [6], and increase in F&V intake.

The use of game elements to change eating behavior has gained more attention over the last two decades [10–12]. Games created with the intention of developing skills and knowledge are classified as *serious games*. Serious games were initially defined by Abt [13] as games that " … *have an explicit and carefully thought-out educational purpose and are not intended to be played primarily for amusement. This does not mean that serious games are not, or should not be, entertaining*". Playing games is usually associated with fun social interactions of a competitive nature and is driven by both intrinsic and extrinsic motivation [14,15], providing a hands-on approach. The latter has been found more effective in increasing vegetable consumption in children compared to educational programs [6]. Thus, specially designed games might be useful tools for motivating and encouraging exploration of a variety of foods, including that of F&V, and to further promote a change in eating behavior.

Games have demonstrated potential for increasing children's F&V consumption [16,17], while studies on the effect of games on adults are scarce and show only little or no effect [18,19]. Investigation into the effect of games on families does not exist to the knowledge of the authors of this study, constituting a gap in knowledge. This gap is particularly interesting as efforts made to change eating behavior have been found to be more efficient when directed at the family level rather than at the individual level [20], since parental food habits is one of the most important determinants of children's food choice and behavior [21].

Thus, the aim of this pilot study was to investigate if a specially developed serious game could improve food behavior in relation to fruit and vegetables in families with children aged 5 to 13 years. Food behavior was investigated through measures related to the game content: food neophobia and willingness to taste, food vocabulary used to describe F&V, and qualitative measures.

2. Material and Methods

2.1. Recruitment and Randomization

Sixteen families were recruited through social media and a newsletter shared by the project Taste for Life (a research and communication collaboration of scientists in Denmark with focus on taste, www.taste-for-life.org) to participate in the pilot study. Inclusion criteria were no F&V allergies and address in or around the area of Copenhagen for logistic reasons. Most participating families consisted of two children and two parents. Some families contained one or two children in the target age group and one child outside of the target age group, who participated in the game but not in the tests. The families were randomly assigned to either a game group or a non-game. Two families (one game and one non-game family) dropped out of the study before the baseline test; one for unknown reasons and another due to illness. The game-group and non-game-group each contained seven families at the beginning of the intervention. The study complied with the Helsinki declaration. After reviewing the study protocol, the study was found not to require ethical approval (j.nr. 19007287). The data collection and handling plan was approved by the institutional GDPR office (j.nr.: 514-0120/19-5000). Parents gave written, informed consent on behalf of themselves and their children, and children agreed to participate and for data to be used for scientific publications.

2.2. Intervention Material

Developing a game, which unites fitting motivators, a fitting social situation, and mere exposure to novel or disliked foods through sensory interactions, have the potential to be a successful strategy to encourage food exploration and possibly change eating behavior in families.

A serious game was developed for the purpose of this study and was called *The Kingdom of Taste*. The game is played by up to five players and is composed of:

1. One game board with 30 boxes marked on it of which 23 contains a task or action to be done;
2. 88 food cards (with names and pictures of F&V, works as point cards);
3. 5 colored game pieces;
4. One die;
5. One booklet containing an illustrated backstory and the rules;
6. Parental instructions with examples/suggestions on how to solve the different types of tasks;
7. 6 cups with lids (used to contain and hide taste samples of F&V to be used in the game).

Six different F&V are to be used during the game. The F&V are cut into appropriate pieces, one for each player, and placed in the six cups and covered with the lids. The lids were included to add an additional element of surprise and excitement for the players, as they would not see which F&V they were to taste, before landing on a taste task. This could potentially change the level of arousal and the participant's optimal complexity of foods, as described by Dember and Earl [22], before uncovering and thereby affect willingness to taste the hidden F&V.

The game is typically played by 3–5 players (1–3 children and 2 parents from the participating families) and takes 30–60 min. The board game is centered around a story of a chef who has forgotten to purchase F&V for a dinner party at the castle. The chef asks the players to help him collect as many F&V (point cards) as possible on their way from the village to the castle. To collect F&V, the players have to solve different tasks present on the game board. The tasks fall within three categories: (1) descriptive tasks where F&V are to be described with regard to flavor, appearance, and associations; (2) taste tasks where the players has the opportunity of tasting up to six different and unknown F&V; and (3) creativity tasks related to preparation, cooking techniques, and construction of meals. The tasks are represented on the game board as three distinctive zones as shown in Figure 1. The tasks are created to increase familiarity of a large variety of F&V, both through descriptive tasks and through tastings. Mere exposure to the F&V through pictures, words, and tastings could potentially increase affection of these [23]. Creative meal planning is a part of the game in the last zone and as the game is finalized by each player composing a three-course meal with his/her collected F&V card (points). Sparking exploration and interest in meal composition could inspire players to bring this creativity to the kitchen and further affect food behavior. The game aimed at obtaining a suitable level of difficulty for the target group, in accordance with the Theory of Flow, which describes how the relationship between skill level and posed challenges needs to be balanced to achieve a state of flow; i.e., when the challenge a person is faced with is not too difficult nor too easy to solve [24,25]. Before the pilot test, the game was tested by five families with children aged 4 to 9 years and one school class with students aged 11 to 12 years. The families received all necessary materials (except F&V, which they were to provide themselves with the possibility of receiving compensation for their purchases) and a questionnaire with questions regarding the game elements, age group, entertainment, etc., to be filled out after having tested the game. The game was modified according to this feedback.

The game was used as intervention material for the game-families.

The non-game-families were provided with a representative selection of the three categories of tasks present on the board game, including tastings of F&V, but without the game context. The non-game material was comprised of a sheet of task instructions, 30 food cards (with names of the F&V and no pictures), one parental instruction with examples/suggestions on how to solve the tasks, and containers without lids for taste samples. Lids were not included in order to limit any game element that could create additional excitement during a task.

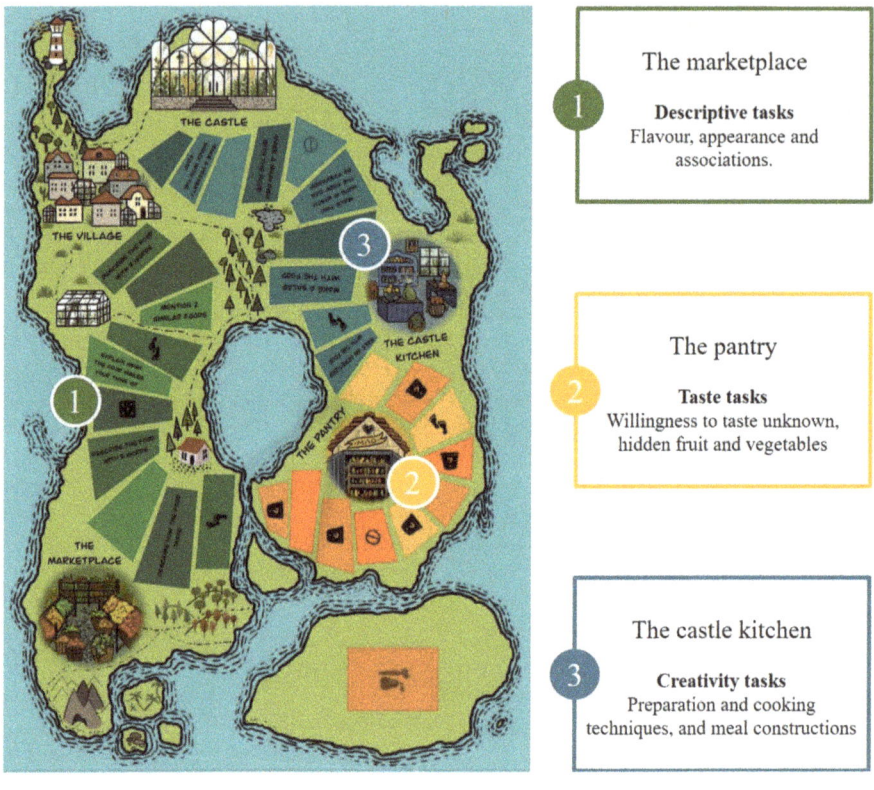

Figure 1. The Kingdom of Taste and an overview of the three zones and their distinctive tasks.

2.3. Study Design

The study timeline consisted of a baseline test, a three-week intervention period, and a follow-up test. The families were instructed to perform their designated assignments at home once a week during the three-week intervention period; i.e., the game-families were to play the serious game, and the non-game-families were to perform similar tasks without the game element a total of three times. F&V for the home assignments were delivered to all families (both game and non-game families) once a week during the intervention period, at their home address.

Table 1 provides an overview of the taste samples used at the home assignments. The F&V for taste samples were chosen based on the theory of *Zone of Proximal Development* [26], as this theory has recently been used to explain flavor preference development in children [27]. The theory of the Zone of Proximal Development is originally a model with three levels (Zone of Actual Development, Zone of Proximal Development, and Zone of Insurmountable Difficulty) describing children's cognitive development as a result of social interaction between individuals with different skill levels [26]. In a food context, The Zone of Actual Development represents foods that are familiar, liked, and considered to be safe to eat for the child on his/her own, whereas the Zone of Proximal Development represents foods that are considered exiting, unknown, and associated with some degree of uncertainty, which the child is only able or willing to taste under adult guidance and support [27]. F&V choices aimed at having two F&V belonging to the Zone of Actual Development (upper two rows in Table 1) and four F&V in the Zone of Proximal Development (lower four rows in Table 1).

Table 1. Overview of the taste samples used for the home assignments.

Week 1	Week 2	Week 3
Apple	Banana	Cucumber
Carrot	Tomato	Pear
Fennel	Passion fruit	Dried goji berries
Water chestnut [a]	Enoki mushrooms	Bamboo shoots [a]
Jerusalem artichoke	Onion sprouts	Turmeric root
Green olives [a]	Nashi pear	Cherimoya

[a] Conserved in brine.

At the end of the follow-up session, all families received a 500 DKK (75 USD) gift card of their choice as a thank-you-gift for their participation in the study, and the non-game-families further received a *Kingdom of Taste* game.

2.4. Questionnaire Design and Test Protocol

Baseline and follow-up tests were performed at the university with a maximum of two families present in the same room at a time placed in far ends of the room, never mixing families from different intervention groups. Each test took approximately one hour.

Mixed methods were applied for the data collection of this study in order to obtain a fuller insight into the intervention effects, as a combination of quantitative and qualitative methods can provide insights that may be missed when only using one of them [28]. The choice of using mixed methods was further based on the expectation that food behavior is a complex concept, which is possibly difficult to measure by current quantitative tools. The questionnaire developed for the baseline test consisted of three quantitative parts: (1) A Danish version of the six-item version of the original food neophobia scale (FNS) [29], first used in [30]; (2) a box for describing the presented F&V (a measure of food vocabulary, single words only); and (3) willingness to taste the presented F&V (yes/no), including liking measured on a 7-point hedonic smiley scale and stating familiarity and frequency of consumption to provide an idea of the level of preliminary knowledge about the F&V used in the tests. The questionnaire was to be filled out individually, though the younger children had the opportunity to receive assistance either from one of the two first authors of this article or their parents.

The follow-up test consisted of the same quantitative tasks as the baseline test to measure change during the intervention period, but further included qualitative questions for the parents to answer. The qualitative questionnaire consisted of open-ended questions regarding observed changes in food behavior at home during the intervention period; changes in willingness to taste, how they discussed F&V, and changes in the children's engagement with F&V.

The F&V used at the baseline and the follow-up test were the same; banana, carrot, broccoli, papaya, prune, and caper berry, which were chosen based on the same considerations as the taste samples for the home assignments. The order of the F&V was randomized and varied between all the families at the two test sessions. The F&V were placed on two plates, one plate with taste samples and another plate with the F&V in its true shape (uncut, except for the broccoli and papaya which were cut in half), for the participants to use as a visual tool when answering the questions. The F&V were presented one at a time. Additional materials present were pens, paper plates, napkins, crispbread, cups, and water.

2.5. Data Analysis

All statistical data analyses were conducted using R-studio statistical free software (version 1.1.456, Boston, United States) [31]. Graphs were made using Microsoft Office Excel (2016) and Microsoft Office PowerPoint (2016).

The participants were divided into groups according to treatment and age group: game-children (GC), non-game-children (nGC), game-parents (GP), and non-game-parents (nGP). Baseline differences between GC vs. nGC and GP vs. nGP were tested for by conducting a Mann–Whitney U test for age, gender, food neophobia, liking, and word count, and Fisher's exact test was used to test for baseline differences in willingness to taste.

A McNemar test tests if two response variables are significantly different from each other within a study sample and was used for testing significant differences in willingness to taste (yes/no) between baseline and follow-up within each of the four groups. A linear mixed model tested for differences within each of the four groups between baseline and follow-up in the FNS score, liking, and word count. The collected words were both analyzed as total word count as well as count within the word-categories *hedonic*, *descriptive*, and *other*. The model was further used to test the difference in change found between the treatments in both age groups (GC vs. nGC and GP vs. nGP) for the same measures. Residuals of the linear model not following a normal distribution were transformed by a log-transformation.

A Cronbach's alpha test was run on the FNS scores in each of the two age groups to test reliability. The test was run on data from baseline and follow-up test separately.

The qualitative feedback collected at the follow-up test was analyzed by using a combination of pre-set and emerging codes (willingness to taste, food language, food engagement, game related) with individual emerging sub-codes.

3. Results

Two non-game-families dropped out of the study just before the follow-up test; one due to illness and another due to scheduling issues. Seven game-families and five non-game-families completed the follow-up test. Three children who participated in the baseline test did not participate in the follow-up test due to illness. A total of 12 families and 39 participants completed the entire study; 22 in the game-group and 17 in the non-game-group. Table 2 shows the age and gender distribution in the two groups. No differences were found in age or gender distribution when comparing the treatments in both age groups.

Table 2. Age and gender distribution of participants who completed both baseline and follow up test.

	Game Group (n = 22)	Non-Game Group (n = 17)
	Children	
Number of children (n)	10	8
Age (mean ± SEM, range)	9 ± 0.9 (5–13)	8 ± 0.6 (6–10)
Gender (female, n (%))	5 (50%)	4 (50%)
	Parents	
Number of parents (n)	12	9
Age (mean ± SEM, range)	40 ± 0.1 (35–47)	38 ± 0.8 (35–41)
Gender (female, n (%))	6 (50%)	5 (55.6%)

Children (n = 18) and parents (n = 21).

3.1. Quantitative Measures

3.1.1. Food Neophobia, Willingness to Taste, and Liking

No significant differences were found at baseline between the treatments in both age groups in FNS score. All groups showed a decrease in FNS score from baseline to follow-up test, but significant reductions in FNS score were only found in nGC, GP, nGP but not in GC, as shown in Figure 2. Of the 10 GC, seven showed a decrease, one remained unchanged and two showed an increase in food neophobia at follow-up.

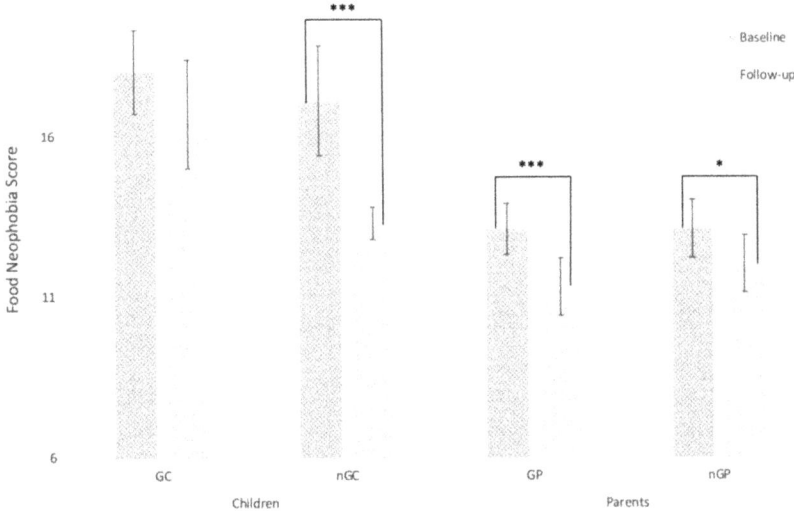

Figure 2. Mean (±SEM) range of food neophobia scale (FNS) score at baseline and follow up. Abbreviations: Game-children (GC), non-game-children (nGC), game-parents (GP), non-game-parents (nGP). Significance level estimated by a linear mixed model. Significance levels: *** $p < 0.001$, ** $p < 0.01$, * $p < 0.05$.

Cronbach's Alpha was calculated for the FNS score of the children and the parents separately. At baseline $\alpha = 0.64$ for both the children and parents, and at follow-up $\alpha = 0.8$ and 0.7 for children and adults, respectively. These sizes indicate consistency.

No significant difference in willingness to taste was found between treatments and age groups at baseline or between baseline and follow-up in any of the groups, and only minor and scattered changes in liking between baseline and follow-up were observed as seen in Table 3.

Table 3. Mean (SEM) of liking of the six fruit and vegetables (F&V) at baseline and follow-up (1 = super bad; 2 = really bad; 3 = bad; 4 = neither good nor bad; 5 = good; 6 = really good; 7 = super good).

		Children				Parents				
		GC		nGC		GP		nGP		
		Mean (SEM)	p^a	Mean (SEM)	p^a	Diff. p^b	Mean (SEM)	p^a	Mean (SEM)	p^a	Diff. p^b
Carrot	Baseline	5.6 (0.3)		6.1 (0.4)			6.3 (0.2)		5.9 (0.4)		
	Follow-up	5.5 (0.4)		5.8 (0.5)			5.9 (0.3)		5.6 (0-3)		
Banana	Baseline	6.3 (0.3)		6.7 (0.2)			6.3 (0.3)	***	6.4 (0.4)		
	Follow-up	6.3 (0.3)		5.5 (0.9)			5.8 (0.3)		6.3 (0.3)		
Broccoli	Baseline	4.7 (0.4)		4.3 (1.0)			5.6 (0.2)		5.4 (0.2)		
	Follow-up	5.0 (0.4)		4.5 (0.8)			5.7 (0.3)		5.4 (0.5)		
Papaya	Baseline	3.6 (0.3)	*	2.9 (0.3)	***		4.0 (0.3)		2.9 (0.4)	***	
	Follow-up	4.3 (0.4)		4.4 (0.5)			4.6 (0.3)		4.9 (0.3)		
Prune	Baseline	5.0 (0.5)		5.2 (0.7)			5.1 (0.4)		4.8 (0.5)	*	*
	Follow-up	5.0 (0.6)		5.1 (0.6)			5.0 (0.3)		5.4 (0.4)		
Caper berry	Baseline	3.1 (1.0)		2.3 (1.0)	*		4.5 (0.4)		3.6 (0.6)		
	Follow-up	4.2 (1.2)		2.6 (0.8)			4.7 (0.4)		4.0 (0.7)		

Significance level estimated by a linear mixed model. Abbreviations: Game-children (GC), non-game-children (nGC), game-parents (GP), non-game-parents (nGP). Significance levels: *** $p < 0.001$, ** $p < 0.01$, * $p < 0.05$. [a] p-value shows significant level of change from baseline to follow-up in the groups. [b] p-value shows significant level of difference in change from baseline to follow-up between CG and nCG and between GP and nGP.

3.1.2. Food Vocabulary Used by Families to Describe F&V

Food vocabulary was measured through counting the number of single words used to describe a given F&V, and categorized them in one of three word categories: *Hedonic* (e.g., "delicious"), *descriptive* (e.g., "green") or *other* (e.g., "monkey"). Only a few significant changes in number of words used to describe the presented F&V was found. When a significant change was present, it was characterized as an increase in word count in the non-game-group and a decrease in the game-group, with no general tendency of specific word groups increasing or decreasing more than others (Table S1). The changes in words were not specifically connected to any of the three word-categories hedonic, descriptive, or other.

3.2. Qualitative Measures

3.2.1. Perceived Change in Food Behavior

Food behavior was measured as willingness to taste, food language, and food engagement in the qualitative questionnaire. All 12 families reported an increase in willingness to taste in the qualitative questionnaire. Six families, four game and two non-game, expressed that their food language had changed over the course of the intervention period. Eight families, five game and three non-game, indicated that they have been having food-related conversations during the intervention period. Nine families, five game and four non-game, reported an increase in the children's food engagement on one or more parameters: increased interest in food, cooking, or meal planning. When summarizing the qualitative results, parents reported improved food behavior independently on the presence of a game element.

3.2.2. Motivational Effect of the Game Element

Six of the seven game-families commented on the use of a game to increase willingness to taste. Four of them reported how the game/competitive element in the game increased their children's willingness to taste the F&V in the home assignment, as expressed by one mother: *"The game/competitive element in the game caused our children to not want to lose and (they) tasted almost everything the last couple of weeks"*. Two of the game families further commented that the taste tasks were the most exciting part of the game. The mother of one game-family wrote: *"During the home assignments it was obvious that the children were looking forward to tasting the food, and that the best part was when someone landed on a taste task"*. Two game families further reported how their children had requested to play the game during the intervention period.

4. Discussion

4.1. Food Neophobia and Willingness to Taste

Several studies have found food neophobia to decrease from childhood to adulthood [32–34]. Based on this knowledge, the lower level of food neophobia in the parents in comparison to the children was expected.

FNS have been used to measure the effect of sensory education on food behavior, showing lower scores after intervention [35,36] but not always significantly [35]. All four groups in this study showed a decrease in FNS after intervention either significantly (GP, nGP, and nGP, $p < 0.05$) or non-significantly (GC) corresponding with existing literature. Whether the change in FNS scores is persistent is unknown, as long-term effects were not investigated in this study, but the change indicates the existence of subjective perceptions of change among the participants, at least during the intervention period. This perception of change may result from the participants' own observations of behavioral changes, such as increased courage to try new foods or being less particular about which foods to eat during and after the completion of the home assignments. This indicates that continuous use of the home assignments may potentially change food neophobia persistently, as a result of increasing willingness to try foods and thereby increase exposure to disliked and novel foods, potentially giving rise to the effect of mere exposure [23].

All 12 families reported that they had experienced an increase in willingness to taste, independent of treatment, supporting the decrease in FNS scores and indicating that the serious game did not provide an additional effect over the tasks performed without the game element.

The game-families generally ascribed the increase in willingness to taste to the competitive element of the game due to its motivational effect. Overcoming a personal boundary of tasting something unknown or novel might function as an intrinsic motivation for the participants, caused by feelings of satisfaction and joy of self-accomplishments, or due to enjoyment of playing the game [14]. As the game further gives rise to extrinsic motivation through the possibility of earning points, winning, and receiving feedback and praise from other players, the participants might further be more motivated to engage [14]. The combination of both intrinsic and extrinsic motivations thereby seems to have resulted in a high degree of willingness to taste during the home assignments in the game-families. The game-families only reported a positive outcome of using extrinsic motivation to get their children to taste the F&V in the game, but previous studies have indicated negative outcomes, as reviewed by DeCosta et al. [6]. Using extrinsic motivation, may have an undermining effect on intrinsic motivation [37], as e.g., parental prompting and restriction of food intake have been found to cause children to override their internal cues of hunger, satiety, and pleasure [6], which could lead to overeating or other negative consequences. These findings could indicate potential negative consequences of using a game to improve food behavior and willingness to taste although this was not indicated by the results of this study. A potential explanation could be the more positive type of extrinsic motivation found in the game compared to a normal eating situation, such as the possibility of gaining rewards (point cards, praises, and cheers) and the wish to win.

In the non-game-families, several of the parents reported that they were impressed by how many of the novel F&V their children were willing to taste during the home assignment. The intrinsic motivation of self-accomplishment might likewise have occurred in the non-game-families during the home assignment. The surprise from the parents' side, that their children were willing to taste the large variety of F&V presented, could also be an example of the discrepancy in expected pickiness between children and parents found by the Danish Agriculture and Food Council [38], as parents perceive their children to be pickier than the children themselves are. The children could have been willing to taste such F&V before the intervention period but may not have been served it due to the parents' expectations of their refusal to taste it. In a review by Scaglioni et al. [21], parental food habits were shown to be one of the most important determinants of children's food choice and behavior. Together with the gap between parental and child beliefs about picky eating, this could be part of the reason why the F&V consumption of European children does not meet the recommendations [2,3]. The children are to a large extent limited in their F&V selection to what is available in the kitchen at home—and what is available and served at home might be limited to what the parents believe to be what their children like [7]. The F&V used in this study were selected to be a mix of well-known and novel stimuli and thereby expose the families to F&V other than what they usually eat. Simply tasting and experiencing novel F&V could be a way to enlighten parents of their children's higher willingness to taste and eat new F&V than what they believe and thereby be a motivation to incorporate such new foods in the kitchen, which will likely lead to increased F&V intake.

The taste samples used in the game-group were kept a secret until the point of tasting (hidden in a container with lid), whereas the samples were visible for the non-game-families from the beginning of their home assignment (placed in a container without lid). This additional element of secrecy present in the game-families' assignment may have increased the level of arousal before the reveal of the F&V [22]. Even if the F&V hidden were well-known or at least known to some degree, the participants would not know before opening the container in which they were hidden. The anticipation of what was hidden could possibly increase the arousal, in contrast to the non-game-group where the participants were able to see the F&V before engaging in tasting.

No changes in willingness to taste were found, which does not align with the reduction in FNS scores and the qualitative perception of increased willingness to taste. This lack of difference in willingness to taste could be caused by the high willingness present at the baseline test. Using willingness to taste might thereby not be the best measure for investigating a change in courage to taste different foods, when the stimuli is mostly well-known F&V and when the participants are not neophobic. Other studies have found varying effects of using willingness to taste, ranging from positive effects [36] and temporary effects [35] to no change [39]. This line of thought was recently shared by Olsen [40], who suggests that the focus in this area of research is too narrow and could benefit from using a broader specter of outcome measures, including qualitative ones. If this is the case, the varying effects of sensory education on willingness to taste [35,36,39] may be explained by the inadequacy of the measurement approach rather than the sensory education itself. Other approaches have been made in an attempt to develop a behavioral food neophobia measure for children, such as using wiliness to taste where the children were to taste an unknown food based on their own previous indication of willingness [35], and correlating it with the FNS, but the correlations found between the two tests were generally weak [35,41]. The poor correlation between the FNS and the behavioral food neophobia tests indicates that the two tests may measure two different things. More research into how to effectively measure these, which are considered closely related concepts, is required in order to perform this kind of studies.

The difficulties of using willingness to taste as a behavioral measure of food neophobia may indicate that willingness to taste is a far more complex concept than simply a yes/no question. It may be assumed that different levels of novelty and resistance towards certain foods exist, which may mean that the action of tasting a novel food is rejected but does not necessarily mean that other forms of interactions with the novel food are rejected. Such other interactions could potentially result in willingness to taste at a later time point because of increased familiarity [42]. This speculation is supported by the findings of Dazeley and Houston-Price [43] and Coulthard and Sealy [10], who both found that non-taste sensory interaction increased children's tasting afterwards.

4.2. Food Vocabulary Used by Families to Describe F&V

The limited changes in word count when describing the F&V are in accordance with previous studies, where 11- to 13-year old children showed a decrease in number of words used to describe bread in both an intervention and control group after sensory education [44]. Mustonen et al. [44] expected the lower number of words to be partly due to restlessness in the children during the follow-up test, which was also observed in this study in several children. Likewise, several parents showed signs of restlessness and appeared to use less time on this task at the follow-up test. As the baseline and follow-up test questionnaires were identical, an explanation could be that the writing tasks at follow-up test perhaps were perceived as tedious and not as exciting and fun as tasting the unknown F&V. This speculation is backed up by the qualitative data, where the tasting part was described by two families to be the best part of the game. The tendency to an increase in word count in the control groups and decrease in the intervention groups could indicate that the game element was interfering with the descriptive tasks. The game players might have been eager to move on to other parts of the game that they found more fun, as indicated by some of the game-families, as described in Section 4.4. Focus of the non-game-families, on the other hand, may have been more on the task itself, as there were no game elements. Due to the simpler nature and the limited number of tasks (each participant only having to answer four questions per session), more effort may have been put into solving the non-game. If the outcome is to achieve a more nuanced food language through increasing vocabulary and ability to describe F&V, better results might be achieved by completing the tasks without a game element.

4.3. Qualitative Measures

The qualitative feedback received form the parents showed a positive improvement in food behavior in both groups, indicating that the specific tasks (describing, tasting, and being creative with

F&V) present in both the game and non-game assignments possibly are sufficient on their own to improve food behavior. It is not possible to tell which element of the home assignment caused the improvements seen in both groups or if it was a collaborative effect.

Both the game tasks and the non-game tasks caused the families to designate time specifically to explore F&V by sensory and mental interactions together which may be a contributing factor to why a positive effect was found in both groups. The positive effect of designating time to these types of tasks has also been found in other studies [10,43,45]. The social situation can also affect willingness to taste through listening to others' reflections and expectations and observing their behavior towards the F&V [46,47].

4.4. Can Serious Games Improve Food Behaviour in Families?

The results of this pilot study do not show any additional effect of using a serious game to improve food behavior in families compared to performing similar non-game tasks, despite the fact that other studies [10,48] have found an effect of physical games on vegetable consumption in children, indicating a potential effect of games. As this pilot study failed to show an effect, further research into this specific segment and topic should be done in order to fully understand the possible outcomes. Conducting a similar study on a larger scale with increased intervention time is recommended in order to investigate if long-term use of the intervention materials would show additional differences between the groups. The additional motivators [14,15] of the game may give rise to continuous use of the game as indicated in the qualitative feedback where the GC requested to play the game during the intervention period. Such continuous use would result in continuous exposure to F&V and here potentially facilitate long-term effects through mere exposure [23]. On the contrary, the non-game tasks may become more tedious in the long run due to fewer motivators. This speculation was substantiated in the qualitative feedback by several of the parents in the game group, mentioning the game as an important motivator. Two game-families reported how their children had requested to play the game again, substantiating the motivational effects of a game.

On the other hand, it is still worth considering the possibility of a long-term effect of the non-game tasks as well, as they are less confined to a specific situation (a game situation), and therefore may be more easily incorporated into a busy lifestyle. Although playing *The Kingdom of Taste* has the potential to be more motivating over time, the non-game tasks may become integrated into the family's food habits more effortlessly and thereby constitute easy and accessible tools to introduce novel foods. If elements of the home assignments are adopted as new habits in everyday meal situations, rather than requiring the family to set aside time specifically to do the tasks in the format used in this study, the positive effect may occur more automatically and effortlessly [49]. The results of the simple tasks performed by the non-game-families in this study are an example of how little effort it takes to improve food behavior. It seems that it is a matter of making a habit of tasting and discussing ingredients, flavors, etc., of F&V together in an explorative manner—leading to a continuous introduction to and integration of novel F&V, which could cause a shift in food choice and behavior. Ultimately, this could result in overcoming the limiting factors faced by parents of introducing novel vegetables [7]. These speculations on turning the elements of the home assignments into everyday habits are not substantiated by the collected data, as long-term effects were not investigated, causing a need for further research.

4.5. Strengths and Limitations

The use of mixed methods in this study constituted a strength, as the qualitative data provided insights that would otherwise not have been discovered through the quantitative data, markedly changing the discussion and conclusion of the study. The major limitation to the study was the small sample size, which over the course of the intervention period was reduced from 49 to 39 individuals, and as mentioned previously, it would be valuable to conduct a similar study with increased sample size and time span. Another limitation was that the families were recruited from a small geographical area in or around Copenhagen, potentially limiting the diversity of family lifestyles and social and environmental surroundings. Copenhagen has a large percentage of people with high educational levels compared to other parts of Denmark, which is expectedly reflected in this study sample and can have caused a bias as educational levels have been found to correlate to diets and health. Furthermore, as participating families were recruited through social media and newsletters by Taste for Life, they can be expected to have a higher interest in food than the general population, which implies that results may not extrapolate to all families. Different family compositions (varying from two parents and three children to two parents and one child) and children's age will likely have an impact on the effect of the game concerning level of help provided and adaptation of tasks. Another limitation arises from the younger children being able to receive help from their parents or the experimenter to fill in the test questionnaire. Although parents were requested not to help their children with anything other than writing, it is uncertain whether patents fully complied with the instructions, and they may also have suggested responses to their children. This could potentially cause a difference between children able to write by themselves and children not able to write by themselves. It is not possible to know if the children, who requested to play the game again, did it to gain attention from their parents or if it was because they wanted to play the game. Due to the limited period of time available to complete the study, it was not possible to measure if the effect of the intervention was persistent over time. It is recommended that future studies contain a control group with no tasks or tasting of F&V to be able to measure any possible differences in effect between using the game and not doing any tasks.

5. Conclusions

In conclusion, most families reported improved food behavior towards F&V in the children—regardless of the presence of a serious game. This indicates that designating time as a family to taste and discuss attributes and handling of F&V is enough to improve food behavior. However, the quantitative results were not as clear, as most measures showed no or limited change. A decrease in food neophobia score was seen in all four groups; however, it was only significant for the parental groups and the non-game-children, indicating no difference between the treatment groups. The lack of complete alignment between the quantitative and qualitative results raises the question of whether current quantitative measures are capable of truly reflecting concepts as complex as willingness to taste and food behavior. Based on these findings, conducting a similar study of larger scale to investigate if these results are persistent is recommended. Results of such a study could be used to consider if future research in this area should initially focus on developing new and better ways of measuring the complex concepts within this field of study by adopting a broader approach of both quantitative and qualitative measures.

6. Future Perspectives

Based on the discussion of appropriate measures to investigate a change in food behavior, a better approach may be to evaluate the journey towards willingness to taste, instead of the end point (tasting). The authors of this article therefore suggest that *food exploration* could serve as a new concept, which through both quantitative and qualitative measures allows the assessment of many different ways of interacting with novel food. Exploring foods can take place in several ways, both as a sensory interaction (tactile, olfactory, visual, auditory, gustatory) or as a mental interaction (e.g., using one's imagination to compose a meal, associating one food with another food, memory, etc.). Examples of exploring a novel or disliked food could for instance be a sensory-based description of a food based on flavor and appearance or a combination of sensory and mental interaction, as seen in the study by Coulthard and Sealy [10], where pre-school children created pictures using F&V. The concept of food exploration acknowledges the existence of different levels of novelty and resistance towards certain foods. If a person is not comfortable with tasting a novel food, he or she might be comfortable with interacting with the food in other ways. Engaging in non-taste sensory or mental interaction with foods might give rise to willingness to taste at a later time point.

Supplementary Materials: The following are available online at http://www.mdpi.com/2072-6643/12/5/1415/s1. Table S1: Mean (SEM) number of words used to describe the six F&V in the baseline and follow-up test and significance in difference for the treatment and age groups.

Author Contributions: Conceptualization and methodology, S.S., A.S. and A.O.; data collection, and data analyses, S.S. and A.S., interpretation of data, S.S., A.S and A.O., writing of the manuscript, S.S., review and editing, S.S. and A.O., supervision and funding acquisition, A.O. All authors have read and agreed to the published version of the manuscript.

Funding: This study was part of the "Taste for Life" project, which is financed by Nordea-fonden. The foundation had no involvement in the work.

Acknowledgments: We would like to thank Cathrine Terkelsen for her help and guidance with working with children and qualitative data in this project, Anna Skouw Nielsen for illustrating the game board and the booklet, and Peter Willer Hansen for producing the physical elements of the game.

Conflicts of Interest: All authors declare that there are no conflicts of interest regarding the publication of this paper.

References

1. World Health Organization. *Global Health Risks—Mortality and Burden of Disease Attributable to Selected Major Risks*; World Health Organization: Geneva, Switzerland, 2009.
2. Yngve, A.; Wolf, A.; Poortvliet, E.; Elmadfa, I.; Brug, J.; Ehrenblad, B.; Franchini, B.; Haraldsdóttir, J.; Krølner, R.; Maes, L.; et al. Fruit and Vegetable Intake in a Sample of 11-Year-Old Children in 9 European Countries: The Pro Children Cross-Sectional Survey. *Ann. Nutr. Metab.* **2005**, *49*, 236–245. [CrossRef] [PubMed]
3. Lynch, C.; Kristjansdottir, A.G.; te Velde, S.J.; Lien, N.; Roos, E.; Thorsdottir, I.; Krawinkel, M.; de Almeida, M.D.V.; Papadaki, A.; Ribic, C.H.; et al. Fruit and vegetable consumption in a sample of 11-year-old children in ten European countries—The PRO GREENS cross-sectional survey. *Public Health Nutr.* **2014**, *17*, 2436–2444. [CrossRef]
4. World Health Organization. *Diet, Nutrition and the Prevention of Chronic Diseases. Joint WHO/FAO Expert Consultation*; WHO Technical Report Series No. 916; World Health Organization: Geneva, Switzerland, 2003.
5. Nicklaus, S.; Issanchou, S. Children and food choice. In *Understanding Consumers of Food Products*; Elsevier: Amsterdam, The Netherlands, 2007; pp. 329–358. [CrossRef]
6. DeCosta, P.; Møller, P.; Frøst, M.B.; Olsen, A. Changing children's eating behaviour—A review of experimental research. *Appetite* **2017**, *113*, 327–357. [CrossRef] [PubMed]
7. The Danish Meal Partnership. *U & A om Grøntsager*; The Danish Meal Partnership: Copenhagen, Denmark, 2017.
8. Raggio, L.; Gámbaro, A. Study of the reasons for the consumption of each type of vegetable within a population of school-aged children. *BMC Public Health* **2018**, *18*, 1163. [CrossRef] [PubMed]
9. Birch, L.L.; Fisher, J.O. Development of eating behaviors among children and adolescents. *Pediatrics* **1998**, *101 Pt 2*, 539–549.
10. Coulthard, H.; Sealy, A. Play with your food! Sensory play is associated with tasting of fruits and vegetables in preschool children. *Appetite* **2017**, *113*, 84–90. [CrossRef]
11. Dias, M.; Agante, L. Can advergames boost children's healthier eating habits? A comparison between healthy and non-healthy food. *J. Consum. Behav.* **2011**, *10*, 152–160. [CrossRef]
12. Lakshman, R.R.; Sharp, S.J.; Ong, K.K.; Forouhi, N.G. A novel school-based intervention to improve nutrition knowledge in children: Cluster randomised controlled trial. *BMC Public Health* **2010**, *10*, 123. [CrossRef]
13. Abt, C. *Serious Games*; Viking Press: New York, NY, USA, 1970.
14. Ryan, R.M.; Deci, E.L. Intrinsic and Extrinsic Motivations: Classic Definitions and New Directions. *Contemp. Educ. Psychol.* **2000**, *25*, 54–67. [CrossRef]
15. Ryan, R.M.; Rigby, C.S.; Przybylski, A. The Motivational Pull of Video Games: A Self-Determination Theory Approach. *Motiv. Emot.* **2006**, *30*, 344–360. [CrossRef]
16. Folkvord, F.; Anastasiadou, D.T.; Anschütz, D. Memorizing fruit: The effect of a fruit memory-game on children's fruit intake. *Prev. Med. Rep.* **2017**, *5*, 106–111. [CrossRef] [PubMed]

17. Jones, B.A.; Madden, G.J.; Wengreen, H.J. The FIT Game: Preliminary evaluation of a gamification approach to increasing fruit and vegetable consumption in school. *Prev. Med. (Baltim.)* **2014**, *68*, 76–79. [CrossRef] [PubMed]
18. Bannai, Y.; Kosaka, T.; Aiba, N. Food Practice Shooter: A Serious Game with a Real-World Interface for Nutrition and Dietary Education. In *Human Interface and the Management of Information in the Information and Knowledge Design and Evaluation—16th International Conference, HCI International 2014 Heraklion, Crete, Greece, June 22–27, 2014 Proceedings, Part I*; LNCS 3196; Springer: Cham, Switzerland, 2014; pp. 139–147. [CrossRef]
19. Tikka, P.; Laitinen, M.; Manninen, I.; Oinas-Kukkonen, H. Reflection through Gaming: Reinforcing Health Message Response through Gamified Rehearsal. In Proceedings of the 13th International Conference, PERSUASIVE 2018, Waterloo, ON, Canada, 18–19 April 2018; pp. 200–212. [CrossRef]
20. Gruber, K.J.; Haldeman, L.A. Using the family to combat childhood and adult obesity. *Prev. Chronic Dis.* **2009**, *6*, A106. [PubMed]
21. Scaglioni, S.; De Cosmi, V.; Ciappolino, V.; Parazzini, F.; Brambilla, P.; Agostoni, C. Factors Influencing Children's Eating Behaviours. *Nutrients* **2018**, *10*, 706. [CrossRef] [PubMed]
22. Dember, W.N.; Earl, R.W. Analysis of exploratory, manipulatory, and curiosity behaviors. *Psychol. Rev.* **1957**, *64*, 91–96. [CrossRef] [PubMed]
23. Zajonc, R.B. Mere Exposure: A Gateway to the Subliminal. *Curr. Dir. Psychol. Sci.* **2001**, *10*, 224–228. [CrossRef]
24. Shernoff, D.J.; Csikszentmihalyi, M.; Schneider, B.; Shernoff, E.S. Student Engagement in High School Classrooms from the Perspective of Flow Theory. In *Applications of Flow in Human Development and Education*; Springer: Dordrecht, The Netherlands, 2014; pp. 475–494. [CrossRef]
25. Csikszentmihalyi, M. *Beyond Boredom and Anxiety*, 1st ed.; Jossey-Bass Publishers: San Francisco, CA, USA, 1975; p. 231.
26. Vygotsky, L. *Mind in Society: The Development of Higher Psychological Processes*; Cole, M., John-Steiner, V., Scribner, S., Souberman, E., Eds.; Harvard University Press: Cambridge, MA, USA; London, UK, 1978; p. 159.
27. Schneider, M.; Rymann, E. *Sådan Smager Børn—Den Videnskabelige Forklaring på, Hvad Dit Barn Vælger at Spise og Hvorfor*, 1st ed.; Gyldendal: Copenhagen, Denmark, 2018; p. 152.
28. Johnson, R.B.; Onwuegbuzie, A.J. Mixed Methods Research: A Research Paradigm Whose Time Has Come. *Educ. Res.* **2004**, *33*, 14–26. [CrossRef]
29. Pliner, P.; Hobden, K. Development of a scale to measure the trait of food neophobia in humans. *Appetite* **1992**, *19*, 105–120. [CrossRef]
30. Hausner, H.; Olsen, A.; Møller, P. Mere exposure and flavour–flavour learning increase 2–3 year-old children's acceptance of a novel vegetable. *Appetite* **2012**, *58*, 1152–1159. [CrossRef]
31. R Studio Team. *RStudio: Integrated Development for R*; RStudio, Inc.: Boston, MA, USA, 2020.
32. Pelchat, M.L.; Pliner, P. "Try it. You'll like it". Effects of information on willingness to try novel foods. *Appetite* **1995**, *24*, 153–165. [CrossRef]
33. McFarlane, T.; Pliner, P. Increasing Willingness to Taste Novel Foods: Effects of Nutrition and Taste Information. *Appetite* **1997**, *28*, 227–238. [CrossRef] [PubMed]
34. Pliner, P.; Loewen, E.R. Temperament and Food Neophobia in Children and their Mothers. *Appetite* **1997**, *28*, 239–254. [CrossRef] [PubMed]
35. Reverdy, C.; Chesnel, F.; Schlich, P.; Köster, E.P.; Lange, C. Effect of sensory education on willingness to taste novel food in children. *Appetite* **2008**, *51*, 156–165. [CrossRef] [PubMed]
36. Mustonen, S.; Tuorila, H. Sensory education decreases food neophobia score and encourages trying unfamiliar foods in 8–12-year-old children. *Food Qual. Prefer.* **2010**, *21*, 353–360. [CrossRef]
37. Deci, E.L.; Koestner, R.; Ryan, R.M. A meta-analytic review of experiments examining the effects of extrinsic rewards on intrinsic motivation. *Psychol. Bull.* **1999**, *125*, 627–668. [CrossRef]
38. Danish Agriculture & Food Council. *Kræsne Børn? Forældre og Børn er Uenige*; Danish Agriculture & Food Council: Copenhagen, Denmark, 2017.
39. Battjes-Fries, M.C.E.; Haveman-Nies, A.; Zeinstra, G.G.; van Dongen, E.J.I.; Meester, H.J.; van den Top-Pullen, R.; van't Veer, P.; de Graaf, K. Effectiveness of Taste Lessons with and without additional experiential learning activities on children's willingness to taste vegetables. *Appetite* **2017**, *109*, 201–208. [CrossRef]

40. Olsen, A. Reflections on current practice for taste learning in children. *Int. J. Gastron. Food Sci.* **2019**, *15*, 26–29. [CrossRef]
41. Pliner, P. Development of Measures of Food Neophobia in Children. *Appetite* **1994**, *23*, 147–163. [CrossRef]
42. Cooke, L. The importance of exposure for healthy eating in childhood: A review. *J. Hum. Nutr. Diet* **2007**, *20*, 294–301. [CrossRef]
43. Dazeley, P.; Houston-Price, C. Exposure to foods' non-taste sensory properties. A nursery intervention to increase children's willingness to try fruit and vegetables. *Appetite* **2015**, *84*, 1–6. [CrossRef]
44. Mustonen, S.; Rantanen, R.; Tuorila, H. Effect of sensory education on school children's food perception: A 2-year follow-up study. *Food Qual. Prefer.* **2009**, *20*, 230–240. [CrossRef]
45. Nederkoorn, C.; Theiβen, J.; Tummers, M.; Roefs, A. Taste the feeling or feel the tasting: Tactile exposure to food texture promotes food acceptance. *Appetite* **2018**, *120*, 297–301. [CrossRef] [PubMed]
46. Salvy, S.-J.; Vartanian, L.R.; Coelho, J.S.; Jarrin, D.; Pliner, P.P. The role of familiarity on modeling of eating and food consumption in children. *Appetite* **2008**, *50*, 514–518. [CrossRef] [PubMed]
47. Barthomeuf, L.; Droit-Volet, S.; Rousset, S. How emotions expressed by adults' faces affect the desire to eat liked and disliked foods in children compared to adults. *Br. J. Dev. Psychol.* **2012**, *30*, 253–266. [CrossRef]
48. Coulthard, H.; Ahmed, S. Non taste exposure techniques to increase fruit and vegetable acceptance in children: Effects of task and stimulus type. *Food Qual. Prefer.* **2017**, *61*, 50–54. [CrossRef]
49. Kahneman, D. A perspective on judgment and choice: Mapping bounded rationality. *Am. Psychol.* **2003**, *58*, 697–720. [CrossRef]

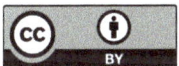

© 2020 by the authors. Licensee MDPI, Basel, Switzerland. This article is an open access article distributed under the terms and conditions of the Creative Commons Attribution (CC BY) license (http://creativecommons.org/licenses/by/4.0/).

MDPI
St. Alban-Anlage 66
4052 Basel
Switzerland
Tel. +41 61 683 77 34
Fax +41 61 302 89 18
www.mdpi.com

Nutrients Editorial Office
E-mail: nutrients@mdpi.com
www.mdpi.com/journal/nutrients

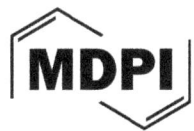

www.ingramcontent.com/pod-product-compliance
Lightning Source LLC
LaVergne TN
LVHW070206100526
838202LV00015B/2004